PSYCHOPATHOLOGY

Psychopathology

From Science to Clinical Practice

Edited by

LOUIS G. CASTONGUAY
THOMAS F. OLTMANNS

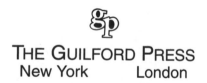

THE GUILFORD PRESS
New York   London

© 2013 The Guilford Press
A Division of Guilford Publications, Inc.
72 Spring Street, New York, NY 10012
www.guilford.com

Printed in the United States of America

This book is printed on acid-free paper.

Last digit is print number: 9 8 7 6 5 4 3 2

The authors have checked with sources believed to be reliable in their efforts to provide
information that is complete and generally in accord with the standards of practice that
are accepted at the time of publication. However, in view of the possibility of human
error or changes in behavioral, mental health, or medical sciences, neither the authors,
nor the editors and publisher, nor any other party who has been involved in the preparation or publication of this work warrants that the information contained herein is in
every respect accurate or complete, and they are not responsible for any errors or omissions or the results obtained from the use of such information. Readers are encouraged
to confirm the information contained in this book with other sources.

Library of Congress Cataloging-in-Publication Data

Psychopathology : from science to clinical practice / edited by Louis G. Castonguay,
Thomas F. Oltmanns.
    pages cm
Includes bibliographical references and index.
ISBN 978-1-4625-0803-7 (hardcover : alk. paper)
1. Psychology, Pathological.   I. Castonguay, Louis Georges, editor of compilation.
II. Oltmanns, Thomas F., editor of compilation.
RC454.P7863 2013
616.89—dc23

2012042843

About the Editors

Louis G. Castonguay, PhD, is Professor of Psychology at Penn State University. Dr. Castonguay's work and research focus on different aspects of the process of change and training, especially in the context of psychotherapy integration. He has also conducted studies on the efficacy of new integrative treatments for depression and generalized anxiety disorder, as well as effectiveness research aimed at better understanding and possibly improving psychotherapy as practice in natural settings. Furthermore, he has been involved in the development of several Practice Research Networks, with the goal of fostering an active collaboration between researchers and clinicians in conducting clinically relevant and scientifically rigorous studies of psychotherapy. Dr. Castonguay has contributed to more than 150 publications (including five coedited books), and received several awards, including the Distinguished Psychologist Award from Division 29 of the American Psychological Association Division of Psychotherapy for lifetime contributions to the field of psychotherapy. He is currently serving on the steering committee of the Society for the Exploration of Psychotherapy Integration, and served as president of both the North American Society for Psychotherapy Research and the International Society for Psychotherapy Research.

Thomas F. Oltmanns, PhD, is the Edgar James Swift Professor of Psychology in Arts and Sciences and Professor of Psychiatry at Washington University in St. Louis, where he is also Director of Clinical Training in Psychology. His early research studies were concerned with the role of cognitive and emotional factors in schizophrenia. With grant support from the National Institute of Mental Health, Dr. Oltmanns's lab is currently conducting a prospective study of the trajectory and impact of personality disorders in middle-aged and older adults. He has served on the board of directors of the Association for Psychological Science and as president of both the Society for Research in Psychopathology and the Society for a Science of Clinical Psychology. Dr. Oltmanns is a recipient of awards for outstanding teaching from Washington University in St. Louis and the University of Virginia. In 2011, he received the Toy Caldwell-Colbert Award for Distinguished Educator in Clinical Psychology from the Society of Clinical Psychology, Division 12 of the American Psychological Association. His other books include *Abnormal Psychology* (coauthored with Robert E. Emery), *Case Studies in Abnormal Psychology* (coauthored with Michele T. Martin, John M. Neale, and Gerald C. Davidson), *Schizophrenia* (coauthored with John M. Neale), and *Delusional Beliefs* (coedited with Brendan A. Maher).

Contributors

Jonathan S. Abramowitz, PhD, Department of Psychology, University of North Carolina at Chapel Hill, Chapel Hill, North Carolina

Allison J. Applebaum, PhD, Memorial Sloan-Kettering Cancer Center, New York, New York

Evelyn Attia, MD, Department of Psychiatry, Weill Medical College, Cornell University, and Department of Psychiatry, Columbia University, New York, New York

Jacques P. Barber, PhD, ABPP, Derner Institute of Advanced Psychological Studies, Adelphi University, Garden City, New York

Richard A. Bryant, PhD, School of Psychology, University of New South Wales, Sydney, New South Wales, Australia

Louis G. Castonguay, PhD, Department of Psychology, The Pennsylvania State University, University Park, Pennsylvania

Elise M. Clerkin, PhD, Department of Psychology, Miami University, Oxford, Ohio

Paul F. Crits-Christoph, PhD, Department of Psychiatry, University of Pennsylvania, Philadelphia, Pennsylvania

Deborah R. Glasofer, PhD, Department of Psychiatry, Columbia University, New York, New York

Marvin R. Goldfried, PhD, Department of Psychology, Stony Brook University, Stony Brook, New York

Sheri L. Johnson, PhD, Department of Psychology, University of California, Berkeley, Berkeley, California

Jutta Joormann, PhD, Department of Psychology, University of Miami, Coral Gables, Florida

Terence M. Keane, PhD, Behavioral Sciences Division, National Center for PTSD, Department of Psychiatry, Boston University School of Medicine, and Research Service, VA Boston Healthcare System, Boston, Massachusetts

Ann M. Kring, PhD, Department of Psychology, University of California, Berkeley, Berkeley, California

Joelle LeMoult, PhD, Anxiety Treatment and Research Centre, St. Joseph's Healthcare, Hamilton, Ontario, Canada

Jeffrey J. Magnavita, PhD, ABPP, Glastonbury Psychological Associates, P.C., Glastonbury, Connecticut

Andrew McAleavey, MS, Department of Psychology, The Pennsylvania State University, University Park, Pennsylvania

Michelle G. Newman, PhD, Department of Psychology, The Pennsylvania State University, University Park, Pennsylvania

Thomas F. Oltmanns, PhD, Department of Psychology, Washington University in St. Louis, St. Louis, Missouri

Michael W. Otto, PhD, Department of Psychology, Boston University, Boston, Massachusetts

Robert O. Pihl, PhD, Department of Psychology, McGill University, Montreal, Quebec, Canada

Kathleen M. Pike, PhD, Department of Psychiatry and Department of Counseling and Clinical Psychology, Columbia University, New York, New York

Abigail D. Powers, MA, Department of Psychology, Washington University in St. Louis, St. Louis, Missouri

David A. Sbarra, PhD, Department of Psychology, University of Arizona, Tucson, Arizona

Lynne Siqueland, PhD, private practice, Plymouth Meeting, Pennsylvania

David A. Smith, PhD, Department of Psychology, University of Notre Dame, Notre Dame, Indiana

Craig Steel, PhD, Department of Psychology, School of Psychology and Clinical Language Sciences, University of Reading, Reading, United Kingdom

Sherry H. Stewart, PhD, Department of Psychology, Dalhousie University, Halifax, Nova Scotia, Canada

Lauren E. Szkodny, MS, Department of Psychology, The Pennsylvania State University, University Park, Pennsylvania

Bethany A. Teachman, PhD, Department of Psychology, University of Virginia, Charlottesville, Virginia

Mark A. Whisman, PhD, Department of Psychology, University of Colorado at Boulder, Boulder, Colorado

Til Wykes, PhD, Institute of Psychiatry, King's College London, London, United Kingdom

Preface

This book is aimed at reviewing our current empirical knowledge about some of the most common forms of psychopathology and weaving what we know from this "basic" research into clinical practice. It is designed to serve as both a graduate course text and as a reference book for practicing clinicians.

Virtually all mental health professionals have taken a course in psychopathology. We would guess that most of the graduate courses offered on this topic, like the ones that we teach at Penn State University and Washington University, have two foci: description of particular disorders (in terms of symptoms and characteristics related to their clinical picture) and etiology (variables that are involved in the cause or maintenance) of these clinical problems. Unfortunately, the clinical implications of this research typically receive little consideration. Courses often fail to explain how basic research can inform clinicians by enriching their case formulations, expanding the targets of their treatments, and increasing their repertoire of interventions. This is a lost opportunity to facilitate the integration of science and practice, the time-honored and elusive challenge of our field.

By expending more effort on drawing clinical implications, courses on psychopathology could enhance the ability of current and future clinicians to use rigorously investigated, clinically relevant knowledge to help them decide what to do (or avoid doing) when working with clients who suffer from specific clinical problems. Using research on depression, for example, helpful guidelines can be derived from the findings showing that different ways of coping with stress might explain gender differences in depression rates, that increases in the incidence of depression over the last several decades may point to a crucial need in humans for attachment and communication, and that depressed people tend to provoke anger and frustration in others. These are just a few examples of basic findings that can help clinicians to better assess and treat major depression. At a broader level, the delineation of clinical guidelines based on psychopathology research is likely to open a new pathway toward reducing the gap between science and practice.

This book has been designed to address more fully the empirical and clinical interests of graduate students and experienced practitioners. To reach this compelling but difficult end, each chapter has been coauthored by a combination of scholars, some of them recognized for their expertise in psychopathology, others for their research in psychotherapy, and many for their contributions to both of these fields of knowledge. For each chapter, our goal was to create a team of influential authors who have approached the same clinical disorder from different perspectives and who were willing to engage in an innovative and collaborative writing project that could lead to new ways of thinking about psychopathology and clinical practice.

For the sake of clinical relevance, we included chapters that are concerned with disorders and other problems that meet three criteria: (1) they have a moderate to high level of prevalence in the general population; (2) they have a moderate to high prevalence in treatment settings; and (3) they are the focus of a substantial research literature. Several disorders (e.g., dissociative identity disorder, somatoform disorders, and gender identity disorder) are not discussed in the current book because they are not encountered frequently in clinical practice, or there is not enough basic research on which to build an effective case formulation and treatment plan. The clinical problems covered in this book are depression, generalized anxiety disorder, panic disorder and phobias, obsessive–compulsive disorder, posttraumatic stress disorder, eating disorders, substance use disorders, personality disorders, bipolar disorder, psychotic disorders (positive and negative symptoms), and marital and relationship discord.

Each chapter provides a solid descriptive and etiological grounding to understand psychopathology within the perspective of our current knowledge. They each present an up-to-date survey on issues related to typical symptoms, clinical features (e.g., interpersonal, social, occupational, health, sleep, and sexual problems), course (e.g., onset, duration, outcome, relapse), epidemiology (e.g., prevalence, gender and cross-cultural differences), comorbidity, and etiology (i.e., vulnerability factors involved in cause, maintenance, recurrence, and/or relapse). The authors have derived clinical implications from the research findings they reviewed, anticipating the readers' question: How is this relevant for understanding and treating my clients? Interestingly, because these clinical implications are drawn from basic research in psychopathology, they are not restricted to any one theoretical model underlying current forms of psychotherapy.

In addition, all of the chapters on specific clinical problems identify psychosocial (and medical) treatments that have been empirically validated for their respective problems. While these psychosocial interventions have been linked to particular models of therapy, the authors have also derived general principles of change from these treatments—formulating them in a way that is not necessarily tied to the specific techniques or terminology associated with a particular approach to therapy. As such, and like the clinical implications of basic research, these principles of change provide guidelines that could be assimilated (sometimes after specialized training) in the practice of clinicians, irrespective of their preferred theoretical orientation.

The chapters on specific clinical problems are preceded by an overview of general issues in psychopathology, as well as their relevance for the conceptualization, assessment, and treatment of patients. The last chapter attempts to identify similarities among different clinical problems by examining clinical and etiological issues that cut across diagnostic labels, and by providing general recommendations that may improve their assessment and treatment.

We believe this book will allow students to more fully appreciate the fundamental need to integrate science and practice in their training. In line with the current emphasis on evidence-based practice, this book is also likely to be viewed as a relevant resource by experienced practitioners, as it will allow them to conduct therapy while being informed by psychopathological research. It should also be a valuable guide for investigators doing basic research on psychopathology because it highlights issues from clinical practice that have an important bearing on issues and problems that researchers could address.

Both of us are working within two different scientific and professional traditions—one might say that we belong to different communities of knowledge (see Castonguay, 2011). In fact, we started to work on this book at the beginning of our respective presidential mandates of the Society for Psychotherapy Research and the Society for Research in Psychopathology. We both firmly believe that one way of increasing our understanding of complex phenomena such as psychopathology and psychotherapy is to foster connections between different domains of knowledge. We are also convinced that such connections are most fruitful when they represent a two-way approach. Many hypotheses that have guided scientific studies of psychopathology have been derived from clinical experience. Conversely, many findings from basic research have been extended to the realm of clinical practice. We hope this book will build further connections in order to help us, as a field, better understand and reduce psychological suffering.

LOUIS G. CASTONGUAY
THOMAS F. OLTMANNS

REFERENCE

Castonguay, L. G. (2011). Psychotherapy, psychopathology, research and practice: Pathways of connections and integration. *Psychotherapy Research, 21*, 125–140.

Contents

CHAPTER 1

General Issues in Understanding and Treating Psychopathology

Thomas F. Oltmanns
Louis G. Castonguay

The practice of any mental health profession (clinical and counseling psychology, psychiatry, social work) depends heavily on the ability to recognize and conceptualize various forms of mental disorder. Therapists, irrespective of their professional background and theoretical orientation, must be aware of the varied manifestations of psychopathology. They also have to understand many forms of vulnerability that set the stage for the development and maintenance of commonly occurring mental disorders, which eventually touch all of our lives, either directly or indirectly. In countries like the United States, mental disorders are the second leading cause of disease-related disability and mortality, ranking slightly behind cardiovascular conditions and slightly ahead of cancer (López, Mathers, Ezzati, Jamison, & Murray, 2006).

The individual chapters in this book provide truly unique reviews of the professional literature concerned with specific forms of psychopathology. Each is written by a team of scholars that includes recognized experts in the treatment of the condition, as well as leaders in the scientific study of the causes of the disorder. They have worked together to produce a creative synthesis describing the nature of the disorder (e.g., symptoms, course, epidemiology, and etiology) and the treatment implications that follow from this knowledge (assessment, case formulation, and/or principles of change). These chapters represent classic examples of the thoughtful integration of science and practice: Clinical experience raises important research questions, and evidence from scientific studies leads to the development and evaluation of improved treatment procedures. In this opening chapter, we discuss several basic issues that lay the foundation for subsequent chapters discussing specific types of psychopathology.

DEFINING MENTAL DISORDERS

Any systematic review of what is known about psychopathology first requires attention to how the construct of "mental disorder" is defined. Should some (if not all) mental disorders be conceptualized (completely or in part) as diseases, character flaws, deficits, or problems of living? How are mental disorders distinguished from behaviors that are simply idiosyncratic, eccentric, or out of favor within a particular culture? These questions determine, sometimes explicitly but most often implicitly, how a mental health professional will respond to a particular client or patient, including issues such as whether the person should receive treatment, and what kind of treatment should be provided. Many attempts have been made to define abnormal behavior, but none is entirely satisfactory. No one has provided a universal definition that can account for all situations in which the concept of mental disorder is invoked (Pilgrim, 2005; Zachar & Kendler, 2007).

Arguably, one of the most influential and widely invoked definitions of "mental disorder" was proposed by Wakefield (1992, 2010). According to his argument, a behavioral condition should be considered a mental disorder if, and only if, it meets two criteria:

1. The condition results from the inability of some internal mechanism (mental or physical) to perform its natural function. In other words, something inside the person is not working properly. Examples of such mechanisms include those that regulate levels of emotion, and those that distinguish between real auditory sensations and imagined ones.
2. The condition causes some harm to the person as judged by the standards of the person's culture. These negative consequences are measured in terms of the person's own subjective distress or difficulty performing expected social or occupational roles.

Using Wakefield's terms, mental disorders are defined as "harmful dysfunctions." One element ("dysfunction") of this definition is an attempt to incorporate (as much as it is possible) an objective evaluation of behavior. Wakefield argues that internal processes (e.g., cognition and perception) have a natural function, and that this function is to allow an individual to perceive the world in ways that are shared with other people and to engage in rational thought, problem solving, and adaptive behavior. The dysfunctions in mental disorders are assumed to be the product of disruptions of thought, feeling, communication, perception, and motivation.

This view of mental disorder also recognizes that all types of dysfunction do not lead to a disorder. Only dysfunctions that result in significant harm to the person are considered to be disorders. There are, for example, many types of physical dysfunction, such as albinism, reversal of heart position, and fused toes, that clearly represent a significant departure from the way that some biological process ordinarily functions. These conditions are not considered to be disorders, however, because they are not necessarily harmful to the person.

By definition, mental disorders are harmful to the person's adjustment. They typically affect family relationships, as well as success in educational and occupational activities. There are, of course, other types of harm associated with mental disorders. These include subjective distress, such as high levels of anxiety or depression, as well as more tangible outcomes, such as suicide.

The definition of abnormal behavior presented in the *Diagnostic and Statistical Manual of Mental Disorders* (DSM-5; American Psychiatric Association, 2013), which in the United States is considered a standard diagnostic system, incorporates many of the factors we have already discussed. According to this definition, a "mental disorder" is "a syndrome characterized by clinically significant disturbance in an individual's cognition, emotion regulation, or behavior that reflects a dysfunction in the psychological, biological, or developmental processes underlying mental functioning" (p. 20). The manual also notes that mental disorders are associated with subjective distress or impairment in social functioning. DSM-5 also excludes several conditions from consideration as mental disorders. These include (1) an expectable or culturally sanctioned response to a particular event (e.g., death of a loved one); (2) socially deviant behavior (e.g., the actions of political, religious, or sexual minorities); and (3) conflicts that are between the individual and society (e.g., voluntary efforts to express individuality).

The DSM definition places primary emphasis on the consequences of certain behavioral syndromes. Accordingly, mental disorders are defined by clusters of persistent, maladaptive behaviors that are associated with personal distress, such as anxiety or depression, or with impairment in social functioning, such as job performance or personal relationships. This definition, therefore, recognizes the concept of dysfunction, and it spells out ways in which the harmful consequences of a disorder might be identified.

The practical boundaries of abnormal behavior are defined by the list of disorders included in DSM. Therefore, the manual provides a simplistic, though practical, explanation of how someone's behavior might be considered pathological: It would be considered abnormal if the person's experiences fit the description of one of the forms of mental disorder listed in the diagnostic manual. Conceptually, however, it could be argued that a valid and adequate description of a mental disorder, such as major depression, cannot be restricted to its symptomatic picture. In order to define and understand major depression, it is necessary to consider a description of other clinical features (e.g., marital and health problems with which it is frequently associated), as well as a number of additional issues, such as its typical course (onset, duration, recurrence, relapse), prevalence (across gender and culture), patterns of comorbidity, and vulnerability factors.

Mental disorders are actually best conceived as "hypothetical constructs" (Morey, 1991; Neale & Oltmanns, 1980), which simply are abstract, explanatory devices. In the case of behavioral disorders, a hypothetical construct (i.e., a particular mental disorder) is an internal event whose existence is inferred on the basis of observable behaviors and the context in which they occur. The construct itself cannot be directly observed, but it is tied to overt referents that can be observed. For example, we cannot measure major depression directly, but we can see that the person no longer enjoys formerly pleasurable activities, has withdrawn from social contacts, is sleeping more than usual, has lost his or her appetite, and frequently talks about feeling worthless. Beyond these specific symptoms, the utility of a hypothetical construct ultimately depends on the extent to which it enters into relationships with other constructs and observable events (interrelated dimensions of human functioning). With this approach, a mental disorder is therefore defined by more than simply the diagnostic criteria identified in a diagnostic manual.

Clinically, this approach to defining a disorder (e.g., major depression) does not imply that clinicians should disregard "official" diagnostic criteria. Rather, it suggests that in order to conduct more comprehensive assessments and case formulations of their clients, as well as to identify a more complete list of potential targets for intervention, therapists should complement their diagnostic (DSM-based) evaluation with a careful consideration of nonsymptomatic factors that have been empirically associated with this disorder. One of our goals in this book is to provide a review of research on the factors that appear to contribute to the nature of each of the several specific forms of psychopathology.

EPIDEMIOLOGY

Basic understanding of mental disorders requires data about the frequency with which these disorders occur. Moreover, important clinical, organizational, and social decisions can be based on epidemiological information, such as whether the frequency of a disorder has increased or decreased during a particular period, whether it is more common in one geographic area than in another, and whether certain types of people—based on factors such as gender, race, and socioeconomic status—are at greater risk than other types for the development of the disorder. Health administrators often use such information to make decisions about the allocation of resources for professional training programs, treatment facilities, and research projects. As described in this book, answers to such questions have also provided insights and generated further research on possible risk factors for specific disorders.

How prevalent are the various forms of abnormal behavior? One important dataset regarding this question comes from a large-scale study known as the *National Comorbidity Survey Replication* (NCS-R) conducted between 2001 and 2003 (Kessler et al., 2005; Kessler, Merikangas, & Wang, 2007). Members of this research team interviewed a nationally representative sample of approximately 9,000 people living in the continental United States. Questions were asked pertaining to several (but not all) of the major disorders listed in DSM-IV (American Psychiatric Association, 1994). The NCS-R found that 46% of the people they interviewed received at least one *lifetime* diagnosis (meaning that they met the criteria for one of the disorders assessed at some point during their lives), with first onset of symptoms usually occurring during childhood or adolescence. This proportion of the population is much higher than many people expect, and it underscores the point we made at the beginning of this chapter: All of us can expect to encounter the challenges of a mental disorder—either for ourselves or for someone we love—at some point during our lives.

Figure 1.1 illustrates some results from this study using 12-month prevalence rates—the percentage of people who had experienced each disorder during the most recent year. The most prevalent specific types of disorder were major depression (17%) and alcohol abuse (13%). Various kinds of anxiety disorders were also relatively common. Substantially lower lifetime prevalence rates were found for obsessive–compulsive disorder and bipolar disorder, which each affect approximately 2% of the population. These lifetime prevalence rates are consistent with data reported by earlier epidemiological studies of mental disorders.

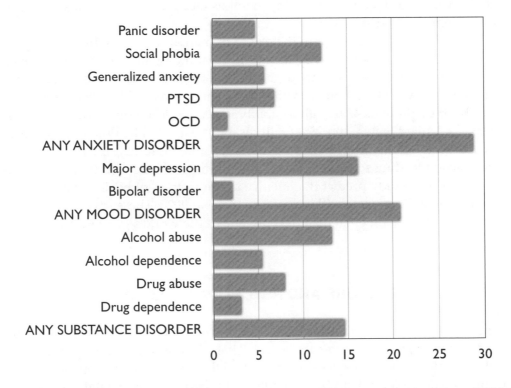

FIGURE 1.1. Twelve-month prevalence rates for various mental disorders (NCS-R data). Data from Kessler, Merikangas, and Wang (2007). *Note.* PTSD, posttraumatic stress disorder; OCD, obsessive–compulsive disorder. The NCS-R used DSM-IV definitions of mental disorders. Thus, PTSD and OCD were still considered forms of anxiety disorder, and the distinction between substance dependence and substance abuse was still recognized.

Although many mental disorders are quite common, they are not always seriously debilitating. The NCS-R investigators assigned each case a score with regard to severity, based on the severity of symptoms, as well as the level of occupational and social impairment that the person experienced. Averaged across all of the disorders diagnosed in the past 12 months, 40% of cases were rated as "mild," 37% as "moderate," and only 22% as "severe." Mood disorders were the most likely to be rated as severe (45%), while anxiety disorders were less likely to be rated as severe (23%). These findings have important clinical (and social) implications, as they suggest that not all individuals meeting criteria of a diagnosis may need immediate treatment. At the same time, it is worth noting that interventions (of varied length and intensity) might be beneficial for some individuals suffering from low-level distress and impairment, as subclinical levels of symptoms can, for some disorders, signal the eventual emergence of acute and severe symptoms.

Epidemiological studies such as the NCS-R have consistently found gender differences for many types of mental disorder: Major depression, anxiety disorders, and eating disorders are more common among women; alcoholism and antisocial personality disorders are more common among men. Patterns of this sort are highlighted throughout the chapters in this book as clues for possible causal mechanisms in some of these disorders.

Epidemiologists also measure the extent of mental disorders' impact on people's lives. In a study sponsored by the World Health Organization (WHO), López et al. (2006) compared the impact of more than 100 forms of disease and injury throughout the world. Although mental disorders are responsible for only 1% of all deaths, they produce 47% of all disability in economically developed countries, such as the United States, and 28% of all disability worldwide. When their impact is measured by combining indices of mortality and disability, mental disorders are the second leading source of disease burden in developed countries. Investigators in the WHO study predict that relative to other types of health problems, the burden of mental disorders will increase by the year 2020. These surprising results indicate strongly that mental disorders are one of the world's greatest health challenges.

CULTURE AND PSYCHOPATHOLOGY

As the evidence regarding the global burden of disease clearly documents, mental disorders affect people all over the world. That does not mean the symptoms of psychopathology and the expression of emotional distress take the same form in all cultures. Epidemiological studies comparing the frequency of mental disorders in different cultures suggest that some disorders, such as schizophrenia, show important consistencies in cross-cultural comparisons. They are found in virtually every culture that social scientists have studied. Other disorders, such as bulimia nervosa, are more specifically associated with cultural factors, as revealed by comparisons of prevalence in different parts of the world and changes in prevalence over generations. Almost 90% of patients with bulimia are women. Within the United States, the incidence of bulimia is much higher among university women than among working women, and it is more common among younger women than among older women. The prevalence of bulimia is much higher in Western nations than in other parts of the world. Furthermore, the number of cases increased dramatically during the latter part of the 20th century (Keel & Klump, 2003). As discussed later in this book, these patterns suggest that holding particular sets of values related to eating and to women's appearance is an important ingredient in establishing risk for development of an eating disorder.

The strength and nature of the relationship between culture and psychopathology varies from one disorder to the next. Several general conclusions can be drawn from cross-cultural studies of psychopathology (Draguns & Tanaka-Matsumi, 2003), including the following points:

- All mental disorders are shaped, to some extent, by cultural factors.
- No mental disorders are entirely due to cultural or social factors.
- Psychotic disorders are less influenced by culture than are nonpsychotic disorders.
- The symptoms of certain disorders are more likely to vary across cultures than are the disorders themselves.

Clinicians must consider the influence of cultural factors in both the expression and recognition of symptoms of mental disorders. People express extreme emotions in ways that are shaped by the traditions of their families and other social groups to which they belong. Intense, public displays of anger or grief might be expected in one culture but be considered signs of disturbance in another. Interpretations of emotional distress and other symptoms of disorder are influenced by the explanations that a person's culture assigns to such experiences. Religious beliefs, social roles, and sexual identities all play an important part in constructing meanings that are assigned to these phenomena (Hwang, Myers, Abe-Kim, & Ting, 2008). The most obvious clinical implication one can derive from these important issues is that the accuracy and utility of a clinical diagnosis depend on more than a simple count of the symptoms that appear to be present. They also hinge on the clinician's ability to consider the cultural context in which the problem appeared. This is a particularly challenging task when the clinician and the person with the problem do not share the same cultural background.

Clinicians can also become sensitized to the importance of cultural issues by considering cultural concepts of distress, patterns of erratic or unusual thinking and behavior that have been identified in diverse societies around the world and do not fit easily into the other diagnostic categories. A list of these syndromes is included in the appendix of DSM-5. They have also been called "culture-bound syndromes" because they are considered to be unique to particular societies, particularly in non-Western or developing countries. Their appearance is easily recognized and understood to be a form of abnormal behavior by members of certain cultures, but they do not conform to typical patterns of mental disorder seen in the United States or Europe. Cultural concepts of distress have also been called "idioms of distress." In other words, they represent a manner of expressing negative emotion that is unique to a particular culture and cannot be easily translated or understood in terms of its individual parts.

One syndrome of this type is a phenomenon known as *ataques de nervios*, which has been observed most extensively among people from Puerto Rico and other Caribbean countries (Lewis-Fernández et al., 2002; San Miguel et al., 2006). Descriptions of this experience include four dimensions, in which the essential theme is loss of control—an inability to interrupt the dramatic sequence of emotion and behavior. These dimensions include emotional expressions (an explosion of screaming and crying, coupled with overwhelming feelings of anxiety, depression, and anger), bodily sensations (including trembling, heart palpitations, weakness, fatigue, headache, and convulsions), actions and behaviors (dramatic, forceful gestures that include aggression toward others, suicidal thoughts or gestures, and trouble eating or sleeping), and alterations in consciousness (marked feelings of "not being one's usual self," accompanied by fainting, loss of consciousness, dizziness, and feelings of being outside of one's body).

Ataques are typically provoked by situations that disrupt or threaten the person's social world, especially the family. Many *ataques* occur shortly after the person learns unexpectedly that a close family member has died. Others result from an imminent divorce or occur after a serious conflict with a child. Women are primarily responsible for maintaining the integrity of the family in this culture, and they are also more likely than men to experience *ataques de nervios*. Puerto Rican women from poor and working-class families define themselves largely in terms of their success in building and maintaining a cohesive family life. When this social role is threatened, an *ataque* may result. This response to threat or conflict—an outburst of powerful, uncontrolled negative emotion—expresses suffering, while simultaneously providing a means for coping with the threat. It serves to signal the woman's distress to important other people and to rally needed sources of social support.

What is the relation between cultural concepts of distress and the formal categories listed in DSM or the *International Classification of Diseases* (ICD)? The answer is unclear and also varies from one syndrome to the next. Are they similar problems that are simply given different names in other cultures? Probably not, at least not in most instances (Guarnaccia & Pincay, 2008). In some cases, people who exhibit behavior that would fit the definition of a culture-bound syndrome would also qualify for another diagnosis, if diagnosed by a clinician trained in the use of the diagnostic manual (Tolin, Robison, Gaztambide, Horowitz, & Blank, 2007). But not everyone who displays the culture-bound syndrome meets criteria for another mental disorder, and of those who do, not all would receive the same diagnosis.

The DSM's glossary on cultural concepts of distress has been praised as a significant advance toward integrating cultural considerations into the classification system (López & Guarnaccia, 2000). It has also been criticized for its ambiguity. The most difficult conceptual issue involves the boundary between culture-bound syndromes and categories found elsewhere in the diagnostic manual. Some critics have argued that they should be fully integrated, without trying to establish a distinction (Hughes, 1998). Others have noted that if culturally unique disorders must be listed separately from other, "mainstream" conditions, then certain disorders now listed in the main body of the manual—especially eating disorders, such as bulimia—should actually be listed as culture-bound syndromes. Like *ataques de nervios*, bulimia nervosa is a condition that is found primarily among a limited number of cultures (Keel & Klump, 2003). "Dissociative amnesia"—the inability to recall important personal information regarding a traumatic event—also resembles culture-bound syndromes, because it appears to be experienced only by people living in modern, developed cultures (Pope, Poliakoff, Parker, Boynes, & Hudson, 2007).

Though it is imperfect, the DSM-5's list of cultural concepts of distress raises important conceptual and clinical implications. The fact that some diagnostic categories that are familiar to most mental health professionals working in Western or developed countries are unique to their cultural environment helps to challenge the frequently held assumption that culture shapes only conditions that appear to be exotic in faraway lands. At a more direct, clinical level the glossary serves to make clinicians more aware of the extent to which their own views of what is normal and abnormal have been shaped by the values and experiences of their own culture (Mezzich, Berganza, & Ruiperez, 2001).

CLASSIFICATION OF PSYCHOPATHOLOGY

One might argue that efforts to classify mental disorders are as important and have raised as much controversy as efforts to define them. Despite many tribulations and debates associated with the classification of psychopathology, this process has served several purposes. A classification system helps clinicians to (1) identify (as accurately and comprehensively as possible) their clients' problems, and (2) formulate a plan of intervention that is most likely to be effective for these difficulties. A classification system also serves an important role in the search for new knowledge. The history of medicine is filled with examples of problems that were recognized long before they could be treated successfully. The classification of a specific set of symptoms has often laid the foundation for research that eventually identified a cure or a way of preventing the disorder.

Modern classification systems in psychiatry were introduced shortly after

World War II. During the 1950s and 1960s, psychiatric classification was widely criticized. One major criticism focused on the lack of consistency in diagnostic decisions (Nathan & Langenbucher, 2003). Independent clinicians frequently disagreed with one another about the use of diagnostic categories. Objections were also raised from philosophical, sociological, and political points of view. For example, some critics charged that diagnostic categories in psychiatry would be more appropriately viewed as "problems in living" than as medical disorders (Szasz, 1963). Others were concerned about the negative impact of using diagnostic labels. In other words, once a psychiatric diagnosis is assigned, the person so labeled might experience discrimination of various kinds, and also find it more difficult to establish and maintain relationships with other people. These are all serious problems that continue to be the topic of important, ongoing discussions involving mental health professionals, as well as patients and their families. Debates regarding these issues did fuel important improvements in the diagnosis of mental disorders, including emphasis on the use of detailed criterion sets for each disorder.

Currently, two diagnostic systems for mental disorders are widely recognized. We have already mentioned DSM-5, which is published by the American Psychiatric Association. The other—the ICD—is published by the World Health Organization. Both systems were first developed shortly after World War II and have been revised several times. The World Health Organization's manual is in its 10th edition and is therefore known as ICD-10. Deliberate attempts are made to coordinate the production of the DSM and ICD manuals. Most of the categories listed in the manuals are identical, and the criteria for specific disorders are usually similar. More than 200 specific diagnostic categories are described in the current edition of DSM. Interestingly, under both systems (DSM and ICD), a person can be assigned more than one diagnosis if he or she meets criteria for more than one disorder.

Most of the available data regarding the etiology and treatment of mental disorders are based on criteria set forth in DSM-IV. Changes in DSM-5 are intended to address perceived shortcomings in these diagnostic criteria. Nevertheless, until empirical studies have been done using the DSM-5 criterion sets, we will not have a solid evidence base from which to draw conclusions about presenting problems, possible etiological mechanisms underlying them, or treatments designed to target them. Until that dataset is established, our work as researchers and clinicians will have to continue to refer to DSM-IV. Thus, in the chapters to come, you will see authors referring to *both* editions of the DSM.

EVALUATION OF PSYCHIATRIC CLASSIFICATION

The most important issue in the evaluation of a diagnostic category is whether it is *useful* (Kendell & Jablensky, 2003). By knowing that a person fits into a particular group or class, do we learn anything meaningful about that person? For example, is the person who fits the diagnostic criteria for schizophrenia likely to improve when he or she is given antipsychotic medication? Or is that person likely to have a less satisfactory level of social adjustment in 5 years than a person who meets diagnostic criteria for bipolar mood disorder? Does the diagnosis tell us anything about the factors or circumstances that might have contributed to the onset of this problem? These questions are concerned with the validity of the diagnostic category.

Validity is, in a sense, a reflection of the success that has been achieved in understanding the nature of a disorder. Have important facts been discovered? Systematic studies aimed at establishing the validity of a disorder may proceed in a sequence of phases (Robins & Guze, 1989). After a clinical description has been established, diagnostic categories are refined and validated through a process of scientific exploration. Unfortunately, relatively few of the disorders listed in the official diagnostic manual are supported by an extensive set of research evidence supporting all possible aspects of validity.

It may be helpful to think of different forms of validity in terms of their relationship in time with the appearance of symptoms of the disorder. "Etiological validity" is concerned with factors that contribute to the onset of the disorder. These are things that have happened in the past. Was the disorder regularly triggered by a specific set of events or circumstances? Did it run in families? The ultimate question with regard to etiological validity is whether there are any specific causal factors that are regularly, and perhaps uniquely, associated with this disorder. If we know that a person exhibits the symptoms of the disorder, do we in turn learn anything about the circumstances that originally led to the onset of the problem?

"Concurrent validity" is concerned with the present time and with correlations between the disorder and other symptoms, circumstances, and test procedures. Is the disorder currently associated with any other types of behavior, such as performance on psychological tests? Do precise measures of biological variables, such as brain structure and function, distinguish reliably between people who have the disorder and those who do not? Clinical studies aimed at developing a more precise description of a disorder also fall into this type of validity.

"Predictive validity" is concerned with the future and with the stability of the problem over time. Will it be persistent? If it is short lived, how long will an episode last? Will the disorder have a predictable outcome? Do people with this problem typically improve if they are given a specific type of medication or a particular form of psychotherapy?

The overall utility of a diagnostic category depends on the body of evidence that accumulates as scientists seek answers to questions raised by these multiple forms of validity ("reliability," or consistency of the diagnostic decisions, is also crucial, as it precedes validity). At this point in time, some disorders included in the diagnostic manual are based on a much more extensive foundation of evidence than others. Thus, more research needs to confirm and enhance the validity (thus, the utility) of our current diagnostic categories. Such research should be conducted in parallel with other efforts (conceptual and empirical) to address serious criticism directed toward the diagnostic manual.

LIMITATIONS OF AND POSSIBLE IMPROVEMENTS TO DSM

Developing each edition of DSM involves a tremendous amount of work (with regard to both theory and research), and each new edition represents an improvement over previous ones (see Widiger, Frances, Pincus, Davis, & First, 1991). Nevertheless, several enduring issues remain to be resolved. One fundamental question that applies to every disorder involves the boundary between normal and abnormal behavior. The definitions included in the DSM-5 are often vague with regard to this threshold (Widiger & Clark, 2000). The manual is based on a categorical approach to classification, but most of the symptoms that define the disorders are actually dimensional in nature. Depressed mood, for example, can vary continuously, from the complete absence of depression to moderate levels of depression, on up to severe levels of depression. The same issue applies to symptoms of anxiety disorders, eating disorders, and substance use disorders. These are all continuously distributed phenomena, and there is not a bright line that divides people with problems from those who do not have problems.

The absence of a specific definition of social impairment is another conceptual and clinical issue that has plagued the current diagnostic manual. Most disorders in DSM include the requirement that a particular set of symptoms causes "clinically significant distress or impairment in social or occupational functioning." However, no specific measurement procedures are provided to make this determination. Mental health professionals must rely on their own subjective judgment of a person's symptoms to decide how distressed or how impaired a person must be in order to qualify for a diagnosis. There is an important need for more specific definitions of these concepts, and better measurement tools are needed for their assessment.

In addition, criticisms of the current classification system have emphasized broad conceptual issues. Some clinicians and investigators have argued that the syndromes defined in the DSM do not represent the most useful ways to think about psychological problems, in terms of either planning current treatments or designing programs of research. For example, it might be better to focus on more homogeneous dimensions of dysfunction, such as anxiety or angry hostility, rather than on syndromes (groups of symptoms) (Smith & Combs, 2010). Clinically and empirically, this raises questions such as the following: Should we design treatments for people who exhibit distorted, negative ways of thinking about themselves, regardless of whether their symptoms happen to involve a mixture of depression, anxiety, or some other pattern of negative emotion or interpersonal conflict? No definite answer is available at this point in time. It would certainly be premature to cut off consideration of these alternatives just because they address problems in a way that deviates from the official diagnostic manual. In our current state of uncertainty, diversity of opinion should be encouraged, particularly if it is grounded in cautious skepticism and supported by rigorous scientific inquiry.

From an empirical and clinical point of view, the DSM is hampered by a number of problems that suggest it does not classify clinical problems into syndromes in the simplest and most beneficial way (Helzer, Kraemer, & Krueger, 2006). One of the thorniest issues involves "comorbidity," which is defined as the simultaneous appearance of two or more disorders in the same person. Comorbidity rates are very high for mental disorders as defined in the DSM system (Eaton, South, & Krueger, 2010). For example, in the National Comorbidity Survey, among those people who qualified for at least one diagnosis at some point during their lifetime, 56% met the criteria for two or more disorders. A small subgroup, 14% of the sample, actually met the diagnostic criteria for three or more lifetime disorders. That group of people accounted for almost 90% of the *severe* disorders in the study.

There are several ways to interpret comorbidity (Krueger, 2002). Some people may independently develop two separate conditions. In other cases, the presence of one disorder may lead to the onset of another. Unsuccessful attempts to struggle with prolonged alcohol dependence, for example, might lead a person to become depressed. Neither of these alternatives creates conceptual problems for the DSM; it makes sense that some people have more than one disorder and that one disorder can lead to another. Unfortunately, the high rates of comorbidity that have been observed empirically suggest that these explanations account for a small proportion of overlap between categories. In a large proportion of cases, the overlapping manifestations of more than one disorder do not seem to reflect clearly distinct diagnostic constructs.

Major clinical problems associated with comorbidity can arise when a person with a mixed pattern of symptoms, usually of a severe nature, simultaneously meets the criteria for more than one disorder. Consider, for example, a client who was treated by one of the authors (T. F. O.) of this chapter. This man experienced a large number of diffuse problems associated with anxiety, depression, and interpersonal difficulties. According to the DSM system, he would have met the criteria for major depressive disorder, generalized anxiety disorder, and obsessive–compulsive disorder, as well as three types of personality disorder. It might be said, therefore, that he suffered from at least six types of mental disorder. But is that really helpful? Is it the best way to think about his problems? Would it be more accurate to say that he had a complicated set of interrelated problems that were associated with worrying, rumination, and the regulation of high levels of negative emotion, and that these problems constituted one complex and severe type of disorder?

The comorbidity issue is related to another limitation of the DSM: the failure to make better use of information regarding the course of mental disorders over time. More than 100 years ago, when schizophrenia and bipolar mood disorder were originally described, the distinction between them was based heavily on observations regarding their long-term course. Unfortunately, most disorders listed in the DSM are defined largely in terms of snapshots of symptoms at particular points in time. Diagnostic decisions are seldom based on a comprehensive analysis of the way that a person's problems evolve over time. If someone meets the criteria for more than one disorder, does it matter which one came first? Is there a predictable pattern in which certain disorders follow the onset of others? What is the nature of the connection between childhood disorders and adult problems? Our knowledge of mental disorders would be greatly enriched if greater emphasis were placed on questions regarding lifespan development (Buka & Gilman, 2002; Oltmanns & Balsis, 2011).

These issues are being considered by the experts who develop each new edition of the DSM and ICD. Of course, all of them will not be solved immediately. Attempts to provide solutions to these problems and limitations will ensure that the classification system will continue to be revised. As before, these changes will be driven by the interaction of clinical experience and empirical evidence. Students, clinicians, and research investigators should all remain skeptical when using this classification system and its successors. At the same time, the complexity of psychopathology and its treatment should encourage all scholars and providers in the field of mental health to pay close attention to our current knowledge, and to derive from it new and creative ways to think about and intervene with mental disorders. The following chapters in this book have been written with this goal in mind.

REFERENCES

American Psychiatric Association. (1994). *Diagnostic and statistical manual of mental disorders* (4th ed.). Washington, DC: Author.

American Psychiatric Association. (2013). *Diagnostic and statistical manual of mental disorders* (5th ed.). Arlington, VA: Author.

Buka, S. L., & Gilman, S. E. (2002). Psychopathology and the lifecourse. In J. E. Helzer & J. J. Hudziak (Eds.), *Defining psychopathology in the 21st century* (pp. 129–142). Washington, DC: American Psychiatric Press.

Draguns, J. G., & Tanaka-Matsumi, J. (2003). Assessment of psychopathology across and within cultures: Issues and findings. *Behaviour Research and Therapy, 41,* 755–776.

Eaton, N. R., South, S. C., & Krueger, R. F. (2010). The meaning of comorbidity among common mental disorders. In T. Millon, R. F. Krueger, & E. Simonsen (Eds.), *Contemporary directions in psychopathology: Scientific foundations of the DSM-V and ICD-11* (pp. 223–241). New York: Guilford Press.

Guarnaccia, P., & Pincay, I. M. (2008). Culture-specific diagnoses and their relationship to mood disorders. In S. Loue & M. Sajatovic (Eds.), *Diversity issues in the diagnosis, treatment and research of mood disorders* (pp. 32–53). New York: Oxford University Press.

Helzer, J. E., Kraemer, H. C., & Krueger, R. F. (2006). The feasibility and need for dimensional psychiatric diagnoses. *Psychological Medicine: A Journal of Research in Psychiatry and the Allied Sciences, 36*(12), 1671–1680.

Hughes, C. C. (1998). The glossary of culture-bound syndromes in DSM-IV: A critique. *Transcultural Psychiatry, 35,* 413–421.

Hwang, W., Myers, H. F., Abe-Kim, J., & Ting, J. Y. (2008). A conceptual paradigm for understanding culture's impact on mental health. *Clinical Psychology Review, 28,* 211–227.

Keel, P. K., & Klump, K. L. (2003). Are eating disorders culture-bound syndromes?: Implications for conceptualizing their etiology. *Psychological Bulletin, 129,* 747–769.

Kendell, R., & Jablensky, A. (2003). Distinguishing between the validity and utility of psychiatric diagnoses. *American Journal of Psychiatry, 160,* 4–12.

Kessler, R. C., Demier, O., Frank, R. G., Olfson, M., Pincus, H., Walters, E. E., et al. (2005).

Prevalence and treatment of mental disorders, 1990 to 2003. *New England Journal of Medicine, 352*, 2515–2523.

Kessler, R. C., Merikangas, K. R., & Wang, P. S. (2007). Prevalence, comorbidity, and service utilization for mood disorders in the United States at the beginning of the twenty-first century. *Annual Review of Clinical Psychology, 3*, 137–158.

Krueger, R. F. (2002). Psychometric perspectives on co-morbidity. In J. E. Helzer & J. J. Hudziak (Eds.), *Defining psychopathology in the 21st century* (pp. 41–54). Washington, DC: American Psychiatric Press.

Lewis-Fernández, R., Guarnaccia, P. J., Martínez, I. E., Salmán, E., Schmidt, A., & Liebowitz, M. (2002). Comparative phenomenology of *ataques de nervios,* panic attacks, and panic disorder. *Culture, Medicine and Psychiatry, 26*, 199–223.

López, S. R., & Guarnaccia, P. J. (2000). Cultural psychopathology: Uncovering the social world of mental illness. *Annual Review of Psychology, 51*, 571–598.

López, A. D., Mathers, C. D., Ezzati, M., Jamison, D. T., & Murray, C. J. L. (2006). *Global burden of disease and risk factors.* Washington, DC: World Bank and Oxford University Press.

Mezzich, J. E., Berganza, C. E., & Ruiperez, M. A. (2001). Culture in DSM-IV, ICD-10, and evolving diagnostic systems. *Psychiatric Clinics of North America, 24*, 407–419.

Mezzich, J. E., Kirmayer, L. J., Kleinman, A. A., Fabrega, H., Parron, D. L., Good, B. J., et al. (2008). The place of culture in DSM-IV. In J. E. Mezzich, G. Caracci, J. E. Mezzich, & G. Caracci (Eds.), *Cultural formulation: A reader for psychiatric diagnosis* (pp. 167–181). Lanham, MD: Aronson.

Morey, L. C. (1991). Classification of mental disorders as a collection of hypothetical constructs. *Journal of Abnormal Psychology, 100*, 289–293.

Nathan, P. E., & Langenbucher, J. (2003). Diagnosis and classification. In G. Stricker, T. A. Widiger, & I. B. Weiner (Eds.), *Handbook of psychology: Clinical psychology* (Vol. 8, pp. 3–26). New York: Wiley.

Neale, J. M., & Oltmanns, T. F. (1980). *Schizophrenia.* New York: Wiley.

Oltmanns, T. F., & Balsis, S. (2011). Personality pathology in later life: Questions about the measurement, course, and impact of disorders. *Annual Review of Clinical Psychology, 7*, 321–349.

Pilgrim, D. (2005). Defining mental disorder: Tautology in the service of sanity in British mental health legislation. *Journal of Mental Health, 14*, 435–443.

Pope, H. G., Poliakoff, M. B., Parker, M. P., Boynes, M., & Hudson, J. I. (2007). Is dissociative amnesia a culture-bound syndrome?: Findings from a survey of historical literature. *Psychological Medicine, 37*, 225–233.

Regier, D. A, Narrow, W. E., Kuhl, E. A., & Kupfer, D. J. (2009). The conceptual development of DSM-5." *American Journal of Psychiatry, 166*, 645–650.

Robins, E., & Guze, S. (1989). Establishment of diagnostic validity in psychiatric illness. In L. N. Robins & J. E. Barrett (Eds.), *The validity of psychiatric diagnosis* (pp. 177–197). New York: Raven Press.

San Miguel, V. E. F., Guarnaccia, P. J., Shrout, P. E., Lewis-Fernandez, R., Canino, G. J., & Ramirez, R. R. (2006). A quantitative analysis of *ataque de nervios* in Puerto Rico: Further examination of a cultural syndrome. *Hispanic Journal of Behavioral Science, 28*, 313–330.

Smith, G. T., & Combs, J. (2010). Issues of construct validity in psychological diagnoses. In T. Millon, R. F. Krueger, & E. Simonsen (Eds.), *Contemporary directions in psychopathology: Scientific foundations of the DSM-V and ICD-11* (pp. 205–222). New York: Guilford Press.

Szasz, T. (1963). *Law, liberty, and psychiatry: An inquiry into the social uses of mental health practices.* New York: Macmillan.

Tolin, D. F., Robison, J. T., Gaztambide, S., Horowitz, S., & Blank, K. (2007). *Ataques de nervios* and psychiatric disorders in older Puerto Rican primary care patients. *Journal of Cross-Cultural Psychology, 38*, 659–669.

Wakefield, J. C. (1992). The concept of mental disorder: On the boundary between biological facts and social values. *American Psychologist, 47,* 373–388.

Wakefield, J. C. (2010). Taking disorder seriously: A critique of psychiatric criteria for mental disorders from the harmful-dysfunction perspective. In T. Millon, R. F. Krueger, & E. Simonsen (Eds.), *Contemporary directions in psychopathology: Scientific foundations of the DSM-V and ICD-11* (pp. 275–300). New York: Guilford Press.

Widiger, T. A., & Clark, L. A. (2000). Toward DSM-5 and the classification of psychopathology. *Psychological Bulletin, 126,* 946–963.

Widiger, T. A., Frances, A. P., Pincus, H. A., Davis, W. W., & First, M. B. (1991). Toward an empirical classification for the DSM-IV. *Journal of Abnormal Psychology, 100,* 280–288

Zachar, P., & Kendler, K. S. (2007). Psychiatric disorders: A conceptual taxonomy. *American Journal of Psychiatry, 164,* 557–565.

CHAPTER 2

Depression

Joelle LeMoult
Louis G. Castonguay
Jutta Joormann
Andrew McAleavey

It is estimated that 16% of the general population experiences clinically significant depression (Kessler, Tat Chiu, Demler, & Walters, 2005). In addition to their
impact on affected individuals and their families, depressive disorders place a burden of almost $50 billion per year on the American economy, accounting for over
20% of costs for all mental illness (Stewart, Ricci, Chee, Hahn, & Morganstein, 2003).
In fact, compared to other physical and mental disorders, depression is the leading
cause of disability worldwide according to the World Health Organization (López
& Murray, 1998). Given the substantial personal and societal costs of this disorder,
efforts to identify vulnerability factors and effective interventions for depression
are particularly important.

Our goal in this chapter is to present basic psychopathology research in depression and to discuss treatment implications of these findings. Though all depressive disorders share similar features, there are some important differences between
diagnostic categories that are not covered in this chapter. Instead we focus here on
depressive symptoms in general and major depressive disorder (MDD) in particular, rather than bipolar or dysthymic disorders. We first address descriptive issues
related to depression: its symptoms, associated clinical features, course and outcome, prevalence, and comorbidity. We then discuss its etiology.

Considering the extensive research on factors that may have a role in the onset,
maintenance, recurrence, and relapse of depression (see Gotlib & Hammen, 2009,
for a survey of this literature), in this chapter we pay only selective attention to
potential determinants of this disorder. Specifically, we have decided to focus the

etiology section on novel empirical findings. This is a timely and important task because, even though effective depression treatments exist, these interventions have undergone few changes in the past decades, and rates of recurrence of depression are still high even after successful treatment.

Cognitive-behavioral therapy (CBT), for example, is currently one of the most empirically supported and effective treatments for this emotional disorder. It is fascinating to see, however, that CBT for depression has undergone few changes in the last 50 years, and that the theoretical foundations of this treatment are still largely rooted in Beck's cognitive theory of depression, proposed in the 1960s. This is all the more surprising given the impressive increase in depression research in recent years, which has led to important improvements in models of depression, including cognitive models, regarding the risk for the onset and maintenance of this disorder. This is not by any means unique to CBT; Joiner and Timmons (2009) note that proponents of interpersonal psychotherapy (IPT) have also failed to incorporate a number of basic findings from interpersonal research.

Among the lines of research emphasized in the etiology section are those that address the role of automatic processes (e.g., cognitive inhibition), emotional regulation processes (e.g., distraction), and biological markers (e.g., dysfunctional neuroendocrine responses to stress). These aspects of depression are not addressed directly in our current treatments; neither are they assessed as potential changes resulting from such treatments. Yet because they have been identified as potential determinants of depression, it may be useful to develop interventions that target these processes. Furthermore, because these basic processes have not been tied to a particular model of psychotherapy, the use of strategies to address them may improve the impact of therapy, irrespective of clinicians' orientation (although the specific interventions and/or ways to use them may vary from one orientation to another).

We summarize some of these recent developments in our understanding of depression and outline implications for treatment later in the chapter. First, as we announced earlier, we address its phenomenology.

PHENOMENOLOGY

Typical Symptoms

The main symptoms of MDD are (1) dysphoria or sustained sadness and (2) anhedonia. These major symptoms are frequently accompanied by other symptoms, such as weight/appetite disturbance, sleep disturbance, psychomotor agitation/retardation, fatigue or loss of energy, feelings of worthlessness or guilt, diminished concentration, and thoughts of suicide or death. Various subtypes of depression have been proposed (e.g., MDD with melancholic features; American Psychiatric Association, 2013), but the utility of these subtypes to research and treatment remains to be established.

The diagnostic criteria put much emphasis on vegetative or somatic symptoms of depression, but it should be kept in mind that these symptoms are not specific to depression and can be found in many disorders, such as generalized anxiety disorder (GAD). There is evidence, however, to support the view that these symptoms are important to diagnosis but may not be central to the disorder. Buchwald and Rudick-Davis (1993) found that the presence of vegetative symptoms is more telling in a diagnosis of depression than the presence of other symptoms. Using a more complete analytic strategy, Mitchell, Goodwin, Johnson, and Hirschfeld (2008) found that somatic symptoms, when present, have high rule-in value for diagnosis but were too rare in the outpatient sample used in their study to provide adequate classification on their own. Instead, according to these authors, mood and emotional symptoms were most clinically useful overall. This suggests that somatic symptoms play a role in depression but may not be central to the disorder in all cases.

What really seems to define depression is that it is a disorder of mood or affect. As a consequence, many newer etiological models of depression emphasize difficulties in emotion regulation as a central feature of the disorder (Joormann, Siemer, & Tran, 2011; Nolen-Hoeksema, Wisco, & Lyubomirsky, 2008). We discuss this aspect in more detail in the section of this chapter on etiology.

Associated Clinical Features

Depressed individuals frequently present with a number of important clinical features. For instance, research indicates that anger or hostility is often a characteristic of depression (e.g., Fava & Rosenbaum, 1999). Importantly, it seems that irritability is correlated with higher severity of depression (Perlis et al., 2005) and represents an additional risk within this population rather than representing a subtype of irritable depression. Others have also found that anger distinguished those with a history of a suicide attempt from those without one (Jandl, Steyer, & Kaschka, 2010; Perlis et al., 2005). Anger also appears to characterize depressed individuals' relationships with others, such as friends, strangers, college roommates, therapists, and spouses (Coyne, Burchill, & Stiles, 1991; Joiner, 2002). It is notable in this context that irritability is listed in the DSM as a symptom of depression in children and adolescents, but not in adults.

Interpersonal problems associated with depression are not restricted to hostility. Depressed individuals have been found to have social skills deficits, as well as to seek both excessive reassurance and aversive feedback (Joiner & Timmons, 2009). As we discuss below, seeking these two types of reactions from others has been identified as a risk factor for depression. Considering such interpersonal difficulties, it is not surprising that depression has been associated with elevated levels of marital dissatisfaction and discord (which, as also discussed in the section on etiology, is perceived as both cause and consequences of depression; Davila, Stroud, & Starr, 2009; Joiner & Timmons, 2009).

The most serious associated feature of MDD is increased risk for suicide. While completed suicide remains an extremely rare event, its consequences are dire. Beautrais et al. (2006) interviewed serious suicide survivors soon after their attempts and found that of any psychiatric disorders, mood disorders were associated with the highest increased likelihood of attempting suicide. Likelihood of attempting suicide increases with depression severity, and acute and intense negative mood tends to precede attempts (Berman, 2009).

Persons with depression also display significant impairment in role performance across domains of functioning. Individuals with depression may experience inability to achieve orgasm (or erections in men), which may exacerbate relationship or marital problems. It is frequently noted that occupational difficulties including reduced work performance co-occur with depressive episodes (e.g., Mintz, Mintz, Arruda, & Hwang, 1992), and that these largely disappear with remission (Kessler & Frank, 1997).

It should be kept in mind as well that general medical conditions are frequently comorbid with MDD, and that depression can precede and follow onset of medical conditions. While there does not seem to be consensus regarding whether (or which) medical conditions predict occurrence of depressive episodes, numerous prospective studies have shown that depression increases the likelihood of physical illness (e.g., Salaycik et al., 2007). When medical conditions (commonly including prostate cancer, breast cancer, and cardiovascular disease) co-occur with depression, the course of the medical condition will likely lengthen, and the medical condition may complicate treatments for depression (Carney, Freedland, Rich, & Jaffe, 1995; Freedland & Carney, 2009). Evidence suggests that the rate of death for people over age 55 increases three to four times with depression, and that likelihood of death may substantially increase during the first year in a nursing home when an individual suffers from depression (American Psychiatric Association, 2000, 2013).

It should also be noted that cognitive factors are associated with depression. As described in the section on etiology, however, while some of them have been identified as risk factors (e.g., bias information processing), others (negative thoughts, dysfunctional attitudes) appear as features or symptoms of current depression episodes.

Epidemiology

Depression is highly prevalent, with lifetime prevalence rates varying between 10 and 25% for women and between 5 and 12% for men (American Psychiatric Association, 2000). Prevalence rates differ considerably by age group, with the prevalence in the 18- to 29-year-old range three times higher than the prevalence in individuals 60 years old or older (American Psychiatric Association, 2013). Interestingly, there has been a steady increase in prevalence rates of depression since World War II (Kessler, Berglund, et al., 2005). Although there are some discrepancies, most studies find that prevalence rates differ between whites, Hispanics, and blacks (Blazer, Kessler, McGonagle, & Swartz, 1994). Similarly, there seems to be evidence from several epidemiological studies (e.g., the National Comorbidity Survey, National Comorbidity Survey Replication, National Survey of Families and Households) that higher rates of depression are found in people living in poverty and those with less education (Kessler et al., 2003). There are, of course, exceptions to these findings, but this seems to be the overall trend. It is also important to note that the manifestation of depression symptoms also varies across cultures and ethnic groups. For instance, somatic complaints are more common in some non-Western populations, which can dramatically influence how clients from these cultures present their complaints in treatment (American Psychiatric Association, 2013).

Another important finding is that women are 1.5 to 3 times as likely as men to experience depressive episodes (American Psychiatric Association, 2013). A critical explanation of this finding refers to differences in emotion regulation that make women more prone than men to respond to critical life events with depressive episodes (Nolen-Hoeksema et al., 2008). We come back to this explanation later in the chapter, when we discuss etiological models of the disorder.

Course and Outcome

The first onset of a major depressive episode can occur at any age, with median age of first onset at approximately 32 years (Kessler, Berglund, et al., 2005). An earlier age of onset has been associated with greater impairment in a number of domains (e.g., social and occupational functioning, quality of life, suicide attempts, recurrence) than experiencing the first episode as an adult (e.g., Zisook et al., 2007). Importantly, approximately 50% of individuals who later develop depression report a number of depressive symptoms even before their first episode. Put another way, subclinical forms of depression are very common and may predict onset of clinical episodes of the disorder (Kessler, Zhao, Blazer, & Swartz, 1997).

Moreover, depression can be both a chronic and a recurrent disorder. More than 70% of people with depression have recurring episodes (Kessler et al., 1997), and the chance of onset of another episode of depression increases with every episode a person experiences. To clarify, whereas 60% of individuals who have experienced one episode of depression will experience a second in their lifetime, 70% of those who have experienced two episodes, and 90% of those who have experienced three episodes will have an additional episode of depression (Keller & Boland, 1998). The typical time to recovery from any given depressive episode ranges from 3 to 6 months; however, a proportion of individuals continue to meet criteria for a depressive episode a year after initial diagnosis (Kendler, Walters, & Kessler, 1997).

Fortunately, a number of psychological (and pharmacological; see Nemeroff & Schatzberg, 2002, for a review) treatments have received empirical support for their efficacy. In a recent review, Follette and Greenberg (2006) categorized three treatments as "well-established" (behavior therapy, cognitive therapy, and IPT); two as "probably efficacious" (short-term psychodynamic therapy, process–experiential therapy); and one (mindfulness therapy) as "experimental," based on promising initial results. Follette and Greenberg also derived from the treatment manuals attached to these psychological therapies six principles of change that could guide evidence-based practice for depression: (1) challenging cognition and behavior; (2) increasing positive reinforcements and decreasing negative reinforcements (for avoidant and depressive behavior) in the client's life; (3) improving the client's interpersonal functioning; (4) improving marital, family and social environment; (5) fostering emotional awareness, acceptance, and regulation; and (6) providing a treatment that is both structured and focused.

Even though initial success rates are high, relapse rates also remain high and suggest that our long-term treatment effects are not even close to what we would hope for (Keller & Boland, 1998). For example, while Hollon, Stewart, and Strunk (2006) reported less than 5% relapse rates 6 months after CBT for most anxiety disorders, they reported a relapse rate (within the same time frame) of almost 20% after discontinuing cognitive therapy for depression (despite the fact that booster sessions were included in the depression but not in the anxiety treatment protocol). Furthermore, the rate of relapse may be worst for individuals who do not fully benefit from treatment. In a study with outpatient depressed patients treated with 16 weeks of CBT, Thase et al. (1992) found that only 9% of complete responders relapsed over 1-year follow-up, compared to 52% of the partial responders.

Comorbidity

Comorbidity among psychiatric disorders has received increasing attention in both clinical research and practice. The presence of comorbidity is now frequently accepted as the rule rather than the exception. Moreover, the presence of comorbidity has important implications for the course, prognosis, and treatment of illness.

Prevalence

Recent results from the National Comorbidity Survey Replication indicate that 45% of individuals with psychopathology meet criteria for more than one disorder (Kessler, Berglund, et al., 2005). Of those with MDD, the percentage of people with comorbidity increases to 76%. There are particularly high correlations between MDD and dysthymia, GAD, social anxiety disorder (SAD), and agoraphobia. Within an outpatient sample, 50.6% of individuals with depression had a comorbid anxiety disorder, with the most common comorbid disorder being SAD (Fava et al., 2000), and estimates of the concordance between rates of lifetime MDD and alcohol or drug dependence are as high as 44% (Miller, Klamen, Hoffmann, & Flaherty, 1996). The prevalence of depression increased from approximately 5.0% in youth who abstained from alcohol to 23.8% in youth who used alcohol at least weekly (Kandel et al., 1997). Personality disorders, especially borderline personality disorder, are also highly associated with depression (Lenzenweger, Lane, Loranger, & Kessler, 2007).

Course

The onset, frequency, and duration of depression are influenced by the presence of comorbid psychiatric disorders. Depressed individuals with comorbid anxiety disorders, for example, tend to be younger during the assessed episode (Fava et al., 2000). Comorbidity of depression and anxiety disorders is also associated with an earlier onset of first depressive episode and longer depressive episodes compared to the presence of depression alone (see Emmanuel, Simmonds, & Tyrer, 1998, for a meta-analysis). Interestingly, research has indicated a temporal sequence in anxiety and depression in which anxiety disorders are more likely to present first. In several epidemiological studies, the onset of SAD preceded the onset of MDD in approximately 70% of comorbid cases (e.g., Fava et al., 2000). Importantly, anxious children are at increased risk for developing depression during adolescence. In the year after first onset of an anxiety disorder, for example, the risk of a major depressive episode increases greatly, with odds ratios ranging from 6.5 for SAD to 62.0 for GAD (Kessler et al., 1996, 2008). Moreover, baseline incidences of a major depressive episode predicted the onset of subsequent GAD. Similar to the temporal order of depression and anxiety disorders, the majority of longitudinal epidemiological data indicate strong evidence for substance use or abuse leading to depression; however, other studies have also suggested that MDD might be a precursor to substance use disorders (Armstrong, & Costello, 2002; Rao & Chen, 2008). In addition, the presence of substance use disorders is associated with more prolonged and recurrent depressive episodes.

Underlying Mechanisms

The co-occurrence of depression and other psychiatric disorders has been explained by a variety of factors, including cognitive biases, biological dysregulation, and coping strategies. Depressed individuals with a comorbid anxiety disorder show more differential biases in their attention and memory than do those without comorbidity (Dannlowski et al., 2006), as detailed in the section on etiology below. Biased processing of negative information may place some individuals at risk for both depression and anxiety disorders. In addition, models have pointed to the fact that some anxiety disorders (e.g., SAD or agoraphobia) may result in decreased social support, which places individuals at greater risk for the onset of a depressive episode following stress. With regard to the co-occurrence of depression and substance use, researchers have suggested chronic substance use may lead to neurobiological changes that increase vulnerability for depression (e.g., Rao, Hammen, & Poland, 2009). For example, Rao and colleagues suggest that increased risk for substance use disorders in depressed individuals might be partially accounted for by increased activation in the hypothalamus–pituitary–adrenal (HPA) axis. Other models highlight the possibility that substance use may be an attempt to improve mood in the absence of more adaptive emotion regulation strategies.

Impairment

When comorbidity is present, it is strongly related to the severity of symptom presentation. Comorbidity of depression and anxiety, in particular, has been associated with more severe complaints, increased behavioral avoidance, greater impairment in social and occupational functioning, higher risk of suicide, and higher utilization of mental health services (see the meta-analysis by Emmanuel et al., 1998). Of the anxiety disorders, the presence of depression with comorbid SAD or GAD is associated with particularly poor outcomes. Comorbidity of SAD and MDD is generally associated with increased risk for suicidality and alcohol dependence (e.g., Kessler, Stang, Wittchen, Stein, & Walters, 1999). Data from two separate epidemiological studies indicated that the presence of depression and comorbid GAD affected perceptions of mental health and high levels of work impairment, over and above that of depression alone (Kessler, DuPont, Berglund, & Wittchen, 1999). The co-occurrence of addictive disorders and depression is also associated with greater impairment. It has been associated with more severe substance-related problems; increased frequency of behavioral problems; and more severe impairment in family, school, and legal domains (see Rao & Chen, 2008, for a review).

Clinical Implications

Basic findings related to the phenomenology and descriptive nature of depression can lead to a number of clinical implications that are likely to be relevant to therapists, irrespective of their theoretical orientation. To begin with, while psychopathology research indicates that depressive affect and diminished pleasure are the most characteristic features of this disorder, it also suggests that the presence of somatic symptoms may be indicative of severe depression. There are at least two reasons for encouraging therapists to assess these somatic symptoms when evaluating their clients' difficulties and progress: (1) because of their relatively low base rate, and (2) because these symptoms do not always get as much emphasis in the psychotherapy literature as psychological symptoms such as feelings of worthlessness, self-reproach, and guilt. For these reasons, vegetative or somatic features of depression may not always be on the therapist's "radar" despite their diagnostic and prognostic relevance.

It is also important for therapists to keep in mind that even though anger is not part of the diagnostic criteria, it is likely to be present and manifest in the therapeutic relationship with a depressed client. Since the psychotherapeutic setting can be viewed as a "microscope" (Goldfried & Davison, 1976) of the client's ways of reacting with others, we can predict from basic research that a number of depressed clients will express frustration toward treatment and/or therapists, and that therapists may experience irritation at some of their depressed clients. When such negative emotions and interactions emerge, clinical astuteness is required to discern how much of this is primarily a manifestation the client's disorder and how much is a reflection of an alliance rupture (e.g., a lack of fit between the client's needs and the treatment implemented by the therapist, or the result of empathic failures on the part of the clinician).

Irrespective of the causes of the client's anger or hostile transactions (and, of course, these causes are likely to be multiple and certainly not irreconcilable), focusing on such negative processes may lead to important therapeutic change. Potential growth opportunities include increasing the client's awareness of the negative impact he or she can have on others, as well as providing a model of how to recognize and discuss one's negative emotion and their contributions to the dynamic of the relationship (which scholars such as Safran and Segal [1990] have referred to as "meta-communication"). As we discuss later in this chapter, a number of other interpersonal issues related to the onset and maintenance of depression may well deserve to be foci of treatment.

One issue that definitely deserves therapists' attention when working with depressed clients is the risk of suicide. A number of factors have been associated with suicidal acts and completions, such as comorbid substance abuse, older age, white ethnicity, and access to lethal means. In addition, certain factors are particularly associated with suicide in depressed individuals, including anxiety, panic attacks, anhedonia, alcohol use, difficulty concentrating, and global insomnia (Sommers-Flanagan & Sommers-Flanagan, 1995). These should be carefully assessed before and during treatment with depressed clients.

Therapists also need to assess (before and during treatment) nonsymptomatic aspects of client functioning, such as work performance and satisfaction, sexual functioning, health problems, and health care behavior. Interventions typically used in effective forms of treatments may lead to a decrease of the symptoms of depression, but they may not directly or immediately have an impact on these other dimensions, which, of course, can have crucial effects on a person's quality of life. Unless these are addressed by longer treatments, specific therapeutic skills, and/or referral to other services, the scope and depth of the therapist's interventions may be limited. While clients may feel better about themselves and have more gratifying relationships with significant others at the end of a short-term therapy, they may well have a recurrence of depression if they continue to be confronted with serious occupational and health difficulties—as suggested by basic research on some of the stressors associated with depression (see below).

Interestingly, clinicians (perhaps especially those in training) should be aware that once they are competent in the implementation of effective treatments for depression, their expertise is likely to be extremely relevant for specific populations and settings, such as medical patients, nursing homes, and workplaces—populations with high rates of depression and negative outcome associated with depressive disorders. As such, behavioral medicine techniques, community-oriented interventions, and behavioral activation (e.g., problem solving, motivational strategies) are likely to be useful parts of their skills repertoire, again, irrespective of their theoretical orientations.

In line with increasing the specificity of psychological treatments for depression, clinicians would be wise to familiarize themselves with cultural differences in the manifestation and report of depressive symptoms. This has clear implications for the possibility of over- or underdiagnosing individuals due to cultural insensitivity, and could also have important meanings for treatment process. For instance, establishing a shared understanding of the causes of somatic symptoms may be key in building a therapeutic alliance, and provide a focus for monitoring treatment progress.

Basic psychopathology research also suggests that clinicians would be well advised to ask when clients had their first depressive episode, as well as to assess for other disorders frequently associated with depression (e.g., anxiety, substance abuse, and personality disorders). As mentioned earlier, both early onset of depression and comorbidity have been linked with more impairment. Because depressed clients with higher levels of impairment have also been shown to improve more with longer therapy than with shorter therapy (Beutler, Blatt, Alimohamed, Levy, & Angtuago, 2006), therapists should expect that an a priori limited number of sessions (e.g., the ones typically involved in research clinical trials) may not be sufficient for these clients. A recent study (Fournier et al., 2008) also suggests that when individuals with moderate to severe depression present with a personality disorder comorbidity, antidepressants should be considered as a first line of attack (at least compared to cognitive therapy).

Because basic research demonstrates that people experience a number of symptoms before suffering from a full episode of depression, and because having such an episode is a strong predictor of future recurrences, "subthreshold" levels of depression should be considered by therapists (and managed health care agencies) as high priority for intervention. Also, considering the strong relationship between the number of previous episodes and the likelihood of future episodes (e.g., 90% of those who have three episodes will have a fourth one), it is crucial for clinicians to assess their clients' past episodes of major depression. Since repeated episodes may indicate extreme vulnerability, therapists should expect that stronger (more intense, longer) doses of treatment might be necessary to foster restoration and/or consolidation of adaptive ways of functioning than the amount of therapeutic attention typically delivered in current empirically supported treatment (EST) for depression. Irrespective of the length and intensity of the treatment required, the data also suggests treatment should continue until the symptoms are fully abated; failure to do this may predict relapse.

Furthermore, since the data also indicate that a substantial number of depressed individuals without treatment do not experience remission from their symptoms for up to a year, treatment should not be delayed because of the conviction that depression tends to go away by itself. This recommendation for treatment can and should be made strongly by therapists, governmental agencies, and managed health care organizations because the research clearly shows that several types of psychological (and pharmacological) therapy work. The evidence supporting treatment of different orientations (cognitive, behavioral, interpersonal, psychodynamic, and experiential) for depression means that it may be clinically unsound for trained clinicians not to use ESTs, or at least treatments that are conceptually and clinically close to (or based on) the specific treatments that have been validated.

Moreover, while these treatments represent a wide variety of approaches, scholars have been able to identify principles of change (or general strategies of interventions) that cut across several of them, and may be fairly seamlessly incorporated into most forms of psychological treatments. As a source of clinically relevant information, these principles are precise enough to guide the focus of clinicians' interventions without being restricted to a narrow and orientation-specific set of prescribed procedures (see Castonguay & Beutler, 2006). There are, for example, many techniques (e.g., interpretation, cognitive restructuring) that therapists can use to challenge client appraisals of self and others, all with similar aims (Goldfried, 1980). In addition, principles of change can help therapists to increase their repertoire of interventions if the treatments they typically conduct with their depressed clients do not systematically target dimensions of functioning that may be involved in the cause or maintenance of depression. For example, in addition to using effective techniques to address "internal" or intrapersonal issues (e.g., exploring a client's emotions or challenging distorted cognitions), experiential, psychodynamic, and cognitive-oriented therapists should also assess and (if necessary) address interactional issues that are frequently associated with depression, such as social isolation, interpersonal skills deficits, and dysfunctional marital or familial relationships. In addition, and as described elsewhere, such empirically anchored principles (along with principles of change related to relationship and participant variables) have provided the foundation for training guidelines to prevent or reduce harmful effects in therapy (Castonguay, Boswell, Constantino, Goldfried, & Hill, 2010).

As mentioned earlier, however, not all depressed clients benefit from therapy, and many who do benefit fail to retain their therapeutic gains after the completion of treatment. There is clearly room for improvement with respect to our current attempt to deal with this debilitating and costly disorder. The best strategy to improve our effectiveness, however, is not likely to encourage clinicians or researchers to devise completely new forms of therapy: Reinventing the wheel is not likely to lead to a panacea. Instead, a more fruitful strategy (but by no means the only one) is to build upon and improve already established and supported treatments. This could be done, for instance, by modifying such treatments based on the findings of psychotherapy process research. As a case in point, preliminary but promising evidence suggests that by adding interpersonal and humanistic interventions aimed at repairing alliance ruptures (a process robustly linked to worse outcome in depression treatment) may improve the efficacy of cognitive therapy for depression (Castonguay et al., 2004; Constantino et al., 2008; Safran & Muran, 2000). Another strategy based on research is prescriptively to use effective treatment based on what appears to work best for particular clients, such as using nondirective interventions with highly resistant client and intervening more ways with depressed clients who are less resistant (see Beutler, Consoli, & Lane, 2005). Another possible (not incompatible) way to improve clinicians' effectiveness is to consider basic findings that are relevant for their understanding and treatment of depressed clients. The delineation of clinical implications of psychopathology research in this chapter (as in chapters in this volume on other disorders), of course, attempts to offer such guidelines.

As most clinicians are already aware, depression is one of the most common problems encountered in clinical practice. Interestingly, and perhaps alarmingly, research has shown that the prevalence of depression has been climbing sharply over recent decades. According to Seligman (1989), this increase points to social/ environmental determinants of depression. Contrasting a 10-fold increase in prevalence observed in the general population with the rate of depression in some "nonmodern" cultures (e.g., Amish), he argued that something in contemporary society causes depression: a focus on individualism rather than on the common good. It might also be that the lack of commitment to common projects has robbed individuals of buffers against depression when confronted with personal difficulties or failures. Our overinvolvement in activities aimed at increasing our individualistic accomplishments, wealth, and comfort might well make it more difficult to reach out and obtain help and support from others when we experience serious difficulties in our lives. What this implies with regard to clinical practice is that irrespective of their orientation, clinicians should help clients renew or create meaningful relationships. They should encourage clients and/or teach them skills to open themselves appropriately and safely to others, as well as to get involved in purposeful and/or pleasurable activities with others.

These clinical implications (i.e., improving client's interpersonal functioning, as well as improving marital, family, and social environment) that emerge from purely basic research are consistent with some of the principles of change derived from another domain of research mentioned earlier: EST. Such convergences of findings across different domains of research may not be a surprise considering the core aspects of human functioning to which they appear to be linked. As argued by MacLean (1985), communication and attachment are two of the evolutionary developments that differentiate not only humans but also all mammals from reptiles. Denying or not attending to such ways of being forces ourselves and our clients to fight a losing evolutionary battle!

Helping clients to be more engaged interpersonally, however, may be more difficult with some than with others. Individuals (let alone cultures) vary in terms of agency and communion needs or tendencies. As described by Bonanno and Castonguay (1993), when conducting therapy with agency-oriented people, it might be best initially to focus on intrapersonal or individualistic issues, so that the tasks and goals of therapy may be more synchronized with individuals' typical ways of coping with life difficulties. With the development of a stronger therapeutic alliance, however, we may begin to focus more on what are likely to be deficits in the interpersonal functioning of these individuals.

ETIOLOGY

As we mentioned early in the chapter, the extent of the empirical literature on potential determinants of depression prevents us from providing a comprehensive review of vulnerability factors for this disorder. Among the most obvious omissions in the following subsections are basic findings related to some biological models (e.g., neurochemical abnormalities, genetic disposition) and learning (e.g., operant and vicarious conditioning) that have been associated with depression (for reviews see Burke, Davis, Otte, & Mohr, 2005; Johnson, Joormann, LeMoult, & Miller, 2009; Sullivan, Neale, & Kendler, 2000). These well-established vulnerability factors have provided a foundation for some of the currently supported treatments (pharmacological or psychological). As we also mentioned, however, our goal is to focus primarily on newer, basic findings and/or etiology research that has not been sufficiently incorporated in our current treatments.

Cognitive Theories

Cognitive models of depression posit that depressed individuals exhibit cognitive biases in all aspects of information processing, including memory, attention, and interpretation (Mathews & MacLeod, 2005), which increase the risk for onset and maintenance of depressive episodes. Although empirical results for some of these biases are mixed, others have been clearly associated with depression and could have important treatment implications.

Memory

Overall, there is strong evidence for biased memory in depression (Mathews & MacLeod, 2005). In fact, better recall of negative, relative to positive, information represents perhaps the most robust cognitive finding associated with major depression. Memory biases are found most consistently in free recall and explicit memory tasks. For example, when attempting consciously to recall details of past events or recently viewed words from a specific learning experience, individuals with depression are more likely than nondepressed controls to recall negative or unpleasant information.

Additional evidence that individual differences in memory play an important role in depression comes from research on overgeneral memory (Williams et al., 2007). These studies show that depressed participants respond to positive and negative cues with memories that summarize a category of similar events. For example, when asked to describe a specific positive memory, nondepressed controls are able to provide specific details of a past event (e.g., "the day my family went to Lake Michigan"); however, individuals with depression recall a more general period in time (e.g., fifth grade). Importantly, this research has demonstrated that overgeneral memories are associated with poor problem solving, difficulty imagining specific future events, and delayed recovery from episodes of depression. Moreover, over-general memories remain stable outside of episodes of the disorder and have been shown to predict later onset of depressive episodes following life events.

Attention

Empirical findings about whether depressed individuals exhibit an attentional bias have been mixed (e.g., see Mogg & Bradley, 2005, for a review). Strikingly, no studies have found a bias in clinically depressed participants when stimuli have been presented subliminally and masked in order to investigate unconscious processing (see Mathews & MacLeod, 2005, for a recent review). Furthermore, no attentional biases were found in participants who had previously been depressed (e.g., Gilboa & Gotlib, 1997). Based on such findings, Williams, Watts, MacLeod, and Matthews (1997) proposed that depressed persons are characterized not by biases in attentional functioning but by biases in postattentional elaboration.

Although this formulation seems plausible, it may be premature to conclude that depressed persons are not characterized by an attentional bias. Recent studies suggest that depressed individuals do not direct their attention to negative information more frequently than do control participants, but once it captures their attention they exhibit difficulties disengaging from it (e.g., Joormann & Gotlib, 2007). Moreover, in their review of the literature, Mogg and Bradley (2005) point out that depressed individuals are more likely to exhibit attentional biases for self-relevant negative stimuli presented for longer durations. In summary, these results suggest that depression is characterized by a selective bias for negative self-relevant information, but this bias does not operate throughout all aspects of selective attention. Depressed individuals may not automatically orient their attention toward negative information in the environment, but once such information has become the focus of their attention, they may have greater difficulty disengaging from it.

Interpretation

Results also have been mixed with regard to whether depression is characterized by an interpretation bias (Lawson, MacLeod, & Hammond, 2002). The strongest evidence that depressed individuals exhibit a negative bias comes from research relying on self-reported interpretations of ambiguous scenarios (e.g., Nunn, Matthews, & Trower, 1997). The reliance on self-report measures, however, has been criticized as being subject to alternative explanations (MacLeod & Mathews, 1991). More recent studies have thus utilized experimental designs that are less subject to response bias effects (Lawson & MacLeod, 1999); however, empirical findings as a result of such designs have been inconsistent. Researchers have found contradictory results when using the same group of participants (Mogg, Bradbury, & Bradley, 2006). Although additional clarification is needed regarding the nature of interpretation biases in depression, biased interpretation toward negative information seems most likely when information is self-referenced and ambiguous.

Inhibition and Cognitive Control

It has been suggested that deficits in cognitive inhibition lie at the heart of memory and attention biases in depression (Joormann, Yoon, & Zetsche, 2007). Depressed individuals have difficulties disengaging from negative material and, consequently, exhibit sustained processing and increased elaboration of negative content. Because the experience of negative mood states and negative life events is associated with the activation of mood-congruent cognitions in working memory, the ability to control the contents of working memory may be critical in differentiating between people who recover easily after experiencing negative affect and those who initiate a vicious cycle of increasingly negative ruminative thinking and deepening sad mood. Using a selective attention task, Joormann and colleagues (2007) reported that depressed participants had difficulties inhibiting negative material. Other evidence for reduced inhibition in depression comes from memory tasks (Joormann & Gotlib, 2008; Power, Dagleish, Claudio, Tata, & Kentish, 2000), which provide further support that depression is associated with difficulties inhibiting negative, irrelevant material.

Moreover, studies examining cognitive aspects of depression are beginning to elucidate the nature of the relations among cognition, emotion regulation, and depression. Findings suggest that inhibition, working memory, and cognitive control are important concepts in understanding the dysfunctional cognitive processes that may underlie sustained processing of negative information and rumination in depression (Joormann et al., 2007). Hasher and Zacks (1988) proposed that the efficient functioning of working memory depends on inhibitory processes that both limit the access of information into working memory and update the contents of working memory by removing information that is no longer relevant. If changes in mood are, in fact, associated with activations of mood-congruent material in working memory, the ability to control the contents of working memory might play an important role in the prevention of rumination and, therefore, in recovery from negative mood (Joormann et al., 2007). Indeed, Hertel (2004) has proposed that depression is characterized by reduced cognitive control that impairs the override of automatic, prepotent response tendencies.

Overall, the literature points to several cognitive biases that may have important treatment implications in depression. For example, evidence suggests that although depressed individuals do not demonstrate an immediate attention bias, they do have trouble disengaging from negative stimuli once it enters into their awareness (e.g., Joormann & Gotlib, 2007). This in turn may lead to the increased elaboration of negative information and contribute to the negative memory biases frequently observed in depression (Mathews & MacLeod, 2005). These intrusive, negative memories are thought to be important contributors to negative mood state and have been linked to symptom severity and persistence (Brewin, Reynolds, & Tata, 1999; Kuyken & Brewin, 1994), making them possible targets for treatment. Moreover, evidence suggests that deficits in cognitive inhibition might underlie the attention and memory biases observed in depression. Such deficits might also contribute to increased elaboration of negative information and rumination (Joormann et al., 2007), which are key contributors to prolonged negative affect. As such, training individuals to control the contents of working memory could interrupt the cognitive mechanisms that contribute to depressive episodes.

Comorbidity and Cognitive Biases

Important differences have been identified in the pattern of cognitive biases depending on whether a comorbid condition is present (e.g., Tarsia, Power, & Sanavio, 2003). For example, whereas non-comorbid depressed participants did not demonstrate a bias in the way they processed emotional words, comorbid depressed and anxious participants were distracted by processing negative words to the extent that it interfered with their ability to process subsequent information (Dannlowski et al., 2006). In addition, differences in attention and memory biases were found between socially anxious participants with and without depression (LeMoult & Joormann, 2010). Compared to non-comorbid participants, those with comorbid social anxiety and depression attended away from angry faces, then subsequently recognized fewer of the angry facial expressions. Gilboa-Schechtman, Erhard-Weiss, and Jeczemien (2002) also found differences in memory biases between non-comorbid anxious individuals and those with comorbid depression. Overall, results suggest that the way individuals process information may depend on the presence of not only depression but also other comorbid diagnoses.

Emotion Regulation in Depression

Recently, depression has often been referred to as a disorder of emotion regulation (ER; Joormann & D'Avanzato, 2010; Gross & Munoz, 1995). Sustained negative affect and persistent reduction in positive affect are the hallmark features of a diagnosis of a major depressive episode. How can we explain that some people respond to what would be considered minor stressors with increasingly negative affect that can spiral into a full-blown depressive episode, while others seem never to become depressed even when they face major adversity? A closer look at the concept of emotion regulation and at mechanisms that allow us to understand individual differences in the important ability to regulate affective states may provide an answer to these questions (Bonanno, 2005). Specifically, it is possible that depression-vulnerable and nonvulnerable people do not differ much in their initial response to a negative life event. Both groups experience sadness and therefore respond with the activation of mood-congruent cognitions and increased accessibility of mood-congruent memories. Depression-vulnerable and nonvulnerable people differ, however, in their ability to recover from this initial response (Teasdale, 1988).

This suggests that we need to examine factors that impair or support this recovery. The construct of ER, which evolved from the more general concept of coping, involves the utilization of behavioral and cognitive strategies to influence the duration, intensity, and experience of affect (Thompson, 1994). Emotions are regulated for a variety of reasons, such as to enhance desirable feelings, maintain social norms, and foster interpersonal relationships (Fischer, Manstead, Evers, Timmer, & Valk, 2004). Recent theories of depression emphasize that increased risk for MDD comes from the use of strategies that fail to down-regulate negative emotions after their initial onset (e.g., Joormann & Gotlib, 2010; Nolen-Hoeksema et al., 2008), which leads to prolonged negative affect (John & Gross, 2004). In response to distress, the use of less effective ER strategies (e.g., rumination, suppression) has been associated with multiple psychological disorders, including depression (Kring & Werner, 2004), whereas effective ER strategies (e.g., distraction, reappraisal) are typically characteristic of healthy psychological functioning (Gross, 1998). Surprisingly few studies have investigated the use and effectiveness of ER strategies in clinical depression. Moreover, most of these studies relied on self-report data and examined people who score high on depression inventories, instead of diagnosed samples. Still, the findings of these studies support the claim that more frequent use of certain strategies (e.g., emotion suppression, rumination, and catastrophizing) and less frequent use of other strategies (e.g., reappraisal, self-disclosure) are related to depression and anxiety symptoms (e.g., Garnefski & Kraaij, 2006). In addition, recent studies suggest that impaired ER not only characterizes currently depressed people but also may be observed after recovery. For example, Ehring, Fischer, Schnülle, Bösterling, and Tuschen-Caffier (2008) found that recovered depressed participants reported greater difficulties than control participants regulating their negative emotions and more frequently used rumination and catastrophizing. Rumination and distraction have received the most attention within the depression literature; however, emerging evidence also points to the important role of suppression, reappraisal, and anger.

Rumination

Rumination, a means of responding to distress by repetitively and passively focusing on symptoms of distress and the potential causes or consequences of these symptoms, is differentiated from negative automatic thoughts by being a *style* of thought rather than just negative *content* (Nolen-Hoeksema et al., 2008). This ER strategy is a particularly salient risk factor for depression because it exacerbates and prolongs depressed mood (see review by Nolen-Hoeksema et al.). Empirical evidence has shown that rumination predicts higher levels of depressive symptoms and onset of major depressive episodes, and mediates the gender difference in depressive symptoms (for a review, see Nolen-Hoeksema et al., 2008). Many studies that experimentally tested the effects of rumination showed that induced rumination leads to sustained negative mood, increased negative cognitions, increased overgeneral autobiographical memory, and decreased problem solving in depressed participants (e.g., Nolen-Hoeksema et al., 2008). Interestingly, healthy controls placed in a negative mood state also experienced prolonged negative affect if instructed to ruminate. Even among control participants, when combined with a negative mood induction, rumination has been shown to affect cortisol production, physiological levels, cognitive processes, and autobiographical memory (e.g., Cui & Huang, 2007; Denson, Fabiansson, Creswell, & Pedersen, 2009). Together these studies provide strong evidence that rumination in the context of either naturally occurring or experimentally induced depressed mood maintains dysphoria, enhances negative thinking, and impairs problem solving. Such evidence also highlights the interconnectedness of cognitive processes, biological functioning, and emotion regulation strategies.

Distraction

In contrast to rumination, distraction involves engaging in positive or neutral activities in order to divert one's thoughts from symptoms of distress and depression (Lyubomirsky, Caldwell, & Nolen-Hoeksema, 1998). For example, one may lower the level of subjective emotion experienced by focusing on thoughts unrelated to the situation (e.g., planning a supermarket shopping list). It is important to differentiate attentional distraction, which involves shifting visual or auditory attention away from emotion-producing stimuli, as discussed earlier, from cognitive distraction described here, which involves shifting one's thoughts away from the emotion or emotion-producing stimuli. Studies have reported that dysphoric, clinically depressed, and recovered depressed people are able to use cognitive distraction to repair an induced negative mood state (Joormann & Siemer, 2004; Joormann, Siemer, & Gotlib, 2007). Indeed, distraction has been associated with adaptive outcomes such as faster physiological recovery from stress (Vickers & Vogeltanz-Holm, 2003), decreased depressed mood (Trask & Sigmon, 1999), and shorter durations of depressive symptoms (Nolen-Hoeksema, Morrow, & Fredrickson, 1993). Depressed participants are less likely to use distraction, however, even though they state that it could help them alleviate their negative affect (Lyubomisky & Nolen-Hoeksema, 1993). Overall, findings suggest that providing specific, neutral or positive, activities or thoughts can take one's mind off of the current negative emotions and alleviate negative moods, including depression and anger (Gerin, Davidson, Christenfeld, Goyal, & Schwartz, 2006; Rusting & Nolen-Hoeksema, 1998). However, see Campbell-Sills and Barlow (2007) and Kross, Ayduk, and Mischel (2005), who point out that persistent distraction serves as an ineffective long-term ER strategy, because it hinders effective problem solving.

Suppression

Both thought suppression and expressive suppression fall under this category. Whereas thought suppression involves not thinking of the emotion-provoking event or stimuli, expressive suppression involves inhibiting the expression of the emotional experience. Ironically, research has shown that thought suppression can lead to increases in the accessibility and frequency of the to-be-suppressed thought (Kircanski, Craske, & Bjork, 2008), and in turn increases in the emotional response (e.g., Wegner & Gold, 1995). Several studies suggest that depressed and recovered depressed people are more likely than control participants to use thought suppression, and that the use of this ER strategy may play an important role in the onset and maintenance of depression (Wenzlaff, Rude, Taylor, Stultz, & Sweatt, 2001). Although studies reveal that participants can successfully engage in expressive suppression when instructed, participants also show greater physiological activation when doing so, suggesting that suppression is an effortful means of regulating emotion (Gross, 1998). Expressive suppression has also been found to be ineffective at regulating negative feelings. In fact, several studies have found that expressive suppression decreases the experience of positive, but not negative, emotions (e.g., Gross & Levenson, 1997; Stepper & Strack, 1993), and the habitual use of this strategy is associated with less well-being and higher levels of depression (Haga, Kraft, & Corby, 2009; Joormann & Gotlib, 2010). Even outside the laboratory, greater use of expressive suppression has been linked to less social support, less social satisfaction, and decreased closeness to others (Srivastava, Tamir, McGonigal, John, & Gross, 2009).

Reappraisal

Reappraisal has increasingly become a focus within the depression literature. This construct refers to the process of changing the way one thinks about a situation in order to alter its emotional impact (John & Gross, 2004). Some people may reappraise a situation by changing their point of view (i.e., taking a third-person rather than first-person perspective), whereas others change their interpretation of the situation (i.e., viewing a difficult task as a challenge rather than as a threat; Ray et al., 2005). Habitual use of this strategy has been associated with adaptive changes in emotions, cognitions, and physiological arousal. For example, reappraisal has been linked to increased well-being, fewer depressive symptoms, increased inhibition of negative material, greater positive autobiographical recall, healthier physiological reactivity to distress, and better interpersonal functioning (Gross & John, 2003; Joormann & Gotlib, 2010). Compared to other ER strategies, such as expressive suppression, reappraisal is associated with the experience of more positive affect and less negative affect (Gross & John, 2003).

Neuroendocrinology

Stressful life events and other psychosocial stressors are robustly associated with the onset, severity, and course of MDD (see review in Hammen, 2005). Dysfunctions in the neuroendocrine system might explain the link between stress and depression, which makes "neuroendocrinology"—the study of interactions between the endocrine and the nervous system—increasingly important. A central component of the neuroendocrine system is the HPA axis, which is central in regulating the hormone cortisol. Cortisol affects many aspects of the body, including metabolism, immune function, and the brain. In addition to being released in response to stressors, it is released spontaneously throughout the day. Spontaneous cortisol production is influenced by sleep–wake cycles, known as "diurnal fluctuations."

Given that functioning of the HPA system is so integrally related to the human stress response, it is not surprising that atypical patterns of both basal HPA functioning and HPA reactivity have been documented in various psychiatric disorders, including depression (e.g., Porter & Gallagher, 2006). From a different perspective, investigating neuroendocrine response in these disorders is important, because it might represent a crucial link to the neurobiological research we describe later. For example, the hippocampus and the prefrontal cortex (PFC) are the brain regions with the highest density of glucocorticoid receptors, and chronic exposure to stressful events that lead to increased cortisol secretion might lead to neurotoxicity in these areas (Sapolsky, 2000). Chronic activation of the HPA axis, which results in high levels of cortisol, can thus disrupt functioning in regions of the brain that are responsible for regulating emotion (e.g., the PFC and the amygdala) and interfere with the ability to cope effectively with stress.

Researchers reported differences in basal HPA activity and diurnal fluctuations of individuals with MDD compared to their nondepressed counterparts. In a review by Burke et al. (2005), studies conducted in the morning found depressed individuals to have lower cortisol levels upon wakening and 30 minutes thereafter. In contrast, studies conducted in the afternoon found elevated cortisol levels in depressed individuals. Some researchers attribute the overproduction of cortisol to faulty negative feedback mechanisms (Porter & Gallagher, 2006). Using techniques such as the dexamethasone suppression test, researchers have found that many patients with depression fail to exhibit the usual suppression of cortisol production after being injected with dexamethasone (e.g., Carroll, 1982). Although common in depression, this finding has not been universal. In a review by Arana, Baldessarini, and Ornsteen (1985), dexamethasone nonsuppression was more commonly found in individuals with psychotic depression and predicted a more severe course.

Public-speaking and cognitive stress challenges have been used as alternative and more natural methods to test the entire HPA system. In a recent meta-analysis,

Burke et al. (2005) reported that depressed individuals exhibit less cortisol reactivity in response to stress and slower cortisol recovery poststress compared to nondepressed individuals. They also reported that the higher the cortisol levels at baseline, the less cortisol produced after the stressor. Blunted cortisol stress reactivity and prolonged poststress recovery was most pronounced in older and more severely depressed participants. Whereas some studies have reported that HPA axis abnormalities in depressed individuals are state-dependent and generally ameliorate with clinical remission (e.g., Ribeiro, Tandon, Grunhaus, & Greden, 1993), those remitted participants who continue to show abnormal cortisol responses have a higher rate of relapse (e.g., Aubry et al., 2007; Zobel et al., 2001).

One concern is that HPA axis dysfunction could reflect the cumulative effect of depressive episodes and related experiences. To test this, investigators have assessed HPA axis functioning in samples of depressed children and, more recently, in samples of children who are at elevated risk for depression. For example, although differences between depressed and nondepressed adolescents in levels of evening cortisol secretion were not found, elevations in evening cortisol levels within the sample of depressed adolescents predicted a recurrent course of the disorder at a 7-year follow-up assessment (Rao et al., 1996; Mathew et al., 2003). In addition, numerous studies have found elevated cortisol secretion in response to acute stressors in depressed children (e.g., Granger, Weisz, McCracken, Ikeda, & Douglas, 1996; Watamura, Donzella, Alwin, & Gunnar, 2003), and cortisol abnormalities in healthy children and adolescents at risk for depression (e.g., Mannie, Harmer, & Cowen, 2007). Other studies, however, have found no differences in waking salivary cortisol levels when comparing people with and without a depressed relative (e.g., Le Masurier, Cowen, & Harmer, 2007). Hence, relatives of depressed persons may vary in degree of cortisol dysregulation, and when they do evidence cortisol dysregulation, this appears to predict symptoms over time (Goodyer, Herbert, Tamplin, & Altham, 2000).

Neuroimaging

Brain areas and neural circuits associated with the generation and regulation of emotional states have received increasing attention in research on affective disorders (see Davidson, Pizzagalli, & Nitschke, 2002, for a review). Over the past decade, theorists have posited that emotional behavior is linked to the functioning of two neural systems, a ventral system and a dorsal system. The ventral system involves brain regions that are important for identifying the emotional significance of a stimulus and producing affect; the dorsal system is important for executive function, including selective attention, planning, and effortful regulation of affective states. Adaptive emotional behavior is posited to depend on the integrity and balanced interaction of these systems (Ochsner & Gross, 2005).

Although the ventral system includes many different brain structures, the vast majority of mood disorders research on this system focuses on the amygdala and the subgenual anterior cingulate cortex (ACC). The dorsal region that has received the most attention is the PFC, with particular focus on the dorsolateral PFC (DLPFC), and some focus on the ventromedial PFC (VMPFC). Although we focus on these regions, it is worth noting that these brain regions interact with many different divisions of the ACC, the PFC, and other brain regions in important ways that have repercussions for understanding emotion. The function of these regions has received a great deal of attention in the past decade. The amygdala has been shown to play a prominent role in emotionally mediated attention, in assigning emotional significance to stimuli, and in memory of emotionally significant events. The subgenual ACC appears to mediate subjective experience of emotion and emotional reaction to stimuli, particularly in guiding reward-seeking behavior (Pizzagalli et al., 2004). The DLPFC appears to be involved in the regulation of emotion (Drevets, 2000). For example, it appears to diminish amygdala activity in response to an emotion challenge (Siegle, Steinhauer, Thase, Stenger, & Carter, 2002).

Beyond the ventral and dorsal regions just described, given the importance of reward responsivity in MDD (Kasch, Rottenberg, Arnow, & Gotlib, 2002), researchers have begun to attend to areas implicated in the anticipation and response to reward, such as the ventral striatum and the nucleus accumbens (e.g., Knutson, Fong, Adams, Varner, & Hommer, 2001), which are also regulated by the PFC (e.g., Phillips, Drevets, Rauch, & Lane, 2003).

Findings from both structural and functional studies provide evidence of imbalanced neural functioning in depression and, in particular, of a hyperactive ventral system (more specifically, the amygdala and subgenual ACC) and a hypoactive dorsal system (DLPFC; see Mayberg, 2002), as well as deficits in areas associated primarily with the processing of rewarding stimuli (Davidson et al., 2002). Here, we discuss the evidence for these deficits, including structural studies, positron emission tomography (PET) studies, and functional magnetic resonance imaging (fMRI) studies of responses to emotion challenges.

Whereas structural studies of the amygdala have yielded inconsistent findings (see Sheline, 2003, for a review), investigators have found abnormal elevations in blood flow, blood oxygenation, and glucose metabolism in the amygdala in depression (Drevets, Bogers, & Raichle, 2002). Indeed, findings of PET studies indicate that increased baseline amygdala activation in depression is positively correlated with depression severity (Abercrombie et al., 1998; Drevets et al., 2002). In addition to being characterized by elevated baseline amygdala activity, several fMRI studies suggest that depressed persons exhibit greater amygdala reactivity to emotional stimuli than do controls, for example, in response to negative facial expressions (e.g., Sheline et al., 2001). Likewise, Siegle et al. (2002) reported increased amygdala activation to negative words in depression. Canli et al. (2005) reported that greater amygdala activation in response to emotional faces predicted recovery from depression in a follow-up assessment. More recently, increased amygdala activation was found during an emotion task among unmedicated depressed persons (Siegle, Thompson, Carter, Steinhauer, & Thase, 2007).

A concern, though, is that much of this research examines the amygdala during episodes of MDD. Increased activation could reflect a state-dependent feature of depression. As noted earlier, studies of at-risk and unaffected family members are particularly important. Increased right amygdala activation to fearful faces has also been found in unaffected persons with a family history of depression in response to the tryptophan depletion paradigms (Sheline et al., 2001) described earlier (van der Veen, Evers, Deutz, & Schmitt, 2007). These findings suggest that amygdala response to emotional stimuli in depression is not just a state marker.

Volume reductions in the subgenual ACC have been associated with depression (e.g., Drevets et al., 1997). In addition, a number of PET studies have reported reduced resting state activity in the subgenual ACC in depressed individuals (e.g., Drevets et al., 1997, 2002). When Drevets (1999) presented adjusted estimates of activity in the subgenual ACC to compensate for the volume loss in this structure associated with depression, he reported that the volume-adjusted activity estimates indicated increased subgenual ACC activity. In addition, Gotlib et al. (2005) found that depressed individuals exhibited greater subgenual ACC activation than did controls in response to emotional faces. Siegle, Carter, and Thase (2006) showed that low reactivity in the subgenual ACC and high reactivity in the amygdala in response to affective words predicted recovery in depressed individuals after CBT.

Depression is also related to structural abnormalities in the DLPFC, such as reduced neuron and glial count and size (e.g., Chana, Landau, Beasley, Everall, & Cotter, 2003). PET studies have consistently found decreased DLPFC activation in depressed compared to healthy individuals (see Drevets, 1998; Mayberg, Keightley, Mahurin, & Brannan, 2004). Studies using tryptophan depletion have reported that individuals who relapse have lower DLPFC activity during relapse than do individual who do not relapse (e.g., Bremner et al., 1997). Recent studies have also found reduced DLPFC response to affective stimuli in depressed compared to healthy controls. Schaefer, Putnam, Benca, and Davidson (2006), for example, reported diminished reactivity of the DLPFC in depressed participants in response to both erotica and positive emotion faces. In a recent study, Siegle, Ghinassi, and Thase (2007) reported that reduced activation in DLPFC during a cognitive task characterized unmedicated depressed participants. Importantly, Hooley, Gruber, Scott, Hiller, and Yurgelun-Todd (2005) reported that compared to control participants, recovered depressed individuals failed to activate the DLPFC while listening to taped criticism from their mothers. This indicates that hypoactivation of the DLPFC is not just related to depressed state.

In regard to regions involved in reward processing, researchers have also found reduced volume in the basal ganglia (the broader structures containing the ventral striatum) among persons with depression (Parashos, Tupler, Blitchington, & Krishnan, 1998). Functional studies also suggest deficits in activation of the ventral striatum. Forbes et al. (2006), for example, reported that depressed children exhibited decreased activation in reward-related brain areas when making reward-related decisions and when receiving reward. Keedwell, Andrew, Williams, Brammer, and

Phillips (2005) found that in the ventral striatum a decreased response to happy stimuli was related to anhedonia in depression. Schaefer et al. (2006) reported that the depression-associated hypoactivation in areas of PFC, basal ganglia, insula, and hippocampus that they observed in response to positive stimuli normalized after successful treatment with antidepressant medication. So far, no studies have investigated activation in reward-related brain areas in healthy relatives of patients diagnosed with depressive disorders.

Interpersonal and Developmental Contributions

Because of the tremendous amount of research on the etiology and maintenance of depression, several volumes on the basic research in this area have been written (e.g., Gotlib & Hammen, 2009). Whereas the emphasis of this chapter is on some recent developments in cognitive and neurological research, it is important to note the substantial developments in our understanding of the interpersonal and developmental processes that contribute to depressive symptoms. We must, for issues of space, resign ourselves to discuss these topics here only briefly.

A substantial number of interpersonal factors have been associated with the onset, maintenance, and/or recurrence of depression across different phases of life. Early risk factors for depression (and related symptoms or problems) include several manifestations of inadequate parenting. Some parental deficits that appear to be related to risk for depression in children (both in youth and adulthood) reflect different types of neglect, such as inattentiveness, withdrawal, emotional unresponsiveness, inconsistent reinforcement, lax enforcement, avoidance of confrontation, and low frequency of positive reinforcement. Other instances of inadequate parenting involve various forms of aggression toward the child, such as overt hostility, intrusiveness, emotional overinvolvement, and overstimulation, as well as physical and sexual abuse. Insecure parent–child attachment and parental conflicts have also been identified as early predictors of depression. Similarly, losing a parent (i.e., death) and having a depressed parent have been associated with depressive disorders (Davila et al., 2009; Goodman & Brand, 2009; Hammen, 2009).

Some of these factors, of course, interact with each other. Impaired parenting, for example, has been found to mediate the relationship between parental depression and child psychological difficulties (Goodman & Brand, 2009; Hammen, 2009). It should also be noted that children's vulnerabilities or problems (biological, cognitive, affective, and/or behavioral) may contribute to parenting difficulties, for instance, by prompting criticism from parents (see Goodman & Brand, 2009; Hammen, 2009). What is clear, however, is that whether their impact is direct or in interaction with other factors, early interpersonal adversities likely contribute to developmental problems (e.g., deficits in emotional regulation, interpersonal skills, and ability to respond to stress) that, as stated by Goodman and Brand (2009), can make children vulnerable to later depression.

Of course, it is not just childhood adverse experiences that can create vulnerability for depression. Major stressful events across the lifespan have also been associated with depression. As reviewed by Monroe, Slavich, and Georgiades (2009), most of the major events that have been linked with the onset of depression are social and/or interpersonal in nature, such as humiliation, social defeat, rejection, social exclusion, and loss. Among the evidence reported by Monroe et al. on the role of social-environmental factors is the finding that depressed individuals who experience major stress prior to the onset of depression have more severe symptoms than depressed people who are not confronted with such stressors (Monroe, Harkness, Simons, & Thase, 2001; Tennant, 2002). Research also suggests that stressful events during depression may interfere with recovery (Mazure, 1998).

We should, of course, mention that stressful events associated with depression are not necessarily (or primarily) interpersonal in nature. Other events, such as occupational failure or job loss (sometimes called agentic stressors), have also been associated with depression from both theoretical and empirical sources. Theoretically, that some individuals may be more vulnerable to depression when facing agentic rather than interpersonal stressors due to personality or cognitive style variables has been hypothesized and empirically investigated for a long time (e.g., Blatt, Quinlan, Chevron, McDonald, & Zuroff, 1982; Clark, Beck, & Brown, 1992). Though sometimes inconsistent, at least some evidence supports the idea that some people may be particularly vulnerable to non-interpersonal stressors (e.g., Mazure, Bruce, Maciejewski, & Jacobs, 2000). In addition, stressful events later in life have also been linked to the early adverse experiences mentioned earlier. For instance, studies suggest that these events may meditate the relationship between parental depression and psychological problems experienced by their children. As argued by Hammen (2009), for instance, the chronic stressful conditions in which depressed individuals live (and contribute to) can be a mechanism of transmission in which parental depression leads to depression in offspring.

Research has also identified a number of interpersonal risk factors for depression that take place specifically after childhood. Among them are romantic difficulties. Depression is indeed associated with the lack of support from (and the betrayal of) one's spouse, couples' difficulty with solving problems, and less satisfaction (and dissolution) in a romantic or marital relationship (Davila et al., 2009). As Davila et al. demonstrated, the relationship between depression and romantic problems is bidirectional. In reference to couple and family relationships, they state, "There is clear and consistent evidence that what happens in people's closest relationships can put them at risk for, or protect them from, depression, and that depression can have substantial negative effects on these relationships" (p. 482). They then eloquently write:

> The very things that are natural aspects of close relationships (e.g., the potential for loss and the need to manage conflict, to be available and supportive, and to negotiate the needs of multiple parties) are the things that can be most depressogenic when not dealt with adaptively, and the aspects of relationships that are often most impaired when people are depressed. (p. 482)

Research evidence also supports the role of specific interpersonal behaviors and style as risk factors for depression. These include excessive reassurance seeking, interpersonal dependency, and adult insecure attachment style (Joiner & Meltalsky, 2001; Joiner & Timmons, 2009; Roberts, Gotlib, & Kassel, 1996). Seeking negative feedback is also linked to both depression and interpersonal rejection. Research on seeking negative feedback is linked to the social-psychological concept of self-verification (Swann, 1983). Numerous studies have demonstrated that depressed individuals prefer to be with (and/or give more credibility to) others who react relatively more negatively to them than with individuals who provide them with positive feedback (e.g., Giesler, Josephs, & Swann, 1996; Swann, Wenzlaff, Krull, & Pelham, 1992). The inferred mechanism is that the desire for safety in having one's view of self confirmed (even when it is negative) is stronger than the disconfirming (but positive) impact that enhancement feedback can have.

There is much more that can be said regarding the social, developmental, and interpersonal causes of depression, and in this section we have only briefly summarized several of the major theories and research paradigms.

Clinical Implications

Several clinical guidelines can be derived from a number of the vulnerability factors described earlier. As previously mentioned, cognitive and affective factors involved in the onset and maintenance of depression are interconnected. Interestingly, research investigating both cognitive bias and emotional regulation suggests that depressed individuals seem to be stuck in maladaptive patterns of automatic reactions. Studies on attention, interpretation, and memory indicate that when depressed, individuals have difficulty disengaging from negative information. Similarly, ER studies show that depressed individuals use strategies that prevent them from recovering from the initial response of sadness and its related mood-congruent thoughts and memories. If these factors do play a causal role in the onset and maintenance of depression, therapeutic interventions that can directly modify them may be particularly promising.

Interestingly, a considerable number of experimental studies suggest that it might be possible to address the deficit of cognitive inhibition found in depressed people by helping them to control the content of their working memory.

Cognitive Bias

Initial studies demonstrate that training dysphoric people to disengage their attention from negative material leads to changes in mood and reduced reactivity to stressful events. In a typical training paradigm, the dot probe is presented more consistently after the non-negative relevant stimuli (rather than follow negative and non-negative stimuli equally), so that participants learn to attend to neutral stimuli. For example, Wells and Beevers (2010) examined the effects of training mild to moderately depressed college students to attend away from dysphoric stimuli. Attention training reduced participants' attention bias toward negative stimuli, which in turn led to a reduction in depressive symptoms. Similar results were also found by Baert, De Raedt, Schacht, and Koster (2010), using a sample of mildly depressed college students; however, attention training did not benefit the group of clinically depressed participants over and above therapy and/or medication. These training paradigms have been extended to show that positive attentional biases can also be trained (Wadlinger & Isaacowitz, 2008). Positive biases had observable effects on subsequent tasks such that participants who had been trained to attend to positive stimuli subsequently looked less at negative images during a stress induction. Moreover, successful attention training toward positive faces has been shown to reduce work-related stress and lower cortisol levels in telemarketers (Dandeneau, Baldwin, Baccus, Sakellaropoulo, & Pruessner, 2007), providing an exciting example of the way modifying cognitive biases may remediate dysfunctions in the neuroendocrine system. Based on these findings, researchers have begun to examine attentional training with clinical samples, but no studies thus far have examined whether modifying cognitive biases in depressed participants leads to improvements in ER.

Recently, researchers have begun to modify interpretive biases in the hope of modifying emotional responding. Mathews and Mackintosh (2000) used ambiguous scenarios to train individuals to make either positive or negative interpretations of ambiguous text. Participants in the negative training condition displayed elevated levels of anxiety, and those in the positive training condition demonstrated decreased symptoms of anxiety, supporting the hypothesis that interpretive biases play a causal role in affecting anxiety levels. The effects of interpretive training have been shown to remain after a 24-hour delay between the training and a subsequent test (Yiend, Mackintosh, & Mathews, 2005), and evidence suggests training people away from negative interpretations can lead to an attenuated anxiety reaction when they watch a distressing television clip (e.g,. Wilson, MacLeod, Mathews, & Rutherford, 2006). Holmes, Lang, and Shah (2009) also found support for the ability of interpretation training to affect emotional responding. Specifically, the authors demonstrated that training positive biases using imagery helped to alleviate a subsequently induced negative mood state. These results suggest that changes in interpretation biases can indeed lead to changes in emotional responding. Again, no studies so far have investigated whether modifying interpretive biases in depression affects emotional responding.

Several cognitive bias modification (CBM) studies have targeted negative memory biases, which are so often found in depression (Mathews & MacLeod, 2005). One study examined the ability to modify negative intrusions following a depressive film using a CBM task (Lang, Moulds, & Holmes, 2009). Those participants who were randomly assigned to the positive CBM condition showed less intrusion and were less aversely impacted by the depressive film than those who were assigned to the negative CBM condition. In addition, Watkins, Baeyens, and Read (2009) targeted the overgeneral memory bias by training participants to become more concrete and specific in their thinking. Dysphoric participants who completed the concreteness training experienced greater increases in concrete thinking and greater decreases in their depressive symptoms than wait-list controls or a bogus concreteness training group. Overall, such findings suggest that it is possible to alter the maladaptive memory biases that place individuals at risk for depression. Such modifications have been linked to changes in mood state; however, additional research is needed to extend these findings to a depressed population.

Researchers have started to investigate the possibility of training cognitive control in depression and of examining the effects of this training on emotion regulation. Joormann, Hertel, LeMoult, and Gotlib (2009), for example, showed that depressed participants can be trained to forget negative material by practicing active suppression, and that they do particularly well when provided with a strategy for how to keep irrelevant material from entering working memory (i.e., by using thought substitutes; Joormann et al., 2009). Brief interventions that target increasing cognitive control in severely depressed outpatients have, in turn, led to significant decreases in both depressive symptoms and rumination (Siegle, Thompson, Carter, Steinhauer, & Thase, 2007), Indeed, work by this group suggests that training in attentional control may be an effective treatment component for depression (Siegle, Ghinassi, et al., 2007). In this training, patients learn to attend selectively to certain sounds, while ignoring irrelevant sounds. After receiving 2 weeks of training, patients exhibited decreases in depressive symptoms compared to patients who received treatment as usual (Siegle, Ghinassi, et al., 2007). Although additional CBM studies with clinically depressed participants are still needed, initial evidence is promising.

Overall, findings suggest that cognitive biases can be modified in relatively short training sessions using easily implemented designs. Modifying cognitive biases has, in turn, been linked to short-term improvements in mood and stress reactivity, which suggests that such training might play an important role in treatment considerations. Future research is needed to extend these investigations to a clinical population, and to investigate the persistence of cognitive changes and mood states over longer durations of time.

Emotion Regulation Strategies

Consistent with some of the studies on cognitive biases, researchers interested in ER have found that rumination on negative events is linked with depression. In contrast, research findings suggest that reappraisal is an effective strategy to change individuals' affect from negative to positive. These findings highlight clear convergence between basic psychopathology research and psychotherapy research. As mentioned earlier, changing client cognitive appraisals has been identified as a principle underlying psychological treatments that work for depression. The basic finding about the positive effect of emotional disclosure (as opposed to the negative impact of emotion suppression) is also consistent with another principle of change indentified earlier (i.e., improving awareness, acceptance, and ER). Interestingly, however, while therapists from different orientations have recognized the importance of changing clients' view of self and others (via various techniques such as reformulation or cognitive restructuring), experiencing and focusing on emotion have been associated with particular forms of EST (e.g., brief psychodynamic, process–experiential, and interpersonal therapies). In fact, psychotherapy process research has shown that cognitive therapists tend more to control and/or reduce client emotion than do psychodynamic therapists (see Blagys & Hilsenroth, 2000). However, in contrast to traditional models underlying CBT (see Messer, 1986), process studies have also shown that the experience and expression of emotion is linked with improvement in CBT (e.g., Castonguay, Goldfried, Wiser, Raue, & Hayes, 1996; Watson & Bedard, 2006). Less surprisingly, emotional activation has also been found to be associated with therapeutic outcome in emotion-focused therapy (EFT; Greenberg & Watson, 2006), an experiential treatment that focuses on the processing and transformation of emotion (see Elliott, Greenberg, & Lietaer, 2004). Thus, both basic and psychotherapy research appear to suggest that therapists might foster clients' improvement by facilitating emotional disclosure, irrespective of their preferred theoretical orientation.

It should be noted that while two of the effective strategies for ER identified in the psychopathology research are consistent with principles of change derived from psychotherapy research, this is not the case for the other effective ER strategy. Distraction, indeed, does not appear to be explicitly emphasized in current EST treatments for depression. The positive effect of this strategy might be viewed as an opportunity to stimulate clinicians and scholars of different orientations to think about creative ways to complement their clinical repertoires with interventions that may help depressed clients to disengage, at appropriate times and places, from rumination and negative emotions. For example, one of the authors of this chapter has learned that blasting Beethoven's Ninth Symphony on his iPod in response to pervasive and recurrent ruminations late at night is not incompatible with (and may actually be a powerful adjunct to) verbally oriented forms of therapy. There are times to explore emotions and examine maladaptive cognitions, but there are also times when we should get our mind away from them.

Stress

Research conducted within both biological and psychological domains of psychopathology have demonstrated that stressful life events have an impact on the onset and maintenance of depression. The obvious implication of such findings is that therapists who are working with depressed clients should be prepared to use interventions to help clients decrease their stress and/or deal more effectively with stressors they encounter in their lives.

Most CBTs for depression include teaching behavioral activation strategies and coping/problem-solving skills to help patients manage ongoing stressors (see

Follette & Greenberg, 2006). However, it is noteworthy that explicit and systematic attention to stress management is a primary focus of a new and promising form of therapy developed by Adele Hayes as an attempt to build upon and increase the efficacy of current ESTs for depression, especially CBT (see Hayes, Feldman, Beevers, Laurenceau, & Cardaciotto, 2007). Because this treatment adds exposure-based principles to CBT, the first phase of treatment is designed to prepare patients to undergo this affectively charged and destabilizing part of therapy. Depressed individuals who seek treatment are frequently experiencing high levels of distress and depletion of resources, and their depressive symptoms and attempts to cope with stressors can generate even more stress (Hammen, 1991). The first stage of this treatment is therefore aimed at helping clients to acquire more equilibrium and stability in their lives. With some stable ground, they can move to the next phase of therapy to activate and emotionally process the key experiences and feelings of worthlessness and defectiveness that fuel the depression. This stabilization phase involves behavioral activation exercises, techniques to recognize and reduce avoidance and rumination, and increasing the health and regularity of sleep, eating, and exercise patterns. Together, the purpose of these interventions is to teach stress management skills and to reduce avoidance, rumination, and stress generation processes that maintain depression. These skills are thought to be critical both to prepare for change and to prevent relapse. There is, of course, no reason to assume that the addition of such stress-regulating strategies should be restricted to CBT-based interventions, because they are not likely to interfere with flexible and competent use of traditional interventions prescribed in any EST-based treatment for depression.

Interestingly, while this treatment represents a new effort to improve the effectiveness of our field, the emphasis on decreasing the client's stress and restoring his or her psychological equilibrium can be traced back to antiquity—when care was provided to restore individual balance of "humors." The theory (or the myth, as Frank [1961] would argue) was different (too much black bile was then believed to cause melancholia), but the interventions are quite similar (perhaps reminding us that many things are not really new under the sun).

Interpersonal Factors

One of the conclusions that can be safely drawn from research on interpersonal vulnerability for depression is that the influence of the past, and especially early relationships with significant others, cannot be denied.

In the clinical literature, the negative and long-standing observation of early adverse relational events can be traced back to Freud's first book (which he published in 1892 with Breuer). While the basic findings reviewed in this chapter do not support Freud's later model of depression (unconscious return of anger at parent turned against the self), they are certainly consistent with his original (and innovative view) that traumatic experiences in childhood can be at the root of later psychopathology. Moreover, the evidence supporting the role of aversive interpersonal events as risks for depression give credence to Alexander and French's (1946) view of the mutative factor in psychotherapy. The client changes, according to these authors, not because he or she acquires insights about previously unconscious conflicts, but because therapy provides him or her with a corrective emotional experience. Therapeutic change takes place, more precisely, when the therapist reacts to the client in a way that is different and thus disconfirms the client's expectations (and fears) of others that he or she derived from the relationship with his or her parents. While the construct of corrective experience emerged from the psychodynamic literature, it is now recognized as factor that cuts across different orientations (Castonguay & Hill, 2012).

There can be no doubt that the relational stance embraced in all form of EST for depression (including CBT; see Castonguay, Constantino, McAleavey, & Goldfried, 2010) sharply contrasts the different form of neglect (e.g., inattentiveness, withdrawal, emotional unresponsiveness) and abuse (e.g., overt hostility, intrusiveness, emotional overinvolvement, overstimulation) that have been frequently experienced by depressed individuals. As such, one could argue that interacting with clients in attentive, engaged, empathic, accepting, affirming, autonomy-granting, calm, structured, and consistent ways (as professed in the writing of leading clinicians of different orientations, such as Carl Rogers, Lorna Benjamin, Marsha Linehan, and Marvin Goldfried), is likely to differ from the way many depressed people have been treated (and therefore expected to be treated) by a person to whom they not only reveal personal material but whom they also view as an authority (a parent-like figure, one might say!). As described elsewhere (see Hill et al., 2012), such disconfirmation of expectations can facilitate the reduction of symptoms, change the view of self and others, and change maladaptive interpersonal patterns.

In contrast, interacting in a hostile and dismissing way might repeat the patterns and prevent change. This is consistent with a number of studies in the psychotherapy literature. For example, after conducting fine-grained analyses of therapist–client transactions of both good and poor outcomes of therapy, Henry, Schacht, and Strupp (1986) found that therapists tended to provide "blaming" and/or complex communications (i.e., seemingly "supportive" statements that also conveyed hostility and/or criticism) in poor outcome cases. In a subsequent study, Henry, Schact, and Strupp (1990) again compared cases with good and poor outcomes, but they used an outcome variable particularly relevant to the construct of corrective experience, or the lack thereof. Based on the theoretical work of Sullivan, and using Benjamin's structured analysis of social behavior, they investigated the client's "introject," which reflects the tendency for people to treat themselves in a manner consistent with how they have been treated by important others (e.g., self-blame consistent with a history of blaming communications on the part of the primary caregiver). Henry at al. (1990) found that in the poor outcome group (i.e., clients who showed no change in negative introject), therapists exercised more disaffiliative interpersonal behaviors (e.g., belittling and blaming, ignoring and neglecting) than in the good outcome group. Within the good outcome condition, therapists displayed an almost complete absence of such negative interpersonal process. These authors also found a significantly positive correlation between the frequency of therapist statements marked by disaffiliative control and hostility and the frequency of patient utterances marked by self-criticism and self-blame. Along the same line, Hilliard, Henry, and Strupp (2000) found that clients with an early interpersonal history of parental hostility reported worse interpersonal process in psychotherapy and experienced worse outcome in symptoms of depression during a controlled clinical trial. One could suggest that the contrast between the early experiences of many depressed clients and the experience of a good relationship with a therapist may mediate (at least in part) the positive link between the working alliance and outcome across different forms of therapy.

In addition to suggesting the importance of adopting an interpersonally warm and involved attitude, one could also argue that basic findings suggest that the therapist should be willing to discuss and/or explore early relationship events (including traumas) and their ramifications relative to the client's relationships with others during the course of his or her life. This is at the core of at least two ESTs: process-experiential (i.e., emotion focused) and short-term psychodynamic therapies. Consistent with the emotion-focused model, the resolution of unfinished business with significant others has been linked with therapeutic change (Elliott et al., 2004). In line with psychodynamic theory, process research has also found that the therapist's accurate interpretation of core relational relationships in the client's life (including the client's wishes and the responses of others) has been linked with positive outcome in this approach (Crits-Christoph & Connolly Gibbons, 2002). Interestingly, however, a focus on past relationships and the pattern of interactions they might have engendered or influenced may also be beneficial in other forms of treatment. For example, while process studies have found that CBT focuses less on developmental and interpersonal issues than does psychodynamic therapy (see Blagys & Hilsenroth, 2000), other investigations suggest that it is helpful when CBT therapists do focus on these issues. For example, Hayes, Castonguay and Goldfried (1996) found that the degree to which CBT therapists focus on attachment with early caregivers predicted not only outcome at the end of treatment but also relapse 2 years after therapy. In addition, Jones and Pulos (1993) found the following interventions to be part of a set of psychodynamic techniques positively associated with improvement: linking patients' feelings or perceptions to situations or behavior of the past; discussing memories or reconstructions of infancy and childhood; the therapist drawing connections between the therapeutic relationship and other relationships; and the therapist identifying recurrent themes in patients' experience or conduct. Also included in the set of psychodynamic techniques that result in positive outcome were interventions aimed at the type of emotional disclosure that, as mentioned earlier, predict improvement in CBT: The therapist emphasizes the patient's feeling to increase the likelihood that he or she experiences them, and draws attention to feelings the patient regards as unacceptable (e.g., anger, envy, or excitement).

Such findings suggest that at times, generating emotional memories in therapy for depression might be helpful, a finding that will not surprise practitioners of CBT for posttraumatic stress disorder and exposure-based psychotherapeutic methods for depression, though this has been often viewed as the domain of psychodynamic therapies. However, considering the presence of memory biases in depression, as well as the dangerous likelihood of triggering rumination and other maladaptive reflective practices, this may not be a good idea in all situations. Instead, it may be that therapists should carefully monitor their use of these techniques, as well as their clients' needs related to early experiences to best navigate these issues.

In addition to the developmental influence of interpersonal events and relationships, basic findings also point out the importance of addressing current interpersonal issues. As mentioned in the clinical implications delineated at the end of the first section of this chapter, research on interpersonal hostility and marital discord provides support to some of the specific principles of change underlying ESTs for depression, in particular interpersonal therapy. Research on interpersonal factors that are involved in the etiology of depression (instead of being part of its phenomenology or associated features) can allow us to be more specific about ways that depressed clients contribute to their depression. When working with depressed clients, therapists should inquire about and, if necessary, attempt to change clients' tendency to seek excessive reassurance and verification of their negative view of self. As pointed out by Joiner and Timmons (2009), such foci of interventions are not explicit parts of current interpersonal therapy. And while they are consistent with principles of change underlying behavior therapy (i.e., "decreasing reinforcement for depressive and avoidant behavior"; Follette & Greenberg, 2006, p. 94), a full recognition of these issues may further improve the efficacy of traditional CT for depression. Hayes et al. (1996) found that relative to interpersonal issues, cognitive therapists tend to focus more on changing patients' cognition about others than on direct interpersonal change. However, they also found that while the latter was linked with positive outcome, the former was predictive of worse outcome. Thus, attempting to foster concrete interpersonal change may well be an important recommendation in many forms of therapy.

CONCLUSION

A large amount of research has been conducted on the psychopathology of depression. Studies investigating its phenomenology have revealed the severity, preponderance, chronicity, and debilitating nature of this disorder. This descriptive research has pointed out several issues that therapists should assess and address (if necessary) when treating depressed persons. Many of these issues are not frequently emphasized in the psychotherapy literature, including low-base-rate somatic symptoms, anger, health and occupational functioning, and onset of the disorder.

Basic research on the etiology of depression has also identified several vulnerability factors (many of them are not covered in this chapter) involved in the onset and/or maintenance of this disorder. Some of these vulnerability factors are in line with the principles of change that underlie currently validated psychological treatments for depression. Several clinical implications that have been derived from the etiological research, however, deserve to be more explicitly and systematically considered as possible ways to improve further some (if not all) of our effective forms of psychotherapy.

Basic research also clearly conveys that the etiology of depression is not restricted to one set of causal or maintaining variables. Depression is likely to have many determinants. In addition, these determinants are interconnected (e.g., Goodman & Brand, 2009), thereby creating complex networks of moderating and mediating influences on client's functioning. Accordingly, rather than restrict their understanding of depression within the confine of a single theory, clinicians are likely to increase their effectiveness by assessing a large number of variables (biological, developmental, emotional, cognitive, behavioral, interpersonal), and to determine which of these variables are likely to play a primary role for each client who experiences depression.

In addition to targeting primary determinants of depression, the therapist's case formulation and treatment plan should take into account how these determinants interact with each other to interfere with the client's optimal level of functioning. While an eclectic or prescriptive approach to depression is likely to be effective (e.g., using social skills techniques with clients whose depression appears to be primarily related to their negative impact on others; using cognitive interventions when a highly functioning individual holds unreasonable standards of living), therapists should also consider (or develop) integrative frameworks that assimilate different dimensions of functioning into broad and cohesive models (e.g., Gotlib & Hammen, 1992). Consistent with both prescriptive and integrative approaches, it is important to keep in mind that improvement in one domain of functioning is likely to have a positive impact on other domains. Adopting a more affiliative way of relating with others not only helps a client to find more fulfillment in relationships, but it is also likely to have an impact on his or her view of self. Therefore, therapists should keep in mind that the use of one set of interventions is likely to have multiple effects. However, it is also important for the therapist to consider that a set of interventions may not have an impact on all potential determinants of depression, and that he or she should broadly assess a client's functioning before terminating therapy, even if substantial changes have been achieved in one dimension of functioning.

REFERENCES

Abercrombie, H. C., Schaefer, S. M., Larson, C. L., Oakes, T. R., Lindgren, K. A., Holden, J. E., et al. (1998). Metabolic rate in the right amygdala predicts negative affect in depressed patients. *NeuroReport, 9,* 3301–3307.

Alexander, F., & French, T. M. (1946). *Psychoanalytic therapy: Principles and applications.* New York: Ronald Press.

American Psychiatric Association. (2000). *Diagnostic and statistical manual of mental disorders* (4th ed., text rev.). Washington, DC: Author.

American Psychiatric Association. (2013). *Diagnostic and statistical manual of mental disorders* (5th ed.). Arlington, VA: Author.

Arana, G. W., Baldessarini, R. J., & Ornsteen, M. (1985). The dexamethasone suppression test for diagnosis and prognosis in psychiatry: Commentary and review. *Archives of General Psychiatry, 42*, 1193–1204.

Armstrong, T. D., & Costello, E. J. (2002). Community studies on adolescent substance use, abuse, or dependence and psychiatric comorbidity. *Journal of Consulting and Clinical Psychology, 70*, 1224–1289.

Aubry, J. M., Gervasoni, N., Osiek, C., Perret, G., Rossier, M. F., Bertschy, G., et al. (2007). The DEX/CRH neuroendocrine test and the prediction of depressive relapse in remitted depressed outpatients. *Journal of Psychiatric Research, 41*, 290–294.

Baert, S., De Raedt, R., Schact, R., & Koster, E. H. W. (2010). Attentional bias training in depression: Therapeutic effects depend on depression severity. *Journal of Behavior Therapy and Experimental Psychiatry, 41*, 265–274.

Beautrais, A. L., Joyce, P. R., Mulder, R. T., Fergusson, D. M., Deavoll, B. J., & Nightingale, S. K. (2006). Prevalence and comorbidity of mental disorders in persons making serious suicide attempts: A case control study. *American Journal of Psychiatry, 153*, 1009–1014.

Berman, A. L. (2009). School-based suicide prevention: Research advances and practice implications. *School Psychology Review, 38*, 233–238.

Beutler, L. E., Blatt, S. J., Alimohamed, S., Levy, K. N., & Angtuago, L. A. (2006). Participants factors in treating dysphoric disorders. In L. Castonguay & L. Beutler (Eds.), *Principles of therapeutic change that work* (pp. 13–63). New York: Oxford University Press.

Beutler, L. E., Consoli, A. J., & Lane, G. (2005). Systematic treatment selection and prescriptive psychotherapy: An integrative eclectic approach. In J. C. Norcross & M. R. Goldfried (Eds.), *Handbook of psychotherapy integration* (2nd ed., pp. 121–143). New York: Oxford University Press.

Blagys, M. D., & Hilsenroth, M. J. (2000). Distinctive features of short-term psychodynamic-interpersonal psychotherapy: A review of the comparative psychotherapy process literature. *Clinical Psychology, 7*, 167–188.

Blazer, D. G., Kessler, R. C., McGonagle, K. A., & Swartz, M. S. (1994). The prevalence and distribution of major depression in a national community samples: The National Comorbidity Survey. *American Journal of Psychiatry, 151*, 979–986.

Blatt, S. J., Quinlan, D. M., Chevron, E. S., McDonald, C., & Zuroff, D. C. (1982). Dependency and self-criticism: Psychological dimensions of depression. *Journal of Consulting and Clinical Psychology, 50*, 113–124.

Bonanno, G. A. (2005). Resilience in the face of potential trauma. *Current Directions in Psychological Science, 14*, 135–138.

Bonanno, G. A., & Castonguay, L. G. (1994). On balancing approaches to psychotherapy: Prescriptive patterns of attention, motivation, and personality. *Psychotherapy: Theory, Research, Practice and Training, 31*, 571–587.

Bremner, J. D., Innis, R. B., Salomon, R. M., Staib, L. H., Ng, C. K., Miller, H. L., et al. (1997). Positron emission tomography measurement of cerebral metabolic correlates of tryptophan depletion-induced depressive relapse. *Archives of General Psychiatry, 54*, 364–374.

Brewin, C. R., Reynolds, M., & Tata, P. (1999). Autobiographical memory processes and the course of depression. *Journal of Abnormal Psychology, 108*, 511–517.

Broderick, P. C. (2005). Mindfulness and coping with dysphoric mood: Contrasts with rumination and distraction. *Cognitive Therapy and Research, 29*(5), 501–510.

Buchwald, A. M., & Rudick-Davis, D. (1993). The symptoms of major depression. *Journal of Abnormal Psychology, 102*, 197–205.

Burke, H. M., Davis, M. C., Otte, C., & Mohr, D. C. (2005). Depression and cortisol responses to psychological stress: A meta-analysis. *Psychoneuroendocrinology, 30,* 846–856.

Campbell-Sills, L., & Barlow, D. H. (2007). Incorporating emotion regulation into conceptualizations and treatments of anxiety and mood disorders. In J. J. Gross (Ed.), *Handbook of emotion regulation* (pp. 542–559). New York: Guilford Press.

Canli, T., Cooney, R. E., Goldin, P., Shah, M., Sivers, H., Thomason, M. E., et al. (2005). Amygdala reactivity to emotional faces predicts improvement in major depression. *NeuroReport, 16,* 1267–1270.

Carney, R. M., Freedland, K. E., Rich, M. W., & Jaffe, A. S. (1995). Depression as a risk factor for cardiac events in established coronary heart disease: A review of possible mechanisms. *Annals of Behavioral Medicine, 17,* 142–149.

Carroll, B. J. (1982). Use of the dexamethasone test in depression. *Journal of Clinical Psychiatry, 43,* 44–50.

Castonguay, L. G., & Beutler, L. E. (2006). Principles of therapeutic change: A task force on participants, relationships, and techniques factors. *Journal of Clinical Psychology, 62,* 631–638.

Castonguay, L. G., Boswell, J. F., Constantino, M. J., Goldfried, M. R., & Hill, C. E. (2010). Training implications of harmful effects of psychological treatments. *American Psychologist, 65,* 34–49.

Castonguay, L. G., Constantino, M. J., McAleavey, A. A., & Goldfried, M. R. (2010). The alliance in cognitive-behavioral therapy. In J. C. Muran & J. P. Barber (Eds.), *The therapeutic alliance: An evidence-based approach to practice and training* (pp. 150–172). New York: Guilford Press.

Castonguay, L. G., Goldfried, M. R., Wiser, S., Raue, P. J., & Hayes, A. H. (1996). Predicting outcome in cognitive therapy for depression: A comparison of unique and common factors. *Journal of Consulting and Clinical Psychology, 64,* 497–504.

Castonguay, L. G., & Hill, C. E. (Eds). (2012). *Transformation in psychotherapy: Corrective Experiences across cognitive behavioral, humanistic, and psychodynamic approaches.* Washington, DC: American Psychological Association Press.

Castonguay, L. G., Schut, A. J., Aikens, D. E., Constantino, M. J., Laurenceau, J.-P., Bologh, L., et al. (2004). Integrative cognitive therapy for depression: A preliminary investigation. *Journal of Psychotherapy Integration, 14,* 4–20.

Chana, G., Landau, S., Beasley, C., Everall, I. P., & Cotter, D. (2003). Two-dimensional assessment of cytoarchitecture in the anterior cingulate cortex in major depressive disorder, bipolar disorder, and schizophrenia: Evidence for decreased neuronal somal size and increased neuronal density. *Biological Psychiatry, 53,* 1086–1098.

Clark, D. A., Beck, A. T., & Brown, G. K. (1992). Sociotropy, autonomy, and life event perceptions in dysphoric and nondysphoric individuals. *Cognitive Therapy and Research, 6,* 635–652.

Constantino, M. J., Marnell, M. E., Haile, A. J., Kanther-Sista, S. N., Woman, K., Zappert, L., et al. (2008). Integrative cognitive therapy for depression: A randomized pilot comparison. *Psychotherapy: Theory, Research, Practice and Training, 45,* 122–134.

Coyne, J. C., Burchill, S. A. L., & Stiles, W. (1991). An interactional perspective on depression. In C. R. Snyder & D. O. Forsyth (Eds.), *Handbook of social and clinical psychology: The health perspective* (pp. 327–349). New York: Pergamon.

Crits-Christoph, P., & Connolly Gibbons, M. B. (2002). Relational interpretations. In J. C. Norcross (Ed.), *Psychotherapy relationships that work* (pp. 285–300). New York: Oxford University Press.

Cui, L., & Huang, M. (2007). Effects of rumination and distraction on negative emotion and autobiographical memory. *Acta Psychologica Sinica, 39,* 78–87.

Dandeneau, S. D., Baldwin, M. W., Baccus, J. R., Sakellaropoulo, M., & Pruessner, J. C. (2007). Cutting stress off at the pass: Reducing vigilance and responsiveness to social threat by manipulating attention. *Journal of Personality and Social Psychology, 93,* 651–666.

Dannlowski, U., Kersting, A., Lalee-Mentzel, J., Donges, U.-S., Arolt, V., & Suslow, T. (2006).

Subliminal affective priming in clinical depression and comorbid anxiety: A longitudinal investigation. *Psychiatry Research, 143,* 63–75.

Davidson, R. J., Pizzagalli, D., & Nitschke, J. B. (2002). The representation and regulation of emotion in depression: Perspectives from affective neuroscience. In I. H. Gotlib & C. L. Hammen (Eds.), *Handbook of depression* (pp. 219–244). New York: Guilford Press.

Davila, J., Stroud, C. B., & Starr, L. R. (2009). Depression in couples and families. In I. H. Gotlib & C. L. Hammen (Eds.), *Handbook of depression* (pp. 467–491). New York: Guilford Press.

Denson, T., Fabiansson, E., Creswell, J., & Pedersen, W. (2009). Experimental effects of rumination styles on salivary cortisol responses. *Motivation and Emotion, 33,* 42–48.

Drevets, W. C. (1998). Functional neuroimaging studies of depression: The anatomy of melancholia. *Annual Review Medicine, 49,* 341–361.

Drevets, W. C. (1999). Prefrontal cortical–amygdalar metabolism in major depression. *Annals of the New York Academy of Science, 877,* 614–637.

Drevets, W. C. (2000). Neuroimaging studies of mood disorders. *Biological Psychiatry, 48,* 813–829.

Drevets, W. C., Bogers, W., & Raichle, M. E. (2002). Functional anatomical correlates of antidepressant drug treatment assessed using PET measures of regional glucose metabolism. *European Neuropsychopharmacology, 12,* 527–544.

Drevets, W. C., Price, J. L., Simpson, J. R., Todd, R. D., Reich, T., Vannier, M., et al. (1997). Subgenual prefrontal cortex abnormalities in mood disorders. *Nature, 386,* 824–827.

Ehring, T., Fischer, S., Schnülle, J., Bösterling, A., & Tuschen-Caffier, B. (2008). Characteristics of emotion regulation in recovered depressed versus never depressed individuals. *Personality and Individual Differences, 44,* 1574–1584.

Elliott, R., Greenberg, L. S., & Lietaer, G. (2004). Research on experiential psychotherapies. In M. J. Lambert (Ed.), *Bergin and Garfield's handbook of psychotherapy and behavior change* (5th ed., pp. 493–539). New York: Wiley.

Emmanuel, J., Simmonds, S., & Tyrer, P. (1998). Systematic review of the outcome of anxiety and depressive disorders. *British Journal of Psychiatry, 34,* 35–41.

Fava, M., Rankin, M. A., Wright, E. C., Alpert, J. E., Nierenberg, A. A., Pava, J., et al. (2000). Anxiety disorders in major depression. *Comprehensive Psychiatry, 41,* 97–102.

Fava, M., & Rosenbaum, J. F. (1999). Anger attacks in patients with depression, *Journal of Clinical Psychiatry, 60,* 21–24.

Fischer, A., H., Manstead, A. S. R., Evers, C., Timmers, M., & Valk, G. (2004). Motives and norms underlying emotion regulation. In P. Philippot & R. S. Feldman (Eds.), *The regulation of emotion* (pp. 187–210). Mahwah, NJ: Erlbaum.

Follette, W., & Greenberg, L. (2006). Technique factors in treating dysphoric disorders. In L. Castonguay & L. Beutler (Eds.), *Principles of therapeutic change that work* (pp. 83–109). New York: Oxford University Press.

Forbes, E. E., May, J. C., Siegle, G. J., Ladouceur, C. D., Ryan, N. D., Carter, C. S., et al. (2006). Reward-related decision-making in pediatric major depressive disorder: An fMRI study. *Journal of Child Psychology and Psychiatry, 47,* 1031–1040.

Fournier, J.C., DeRubeis, R.J., Shelton, R.C., Gallop, R., Amsterdam, J.D., & Hollon, S.D. (2008). Antidepressant medications v. cognitive therapy in people with depression with or without personality disorder. *British Journal of Psychiatry, 192,* 124–129.

Frank, J.D. (1961). *Persuasion and healing.* Baltimore: Johns Hopkins University Press.

Freedland, K. E., & Carney, R. M. (2009). Treatment-resistant depression and mortality after acute coronary syndrome. *American Journal of Psychiatry, 166,* 410–417.

Garnefski, N., & Kraaij, V. (2006). Relationships between cognitive emotion regulation strategies and depressive symptoms: A comparative study of five specific samples. *Personality and Individual Differences, 40,* 1659–1669.

Gerin, W., Davidson, K., Christenfeld, N., Goyal, T., & Schwartz, J. (2006). The role of angry rumination and distraction in blood pressure recovery from emotional arousal. *Psychosomatic Medicine, 68,* 64–72.

Giesler, R. B., Josephs, R. A., & Swann, W. B. (1996). Self-verification in clinical depression: The desire for negative evaluation. *Journal of Abnormal Psychology, 105,* 358–368.

Gilboa, E., & Gotlib, I. H. (1997). Cognitive biases and affect persistence in previously dysphoric and never-dysphoric individuals. *Cognition and Emotion, 11,* 517–538.

Gilboa-Schechtman, E., Erhard-Weiss, D., & Jeczemien, P. (2002). Interpersonal deficits meet cog-nitive biases: Memory for facial expressions in depressed and anxious men and women. *Psychiatry Research, 113,* 279–295.

Goldfried, M. R. (1980). Toward the delineation of therapeutic change principles. *American Psy-chologist, 35,* 991–999.

Goldfried, M. R., & Davison, G. C. (1976). *Clinical behavior therapy.* New York: Wiley.

Goodman, S. H., & Brand, S. R. (2009). Depression and early adverse experiences. In I. H. Gotlib & C. L. Hammen (Eds.), *Handbook of depression* (pp. 249–274). New York: Guilford Press.

Goodyer, I. M., Herbert, J., Tamplin, A., & Altham, P. M. E. (2000). Recent life events, cortisol, dehydroepiandrosterone and the onset of major depression in high-risk adolescents. *British Journal of Psychiatry, 177,* 499–504.

Gotlib, I. H., & Hammen, C. L. (1992). *Psychological aspects of depression: Toward a cognitive-interper-sonal integration.* New York: Wiley.

Gotlib, I. H., & Hammen, C. L. (Eds.). (2009). *Handbook of depression* (2nd ed.). New York: Guilford Press.

Gotlib, I. H., Sivers, H., Gabrieli, J. D. E., Whitfield-Gabrieli, S., Goldin, P., Minor, K. L., et al. (2005). Subgenual anterior cingulate activation to valenced emotional stimuli in major depression. *NeuroReport, 16,* 1731–1734.

Granger, D. A., Weisz, J. R., McCracken, J. T., Ikeda, S. C., & Douglas, P. (1996). Reciprocal influ-ences among adrenocortical activation, psychosocial processes, and the behavioral adjust-ment of clinic-referred children. *Child Development, 67,* 3250–3262.

Greenberg, L. S., & Watson, J. C. (2006). *Emotion-focused therapy for depression.* Washington, DC: American Psychological Asssociation.

Gross, J. J. (1998). The emerging field of emotion regulation: An integrative review. *Review of General Psychology, 2,* 271–299.

Gross, J. J., & John, O. P. (2003). Individual differences in two emotion regulation processes: Implications for affect, relationship, and well-being. *Journal of Personality and Social Psychol-ogy, 85,* 348–362.

Gross, J. J., & Levenson, R. W. (1997). Hiding feelings: The acute effects of inhibiting negative and positive emotion. *Journal of Abnormal Psychology, 106,* 95–103.

Gross, J. J., & Munoz, R. F. (1995). Emotion regulation and mental health. *Clinical Psychology: Sci-ence and Practice, 2,* 151–164.

Haga, S. M., Kraft, P., & Corby, E.-K. (2009). Emotion regulation: Antecedents and well-being outcomes of cognitive reappraisal and expressive suppression in cross-cultural samples. *Journal of Happiness Studies, 10,* 271–291.

Hammen, C. L. (1991). Generation of stress in the course of unipolar depression. *Journal of Abnor-mal Psychology, 96,* 190–198.

Hammen, C. L. (2005). Stress and depression. *Annual Reviews in Clinical Psychology, 1,* 293–319.

Hammen, C. L. (2009). Children of depressed parents. In I. H. Gotlib & C. L. Hammen (Eds.), *Handbook of depression* (pp. 275–297). New York: Guilford Press.

Hasher, L., & Zacks, R, T. (1988). Working memory, comprehension, and aging: A review and new view. In G. H. Bower (Ed.), *The psychology of learning and motivation: Advances in research and theory* (pp. 193–225). New York: Academic Press.

Hayes, A. H., Castonguay, L. G., & Goldfried, M. R. (1996). Effectiveness of targeting the vulnerability factors of depression in cognitive therapy. *Journal of Consulting and Clinical Psychology, 64,* 623–627.

Hayes, A. M., Feldman, G., Beevers, C., Laurenceau, J. P., & Cardaciotto, L. (2007). Discontinuities and cognitive changes in exposure-based cognitive therapy for depression. *Journal of Consulting and Clinical Psychology, 75,* 409–421.

Henry, W. P., Schacht, T. E., & Strupp, H. H. (1986). Structural analysis of social behavior: Application to a study of interpersonal process in differential psychotherapeutic outcome. *Journal of Consulting and Clinical Psychology, 54*(1), 27–31.

Henry, W. P., Schacht, T. E., & Strupp, H. H. (1990). Patient and therapist introject, interpersonal process, and differential psychotherapy outcome. *Journal of Consulting and Clinical Psychology, 58,* 768–774.

Hertel, P. (2004). Memory for emotional and nonemotional events in depression: A question of habit? In R. Daniel & P. Hertel (Eds.), *Memory and emotion* (pp. 186–216). New York: Oxford University Press.

Hill, C. E., Castonguay, L. G., Farber, B. A., Knox, S., Stiles, W. B., Anderson, T., et al. (2012). Corrective experiences in psychotherapy: Definitions, processes, consequences, and research directions. In L. G. Castonguay & C. D. Hill (Eds.), *Transformation in psychotherapy: Corrective experiences across cognitive behavioral, humanistic, and psychodynamic approaches.* Washington, DC: American Psychological Association.

Hilliard, R. B., Henry, W. P., & Strupp, H. H. (2000). An interpersonal model of psychotherapy: Linking patient and therapist developmental history, therapeutic process, and types of outcome. *Journal of Consulting and Clinical Psychology, 68,* 125–133.

Hollon, S. D., Stewart, M. O., & Strunk, D. (2006). Enduring effects for cognitive behavior therapy in the treatment of depression and anxiety. *Annual Review of Psychology, 57,* 285–315.

Holmes, E. A., Lang, T. J., & Shah, D. M. (2009). Developing interpretation bias modification as a "cognitive vaccine" for depressed mood—Imagining positive events makes you feel better than thinking about them verbally. *Journal of Abnormal Psychology, 118,* 76–88.

Hooley, J. M., Gruber, S. A., Scott, L. A., Hiller, J. B., & Yurgelun-Todd, D. A. (2005). Activation in dorsolateral prefrontal cortex in response to maternal criticism and praise in recovered depressed and healthy control participants. *Biological Psychiatry, 57,* 809–812.

Jandl, M., Steyer, J., Kaschka, & W. P. (2010). Suicide risk markers in major depressive disorder: A study of electrodermal activity and event-related potentials. *Journal of Affective Disorders, 123,* 138–149.

John, O. P., & Gross, J. J. (2004). Healthy and unhealthy emotion regulation: Personality processes, individual differences, and life span development. *Journal of Personality, 72,* 1301–1333.

Johnson, S. L., Joormann, J., LeMoult, J., & Miller, C. (2009). Mood disorders: Biological bases. In P. H. Blaney & T. Millon (Eds.), *Oxford textbook of psychopathology* (2nd ed.). New York: Oxford University Press.

Joiner, T. E. (2002). Depression in its interpersonal context. In I. H. Gotlib & C. L. Hammen (Eds.), *Handbook of depression* (pp. 295–313). New York: Guilford Press.

Joiner, T. E., & Metalsky, G. I. (2001). Excessive reassurance-seeking: Delineating a risk factor involved in the development of depressive symptoms. *Psychological Science, 12,* 371–378.

Joiner, T. E., & Timmons, K. A. (2009). Depression in its interpersonal context. In I. H. Gotlib & C. L. Hammen (Eds.), *Handbook of depression* (pp. 322–339). New York: Guilford Press.

Jones, E. E., & Pulos, S. M. (1993). Comparing the process in psychodynamic and cognitive-behavioral therapies. *Journal of Consulting and Clinical Psychology, 61,* 306–316.

Joormann, J., & D'Avanzato, C. (2010). Emotion regulation in depression: Examining the role of cognitive processes. *Cognition and Emotion, 24,* 913–939.

Joormann, J., & Gotlib, I. H. (2007). Selective attention to emotional faces following recovery from depression. *Journal of Abnormal Psychology, 116,* 80–85.

Joormann, J., & Gotlib, I. H. (2008). Updating the contents of working memory in depression: Interference from irrelevant negative material. *Journal of Abnormal Psychology, 117,* 182–192.

Joormann, J., & Gotlib, I. H. (2010). Emotion regulation in depression: Relation to cognitive inhibition. *Cognition and Emotion, 24,* 281–298.

Joormann, J., Hertel, P. T., LeMoult, J., & Gotlib, I. H. (2009). Training forgetting of negative material in depression. *Journal of Abnormal Psychology, 118,* 34–43.

Joormann, J., & Siemer, M. (2004). Memory accessibility, mood regulation, and dysphoria: Difficulties in repairing sad mood with happy memories? *Journal of Abnormal Psychology, 113,* 179–188.

Joormann, J., Siemer, M., & Gotlib, I. H. (2007). Mood regulation in depression: Differential effects of distraction and recall of happy memories on sad mood. *Journal of Abnormal Psychology, 116,* 484–490.

Joormann, J., Siemer, M., & Tran, T. B. (2011). Implicit interpretation biases affect emotional vulnerability: A training study. *Cognition and Emotion, 25,* 546–558.

Joormann, J., Yoon, K. L., & Zetsche, U. (2007). Cognitive inhibition in depression. *Applied and Preventive Psychology, 12,* 128–139.

Kandel, D. B., Johnson, J. G., Bird, H. R., Canino, G., Goodman, S. H., Lahey, B. B., et al. (1997). Psychiatric disorders associated with substance use among children and adolescents: Findinga from the Methods for the Epidemiology of Child and Adolescent Mental Disorders (MECA) study. *Journal of Abnormal Child Psychology, 25,* 121–132.

Kasch, K. L., Rottenberg, J., Arnow, B., & Gotlib, I. H. (2002). Behavioral activation and inhibition systems and the severity and course of depression. *Journal of Abnormal Psychology, 111,* 589–597.

Keedwell, P. A., Andrew, C., Williams, S. C. R., Brammer, M. J., & Phillips, M. L. (2005). The neural correlates of anhedonia in major depressive disorder. *Biological Psychiatry, 58,* 843–853.

Keller, M. B., & Boland, R. J. (1998). Implications of failing to achieve successful long-term maintenance treatment of recurrent unipolar major depression. *Biological Psychiatry, 44,* 438–460.

Kendler, K. S., Walters, E. E., & Kessler, R. C. (1997). The prediction of length of major depressive episodes: Results from an epidemiological sample of female twins. *Psychological Medicine, 27,* 107–117.

Kessler, R. C., Berglund, P., Demler, O., Jin, R., Koretz, D., Merikangas, K., et al. (2003). The epidemiology of major depressive disorder. *Journal of the American Medical Association, 289,* 3095–3105.

Kessler, R. C., Berglund, P., Demler, O., Jin, R., Merikangas, K. R., & Walters, E. E. (2005). Lifetime prevalence and age-of-onset distributions of DSM-IV disorders in the National Comorbidity Survey Replication. *Archives of General Psychiatry, 62,* 593–602.

Kessler, R. C., DuPont, R. L., Berglund, P., & Wittchen, H.-U. (1999). Impairment in pure and comorbid generalized anxiety disorder and major depression at 12 months in two national surveys. *American Journal of Psychiatry, 156,* 1915–1923.

Kessler, R. C., & Frank, R. G. (1997). The impact of psychiatric disorders on work loss days. *Psychological Medicine, 27,* 861–873.

Kessler, R. C., Gruber, M., Hettema, J. M., Hwang, I., Sampson, N., & Yonkers, K. A. (2008). Comorbid major depression and general anxiety disorders in the National Comorbidity Survey follow-up. *Psychological Medicine, 38,* 365–374.

Kessler, R. C., Nelson, C. B., McGonagle, K. A., Edlund, M. J., Frank, R. G., & Leaf, P. J. (1996). The epidemiology of co-occuring addictive and mental disorders: Implications for prevention and service utilization. *American Journal of Orthopsychiatry, 66,* 17–31.

Kessler, R. C., Stang, P., Wittchen, H.-U., Stein, M., & Walters, E. E. (1999). Lifetime comorbidities between social phobia and mood disorders in the US National Comorbidity Survey. *Psychological Medicine, 29,* 555–567.

Kessler, R. C., Tat Chiu, W., Demler, O., & Walters, E. E. (2005). Prevalence, severity, and comorbidity of 12–month DSM-IV disorders in the National Comorbidity Survey Replication. *Archives of General Psychiatry, 62,* 617–627.

Kessler, R. C., Zhao, S., Blazer, D. G., & Swartz, M. (1997). Prevalence, correlates, and course of minor depression and major depression in the National Comorbidity Survey. *Journal of Affective Disorders, 45,* 19–30.

Kircanski, K., Craske, M. G., & Bjork, R. A. (2008). Thought suppression enhances memory bias for threat material. *Behaviour Research and Therapy, 46,* 462–476.

Kirschbaum, C., & Hellhammer, D. H. (1994). Salivary cortisol in psychoneuroendocrine research: Recent developments and applications. *Psychoneuroendocrinology, 19,* 313–333.

Knutson, B., Fong, G. W., Adams, C. M., Varner, J. L., & Hommer, D. (2001). Dissociation of reward anticipation and outcome with event-related fMRI. *NeuroReport, 12,* 3683–3687.

Kring, A. M., & Werner, K. H. (2004). Emotion regulation and psychopathology. In P. Philippot & R. S. Feldman (Eds.), *The regulation of emotion* (pp. 359–385). Mahwah, NJ: Erlbaum.

Kross, E., Ayduk, O., & Mischel, W. (2005). When asking "why" does not hurt. *Psychological Science, 16,* 709–715.

Kuyken, W., & Brewin, C. R. (1994). Intrusive memories of childhood abuse during depressive episodes. *Behaviour Research and Therapy, 32,* 525–528.

Lang, T. J., Moulds, M. L., & Holmes, E. A. (2009). Reducing depressive intrusions via a computerized cognitive bias modification of appraisals task: Developing a cognitive vaccine. *Behaviour Research and Therapy, 47,* 139–145.

Larson, R. J. (2000). Toward a science of mood regulation. *Psychological Inquiry, 11,* 129–141.

Lawson, C., & MacLeod, C. (1999). Depression and the interpretation of ambiguity. *Behaviour Research and Therapy, 37,* 463–474.

Lawson, C., MacLeod, C., & Hammond, G. (2002). Interpretation revealed in the blink of an eye: Depressive bias in the resolution of ambiguity. *Journal of Abnormal Psychology, 111,* 321–328.

Le Masurier, M., Cowen, P. J., & Harmer, C. J. (2007). Emotional bias and waking salivary cortisol in relative of patients with major depression. *Psychological Medicine, 37,* 403–410.

LeMoult, J., & Joormann, J. (2010). Attention and memory biases in social anxiety disorder: The role of comorbid depression. *Cognitive Therapy and Research, 36*(1), 47–57.

Lenzenweger, M. F., Lane, M. C., Loranger, A. W., & Kessler, R. C. (2007). DSM-IV personality disorders in the National Comorbidity Survey Replication. *Biological Psychiatry, 62,* 553–564.

López, A. D., & Murray, C. J. L. (1998). *The global burden of disease.* Cambridge, MA: Harvard School of Public Health.

Lyubomirsky, S., Caldwell, N. D., & Nolen-Hoeksema, S. (1998). Effects of ruminative and distracting responses to depressed mood on the retrieval of autobiographical memories. *Journal of Personality and Social Psychology, 75,* 166–177.

Lyubomirsky, S., & Nolen-Hoeksema, S. (1993). Self-perpetuating properties of dysphoric rumination. *Journal of Personality and Social Psychology, 65,* 339–349.

MacLean, P. D. (1985). Evolutionary psychiatry and the triune brain. *Psychological Medicine, 15,* 219–221.

MacLeod, C., & Mathews, A. (1991). Cognitive–experimental approaches to the emotional disorders. In P. R. Martin (Ed.), *Handbook of behavior therapy and psychological science: An integrative approach* (pp. 116–150). Elmsford, NY: Pergamon.

Mannie, Z. N., Harmer, C. J., & Cowen, P. J. (2007). Increased waking salivary cortisol levels in young people at familial risk of depression. *American Journal of Psychiatry, 164,* 617–621.

Mathews, A., & Mackintosh, B. (2000). Induced emotional interpretation bias and anxiety. *Journal of Abnormal Psychology, 109,* 602–615.

Mathews, A., & MacLeod, C., (2005). Cognitive vulnerability to emotional disorders. *Annual Review of Clinical Psychology, 1,* 167–195.

Mathew, S. J., Coplan, J. D., Goetz, R. R., Feder, A., Greenwald, S., Dahl, R. E., et al. (2003). Differentiating depressed adolescent 24 h cortisol secretion in light of their adult clinical outcome. *Neuropsychopharmacology, 28,* 1336–1343.

Mayberg, H. S. (2002). *Mapping mood: An evolving emphasis on frontal–limbic interactions.* New York: Oxford University Press.

Mayberg, H. S., Keightley, M., Mahurin, R. K., & Brannan, S. K. (2004). *Neuropsychiatric aspects of mood and affective disorders.* Washington, DC: American Psychiatric Publishing.

Mazure, C. M. (1998). Life stressors as risk factors in depression. *Clinical Psychology: Science and Practice, 5,* 291–313.

Mazure, C. M., Bruce, M. L., Maciejewski, P. K., & Jacobs, S. C. (2000). Adverse life events and cognitive–personality characteristics in the prediction of major depression and antidepressant response. *American Journal of Psychiatry, 157,* 896–903.

Messer, S. B. (1986). Behavioral and psychoanalytic perspectives at therapeutic choice points. *American Psychologist, 41,* 1261–1272.

Miller, N. S., Klamen, D., Hoffmann, N. G., & Flaherty, J. A. (1996). Prevalence of depression and alcohol and other drug dependence in addictions treatment populations. *Journal of Psychoactive Drugs, 28,* 111–124.

Mintz, J., Mintz, L. I., Arruda, M. J., & Hwang, S. S. (1992). Treatments of depression and the functional capacity to work. *Archives of General Psychiatry, 49,* 761–768.

Mitchell, P. B., Goodwin, G. M., Johnson, G. F., & Hirschfeld, R. M. A. (2008). Diagnostic guidelines for bipolar depression: A probabilistic approach. *Bipolar Disorders, 10,* 144–152.

Mogg, K., Bradbury, K. E., & Bradley, B. P. (2006). Interpretation of ambiguous information in clinical depression. *Behaviour Research and Therapy, 44,* 1411–1419.

Mogg, K., & Bradley, B. P. (2005). Attentional bias in generalized anxiety disorder versus depressive disorder. *Cognitive Therapy and Research, 29,* 29–45.

Monroe, S. M., Harkness, K., Simons, A. D., & Thase, M. E. (2001). Life stress and the symptoms of major depression. *Journal of Nervous and Mental Disease, 189,* 168–175.

Monroe, S. M., Slavich, G. M., & Georgiades, K. (2009). The social environment and life stress in depression. In I. H. Gotlib & C. L. Hammen (Eds.), *Handbook of depression* (pp. 340–360). New York: Guilford Press.

Nemeroff, C. B., & Schatzberg, A. F. (2002). Pharmacological treatment of unipolar depression. In P. E. Nathan & J. M. Gorman (Eds.), *A guide to treatments that work* (3rd ed., pp. 271–288). New York: Oxford University Press.

Nolen-Hoeksema, S., Morrow, J., & Fredrickson, B. L. (1993). Response styles and the duration of episodes of depressed mood. *Journal of Abnormal Psychology, 102,* 20–28.

Nolen-Hoeksema, S., Wisco, B. E., & Lyubomirsky, S. (2008). Rethinking rumination. *Perspectives on Psychological Science, 3,* 400–424.

Nunn, J.D., Mathews, A., & Trower, P. (1997). Selective processing of concern-related information in depression. *British Journal of Clinical Psychology, 36,* 489–503.

Ochsner, K. N., & Gross, J. J. (2005). The cognitive control of emotion. *Trends in Cognitive Sciences, 9,* 242–249.

Parashos, I. A., Tupler, L. A., Blitchington, T., & Krishnan, K. R. (1998). Magnetic resonance morphometry in patients with major depression. *Psychiatry Research: Neuroimaging, 84,* 7–15.

Perlis, R. H., Fraguas, R., Fava, M., Trivedi, M. H., Luther, J. F., Wisniewski, S. R., et al. (2005). Prevalence and clinical correlates of irritability in major depressive disorder: A preliminary report from the Sequenced Treatment Alternatives to Relieve Depression Study. *Journal of Clinical Psychiatry, 66*(2), 159–166.

Phillips, M. L., Drevets, W. C., Rauch, S. L., & Lane, R. (2003). Neurobiology of emotion perception II: Implications for major psychiatric disorders. *Biological Psychiatry, 54*, 515–528.

Pizzagalli, D. A., Oakes, T. R., Fox, A. S., Chung, M. K., Larson, C. L., Abercrombie, H. C., et al. (2004). Functional but not structural subgenual prefrontal cortex abnormalities in melancholia. *Molecular Psychiatry, 9*, 393–405.

Porter, R., & Gallagher, P. (2006). Abnormalities of the HPA axis in affective disorders: Clinical subtypes and potential treatments. *Acta Neuropsychiatrica, 18*, 193–209.

Power, M. J., Dalgleish, T., Claudio, V., Tata, P., & Kentish, J. (2000). The directed forgetting task: Application to emotionally valent material. *Journal of Affective Disorders, 57*, 147–157.

Rao, U., & Chen, L.-A. (2008). Neurobiological and psychosocial processes associated with depressive and substance-related disorders in adolescents. *Current Drug Abuse Reviews, 1*, 68–80.

Rao, U., Dahl, R. E., Ryan, N. D., Birmaher, B., Williamson, D. E., Giles, D. E., et al. (1996). The relationship between longitudinal clinical course and sleep and cortisol changes in adolescent depression. *Biological Psychiatry, 40*, 474–484.

Rao, U., Hammen, C. L., & Poland, R. E. (2009). Mechanisms underlying the comorbidity between depressive and addictive disorders in adolescents: Interactions between stress and HPA activity. *American Journal of Psychiatry, 166*, 361–369.

Ray, R. D., Ochner, K. N., Cooper, J. C., Robertson, E. R., Gabrieli, J. E. D., & Gross, J. J. (2005). Individual differences in trait rumination and the neural systems supporting cognitive reappraisal. *Cognitive, Affective, and Behavioral Neuroscience, 5*, 156–168.

Ribeiro, S.C., Tandon, R., Grunhaus, L., & Greden, J. F. (1993). The DST as a predictor of outcome in depression: A meta-analysis. *American Journal of Psychiatry, 150*, 1618–1629.

Roberts, J. E., Gotlib, I. H., & Kassel, J. D. (1996). Adult attachment security and symptoms of depression: The mediating roles of dysfunctional attitudes and low self-esteem. *Journal of Personality and Social Psychology, 70*, 310–320.

Rusting, C. L., & Nolen-Hoeksema, S. (1998). Regulating responses to anger: Effects of rumination and distraction on angry mood. *Journal of Personality and Social Psychology, 74*, 790–803.

Safran, J. D., & Muran. J. C. (2000). *Negotiating the therapeutic alliance: A relational treatment guide.* New York: Guilford Press.

Safran, J. D., & Segal, Z. V. (1990). *Interpersonal process in cognitive therapy.* New York: Basic Books.

Salaycik, K. J., Kelly-Hayes, M., Beiser, A., Nguyen, A.-H., Brady, S. M., Kase, C. S., et al. (2007). Depressive symptoms and risk of stroke: The Framingham Study. *American Heart Association Journal, 38*, 16–21.

Sapolsky, R. M. (2000). Glucocorticoids and hippocampal atrophy in neuropsychiatric disorders. *Archives of General Psychiatry, 57*, 925–935.

Schaefer, H. S., Putnam, K. M., Benca, R. M., & Davidson, R. J. (2006). Event-related functional magnetic resonance imaging measures of neural activity to positive social stimuli in pre- and post-treatment depression. *Biological Psychiatry, 60*, 974–986.

Seligman, M. E. (1989). Research in clinical psychology: Why is there so much depression today? In S. Ira (Ed.), *The G. Stanley Hall lecture series: Vol. 9* (pp. 75–96). Washington, DC: American Psychological Association.

Sheline, Y. I. (2003). Neuroimaging studies of mood disorders effects on the brain. *Biological Psychiatry, 54*, 338–352.

Sheline, Y. I., Barch, D. M., Donnelly, J. M., Ollinger, J. M., Snyder, A. Z., & Mintum, M. A. (2001). Increased amygdala responses to masked emotional faces in depressed subjects resolves with antidepressant medication: An fMRI study. *Biological Psychiatry, 50*, 651–658.

Siegle, G. J., Carter, C. S., & Thase, M. E. (2006). Use of fMRI to predict recovery from unipolar depression with cognitive behavior therapy. *American Journal of Psychiatry, 163*, 735–738.

Siegle, G. J., Ghinassi, F., & Thase, M. E. (2007). Neurobehavioral therapies in the 21st century:

Summary of an emerging field and an extended example of cognitive control training for depression. *Cognitive Therapy and Research, 31,* 235–262.

Siegle, G. J., Steinhauer, S. R., Thase, M. E., Stenger, V. A., & Carter, C. S. (2002). Can't shake that feeling: Assessment of sustained event-related fMRI amygdala activity in response to emotional information in depressed individuals. *Biological Psychiatry, 51,* 693–707.

Siegle, G. J., Thompson, W., Carter, C. S., Steinhauer, S. R., & Thase, M. E. (2007). Increased amygdala and decreased dorsolateral prefrontal BOLD responses in unipolar depression: Related and independent features. *Biological Psychiatry, 61,* 198–209.

Sommers-Flanagan, J., & Sommers-Flanagan, R. (1995). Intake interviewing with suicidal patients: A systematic approach. *Professional Psychology: Research and Practice, 26*(1), 41–47.

Srivastava, S., Tamir, M., McGonigal, K. M., John, O. P., & Gross, J. J. (2009). The social costs of emotional suppression: A prospective study of the transition to college. *Journal of Personality and Social Psychology, 96,* 883–897.

Stepper, S., & Strack, F. (1993). Proprioceptive determinants of emotional and nonemotional feelings. *Journal of Personality and Social Psychology, 64,* 211–220.

Stewart, W. F., Ricci, J. A., Chee, E., Hahn, S. R., & Morganstein, D. (2003). Cost of lost productive work time among US workers with depression. *Journal of the American Medical Association, 289,* 3135–3144.

Sullivan, P. F., Neale, M. C., & Kendler, K. S. (2000). Genetic epidemiology of major depression: Review and meta-analysis. *American Journal of Psychiatry, 157,* 1552–1562.

Swann, W. B., Jr. (1983). Self-verification: Bringing social reality into harmony with the self. In J. Suls & A. G. Greenwald (Eds.), *Social psychological perspectives on the self* (pp. 33–66). Hillsdale, NJ: Erlbaum.

Swann, W. B., Wenzlaff, R. M., Krull, D. S., & Pelham, B. W. (1992). Allure of negative feedback: Self-verification strivings among depressed persons. *Journal of Abnormal Psychology, 101*(2), 293–306.

Tarsia, M., Power, M. J., & Sanavio, E. (2003). Implicit and explicit memory biases in mixed anxiety–depression. *Journal of Affective Disorders, 77,* 213–225.

Teasdale, J. D. (1988). Cognitive vulnerability to persistent depression. *Cognition and Emotion, 2,* 247–274.

Tennant, C. (2002). Life events, stress and depression: A review of recent findings. *Australian and New Zealand Journal of Psychiatry, 36,* 173–182.

Thase, M. E., Simons, A. D., McGeary, J., Cahalane, J. F., Hughes, C., Harden, T., et al. (1992). Relapse after cognitive behavior therapy of depression: Potential implications for longer courses of treatment. *American Journal of Psychiatry, 149,* 1046–1052.

Thompson, R. A. (1994). Emotion regulation: A theme in search of definition. *Monographs of the Society for Research in Child Development, 59,* 25–52, 250–283.

Trask, P., & Sigmon, S. T. (1999). Ruminating and distracting: The effects of sequential tasks on depressed mood. *Cognitive Therapy and Research, 23,* 231–246.

van der Veen, F. M., Evers, E. A., Deutz, N. E., & Schmitt, J. A. (2007). Effects of acute tryptophan depletion on mood and facial emotion perception related brain activation and performance in healthy women with and without a family history of depression. *Neuropsychopharmacology, 32,* 216–224.

Vickers, K. S., & Vogeltanz-Holm, N. D. (2003). The effects of rumination and distraction tasks on psychophysiological responses and mood in dysphoric and nondysphoric individuals. *Cognitive Therapy and Research, 27,* 331–348.

Wadlinger, H. A., & Isaacowitz, D. M. (2008). Looking happy: The experimental manipulation of a positive visual attention bias. *Emotion, 8,* 121–126.

Watamura, S. E., Donzella, B., Alwin, J., & Gunnar, M. R. (2003). Morning-to-afternoon increases in cortisol concentrations for infants and toddlers at child care: Age differences and behavioral correlates. *Child Development, 74,* 1006–1020.

Watkins, E., Baeyens, C. B., & Read, R. (2009). Concreteness training reduces dysphoria: Proof-of-principle for repeated cognitive bias modification in depression. *Journal of Abnormal Psychology, 118,* 55–64.

Watson, J. C., & Bedard, D. (2006). Clients' emotional processing in psychotherapy: A comparison between cognitive-behavioral and process-experiential psychotherapy. *Journal of Consulting and Clinical Psychology, 74,* 152–159.

Wegner, D. M., & Gold, D. B. (1995). Fanning old flames: Emotional and cognitive effects of suppressing thoughts of a past relationship. *Journal of Personality and Social Psychology, 68,* 782–792.

Wells, T. T., & Beevers, C. G. (2010). Biased attention and dysphoria: Manipulating selective attention reduces subsequent depressive symptoms. *Cognition and Emotion, 24,* 719–728.

Wenzlaff, R. M., Rude, S. S., Taylor, C. J., Stultz, C., & Sweatt, R. A. (2001). Beneath the veil of thought suppression: Attentional bias and depression risk. *Cognition and Emotion, 15,* 435–452.

Williams, J. M. G., Barnhofer, T., Crane, C., Hermans, D., Raes, F., & Dalgleish, T. (2007). Autobiographical memory specificity and emotional disorder. *Psychological Bulletin, 133,* 122–148.

Williams, J. M. G., Watts, F. N., MacLeod, C., & Mathews, A. (1997). *Cognitive psychology and the emotional disorders* (2nd ed.). New York: Wiley.

Wilson, E. J., MacLeod, C., Mathews, A., & Rutherford, E. M. (2006). The causal role of interpretive bias in anxiety reactivity. *Journal of Abnormal Psychology, 115,* 103–111.

Yiend, J., Mackintosh, B., & Mathews, A. (2005). Enduring consequences of experimentally induced biases in interpretation. *Behaviour Research and Therapy, 43,* 779–797.

Zisook, S., Lesser, I., Stewart, J. W., Wisniewski, S. R., Balasubramani, G. K., Fava, M., et al. (2007). Effect of age at onset on the course of major depressive disorder. *American Journal of Psychiatry, 164,* 1539–1546.

Zobel, A. W., Nickel, T., Sonntag, A., Uhr, M., Holsboer, F., & Ising, M. (2001). Cortisol response in the combined dexamethasone/CRH test as predictor of relapse in patients with remitted depression: A prospective study. *Journal of Psychiatric Research, 35,* 83–94.

CHAPTER 3

Generalized Anxiety Disorder

Michelle G. Newman
Paul F. Crits-Christoph
Lauren E. Szkodny

Generalized anxiety disorder (GAD) has been conceptualized as the "basic" anxiety disorder given its apparent early onset, persistent course, and resistance to change (Brown, Barlow, & Liebowitz, 1994). Accordingly, understanding the etiological and maintaining factors of GAD may have implications for understanding all anxiety disorders (Roemer, Orsillo, & Barlow, 2002).

TYPICAL SYMPTOMS AND ASSOCIATED FEATURES

GAD is characterized by excessive and typically uncontrollable worry, and generally is associated with physical symptoms, such as (1) restlessness or feeling keyed up or on edge, (2) fatigue, (3) concentration difficulties, (4) irritability, (5) muscle tension, (6) sleep disturbance (American Psychiatric Association, 2013). The DSM (both the DSM-IV and the new edition, DSM-5) indicates that a GAD diagnosis may be warranted if worry occurs more days than not for at least 6 months, and at least three physical symptoms are present (American Psychiatric Association, 2000, 2013).

All six of these symptoms reflect central nervous system (CNS) rather than autonomic nervous system (ANS) activity (Borkovec & Newman, 1998). Although the typical age of onset of GAD is unclear, because studies have reported various ages of onset depending on which DSM criteria are used, early age of onset has been associated with self-reported childhood history of fears; inhibited or avoidance behavior; developmental, academic, and social-interactional difficulties; and a disturbed home environment (Hoehn-Saric, Hazlett, & McLeod, 1993). Late age of onset has been found to be related to a greater likelihood of reporting a precipitating stressful event that corresponded with the onset of GAD (Hoehn-Saric et al., 1993).

As noted, a key feature of GAD is worry, which has been defined as "a chain of thoughts and images, negatively affect-laden and relatively uncontrollable . . . an attempt to engage in mental problem-solving on an issue whose outcome is uncertain but contains the possibility of one or more negative outcomes . . . [and] relate[d] closely to the fear process" (Borkovec, Robinson, Pruzinsky, & DePree, 1983, p. 10). The definition was later extended to include anxious apprehension for future negative events (Borkovec, Ray, & Stober, 1998). Although worry is a common cognitive phenomenon, it can become a persistent, daily activity and develop a number of features that make it a disabling source of extreme emotional discomfort, as experienced by individuals with GAD. It is directed at not only major life issues (e.g., health, finances, relationships, work-related matters) but also many minor, day-to-day issues and hassles that others would not perceive as threatening (e.g., household chores). Additionally, pathological worry is closely associated with catastrophizing, leading to mounting levels of anxiety and distress. The key distinction between normal and pathological worry in GAD is pervasiveness and controllability. To illustrate, participants with GAD in both college student (Borkovec et al., 1983) and clinical (Craske, Rapee, Jackel, & Barlow, 1989) samples report more difficulty controlling the onset or termination of their worry than do nonanxious controls.

Associated cognitive features of GAD elucidate the nature and function of worry in this disorder. Worry is predominated by negative verbal thought activity, as demonstrated in both anxious and nonanxious samples (Borkovec & Inz, 1990), such that when people worry, they talk to themselves about negative events they fear may occur in the future (Borkovec et al., 1998). Due to its somatically activating nature, worry is a strategy employed to avoid affective reactivity (Llera & Newman, 2010; Newman & Llera, 2011). For instance, because worry creates distress, it has been shown to reduce the likelihood of further reactivity associated with a fearful event or situation and prevent adequate exposure (e.g., Borkovec & Hu, 1990; Llera & Newman, 2010), thereby hindering emotional processing of aversive stimuli. Additionally, worry, as reflected in a clinical population, represents an attempt to avoid being surprised by negative events or a means to prepare for the worst (e.g., Borkovec & Roemer, 1995).

Furthermore, GAD and worry have a distinctive psychophysiological profile. For example, individuals with GAD do not show typical cardiac reactivity in response to threat as do people diagnosed with other anxiety disorders. Instead, they exhibit a reduction in the range of heart rate variability characterized by a state of autonomic rigidity (e.g., lack of autonomic reactivity; Thayer, Friedman, & Borkovec, 1996). In other words, people with GAD tend to have high stable heart rates and low heart rate variability, often referred to as lack of vagal tone. In an examination of heart rate variability during rest, aversive imagery, and worrisome thinking in analogue GAD (Llera & Newman, 2010; Lyonfields, Borkovec, & Thayer, 1995), induced states of worry created a reduction in vagal tone. This vagal deficiency and the resulting autonomic inflexibility found in GAD are related to pervasive worry, as demonstrated by empirical findings that worry physically reduces vagal tone in nonanxious controls (Holmes & Newman, 2006).

GAD and worry also impact information processing in ways that interfere with learning from experience and contribute to the maintenance of anxious meanings attributed to various stimuli. People with GAD persistently scan their environment for potential danger (e.g., Mathews & MacLeod, 1994), and demonstrate a bias for attending to threat cues and negatively interpreting ambiguous or neutral stimuli. In other words, individuals with GAD constantly detect threat in their surrounding environment. However, since there is no actual danger, as it only exists in their minds in the future, the threat cannot be physically avoided. As long as danger is perceived, individuals with GAD mentally continue to search for ways to avoid it or prepare themselves to cope with it. Thus, worry is a mental response to perceived threat when no behavioral solution exists. It primarily functions as a problem-focused maladaptive coping behavior, a means actively to avoid large increases or shifts in current negative emotions and future consequences (Borkovec & Newman, 1998).

Moreover, research has shown that individuals with GAD exhibit memory biases for mood-congruent threat information, such that they display cognitive avoidance of threats resulting in explicit memory for the material but enhanced implicit memory (e.g., Mathews & MacLeod, 1994), indicating both avoidance and extensive processing of perceived threatening stimuli. In particular, participants with GAD recalled fewer threat words than controls when using an attentional memory task, but they recalled more threat words than controls when using an implicit, or automatic, memory task (e.g., Mathews & MacLeod, 1994). However, this research is potentially limited by the use of nomothetic stimulus sets when examining memory bias in individuals with GAD. Therefore, idiographic, or personally relevant, words have also been used in studies of both implicit and explicit memory biases in GAD. In one such study using personally relevant words (Coles, Turk, & Heimberg, 2007), both implicit and explicit memory biases in individuals with GAD, compared to nonanxious controls, were found. Similarly, in a study in which patients with GAD were required to monitor their daily worry predictions and the rate at which their predicted outcomes actually occurred, the outcomes turned out better than expected 84% of the time (Borkovec, Hazlett-Stevens, & Diaz, 1999). Of the remainder, clients coped better than expected in 78% of the cases. Finally, the core aversive event actually occurred in only 3% of all worries, suggesting that clients with GAD fail to process evidence in their environment that would contradict their fears.

GAD is also associated with significant distress, disability, and impairment in quality of life. The most detailed information on disability and quality-of-life effects of GAD comes from the Epidemiologic Catchment Area (ECA) community survey (Robins & Regier, 1991), one of the largest investigations of the prevalence of mental disorders, and from a multisite survey of psychiatric outpatients (Massion,

Warshaw, & Keller, 1993). The overall picture for GAD is one of significant psychosocial impairment, with 38% of ECA subjects and 71% of outpatients characterizing their emotional health as only fair to poor; 27% and 25%, respectively, were receiving disability payments, and only about 50% were working full-time. Of those who were working, 38% had missed at least 1 week of work in the past year due to their anxiety (Massion et al., 1993). The ECA survey also found a strong correlation between both occupational status and income, and GAD. GAD was associated with a threefold greater likelihood of working at a low occupational level, and a more than a twofold likelihood of earning less than $10,000 per year. Studies suggest that role impairment in those with pure GAD (without comorbidity) is comparable to pure major depressive disorder (MDD), as well as other mood disorders (Grant et al., 2005a; Kessler, Stang, Wittchen, Stein, & Walters, 1999; Wittchen, Carter, Pfister, Montgomery, & Kessler, 2000). Moreover, high rates of suicidality can be found in persons with GAD. In one longitudinal epidemiological study in the United States, young adults (16 to 25 years) diagnosed with GAD had a sixfold increased likelihood of suicidal ideation and a more than twofold greater likelihood of attempted suicide, after researchers controlled for other mental disorders and stressful life events (Boden, Fergusson, & Horwood, 2007).

GAD also has consequences for physical health, with 35% of individuals with GAD in the ECA sample, and 23% of those in the Massion et al. (1993) sample, rating their physical health as only fair to poor. GAD is also associated with a number of comorbid medical problems such as asthma (Goodwin, Jacobi, & Thefeld, 2003), chronic pain conditions (e.g., Von Korff et al., 2005), and irritable bowel syndrome (e.g., Gros, Antony, McCabe, & Swinson, 2009). Furthermore, GAD is a risk factor for coronary heart disease independent of depression (e.g., Barger & Sydeman, 2005; Todaro, Shen, Raffa, Tilkemeier, & Niaura, 2007). One study also showed that the onset of GAD preceded the onset of cardiac illness (Harter, Conway, & Merikangas, 2003). In terms of health care utilization, studies reveal that persons with GAD are among the heaviest users of primary care, specialty clinic, and emergency room resources, contributing substantially to the nonpsychiatric cost associated with anxiety disorders in the United States (e.g., Fogarty, Sharma, Chetty, & Culpepper, 2008; Jones, Ames, Jeffries, Scarinci, & Brantley, 2001). Even individuals who do not meet the full criteria for GAD but have a subthreshold level of GAD symptoms demonstrate significant disability and treatment seeking. Compared to patients with no psychiatric symptoms, pure subthreshold GAD is associated with significantly greater social disability, as well as poorer health ratings (Weiller, Bisserbe, Maier, & Lecrubier, 1998).

Finally, GAD has been associated with interpersonal dysfunction (Crits-Christoph, Gibbons, Narducci, Schamberger, & Gallop, 2005; Newman & Erickson, 2010; Przeworski et al., 2011). Individuals with GAD tend to report a predominance of worrisome thoughts related to relationship concerns (Breitholtz, Johansson, & Öst, 1999; Roemer, Molina, & Borkovec, 1997). They also exhibit a tendency to perceive social threats in their environment (e.g., Mogg, Mathews, & Eysenck, 1992). In a like manner, GAD is more associated with marital discord or dissatisfaction than other anxiety or mood disorders (e.g., Whisman, 1999). Specifically, individuals with GAD, compared to those without GAD, are more likely to have enmeshed relationships or to engage in role reversal, such as a child or adolescent assuming parental responsibility (Cassidy & Shaver, 1999; Cassidy, 1995). With regard to their interpersonal difficulties, people with GAD display disruption in perception of their negative interpersonal impact on others (Erickson & Newman, 2007), which can impact their relationships and maintain interpersonal dysfunction.

Treatment Implications

Individuals with GAD anxiously anticipate and engage in mental attempts to problem-solve and prepare for the occurrence of negative events that might happen. They navigate their world with biased cognitive processes, such that they frequently detect and interpret threat in their environment, even when no threat exists (Mathews & MacLeod, 1994). Their mental experience is dominated by worry, which is elicited by internal or external cues that signal real or imagined danger. Individuals with GAD use worry to figure out how to prevent bad things from happening or to prepare for the worst (Borkovec & Roemer, 1995). They spend a significant amount of time preoccupied with their worrisome thoughts and therefore tend to describe themselves as having been worriers all their lives. Chronic worry becomes a way of life to the point that these individuals may not realize there are treatments available to them. Since many people with GAD might not even seek treatment, dissemination of information about the helpfulness and availability of psychotherapy for GAD is an important first step.

Individuals with GAD spend so much time worrying that they neglect the world around them. Generally anticipating the worst, they only absorb information in accordance with their negative expectations. They do not utilize information available to them via their emotional experience, which can adaptively motivate or guide their behavior (Borkovec, 2002). Additionally, individuals with GAD fail to take advantage of information from their environment that can facilitate learning and subsequent growth (Borkovec, 2002). In their efforts to focus on imagined threat, they are distracted from the here and now, including any information that may be useful and/or make life less stressful. Despite its negative impact, GAD is unique compared to other anxiety disorders, in that worry is inherently reinforcing. Some individuals with GAD hold the superstitious belief that their worry can actually prevent negative things from happening. The relief they experience when the feared event does not occur reinforces their worry. They are firm in their conviction that if they had not engaged in worrisome thinking, the aversive event might have taken place. Other individuals with GAD believe that their motivation hinges upon their worry. Without it, they would no longer be goal-oriented. They feel that they need to be in a constant state of activation, anticipating future catastrophes so they can avoid them, in order to be successful.

Based on empirical findings on the symptoms and clinical features of GAD reviewed earlier, we can make a number of recommendations about how treatment might best proceed with such patients. As worry is a form of negative reinforcement, individuals with GAD need to gain insight that their worry is ultimately maladaptive. Although it is likely to take considerable therapeutic effort for patients with GAD to learn that their worry is not helpful, clinicians should assist them in developing a new perspective. As many individuals with GAD tend to associate their worry with a motivation to succeed, they need to learn to differentiate between emotional distress and drive and ambition. It is important for them to realize that they can still be goal-oriented in the absence of anxiety. The majority of their experience centers on trying to prevent future disasters; thus, their actions are perceived to be externally motivated. Accordingly, treatment should focus on helping them rediscover the intrinsic motivation behind their actions, and come to understand that it is possible to engage in something even when not actively fearing negative consequences. Patients with GAD do not fully experience life, because they are consumed by mentally creating, and subsequently avoiding, new dangers and threats. In order to maximize their potential they need to refrain from attending to external consequences to the extent that they are disengaged from meaningful and rewarding activities. They need to recognize the negative impact their worry has on their well-being. Thus, before beginning to work with clients on decreasing worry, therapists need to help clients see that their worry is neither helpful nor necessary.

Given the potency of worry, it is also important to target and track this cognitive process consistently and not to treat GAD as simply diffuse anxiety. Therefore, self-monitoring is likely to be a beneficial component of therapy, irrespective of the clinician's theoretical orientation. In the treatment of GAD, clinicians need to assist their patients in identifying where and when experiences that are inconsistent with their expectations may have occurred. These patients are constantly attuned to imagined negative events that may happen in the future, so it is necessary for them to return to the present moment. Being in the here and now allows for accurate tracking of information that can assist them when they entertain maladaptive beliefs. When focused on what may happen in the future, people with GAD tend to lose some information available to them that they can use to their benefit in their present environment. Therefore, it is important that clinicians help them actively make an effort to track and observe aspects of the world around them that are inconsistent with their apprehensions. Moreover, individuals with GAD need more adaptive ways to perceive, interpret, and predict events. As they are likely to reject information contrary to their negatively biased organizing cognitions, they generally regard positive experiences as flukes. Therefore, therapists need to teach clients how to change their negative beliefs. Overall, a major goal of therapy is to help these patients shift from inaccurate negative expectations to beliefs that are less anxiety provoking.

In addition to teaching new ways of seeing the world, more recently developed treatments have targeted the predilection of individuals with GAD to avoid emotional processing via worry. Given that emotional processing avoidance may be maintaining the generalized anxiety symptoms, active engagement in emotional processing may be an important component of treatment, particularly the processing of fear (Llera & Newman, 2010; Newman, Castonguay, Borkovec, Fisher, & Nordberg, 2008). However, given that worry precludes such processing, and because worry increases and maintains anxiety and stress, an important therapeutic task is to engage clients in the use of applied relaxation. In a relaxed state, emotional processing is more likely.

Because GAD is associated with impairment in health and occupational functioning, it is recommended that clinicians ascribing to all theoretical orientations assess associated disability at different phases of treatment in order to determine ways in which clients can improve those important aspects of functioning. Similarly, therapists should assess for suicidal ideation, intent, and plan throughout the course of treatment, especially if it has been determined that the patient is at risk for suicide. Moreover, some of the somatic symptoms associated with GAD (e.g., fatigue, sleep disturbance, irritability, difficulties with concentration) can be addressed with specific interventions, such as relaxation and sleep hygiene techniques, and should be incorporated into treatment.

Also, because interpersonal problems are highly associated with GAD, therapists should assess interpersonal difficulties at different phases of therapy, including the end of the treatment. Remaining interpersonal problems at the end of therapy have been linked to poor outcome at follow-up. Thus, addressing such problems before the end of treatment may prevent relapse. Both theory and research evidence have suggested that interpersonal problems (past and current) are linked to the cause and/or maintenance of GAD and, as such, are further addressed in the section on etiology.

The aforementioned recommendations are beneficial in targeting the core cognitive, emotional, and behavioral symptoms of individuals diagnosed with GAD. However, individuals who fall below threshold may still be significantly affected by their GAD symptoms. Although their overall dysfunction may not be as severe as that of individuals with full GAD, their symptoms can be just as debilitating during periods of excessive worry and high anxiety. Therefore, it is important to assess clinically for the presence of subthreshold levels of GAD. Whereas a patient is generally treated within an overall diagnostic and therapeutic framework, including consideration of personality disorders, it may be necessary to consider the patient's needs from an individual standpoint, especially if he or she does not meet criteria for a particular disorder but reports some associated symptoms and stabilization is required.

COURSE AND OUTCOME

The most recent data on the course of GAD suggest that it is a highly chronic illness. Although GAD is marked by a later onset than other anxiety disorders (median onset age was 31; Kessler, Berglund, Demler, et al., 2005), it has a low probability of recovery and a high likelihood of recurrence in cases when recovery takes place. For example, in data from the Harvard–Brown Anxiety Research Program (HARP), a naturalistic prospective study of psychiatric patients, the probability of recovery from GAD over a 12-year period was 58%, and the probability of subsequent recurrence among those who did recover was 45% (e.g., Yonkers, Dyck, Warshaw, & Keller, 2000). A more recent prospective study of primary care patients over a 2-year time period found that the majority of individuals with GAD at baseline continued to experience significant GAD symptoms after 2 years, with a 39% probability of full recovery. Moreover, 52% of those who did experience recovery had a recurrence (Rodriguez et al., 2006). Additional data from controlled treatment studies also indicate that patients with GAD rarely experience full or sustained recovery from symptoms (Brown, Schulberg, Madonia, Shear, & Houck, 1996; Durham, Allan, & Hackett, 1997; Yonkers, Bruce, Dyck, & Keller, 2003).

During the course of their illness, individuals with GAD also do not experience a constant level of symptom severity or impairment. Instead, evidence shows that while experiencing a chronic course, the typical person with GAD shows a fluctuation in symptom severity (e.g., Wittchen, Lieb, Pfister, & Schuster, 2000; Yonkers, Warshaw, Massion, & Keller, 1996). As such, there may be periods of time when the severity of GAD symptoms is below threshold levels, without necessarily indicating recovery. Similarly, individuals with GAD may go from below threshold to threshold levels (Angst, Gamma, Baldwin, Ajdacic-Gross, & Rossler, 2009).

Cognitive-behavioral therapy (CBT) is currently the gold standard treatment for GAD. In a meta-analysis of the extant controlled outcome studies, Borkovec and Ruscio (2001) found that CBT for GAD produces significant improvement that is maintained for up to 2 years following treatment termination. CBT also has been found to generate greater improvement than no treatment, analytic psychotherapy, pill placebo, nondirective therapy, and placebo therapy (e.g., Borkovec & Ruscio, 2001). Although several investigations have not found differences between CBT and either cognitive therapy or behavior therapy alone, others have documented its superiority immediately after treatment or at long-term follow-up, and meta-analyses of studies using common outcome measures indicate that CBT produces the largest effect sizes compared to other therapy and control conditions (Borkovec & Ruscio, 2001). CBT is also well liked by clients and associated with relatively low dropout rates and significant reductions in the need for anxiolytic medication. In addition to showing *statistically* significant improvement, CBT has also demonstrated *clinically* significant improvement. In three of the four interpretable studies that have assessed clinically significant change, CBT showed long-term maintenance or further gains in clinically significant change (Borkovec & Whisman, 1996). CBT interventions include self-monitoring, stimulus control, relaxation, self-control desensitization, and cognitive therapy. As described by Woody and Ollendick (2006) and Newman, Stiles, Janeck, and Woody (2006), these techniques reflect five principles of change (i.e., challenge misconceptions, actively test the validity of erroneous beliefs, use repeated exposure, eliminate avoidance, and improve skills) that can be implemented by various interventions espoused in different approaches).

In terms of pharmacological treatments, benzodiazepines (BZs) and buspirone were the first classes of medications approved by the Food and Drug Administration (FDA) for the treatment of GAD. However, whereas BZs have been the mainstay of short-term anxiolytic treatment, because of rebound anxiety and presence of discontinuation symptoms after only 4–8 weeks of therapy, BZs have been relegated by most physicians to treat only acute anxiety symptoms (Ashton, 1994; Lader & Bond, 1998). In response to BZs only 40% or fewer patients reach remission and about an additional 30% report moderate improvement, with anxiety levels being closer to those of unimproved patients than those of remitting patients (e.g., Shader & Greenblatt, 1993). BZs also carry considerable risk of sedation, motor and cognitive abnormalities, and physical dependency and withdrawal problems (e.g., van Laar, Volkerts, & Verbaten, 2001; Wang, Bohn, Glynn, Mogun, & Avorn, 2001).

Safety concerns regarding BZs provided the impetus for the search of non-BZ anxiolytics, such as the 5-HT$_{1A}$ partial agonists, and antidepressants. Of all 5-HT$_{1A}$ partial agonists studied, only buspirone (Rickels et al., 1982; Volz, Möller, & Sturm, 1994), and not agents such as gepirone (Rickels, Schweizer, DeMartinis, Mandos, & Mercer, 1997), have demonstrated consistent anxiolytic properties. Of the tricyclic antidepressants, imipramine (Kahn et al., 1986; Rickels, Downing, Schweizer, & Hassman, 1993) showed clinical efficacy. In acute double-blind trials, the anxiolytic buspirone consistently demonstrated slower onset and slightly weaker overall antianxiety efficacy compared to various BZs (Rickels, Schweizer, Csanalosi, Case, & Chung, 1988; Scheibe, 1996) and antidepressants (Davidson, DuPont, Hedges, & Haskins, 1999).

Since 1999, a number of studies have documented the efficacy of selective serotonin reuptake inhibitor (SSRI) and serotonin–norepineprhine reuptake inhibitor (SNRI) antidepressants in the treatment of GAD. Venlafaxine XR (extended release) was the first of these drugs to be approved by the FDA for the indication of GAD. In four large-scale studies venlafaxine XR demonstrated significantly better clinical efficacy than placebo after 8 weeks (Davidson et al., 1999; Kelsey, 2000; Rickels, Pollack, Sheehan, & Haskins, 2000; Sheehan, 1999), and after 6 months (Allgulander, Hackett, & Salinas, 2001; Gelenberg et al., 2000) of treatment. Paroxetine was also studied in several GAD trials (Davidson, 2001; McCafferty, Bellew, Zanelli, Iyengar, & Hewett, 2000; Pollack et al., 2001; Rickels et al., 2003) and was also approved by the FDA for the treatment of GAD. Additional SSRI/SNRI medications approved by the FDA for the treatment of GAD include duloxetine and escitalopram.

Despite the efficacy literature on SNRIs and SSRIs in the treatment of GAD, a satisfactory response to short-term treatment occurs for only about 60% of patients, and substantial numbers of these responders have significant residual symptoms.

Consistent with this pattern of significant residual symptoms, low remission rates have been observed for venlafaxine XR (37%; Gelenberg et al., 2000) and paroxetine (36%; Pollack et al., 2001) in the acute phase treatment of GAD. Although continuation and maintenance treatment may prove further to increase response and remission rates, it is equally important to attempt to increase these rates during acute phase short-term treatment in order to improve compliance, relieve suffering and functional impairment, and improve quality of life as quickly as possible. Thus, it is important to test new ways of improving short-term treatment of GAD.

Treatment Implications

Given GAD's chronic fluctuating course, it is recommended that individuals with GAD and subthreshold GAD seek treatment, because it is not likely that GAD symptoms and associated features will permanently resolve themselves over time in the absence of intervention. Although the frequency and intensity of symptoms may decrease unaided, they can resurface to the same degree, especially in response to internal and external stressors. In patients seeking treatment, it can also appear that their GAD symptoms have been successfully treated when assessing at discrete time points. For this reason, clinicians need to be cognizant of the vacillations in GAD symptomatology and the precipitants of that change. Somebody who currently exhibits subthreshold symptoms may be more at risk for developing full-blown GAD. Psychotherapists should use standards employed in epidemiological studies explicitly to track GAD in patients at the symptom level to better understand its ebbs and flows, such as the symptom course indicative of sustained recovery. Also, it is recommended that treatment not be discontinued until clients have shown sustained recovery.

Although data suggest that GAD is a chronic illness, clinicians should also be aware that patients may inaccurately report their symptoms. For instance, if they are feeling anxious in a given moment or for an extended period, they are more likely to report that they have been that way for the past 6 months, thus meeting the chronicity criterion for GAD. Therefore, it is important for therapists to help patients increase their awareness of their patterns of functioning. Likewise, individuals with GAD rarely experience full or sustained recovery. Therefore, it is imperative that therapists approach treatment with realistic expectations and aim not for a "cure" but to help the client to learn how to cope with the disorder. The chronicity and recurrence of GAD also suggests that clients may need long-term therapy, irrespective of treatment approach. Additionally, therapists should incorporate methods to facilitate prediction and prevention of relapses, as well as cope with possible resurgences of the disorder.

In terms of medication options, the consistency of the results reported for venlafaxine XR and paroxetine suggests that today, certainly not only for the short-term (8 weeks) but also for extended (6 months) treatment of GAD, SSRIs and SNRIs seem to be the medication treatment of choice.

EPIDEMIOLOGY

Variations in definition, including subsequent changes to DSM criteria, have interfered with precise prevalence estimates for GAD. However, several epidemiological studies employing large representative samples have approximated actual prevalence rates. Lifetime prevalence of DSM-III-R GAD, excluding comorbid panic and depression, is 3.6% (Kendler, Neale, Kessler, Heath, & Eaves, 1992). The National Comorbidity Survey found a 12-month prevalence of 3.1% and a lifetime prevalence of 5.1% (Wittchen, Zhao, Kessler, & Eaton, 1994). The National Comorbidity Survey Replication study indicates a lifetime prevalence for DSM-IV GAD of 5.7% and a 12-month prevalence of 3.1% (Kessler, Berglund, et al., 2005). Projected lifetime prevalence at age 75 is 8.3%. Based on findings from available epidemiological surveys, most countries around the world appear to have a fairly similar prevalence of GAD.

A number of sociodemographic features are associated with the presence of GAD. First, gender is highly correlated with increased incidence of GAD. Specifically, rates of GAD are approximately two times greater in women than in men in both community (Wittchen et al., 1994) and clinical (e.g., Woodman, Noyes, Black, Schlosser, & Yagla, 1999) samples. Furthermore, the National Comorbidity Survey indicated that previously married respondents had a significantly higher lifetime prevalence of GAD than either married or never-married respondents (Wittchen et al., 1994). Homemakers and other respondents not working outside the home were significantly more likely than other respondents to have GAD; furthermore, prevalence of GAD is related to geographic location, such that incidence is highest in the Northeast United States (Wittchen et al., 1994). Epidemiological surveys in the United States, however, found few differences in the prevalence of GAD among representative ethnic groups (Blazer, Hughes, George, Swartz, & Boyer, 1991; Wittchen et al., 1994). Also, education, religion, living in urban areas, and income were not found to be associated with increased risk of GAD (Wittchen et al., 1994).

Treatment Implications

GAD prevalence rates depend on the current diagnostic criteria. The more rigid the criteria, the less likely individuals are going to be assigned a GAD diagnosis, thereby decreasing the disorder's prevalence rate. However, it is not uncommon for anxious patients to engage in excessive worry or to meet criteria for subthreshold GAD. Therefore, therapists should establish an understanding of the determinants of GAD and related symptomatology, since they are likely to encounter worrisome patients. Although patients may not meet full criteria for GAD, clinicians of all experience levels should not neglect subthreshold GAD symptoms, because the emergence of full GAD may be prevented through early detection of symptoms. Given a patient's sociodemographic features, therapists should be aware that differential risk of GAD may be associated with different determinant stressors, such as divorce or the death of a loved one. Whereas ethnicity, education, religion, and income are not related to increased incidence of GAD, the content of patients' worries may differ depending on their sociodemographic background. Thus, clinicians need to understand the manifestations of GAD within the context of an individual's culture, ethnicity, religion, education, and income level.

COMORBIDITY

An important issue in GAD treatment is comorbidity, which is typically much higher for patients seeking treatment than for persons in the community. However, even in untreated community samples, GAD comorbidity rates are very high. Current comorbidity for GAD has been reported to range from 8 to 22% for dysthymia, 8.6 to 46% for major depression, 10.7 to 27% for social phobia, and 11 to 36% for panic disorder—the four most common comorbid diagnoses (e.g., Brown & Barlow, 1992; Grant et al., 2005b; Wittchen et al., 1994). Judd et al. (1998) reported that 80% of subjects with a lifetime diagnosis of GAD also had a lifetime mood disorder diagnosis, and Grant et al. (2005b) reported that only 10.2% of participants did not have a comorbid mental disorder. Substance abuse and personality disorders constitute two other important categories of comorbidity that may complicate the natural history of the anxiety disorders (e.g., Massion et al., 1993; Noyes et al., 1992). Current alcoholism has been reported in a large community survey to occur at a rate of 11% (Wittchen et al., 1994). Personality disorder comorbidity rates for GAD have been reported in the 30–60% range (e.g., Mavissakalian, Hamann, Abou Haidar, & de Groot, 1993; Noyes et al., 1992).

Such comorbidity occurs both concurrently and sequentially in GAD (Moffitt et al., 2007). In terms of sequential comorbidity, temporal reciprocal comorbidity (i.e., comorbidity can precede or follow GAD) has been found between GAD and alcohol abuse/dependence, GAD and panic disorder, and GAD and major depression (e.g., Grant et al., 2009; Moffitt et al., 2007; Wittchen, Kessler, Pfister, & Lieb, 2000). Moreover, within a given time period, the presence of GAD at time 1 increases the likelihood of the development of a different disorder at time 2. For example, data from the National Comorbidity Replication Study indicated that active GAD better predicted new onsets of subsequent mental disorders than did remitted GAD, even when severity was controlled (Ruscio et al., 2007). In terms of specific disorders, current GAD significantly predicted subsequent panic disorder, posttraumatic stress disorder (PTSD), any mood disorder, and any substance use disorder; even subthreshold levels of GAD significantly predicted new onsets of panic disorder, mood disorders, and substance use disorders (Ruscio et al., 2007). Similarly, in a prospective study, the current risk factors for the development of new episodes of depression in currently nondepressed adults included previous episodes of subthreshold GAD (Barkow et al., 2002).

Because GAD is highly comorbid with other disorders, particularly MDD (Grant et al., 2005b; Kessler, Chiu, Demler, Merikangas, & Walters, 2005) and because there is evidence for a common genetic origin between GAD and MDD (e.g., Kendler, Gardner, Gatz, & Pedersen, 2007), some researchers have questioned whether GAD is a distinct disorder. However, a number of pieces of evidence support the distinctiveness of GAD. For example, GAD appears to be a discrete disorder with fairly good construct validity (e.g., Brown, Chorpita, & Barlow, 1998). In fact, pure lifetime GAD (eventuating in no other diagnosis) has been found to occur at the not inconsiderable rate of 0.5% (Wittchen et al., 1994). Furthermore, nonpure lifetime GAD actually has only modest symptom overlap with the other mental disorder diagnoses with which it is commonly comorbid (Clark, Beck, & Beck, 1994). GAD and MDD are equally likely to be temporally primary (Moffitt et al., 2007), refuting the notion that GAD is simply a prodrome for MDD. In addition, the course of comorbid GAD is unrelated to whether GAD is temporally primary or secondary (e.g., Kessler et al., 2008). In terms of the discrimination between MDD and GAD, studies show differences between the disorders in risk factors (Moffitt et al., 2007), as well as in intertemporal stability that cannot be explained by a common underlying internalizing factor (Fergusson, Horwood, & Boden, 2006).

In addition, although there are common genetic influences between GAD and MDD, the environmental determinants of the two disorders are more distinct (e.g., Kendler, 1996; Kendler et al., 2007). Neuropsychological studies also find differences between the disorders in attentional and memory biases (e.g., Hazen, Vasey, & Schmidt, 2009). Furthermore, whereas pure GAD and pure MDD are equally disabling, disability is substantially increased when the two co-occur, suggesting that the status of GAD as an independent disorder is at least comparable to MDD (e.g., Kessler, 2000; Kessler, Berglund, et al., 2002). There are also striking differences between the two disorders in their underlying neurobiology (Goldberg, 2008; Martin, Nemeroff, & Regier, 2010).

Comorbidity is associated with further impairment. Persons with comorbidity in addition to GAD report more disability days (Hunt, Issakidis, & Andrews, 2002), more interference from symptoms of GAD (Wittchen et al., 1994), and increased likelihood of interpersonal problems (Judd et al., 1998) compared to those with pure GAD. In addition, they pose a greater risk of suicide (e.g., Boden et al., 2007). Moreover, compared to those with pure GAD, those with current comorbid disorders report more hospitalizations, visits to the emergency room, consultations with medical specialists, laboratory tests, medication use, and work absenteeism (Souetre et al., 1994; Wittchen et al., 1994). Studies also suggest that persons with depression and GAD are at greater risk for mortality from coronary heart disease than are those with MDD or GAD alone (Sevincok, Buyukozturk, & Dereboy, 2001). Thus, individuals with comorbid conditions incur more direct and indirect costs than do those with pure GAD (e.g., Souetre et al., 1994).

Several studies have also found that comorbid disorders reduce the likelihood of naturalistic remission from GAD (e.g., Bruce et al., 2005; Kessler, Andrade, et al.,

2002). For example, data from the World Health Organization suggested that simple phobia predicted persistence of GAD (Kessler, Andrade, et al., 2002), and analyses of HARP data showed that comorbid depression or panic disorder was associated with decreased likelihood of remission from GAD (Bruce, Machan, Dyck, & Keller, 2001; Bruce et al., 2005). Similarly, when GAD was secondary to panic disorder or major depression, it was associated with a more severe and chronic course of the primary disorders (e.g., Kessler et al., 1996, 1998). Moreover, when GAD was comorbid to social phobia, it was associated with decreased probability of remission and increased probability of recurrence of the social phobia (Bruce et al., 2005).

Comorbid interpersonal factors such as marital tension (Durham et al., 1997) and comorbid personality disorders (e.g., Massion et al., 2002) have predicted negative CBT treatment outcomes, and higher dropout rate and reduced likelihood of remission. Also, Borkovec, Newman, Pincus, and Lytle (2002) found that CBT failed to make a significant change in most Inventory of Interpersonal Problems—Circumplex (IIP-C) scales at posttherapy, and most clients continued to score at least one standard deviation above normative levels on at least one IIP-C subscale. In the same study, clients endorsing pretherapy interpersonal problems associated with dominance (e.g., Domineering/Controlling, Intrusive/Needy, Vindictive/Self-Centered) responded least favorably to CBT, and such problems left untreated predicted failure to maintain follow-up gains. Such evidence warrants therapy techniques specifically to address interpersonal problems, including the client's contribution to maintaining maladaptive ways of relating with others.

Treatment Implications

GAD is a highly comorbid disorder that either functions as the primary disorder or within the context of other psychopathology, and it can still be a significant problem even when it may not be the primary disorder. Likewise, it is important periodically to assess for the presence of other disorders throughout treatment, even if GAD is the principal diagnosis. This enables clinicians to adjust the treatment plan in accordance with the client's difficulties. Additionally, assessing psychopathology (including personality disorders and interpersonal problems more broadly) at the end of treatment allows clinicians to determine whether therapy had an impact on comorbid disorders. The detection of such problems might call for additional interventions specifically targeting remaining problems, particularly interpersonal problems, because these tended to predict poor outcome after therapy has been completed. Similarly, given the high level of comorbid GAD observed in other disorders, especially depression, it is advantageous for clinicians to assess for GAD at different phases of treatment, even when it is not the primary disorder.

Furthermore, the presence of worrisome thinking that is difficult to control distinguishes GAD from other disorders and suggests the importance of directly targeting a patient's worry. Conceptualization and treatment planning may differ depending on comorbidity, such that one disorder or related symptoms can affect the symptom expression of another disorder. Whereas individuals with GAD are less likely than those with other disorders to engage in behavioral avoidance, a comorbid diagnosis of GAD and panic disorder can alter a patient's pattern of symptoms and may require inclusion of situational exposure techniques. Also, GAD can be associated with symptoms of other disorders in the absence of those disorders. For instance, individuals with GAD occasionally avoid worry triggers. Thus, a thorough assessment of any and all avoidance patterns, even subtle avoidance, is important. Overall, a clinician may approach a patient's GAD symptomatology differently if other diagnoses or associated symptoms and features are present. Because of the interrelationships among GAD and associated disorders, addressing comorbid disorders and symptoms in patients with GAD may be critical to achieving long-term recovery from GAD.

ETIOLOGY

Although many biological, psychological, and social factors are likely to be involved in the predisposition and/or cause of GAD, it is important to keep in mind that the development of GAD is attributed to the complex interplay of genetic, biological, environmental, and psychological vulnerability factors. According to twin studies (Kendler et al., 1992, 1995), GAD is moderately regulated by genetic factors, such that about 30% of the variance is due to heritability. Similarly, heritable traits related to temperament (accounting for 30–50% of the variance), such as neuroticism, negative affectivity, and anxiety, are strongly associated with the presence of anxiety disorders (e.g., Brown et al., 1998; Clark, Watson, & Mineka, 1994). Whereas family studies indicated that the development of GAD is more likely in individuals having a first-degree relative with the disorder (Noyes, Clarkson, Crowe, Yates, & McChesney, 1987), it is difficult to distinguish environmental and genetic factors. Although genetic influences do not represent causal factors in the development of GAD, heritability contributes to a general biological predisposition to anxiety, which interacts with other elements in the emergence of a distinct disorder (e.g., Kendler et al., 1995). An underlying genetic vulnerability to anxiety in general manifests as GAD when the necessary biological, psychological, and environmental elements converge.

Besides theories featuring genetic determinants of anxiety disorders, conditioning and learning theories illuminate important factors in the development and maintenance of anxiety, and therefore likely have a role in the disorder of GAD. Classical conditioning theory suggests that a child comes to fear a conditioned stimulus (CS) following repeated pairings with an aversive unconditioned stimulus (UCS). The CS generates anxiety in the child, since he or she expects it to result in an aversive outcome. Anxious behavior is reinforced and maintained upon avoiding the CS (Mowrer, 1939). Operant conditioning provides another route to the development and maintenance of anxiety, such that parents have been shown to foster anxious behavior via extra attention and reassurance, and assistance with avoidant behavior (Ayllon, Smith, & Rogers, 1970).

Social modeling may also contribute to anxious behavior (Bandura & Menlove, 1968). Likewise, early attachment likely plays a role in the development and maintenance of GAD. To illustrate, Bowlby (1982) suggested that anxiety is a product of insecure attachment, such that when an attachment figure is in some way absent, the child fails to develop a secure base from which to explore his or her environment. Subsequently, he or she may view the world as an unpredictable, uncontrollable, and threatening place, thereby exaggerating the likelihood and negative impact of feared events, and underestimate his or her ability to cope with these events. In support of Bowlby's proposed model, a prospective study found that anxious attachment in infants predicted later development of anxiety disorders (Warren, Huston, Egeland, & Sroufe, 1997). In a retrospective study, anxious parents endorsed less parental care and more overprotection than matched controls (Parker, 1981). Additionally, participants who classified their parents as higher on protection and lower on care exhibited higher trait anxiety than those who did not attribute these traits to their parents.

As noted earlier, individuals with GAD also have cognitive biases. It is possible (although there are no empirical data to support this), that such cognitive biases develop prior to the onset of GAD and serve as risk factors for the disorder. Theoretically, one might imagine a scenario in which a child learns that bad things happen unexpectedly; thus, the child develops a maladaptive strategy to cope with this by repeatedly interpreting ambiguous information as an indication that something bad has happened or will happen, as a means to prepare for the worst. Models of GAD implicate processes such as worry about worry (Wells, 2005), intolerance of uncertainty (Dugas, Buhr, & Ladouceur, 2004), and fear of a negative emotional contrast (i.e., the fear of being disappointed or emotionally caught off guard) as being possible cognitive factors that precede the development of GAD (Newman & Llera, 2011).

Considering the personality correlates of GAD, children with this disorder are more likely to be perfectionists, to seek excessive approval, and to need constant reassurance regarding their worries. They are overly conforming and self-conscious, often possessing a negative self-image. Moreover, anxious children tend to be shy, withdrawn, and lonely (Strauss, Lease, Kazdin, Dulcan, & Last, 1989), and experience difficulty making friends (Strauss, Lahey, Frick, Frame, & Hynd, 1988). Subsequent fear and negative expectations of social situations can interfere with interpersonal functioning. Accordingly, these children may engage in negative interpersonal cycles (Safran & Segal, 1990) in which they influence others' behavior in a manner that serves to reinforce their negative expectations and contributes to the maintenance of their anxiety. In a similar fashion, individuals with GAD are often fearful, expect negative responses from others, and demonstrate a bias toward social threat cues (e.g., Mathews & MacLeod, 1985; Mogg et al., 1992). In an experimental investigation of maladaptive social cognitions, interpersonal behaviors, and emotional regulation in GAD (Erickson & Newman, 2007), participants with GAD exhibited more biased perceptions of their impact on others during an interaction task, tending either to overestimate or underestimate the degree of their negative impact, compared to nonanxious controls.

During childhood, individuals with GAD may have learned that caring for others elicits love, approval, and nurturance. Extending this pattern into adulthood, they are frequently concerned about interpersonal relationships (Breitholtz et al., 1999; Roemer et al., 1997). Thus, worry may function as a means of anticipating the needs of, and threats to, significant others in the pursuit of satisfying interpersonal needs. Given their faulty perception of their social impact on others (Erickson & Newman, 2007), it follows that individuals with GAD would show not only greater interpersonal distress but also greater rigidity in their interpersonal styles across differing situations than nonanxious people (Przeworski et al., 2011). Furthermore, studies indicated that those with GAD scored higher on role-reversed/enmeshed relationships than did nonanxious individuals (Cassidy & Shaver, 1999; Cassidy, 1995). These individuals generally perceive threat in their environment and may therefore feel the need to anticipate and control any potential danger to themselves or their significant others. Conversely, individuals with GAD may also experience greater feelings of unresolved anger toward their primary caregivers (Cassidy & Shaver, 1999; Cassidy, 1995), further exacerbating their interpersonal difficulties.

Treatment Implications

Although many biological, psychological, and social factors are likely to be involved in the predisposition and/or cause of GAD, it is important to keep in mind that the etiology of a disorder does not necessarily have bearing on its maintenance. Whereas people come to behave in certain ways as a result of some developmental or etiological factor, the behavior often persists in the absence of its origin. Often it is difficult to determine how a particular disorder develops, but recovery is possible if maintaining factors are identified and addressed. Therapists should investigate those factors that may contribute to their GAD patients' worrisome and anxious states, especially since these patients tend to engage in behaviors that are perceived to be helpful but ultimately may exacerbate their problem. Additionally, it is important to be watchful of any secondary gains that enable the patients' conditions. For example, GAD is often associated with reassurance-seeking behavior. Individuals with this disorder work themselves into an excessively worried state, then want validation from significant others that they are OK. They learn to associate worry with reassurance, which inadvertently perpetuates their worrisome thinking.

Once GAD maintaining factors have been identified, therapy can center on eliminating those factors. Many of these factors have been targeted in cognitive-behavioral therapy (CBT) protocols. We should mention, however, that CBT techniques such as relaxation, stimulus control, social skills training, and exposure (*in vivo* and imaginal) can be incorporated into treatment, irrespective of the therapist's theoretical approach. As mentioned earlier, these CBT interventions can be viewed as particular manifestations of general principles of change that could be implemented by other techniques typically prescribe in other orientations (cognitive distortions and processes, for instance, can be addressed by the use of confrontation and interpretation, as well as by cognitive restructuring; see Castonguay, 2000; Newman et al., 2006). Similarly, some more recently developed treatments for GAD have also tried to make use of interpersonally focused psychotherapies directed at addressing the high rate of interpersonal problems in GAD (e.g., Crits-Christoph et al., 2005; Newman et al., 2008, 2011), thereby underscoring the importance of integrating therapy techniques in the treatment of GAD. Also, new attention-retraining treatments have been developed explicitly to target cognitive biases (Amir, Beard, Burns, & Bomyea, 2009). It may also be important for therapists of all orientations to pay attention to cognitive biases in patients and to direct them toward evidence that does not substantiate such biases.

CONCLUSION

Worry is a universal experience that enables people to deal with challenging future events. Since this thought style is more abstract and less concrete (less image producing) than other types of thinking (Borkovec & Inz, 1990), it allows for abstract processing of emotional information, thereby facilitating avoidance of reactivity and surprising negative events. Thus, it functions as a strategy to manage the unpredictability and uncontrollability of potentially threatening future events. Nevertheless, the worry experienced by individuals with GAD is a pervasive, uncontrollable daily activity that often elicits emotional discomfort. Although patients with GAD engage in worry as a means to combat potential threat, it serves to exacerbate their anxiety. Accordingly, GAD can be associated with debilitating distress, disability, and impairment in quality of life.

Overall, GAD is a highly chronic and comorbid anxiety disorder whose etiology is linked to a combination of genetic, biological, environmental, and psychological factors. Its core and associated symptoms are the products of the interaction between cognitive, imaginal, and physiological responses to continuously perceived threat (Borkovec & Inz, 1990; Newman & Borkovec, 2002). Although it is the least successfully treated anxiety disorder given its chronicity and pervasiveness (Brown et al., 1994), CBT is an efficacious treatment for GAD. CBT targets each of the aforementioned response systems, and interventions include self-monitoring, stimulus control, relaxation, self-control desensitization, and cognitive therapy. Publication of DSM-5 has brought significant changes to the diagnostic criteria for anxiety disorders, but for GAD worry continues to play a central, prominent role in this disorder's conceptualization (American Psychiatric Association, 2013). Therefore, when treating GAD, clinicians and therapists should assist patients in recognizing the

detrimental impact their worry has on their psychological and emotional functioning, and identifying and tracking their worrisome thinking, as well as underscore
those experiences and aspects in the patients' environment that are inconsistent
with their schemas to remediate maladaptive thought and behavior patterns.

REFERENCES

Allgulander, C., Hackett, D., & Salinas, E. (2001). Venlafaxine extended release (ER) in the treatment of generalised anxiety disorder: Twenty-four-week placebo-controlled dose-ranging
study. *British Journal of Psychiatry, 179*(1), 15–22.

American Psychiatric Association. (2000). *Diagnostic and statistical manual of mental disorders* (4th
ed., text rev.). Washington, DC: Author.

American Psychiatric Association. (2013). *Diagnostic and statistical manual of mental disorders* (5th
ed.). Arlington, VA: Author.

Amir, N., Beard, C., Burns, M., & Bomyea, J. (2009). Attention modification program in individuals with generalized anxiety disorder. *Journal of Abnormal Psychology, 118*(1), 28–33.

Angst, J., Gamma, A., Baldwin, D. S., Ajdacic-Gross, V., & Rossler, W. (2009). The generalized
anxiety spectrum: Prevalence, onset, course and outcome. *European Archives of Psychiatry
and Clinical Neuroscience, 259*(1), 37–45.

Ashton, H. (1994). Guidelines for the rational use of benzodiazepines: When and what to use.
Drugs, 48(1), 25–40.

Ayllon, T., Smith, D., & Rogers, M. (1970). Behavioral management of school phobia. *Journal of
Behavior Therapy and Experimental Psychiatry, 1*(2), 125–138.

Bandura, A., & Menlove, F. L. (1968). Factors determining vicarious extinction of avoidance
behavior through symbolic modeling. *Journal of Personality and Social Psychology, 8*(2, Pt. 1),
99–108.

Barger, S. D., & Sydeman, S. J. (2005). Does generalized anxiety disorder predict coronary heart
disease risk factors independently of major depressive disorder? *Journal of Affective Disorders, 88*(1), 87–91.

Barkow, K., Maier, W., Üstün, T. B., Gänsicke, M., Wittchen, H. U., & Heun, R. (2002). Risk factors
for new depressive episodes in primary health care: An international prospective 12-month
follow-up study. *Psychological Medicine, 32*(4), 595–607.

Blazer, D. G., Hughes, D. C., George, L. K., Swartz, M. S., & Boyer, R. (1991). Generalized anxiety
disorder. In L. N. Robins & D. A. Regier (Eds.), *Psychiatric disorders in America: The Epidemiologic Catchment Area study* (pp. 180–203). New York: Free Press.

Boden, J. M., Fergusson, D. M., & Horwood, L. J. (2007). Anxiety disorders and suicidal behav-
iours in adolescence and young adulthood: Findings from a longitudinal study. *Psychological Medicine, 37*(3), 431–440.

Borkovec, T. D. (2002). Life in the future versus life in the present. *Clinical Psychology: Science and
Practice, 9*(1), 76–80.

Borkovec, T. D., Hazlett-Stevens, H., & Diaz, M. L. (1999). The role of positive beliefs about worry
in generalized anxiety disorder and its treatment. *Clinical Psychology and Psychotherapy, 6*(2),
126–138.

Borkovec, T. D., & Hu, S. (1990). The effect of worry on cardiovascular response to phobic imagery. *Behaviour Research and Therapy, 28*(1), 69–73.

Borkovec, T. D., & Inz, J. (1990). The nature of worry in generalized anxiety disorder: A predominance of thought activity. *Behaviour Research and Therapy, 28*(2), 153–158.

Borkovec, T. D., & Newman, M. G. (1998). Worry and generalized anxiety disorder. In P.

Salkovskis (Ed.), *Comprehensive clinical psychology: Vol. 6. Adults: Clinical formulation and treatment*. Oxford, UK: Pergamon.

Borkovec, T. D., Newman, M. G., Pincus, A. L., & Lytle, R. (2002). A component analysis of cognitive-behavioral therapy for generalized anxiety disorder and the role of interpersonal problems. *Journal of Consulting and Clinical Psychology, 70*(2), 288–298.

Borkovec, T. D., Ray, W. J., & Stober, J. (1998). Worry: A cognitive phenomenon intimately linked to affective, physiological, and interpersonal behavioral processes. *Cognitive Therapy and Research, 22*(6), 561–576.

Borkovec, T. D., Robinson, E., Pruzinsky, T., & DePree, J. A. (1983). Preliminary exploration of worry: Some characteristics and processes. *Behaviour Research and Therapy, 21*(1), 9–16.

Borkovec, T. D., & Roemer, L. (1995). Perceived functions of worry among generalized anxiety disorder subjects: Distraction from more emotionally distressing topics? *Journal of Behavior Therapy and Experimental Psychiatry, 26*(1), 25–30.

Borkovec, T. D., & Ruscio, A. M. (2001). Psychotherapy for generalized anxiety disorder. *Journal of Clinical Psychiatry, 62*(Suppl. 11), 37–45.

Borkovec, T. D., & Whisman, M. A. (1996). Psychosocial treatment for generalized anxiety disorder. In M. R. Mavissakalian & R. F. Prien (Eds.), *Long-term treatments of anxiety disorders* (pp. 171–199). Washington, DC: American Psychiatric Association.

Bowlby, J. (1982). *Attachment and loss: Vol. 1. Attachment* (2nd ed.). New York: Basic Books.

Breitholtz, E., Johansson, B., & Öst, L. G. (1999). Cognitions in generalized anxiety disorder and panic disorder patients: A prospective approach. *Behaviour Research and Therapy, 37*(6), 533–544.

Brown, C., Schulberg, H. C., Madonia, M. J., Shear, M. K., & Houck, P. R. (1996). Treatment outcomes for primary care patients with major depression and lifetime anxiety disorders. *American Journal of Psychiatry, 153*(10), 1293–1300.

Brown, T. A., & Barlow, D. H. (1992). Comorbidity among anxiety disorders: Implications for treatment and DSM-IV. *Journal of Consulting and Clinical Psychology, 60*(6), 835–844.

Brown, T. A., Barlow, D. H., & Liebowitz, M. R. (1994). The empirical basis of generalized anxiety disorder. *American Journal of Psychiatry, 151*(9), 1272–1280.

Brown, T. A., Chorpita, B. F., & Barlow, D. H. (1998). Structural relationships among dimensions of the DSM-IV anxiety and mood disorders and dimensions of negative affect, positive affect, and autonomic arousal. *Journal of Abnormal Psychology, 107*(2), 179–192.

Bruce, S. E., Machan, J. T., Dyck, I., & Keller, M. B. (2001). Infrequency of "pure" GAD: Impact of psychiatric comorbidity on clinical course. *Depression and Anxiety, 14*(4), 219–225.

Bruce, S. E., Yonkers, K. A., Otto, M. W., Eisen, J. L., Weisberg, R. B., Pagano, M., et al. (2005). Influence of psychiatric comorbidity on recovery and recurrence in generalized anxiety disorder, social phobia, and panic disorder: A 12-year prospective study. *American Journal of Psychiatry, 162*(6), 1179–1187.

Cassidy, J. A. (1995). Attachment and generalized anxiety disorder. In D. Cicchetti & S. L. Toth (Eds.), *Emotion, cognition, and representation: Rochester Symposium on Developmental Psychopathology* (Vol. 6, pp. 343–370). Rochester, NY: University of Rochester Press.

Cassidy, J., & Shaver, P. R. (Eds.). (1999). *Handbook of attachment: Theory, research, and clinical applications*. New York: Guilford Press.

Castonguay, L. G. (2000). A common factors approach to psychotherapy training. *Journal of Psychotherapy Integration, 10*(3), 263–282.

Clark, D. A., Beck, A. T., & Beck, J. S. (1994). Symptom differences in major depression, dysthymia, panic disorder, and generalized anxiety disorder. *American Journal of Psychiatry, 151*(2), 205–209.

Clark, L. A., Watson, D., & Mineka, S. (1994). Temperament, personality, and the mood and anxiety disorders. *Journal of Abnormal Psychology, 103*(1), 103–116.

Coles, M. E., Turk, C. L., & Heimberg, R. G. (2007). Memory bias for threat in generalized anxiety disorder: The potential importance of stimulus relevance. *Cognitive Behaviour Therapy, 36*(2), 65–73.

Craske, M. G., Rapee, R. M., Jackel, L., & Barlow, D. H. (1989). Qualitative dimensions of worry in DSM-III-R generalized anxiety disorder subjects and nonanxious controls. *Behaviour Research and Therapy, 27*(4), 397–402.

Crits-Christoph, P., Gibbons, M. B. C., Narducci, J., Schamberger, M., & Gallop, R. (2005). Interpersonal problems and the outcome of interpersonally oriented psychodynamic treatment of GAD. *Psychotherapy: Theory, Research, Practice and Training, 42*(2), 211–224.

Davidson, J. R. T. (2001). Pharmacotherapy of generalized anxiety disorder. *Journal of Clinical Psychiatry, 62*(Suppl. 11), 46–50.

Davidson, J. R., DuPont, R. L., Hedges, D., & Haskins, J. T. (1999). Efficacy, safety, and tolerability of venlafaxine extended release and buspirone in outpatients with generalized anxiety disorder. *Journal of Clinical Psychiatry, 60*(8), 528–535.

Dugas, M., Buhr, K., & Ladouceur, R. (2004). The role of intolerance of uncertainty in etiology and maintenance. In R. Heimberg, D. Mennin, & C. Turk (Eds.), *Generalized anxiety disorder: Advances in research and practice* (pp. 143–163). New York: Guilford Press.

Durham, R. C., Allan, T., & Hackett, C. A. (1997). On predicting improvement and relapse in generalized anxiety disorder following psychotherapy. *British Journal of Clinical Psychology, 36*(1), 101–119.

Erickson, T. M., & Newman, M. G. (2007). Interpersonal and emotional processes in generalized anxiety disorder analogues during social interaction tasks. *Behavior Therapy, 38*(4), 364–377.

Fergusson, D. M., Horwood, L. J., & Boden, J. M. (2006). Structure of internalising symptoms in early adulthood. *British Journal of Psychiatry, 189*(6), 540–546.

Fogarty, C. T., Sharma, S., Chetty, V. K., & Culpepper, L. (2008). Mental health conditions are associated with increased health care utilization among urban family medicine patients. *Journal of the American Board of Family Medicine, 21*(5), 398–407.

Gelenberg, A. J., Lydiard, R. B., Rudolph, R. L., Aguiar, L., Haskins, J. T., & Salinas, E. (2000). Efficacy of venlafaxine extended-release capsules in nondepressed outpatients with generalized anxiety disorder: A 6-month randomized controlled trial. *Journal of the American Medical Association, 283*(23), 3082–3088.

Goldberg, D. (2008). Towards DSM-V: The relationship between generalized anxiety disorder and major depressive episode. *Psychological Medicine, 38*(11), 1671–1675.

Goodwin, R. D., Jacobi, F., & Thefeld, W. (2003). Mental disorders and asthma in the community. *Archives of General Psychiatry, 60*(11), 1125–1130.

Grant, B. F., Goldstein, R. B., Chou, S. P., Huang, B., Stinson, F. S., Dawson, D. A., et al. (2009). Sociodemographic and psychopathologic predictors of first incidence of DSM-IV substance use, mood and anxiety disorders: Results from the Wave 2 National Epidemiologic Survey on Alcohol and Related Conditions. *Molecular Psychiatry, 14*, 1051–1066.

Grant, B. F., Hasin, D. S., Stinson, F. S., Dawson, D. A., Chou, S. P., June Ruan, W., et al. (2005a). Co-occurrence of 12-month mood and anxiety disorders and personality disorders in the US: Results from the National Epidemiologic Survey on Alcohol and Related Conditions. *Journal of Psychiatric Research, 39*(1), 1–9.

Grant, B. F., Hasin, D. S., Stinson, F. S., Dawson, D. A., June Ruan, W., Goldstein, R. B., et al. (2005b). Prevalence, correlates, co-morbidity, and comparative disability of DSM-IV generalized anxiety disorder in the USA: Results from the National Epidemiologic Survey on Alcohol and Related Conditions. *Psychological Medicine, 35*(12), 1747–1759.

Gros, D. F., Antony, M. M., McCabe, R. E., & Swinson, R. P. (2009). Frequency and severity of the symptoms of irritable bowel syndrome across the anxiety disorders and depression. *Journal of Anxiety Disorders, 23*(2), 290–296.

Harter, M. C., Conway, K. P., & Merikangas, K. R. (2003). Associations between anxiety disorders and physical illness. *European Archives of Psychiatry and Clinical Neuroscience, 253*(6), 313–320.

Hazen, R. A., Vasey, M. W., & Schmidt, N. B. (2009). Attentional retraining: A randomized clinical trial for pathological worry. *Journal of Psychiatric Research, 43*(6), 627–633.

Hoehn-Saric, R., Hazlett, R. L., & McLeod, D. R. (1993). Generalized anxiety disorder with early and late onset of anxiety symptoms. *Comprehensive Psychiatry, 34*(5), 291–298.

Holmes, M., & Newman, M. G. (2006). Generalized anxiety disorder. In F. Andrasik (Ed.), *Comprehensive handbook of personality and psychopathology: Vol. 2. Adult psychopathology* (pp. 101–120). New York: Wiley.

Hunt, C., Issakidis, C., & Andrews, G. (2002). DSM-IV generalized anxiety disorder in the Australian National Survey of Mental Health and Well-Being. *Psychological Medicine, 32*(4), 649–659.

Jones, G. N., Ames, S. C., Jeffries, S. K., Scarinci, I. C., & Brantley, P. J. (2001). Utilization of medical services and quality of life among low income patients with generalized anxiety disorder attending primary care clinics. *International Journal of Psychiatry in Medicine, 31*(2), 183–198.

Judd, L. L., Kessler, R. C., Paulus, M. P., Zeller, P. V., Wittchen, H. U., & Kunovac, J. L. (1998). Comorbidity as a fundamental feature of generalized anxiety disorders: Results from the National Comorbidity Study (NCS). *Acta Psychiatrica Scandanavica, 98*(Suppl. 393), 6–11.

Kahn, R. J., McNair, D. M., Lipman, R. S., Covi, L., Rickels, K., Downing, R., et al. (1986). Imipramine and chlordiazepoxide in depressive and anxiety disorders: II. Efficacy in anxious outpatients. *Archives of General Psychiatry, 43*(1), 79–85.

Kelsey, J. E. (2000). Efficacy, safety, and tolerability of venlafaxine XR in generalized anxiety disorder. *Depression and Anxiety, 12*(Suppl. 1), 81–84.

Kendler, K. S. (1996). Major depression and generalised anxiety disorder same genes, (partly) different environments—Revisited. *British Journal of Psychiatry, 168*(Suppl. 30), 68–75.

Kendler, K. S., Gardner, C. O., Gatz, M., & Pedersen, N. L. (2007). The sources of co-morbidity between major depression and generalized anxiety disorder in a Swedish national twin sample. *Psychological Medicine, 37*(3), 453–462.

Kendler, K. S., Neale, M. C., Kessler, R. C., Heath, A. C., & Eaves, L. J. (1992). Generalized anxiety disorder in women: A population-based twin study. *Archives of General Psychiatry, 49*(4), 267–272.

Kendler, K. S., Walters, E. E., Neale, M. C., Kessler, R. C., Heath, A. C., & Eaves, L. J. (1995). The structure of the genetic and environmental risk factors for six major psychiatric disorders in women: Phobia, generalized anxiety disorder, panic disorder, bulimia, major depression, and alcoholism. *Archives of General Psychiatry, 52*(5), 374–383.

Kessler, R. C. (2000). The epidemiology of pure and comorbid generalized anxiety disorder: A review and evaluation of recent research. *Acta Psychiatrica Scandinavica, 102*(Suppl. 406), 7–13.

Kessler, R. C., Andrade, L. H., Bijl, R. V., Offord, D. R., Demler, O. V., & Stein, D. J. (2002). The effects of co-morbidity on the onset and persistence of generalized anxiety disorder in the ICPE surveys. *Psychological Medicine, 32*(7), 1213–1225.

Kessler, R. C., Berglund, P., Demler, O., Jin, R., Merikangas, K. R., & Walters, E. E. (2005). Lifetime prevalence and age-of-onset distributions of DSM-IV disorders in the National Comorbidity Survey Replication. *Archives of General Psychiatry, 62*(6), 593–602.

Kessler, R. C., Berglund, P. A., Dewit, D. J., Ustun, T. B., Wang, P. S., & Wittchen, H. U. (2002). Distinguishing generalized anxiety disorder from major depression: Prevalence and impairment from current pure and comorbid disorders in the US and Ontario. *International Journal of Methods in Psychiatric Research, 11*(3), 99–111.

Kessler, R. C., Chiu, W. T., Demler, O., Merikangas, K. R., & Walters, E. E. (2005). Prevalence, severity, and comorbidity of 12–month DSM-IV disorders in the National Comorbidity Survey Replication. *Archives of General Psychiatry, 62*(6), 617–627.

Kessler, R. C., Gruber, M., Hettema, J. M., Hwang, I., Sampson, N., & Yonkers, K. A. (2008). Comorbid major depression and generalized anxiety disorders in the National Comorbidity Survey follow-up. *Psychological Medicine, 38*(3), 365–374.

Kessler, R. C., Nelson, C. B., McGonagle, K. A., Liu, J., Swartz, M., & Blazer, D. G. (1996). Comorbidity of DSM-III-R major depressive disorder in the general population: Results from the US National Comorbidity Survey. *British Journal of Psychiatry, 168*(Suppl. 30), 17–30.

Kessler, R. C., Stang, P., Wittchen, H. U., Stein, M., & Walters, E. E. (1999). Lifetime comorbidities between social phobia and mood disorders in the US National Comorbidity Survey. *Psychological Medicine, 29*(3), 555–567.

Kessler, R. C., Stang, P. E., Wittchen, H. U., Ustun, T. B., Roy-Burne, P. P., & Walters, E. E. (1998). Lifetime panic–depression comorbidity in the National Comorbidity Survey. *Archives of General Psychiatry, 55*(9), 801–808.

Lader, M. H., & Bond, A. J. (1998). Interaction of pharmacological and psychological treatments of anxiety. *British Journal of Psychiatry, 173*(Suppl. 34), 42–48.

Llera, S. J., & Newman, M. G. (2010). Effects of worry on physiological and subjective reactivity to emotional stimuli in generalized anxiety disorder and nonanxious control participants. *Emotion, 10*(5), 640–650.

Lyonfields, J. D., Borkovec, T. D., & Thayer, J. F. (1995). Vagal tone in generalized anxiety disorder and the effects of aversive imagery and worrisome thinking. *Behavior Therapy, 26*(3), 457–466.

Martin, E. I., Nemeroff, C. B., & Regier, D. A. (2010). The biology of generalized anxiety disorder and major depressive disorder: Commonalities and distinguishing features.. In D. Goldberg, K. S. Kendler, P. Sirovatka, & D. A. Regier (Eds.), *Diagnostic issues in depression and generalized anxiety disorder: Refining the research agenda for DSM-V* (pp. 45–70). Arlington, VA: American Psychiatric Association.

Massion, A. O., Dyck, I. R., Shea, M. T., Phillips, K. A., Warshaw, M. G., & Keller, M. B. (2002). Personality disorders and time to remission in generalized anxiety disorder, social phobia, and panic disorder. *Archives of General Psychiatry, 59*(5), 434–440.

Massion, A. O., Warshaw, M. G., & Keller, M. B. (1993). Quality of life and psychiatric morbidity in panic disorder and generalized anxiety disorder. *American Journal of Psychiatry, 150*(4), 600–607.

Mathews, A., & MacLeod, C. (1985). Selective processing of threat cues in anxiety states. *Behaviour Research and Therapy, 23*(5), 563–569.

Mathews, A., & MacLeod, C. (1994). Cognitive approaches to emotion and emotional disorders. *Annual Review of Psychology, 45*, 25–50.

Mavissakalian, M. R., Hamann, M. S., Abou Haidar, S., & de Groot, C. M. (1993). DSM-III personality disorders in generalized anxiety, panic/agoraphobia, and obsessive–compulsive disorders. *Comprehensive Psychiatry, 34*(4), 243–248.

McCafferty, J. P., Bellew, K., Zanelli, R., Iyengar, M., & Hewett, K. (2000). Paroxetine is effective in the treatment of generalized anxiety disorder: Results from a randomized placebo-controlled flexible dose study. *European Neuropsychopharmacology, 10*(Suppl. 3), 347–348.

Moffitt, T. E., Harrington, H., Caspi, A., Kim-Cohen, J., Goldberg, D., Gregory, A. M., et al. (2007). Depression and generalized anxiety disorder: Cumulative and sequential comorbidity in a birth cohort followed prospectivity to age 32 years. *Archives of General Psychiatry, 64*(6), 651–660.

Mogg, K., Mathews, A., & Eysenck, M. (1992). Attentional bias to threat in clinical anxiety states. *Cognition and Emotion, 6*(2), 149–159.

Mowrer, O. H. (1939). A stimulus–response analysis of anxiety and its role as a reinforcing agent. *Psychological Review, 46*(6), 553–566.

Newman, M. G., & Borkovec, T. D. (2002). Cognitive behavioral therapy for worry and generalized anxiety disorder. In G. Simos (Ed.), *Cognitive behaviour therapy: A guide for the practising clinician* (pp. 150–172). New York: Taylor & Francis.

Newman, M. G., Castonguay, L. G., Borkovec, T. D., Fisher, A. J., Boswell, J., Szkodny, L., et al. (2011). A randomized controlled trial of cognitive-behavioral therapy with integrated techniques from emotion-focused and interpersonal therapies. *Journal of Consulting and Clinical Psychology, 79*(2), 171–181.

Newman, M. G., Castonguay, L. G., Borkovec, T. D., Fisher, A. J., & Nordberg, S. S. (2008). An open trial of integrative therapy for generalized anxiety disorder [Special issue]. *Psychotherapy: Theory, Research, Practice and Training, 45*(2), 135–147.

Newman, M. G., & Erickson, T. M. (2010). Generalized anxiety disorder. In J. G. Beck (Ed.), *Interpersonal processes in the anxiety disorders: Implications for understanding psychopathology and treatment* (pp. 235–259). Washington, DC: American Psychological Association.

Newman, M. G., & Llera, S. J. (2011). A novel theory of experiential avoidance in generalized anxiety disorder: A review and synthesis of research supporting a contrast avoidance model of worry. *Clinical Psychology Review, 31*(3), 371–382.

Newman, M. G., Stiles, W. B., Janeck, A., & Woody, S. R. (2006). Integration of therapeutic factors in anxiety disorders. In L. G. Castonguay & L. E. Beutler (Eds.), *Principles of therapeutic change that work* (pp. 187–202). New York: Oxford University Press.

Noyes, R., Clarkson, C., Crowe, R. R., Yates, W. R., & McChesney, C. M. (1987). A family study of generalized anxiety disorder. *American Journal of Psychiatry, 144*(8), 1019–1024.

Noyes, R., Woodman, C., Garvey, M. J., Cook, B. L., Suelzer, M., Chancy, J., et al. (1992). Generalized anxiety disorder vs. panic disorder: Distinguishing characteristics and patterns of comorbidity. *Journal of Nervous and Mental Disease, 180,* 369–379.

Parker, G. (1981). Parental representations of patients with anxiety neurosis. *Acta Psychiatrica Scandinavica, 63*(1), 33–36.

Pollack, M. H., Zaninelli, R., Goddard, A., McCafferty, J. P., Bellew, K. M., Burnham, D. B., et al. (2001). Paroxetine in the treatment of generalized anxiety disorder: Results of a placebo-controlled, flexible-dosage trial. *Journal of Clinical Psychiatry, 62*(5), 350–357.

Przeworski, A., Newman, M. G., Pincus, A. L., Kasoff, M. B., Yamasaki, A. S., Castonguay, L. G., et al. (2011). Interpersonal pathoplasticity in individuals with generalized anxiety disorder. *Journal of Abnormal Psychology, 120*(2), 286–298.

Rickels, K., Downing, R., Schweizer, E., & Hassman, H. (1993). Antidepressants for the treatment of generalized anxiety disorder: A placebo-controlled comparison of imipramine, trazodone, and diazepam. *Archives of General Psychiatry, 50*(11), 884–895.

Rickels, K., Pollack, M. H., Sheehan, D. V., & Haskins, J. T. (2000). Efficacy of extended-release venlafaxine in nondepressed outpatients with generalized anxiety disorder. *American Journal of Psychiatry, 157*(6), 968–974.

Rickels, K., Schweizer, E., Csanalosi, I., Case, W. G., & Chung, H. (1988). Long-term treatment of anxiety and risk of withdrawal: Prospective comparison of clorazepate and buspirone. *Archives of General Psychiatry, 45*(5), 444–450.

Rickels, K., Schweizer, E., DeMartinis, N., Mandos, L., & Mercer, C. (1997). Gepirone and diazepam in generalized anxiety disorder: A placebo-controlled trial. *Journal of Clinical Psychopharmacology, 17*(4), 272–277.

Rickels, K., Weisman, K., Norstad, N., Singer, M., Stoltz, D., Brown, A., et al. (1982). Buspirone and diazepam in anxiety: A controlled study. *Journal of Clinical Psychiatry, 43*(12, Pt. 2), 81–86.

Rickels, K., Zaninelli, R., McCafferty, J., Bellew, K., Iyengar, M., & Sheehan, D. (2003). Paroxetine treatment of generalized anxiety disorder: A double-blind, placebo-controlled study. *American Journal of Psychiatry, 160*(4), 749–756.

Robins, L. N., & Regier, D. A. (1991). *Psychiatric disorders in America: The Epidemiologic Catchment Area Study.* New York: Free Press.

Rodriguez, B. F., Weisberg, R. B., Pagano, M. E., Bruce, S. E., Spencer, M. A., Culpepper, L., et al. (2006). Characteristics and predictors of full and partial recovery from generalized anxiety disorder in primary care patients. *Journal of Nervous and Mental Disease, 194*(2), 91–97.

Roemer, L., Molina, S., & Borkovec, T. D. (1997). An investigation of worry content among generally anxious individuals. *Journal of Nervous and Mental Disease, 185*(5), 314–319.

Roemer, L., Orsillo, S. M., & Barlow, D. H. (2002). Generalized anxiety disorder. In D. H. Barlow (Ed.), *Anxiety and its disorders* (2nd ed., pp. 477–515). New York: Guilford Press.

Ruscio, A. M., Chiu, W. T., Roy-Byrne, P., Stang, P. E., Stein, D. J., Wittchen, H. U., et al. (2007). Broadening the definition of generalized anxiety disorder: Effects on prevalence and associations with other disorders in the National Comorbidity Survey Replication. *Journal of Anxiety Disorders, 21*(5), 662–676.

Safran, J. D., & Segal, Z. V. (1990). *Interpersonal process in cognitive therapy.* New York: Basic Books.

Scheibe, G. (1996). Four-year follow-up in 40 out-patients with anxiety disorders buspirone versus lorazepam. *European Journal of Psychiatry, 10*(1), 25–34.

Sevincok, L., Buyukozturk, A., & Dereboy, F. (2001). Serum lipid concentrations in patients with comorbid generalized anxiety disorder and major depressive disorder. *Canadian Journal of Psychiatry, 46*(1), 68–71.

Shader, R. I., & Greenblatt, D. J. (1993). Use of benzodiazepines in anxiety disorders. *New England Journal of Medicine, 328*(19), 1398–1405.

Sheehan, D. V. (1999). Venlafaxine extended release (XR) in the treatment of generalized anxiety disorder. *Journal of Clinical Psychiatry, 60*(Suppl. 22), 23–28.

Souetre, E., Lozet, H., Cimarosti, I., Martin, P., Chignon, J. M., Ades, J., et al. (1994). Cost of anxiety disorders: Impact of comorbidity. *Journal of Psychosomatic Research, 38*(Suppl. 1), 151–160.

Strauss, C. C., Lahey, B. B., Frick, P., Frame, C. L., & Hynd, G. W. (1988). Peer social status of children with anxiety disorders. *Journal of Consulting and Clinical Psychology, 56*(1), 137–141.

Strauss, C. C., Lease, C. A., Kazdin, A. E., Dulcan, M. K., & Last, C. G. (1989). Multimethod assessment of the social competence of children with anxiety disorders. *Journal of Clinical Child Psychology, 18*(2), 184–189.

Thayer, J. F., Friedman, B. H., & Borkovec, T. D. (1996). Autonomic characteristics of generalized anxiety disorder and worry. *Biological Psychiatry, 39*(4), 255–266.

Todaro, J. F., Shen, B. J., Raffa, S. D., Tilkemeier, P. L., & Niaura, R. (2007). Prevalence of anxiety disorders in men and women with established coronary heart disease. *Journal of Cardiopulmonary Rehabilitation and Prevention, 27*(2), 86–91.

van Laar, M., Volkerts, E., & Verbaten, M. (2001). Subchronic effects of the GABA-agonist lorazepam and the 5-HT-$_{2A/2C}$ antagonist ritanserin on driving performance, slow wave sleep and daytime sleepiness in healthy volunteers. *Psychopharmacology, 154*(2), 189–197.

Volz, H. P., Möller, H. J., & Sturm, Y. (1994). Generalisierte Angsterkrankungen [Generalized anxiety disorders]. *Psychopharmakotherapie, 4*, 101–106.

Von Korff, M., Crane, P., Lane, M., Miglioretti, D. L., Simon, G., Saunders, K., et al. (2005). Chronic spinal pain and physical–mental comorbidity in the United States: Results from the National Comorbidity Survey Replication. *Pain, 113*(3), 331–339.

Wang, P. S., Bohn, R. L., Glynn, R. J., Mogun, H., & Avorn, J. (2001). Hazardous benzodiazepine regimens in the elderly: Effects of half-life, dosage, and duration on risk of hip fracture. *American Journal of Psychiatry, 158*(6), 892–898.

Warren, S. L., Huston, L., Egeland, B., & Sroufe, L. A. (1997). Child and adolescent anxiety disorders and early attachment. *Journal of the American Academy of Child and Adolescent Psychiatry, 36*(5), 637–644.

Weiller, E., Bisserbe, J. C., Maier, W., & Lecrubier, Y. (1998). Prevalence and recognition of anxiety syndromes in five European primary care settings: A report from the WHO study on

Psychological Problems in General Health Care [Special issue]. *British Journal of Psychiatry, 173*(Suppl. 34), 18–23.

Wells, A. (2005). The metacognitive model of GAD: Assessment of meta-worry and relationship with DSM-IV generalized anxiety disorder. *Cognitive Therapy and Research, 29*(1), 107–121.

Whisman, M. A. (1999). Marital dissatisfaction and psychiatric disorders: Results from the National Comorbidity Survey. *Journal of Abnormal Psychology, 108*(4), 701–706.

Wittchen, H. U., Carter, R. M., Pfister, H., Montgomery, S. A., & Kessler, R. C. (2000). Disabilities and quality of life in pure and comorbid generalized anxiety disorder and major depression in a national survey. *International Clinical Psychopharmacology, 15*(6), 319–328.

Wittchen, H. U., Kessler, R. C., Pfister, H., & Lieb, M. (2000). Why do people with anxiety disorders become depressed?: A prospective–longitudinal community study. *Acta Psychiatrica Scandinavica, 102*(Suppl. 406), 14–23.

Wittchen, H. U., Lieb, R., Pfister, H., & Schuster, P. (2000). The waxing and waning of mental disorders: Evaluating the stability of syndromes of mental disorders in the population. *Comprehensive Psychiatry, 41*(2, Suppl. 1), 122–132.

Wittchen, H. U., Zhao, S., Kessler, R. C., & Eaton, W. W. (1994). DSM-III-R generalized anxiety disorder in the National Comorbidity Survey. *Archives of General Psychiatry, 51*(5), 355–364.

Woodman, C. L., Noyes, R., Jr., Black, D. W., Schlosser, S., & Yagla, S. J. (1999). A 5-year follow-up study of generalized anxiety disorder and panic disorder. *Journal of Nervous and Mental Disease, 187*(1), 3–9.

Woody, S. R., & Ollendick, T. H. (2006). Technique factors in treating anxiety disorders. In L. G. Castonguay & L. E. Beutler (Eds.), *Principles of therapeutic change that work* (pp. 167–186). New York: Oxford University Press.

Yonkers, K. A., Bruce, S. E., Dyck, I. R., & Keller, M. B. (2003). Chronicity, relapse, and illness-course of panic disorder, social phobia, and generalized anxiety disorder: Findings in men and women from 8 years of follow-up. *Depression and Anxiety, 17*(3), 173–179.

Yonkers, K. A., Dyck, I. R., Warshaw, M., & Keller, M. B. (2000). Factors predicting the clinical course of generalised anxiety disorder. *British Journal of Psychiatry, 176*(6), 544–549.

Yonkers, K. A., Warshaw, M. G., Massion, A. O., & Keller, M. B. (1996). Phenomenology and course of generalised anxiety disorder. *British Journal of Psychiatry, 168*(3), 308–313.

CHAPTER 4

Panic Disorder and Phobias

Bethany A. Teachman
Marvin R. Goldfried
Elise M. Clerkin

Go to the heart of danger . . . for there you will find safety.
—OLD CHINESE PROVERB

Four types of anxiety disorder are discussed in this chapter: (1) panic disorder, typified by recurrent attacks that involve the rapid onset of multiple physical symptoms (e.g., shortness of breath and racing heart), as well as fear of future attacks; (2) agoraphobia, characterized by avoidance of situations where anxiety or panic symptoms might occur, especially when escape may be difficult; (3) social phobia (also termed "social anxiety disorder"), which involves intense anxiety or avoidance of interpersonal and/or performance situations fueled by fear of negative evaluation by others; and (4) specific phobias, characterized by excessive fear toward a particular object or situation (e.g., animals), certain natural environments (e.g., heights), and closed spaces.

The anxiety disorders overlap considerably with one another, both in terms of their typical symptoms and the models of etiology to explain their development. Thus, rather than review all of the data for each disorder separately, this chapter highlights those aspects of panic disorder and phobias that are shared, then considers the evidence specific to a given disorder. We outline each disorder's common symptoms and related clinical features, natural course and treatment outcome findings, epidemiological data, and the high rates of comorbidity for panic and phobic disorders. Finally, we review general and specific models of etiology, emphasizing the many shared biological and psychological vulnerability factors across the anxiety difficulties. Throughout the chapter, we raise potential clinical implications that follow from the psychopathology literature, and consider some of the many exciting challenges that arise in helping patients reduce their disabling anxiety symptoms. Note, much of the research cited in this chapter followed diagnostic criteria as defined in the fourth edition (or its text revision) of the *Diagnostic and Statistical Manual of Mental Disorders* (DSM-IV; American Psychiatric Association, 1994, 2000), but we also note where diagnostic criteria have changed in the recently released fifth edition of the manual (DSM-5; American Psychiatric Association, 2013).

TYPICAL SYMPTOMS AND ASSOCIATED CLINICAL FEATURES

The anxiety disorders, including panic disorder and the various phobias, share a number of features, such as avoidance behaviors and excessive fear relative to what others would experience in a given situation. These common features (as we discuss below) have led many researchers to suggest that a dimensional perspective may more appropriately characterize the range of anxiety problems, rather than the current classification system that emphasizes specific categories. Thus, we consider symptom dimensions that are common across panic and phobias, as well as the unique ways these difficulties play out across specific disorders. This focus on both common and disorder-specific features is important from a treatment perspective, because seeing patients with multiple rather than isolated anxiety difficulties is the norm (see Brown, Campbell, Lehman, Grisham, & Mancill, 2001).

Subjective distress that is excessive given the objective danger in the environment is present across anxiety difficulties, on a continuum from diffuse worry and future-oriented anxious apprehension (often present in agoraphobia), to more specific targeted fears (seen in specific and social phobias), to imminent threat and panic (characteristic of panic disorder). Along with the subjective sense of fear, anxious individuals typically strive to make their world feel "safe." These maladaptive strategies to reduce the sense of danger and vulnerability often result in extensive efforts to avoid or escape from the feared situations or feelings, which adds considerably to the impairment in occupational, academic, and social functioning typical of panic and phobias. Similarly, anxious individuals often overrely on cues or signals in their environment that help to reduce their distress at entering feared situations (see Rachman, 1994). For instance, a person with agoraphobia may only go out to the mall if his spouse accompanies him; a person with panic disorder may insist upon always carrying her anxiolytic (anxiety-reducing) medication or water bottle whenever she leaves the house; a person with social phobia may only attend a party after he has consumed three beers.

Along with subjective distress and maladaptive behavior patterns, anxious individuals tend to process information in distorted ways that are thought to increase their beliefs about the world being a dangerous, uncontrollable place and the individual being vulnerable to threat (see Williams, Watts, MacLeod, & Mathews, 1997). In particular, it is common to see cognitive processing biases characterized by preferential processing of cues tied to threat or danger (see review by Mathews & MacLeod, 2005). Examples include people with spider phobias paying selective attention to words or pictures related to spiders (e.g., Watts, McKenna, Sharrock, & Trezise, 1986); individuals who are afraid of dogs being more likely to use ferocity features in classifying dogs than nonphobic individuals (Landau, 1980); people with panic disorder misinterpreting benign changes in bodily sensations as catastrophic signs of illness (e.g., interpreting a slightly racing heart as indicative of an impending heart attack; see Clark, 1986); men who are anxious in situations involving heterosexual interactions being more likely than nonanxious men to classify interactions with women as involving evaluation (Goldfried, Padawer, & Robins, 1984); or people with social phobias judging that they have failed terribly at a social performance (e.g., giving a speech) even though outside observers do not rate the performance nearly as harshly (e.g., Stopa & Clark, 1993).

Just as thinking patterns often become highly geared toward managing perceived threats when individuals become anxious, so too can physiological responding. There is considerable variability in the physiological changes that occur across the anxiety disorders, but some degree of the "fight-or-flight" reaction (initially described by Cannon, 1929) is common to both panic and phobic reactions. The fight-or-flight system involves dramatic surges of autonomic arousal that motivate the individual either to escape or avoid a situation or defend oneself. A freezing response may also occur for some individuals. During the heightened activation of the sympathetic branch of the autonomic nervous system, a series of physical reactions that occur very rapidly help to prepare the body for action. These include increased heart rate, rapid breathing, inhibition of digestive processes, constriction of blood vessels in some parts of the body with dilation of blood vessels for muscles, pupil dilation, endorphin release, and acceleration of reflexes (see Gray & McNaughton, 1996). This response prompts the individual for immediate action and is adaptive when a real danger exists in the environment, but it essentially (mal) functions as a false alarm when no objective danger exists, as occurs in panic and phobias (see Barlow, 2002).

Thus, across a variety of emotional response systems (e.g., subjective distress, behavior, physiology, cognitive processing; see Lang, 1985), we see common signs and consequences of anxious arousal associated with both panic disorder and phobias, pointing to their shared phenomenological presentation. These common features (combined with frequent difficulties in determining the clinical threshold for a given disorder, as well as the high level of comorbidity across them) have led to many questions about the adequacy of a categorical classification system for these disorders (see review in Barlow, 2002, Chapter 9). Simply put, questions have arisen as to whether the current system effectively "carves nature at its joints." However, the heuristic value of categories (e.g., for communication about diagnoses) and advantages conferred by the specificity of categorical criteria for research and clinical decision making make it unlikely that the categories will be fully abandoned any time soon (see Brown & Barlow, 2009).

Taking into consideration the overlap across anxiety disorders also recognizes that the typical symptoms unique to each disorder represent important variation in the ways anxiety pathology manifests across individuals (depending on their particular vulnerability factors and learning experiences). We turn to these specific symptoms next.

Panic Disorder and Agoraphobia

Panic disorder is defined by recurrent and unexpected panic attacks, which are followed by at least 1 month of fear about future panic attacks, concern about the consequences of the attacks (e.g., worries about "going crazy"), or changes in behavior related to the attacks (e.g., avoidance or introduction of extensive safety cues). The term "panic attack" is used frequently by the general public, but it has a specific set of criteria in the context of anxiety pathology: The attack must involve a distinct period of intense discomfort and/or fear that rises to a peak within minutes. It must involve at least four of the following symptoms: "palpitations, pounding heart, or accelerated heart rate; sweating; trembling or shaking; sensations of shortness of breath or smothering; feeling of choking; chest pain or discomfort; nausea or abdominal distress; feeling dizzy, unsteady, light-headed, or faint; chills or heat sensations; paresthesias (numbness or tingling sensations); derealization (feelings of unreality) or depersonalization (being detached from oneself); fear of losing control or going crazy; fear of dying" (list from American Psychiatric Association, 2013, p. 208). Attacks that involve fewer than four symptoms are termed "limited symptom" attacks.

Importantly, panic attacks can occur within the context of many anxiety problems (e.g., a person with social phobia may experience a panic attack before having to give a speech), but in these cases the fear focuses on the negative evaluation by others and expected social embarrassment. In panic disorder, the attacks themselves become a problem, as indicated by the fear of future attacks and altered behavior in response to the attacks. For this reason, panic disorder is often described as a "fear of fear" (Goldstein & Chambless, 1978). It is notable that frequent panic attacks are not actually required for the diagnosis, provided that impairment or fear of future attacks is evident. Furthermore, the occurrence of panic attacks alone is not sufficient to warrant a diagnosis of panic disorder. In fact, the lifetime prevalence of nonclinical panic attacks is ~10–15% in the general population, clearly much higher than the prevalence rate of actual panic disorder (e.g., Wittchen & Essau, 1991). Thus, tracking and reducing how often panic attacks occur are useful in treatment but not the sole goal of treatment; rather, helping people reduce their fear of future attacks and diminish associated avoidance is paramount. Along these lines, simply asking patients to monitor the percentage of time they are worried about becoming anxious can provide the therapist—and the patient—with a useful index of change. This marker is meaningful because, at the outset of treatment, the lives of these patients are often very much about their anxiety; indeed, in most of their waking hours they are preoccupied with concern about becoming anxious.

Panic attacks may be entirely unexpected, in that they seem to come on "out of the blue" (when a person cannot identify a trigger), especially during early stages of the disorder. It has been our clinical experience that more often than not, such uncued attacks occur in situations where the person is unaware of the precipitating factors (e.g., a fleeting thought and emotion). Alternatively, they may be expected, in that an attack is more likely to occur following certain triggers (e.g., when in a crowded place), or when the attack regularly occurs after exposure to a particular situation. Situational events may involve a place, such as a restaurant, but they can also be a physical state or symptom (e.g., when experiencing arousal following caffeine intake), or an emotional circumstance (e.g., during conflict with significant others). Not surprisingly, people often start to avoid situations or feelings that tend to trigger their panic attacks. When this becomes extreme and impairing in its own right, the person may qualify for diagnoses of both "panic disorder" and "agoraphobia." (Note that while DSM-IV combined these diagnostic categories into "panic disorder with agoraphobia," DSM-5 treats them as two separate diagnoses. We discuss them together here because the disorders often co-occur, and because the available empirical evidence derives primarily from researchers following the DSM-IV.)

Agoraphobia involves intense anxiety about at least two situations or places in which escape might be difficult or help unavailable should a panic attack or symptoms occur. The excessive anxiety typically lasts for at least 6 months to qualify for a diagnosis, and the feared situations are then avoided (or endured with extreme distress, or only endured in the presence of a companion). Common situations that trigger agoraphobic avoidance include various modes of transportation (e.g., car, bus), going outside of the home alone, or standing in crowds or lines. Avoidance of internal sensations (known as "interoceptive cues") that make a person fearful is also common. These include sensations associated with caffeine, alcohol, or illegal drugs (e.g., Moran, 1986), as well as sensations associated with normal arousal in response to exercise, sex, eating heavy meals, or strong emotional reactions. Also, while it is possible that the anxiety and avoidance can occur without the individual also having had panic disorder, this is relatively rare in clinical settings (Barlow, 1988).

Given the considerable avoidance behaviors and fear of bringing on panic symptoms that characterize panic disorder and/or agoraphobia, it is not surprising that significant impairment is associated with these disorders. The morbidity associated with panic disorder and agoraphobia cuts across almost all domains of biopsychosocial functioning. The disorders can lead to marked constraining of social activities and related problems in marital functioning (Markowitz, Weissman, Ouellette, Lish, & Klerman, 1989). For instance, couples may have stopped having sexual intercourse because of the patient's fears about experiencing intense physical sensations. In addition, difficulties with driving and related travel fears often lead to considerable dependence on loved ones. Work impairment is also common (Alonso et al., 2004) as the triggers associated with panic become more ubiquitous. In severe cases of agoraphobia, the person may literally be homebound, which clearly limits work opportunities. Substance abuse is also more common among persons with panic disorder and agoraphobia than among those in the general population (Markowitz et al., 1989). Sleep dysregulation is also common and may be tied in part to the frequent occurrence of nocturnal panic attacks (reported by approximately 18–45% of patients with panic disorder; Craske et al., 2002). Patients who experience nocturnal panic attacks, which occur when a person wakes from sleep in a state of panic, show similar panic symptom severity and general impairment to that of panic patients who do not experience nocturnal panic. However, patients with nocturnal panic attacks tend to show lower levels of agoraphobic avoidance, possibly because they have more fearful associations with sleep than with external situational factors.

One of the most serious clinical features connected to panic disorder is the increased risk for suicide attempts (e.g., Weissman, Klerman, Markowitz, & Ouellette, 1989). Although there is some controversy about whether heightened risk for suicidal ideation or attempts is uniquely associated with panic disorder, or just indirectly linked through the high rate of co-occurring disorders (e.g., depression, borderline personality and substance use disorders; see American Psychiatric Association, 2009), there is little doubt that clinicians need to be alert to the increased risk in this population, especially given that comorbidity is the norm rather than the exception. In an early meta-analysis (Harris & Barraclough, 1997), panic disorder was associated with a 10-fold increase in suicide risk, relative to expected rates in the population.

Social Phobia/Social Anxiety Disorder

Social phobia is referred to as "social anxiety disorder" in DSM-5. It is characterized by marked and persistent fears of social interactions or performance situations in which scrutiny by others is possible (American Psychiatric Association, 2013). Individuals with social phobia consistently experience anxiety when confronted with social and/or performance situations, and this disproportionate anxiety typically lasts for at least 6 months to qualify for a diagnosis. While DSM-IV required that adults recognize that their fears are unreasonable or excessive, this criterion is no longer required in DSM-5, given the common tendency by socially phobic individuals to overestimate threat in phobic situations. Typically, individuals with social phobia avoid feared social or performance situations. Less frequently, social situations are not avoided but are endured with considerable dread. Significant anticipatory anxiety is also common.

While early theorists believed that social anxiety was caused by deficits in social skills (see Trower, Bryant, & Argyle, 1978), more recent empirical findings are inconsistent regarding the extent to which individuals with social phobia actually have social skills deficits, particularly among adults (e.g., Stopa & Clark, 1993). What is clear is that compared with healthy control participants, people with social phobia are typically more critical of their social performances, even after accounting for actual differences in social abilities (e.g., Rapee & Lim, 1992). Furthermore, research from Wallace and Alden (1997) indicates that individuals with social phobia often believe that they will be unable to make desired impressions upon others, or that they will fail to live up to others' expectations. This fear is tied to one of the defining symptoms of social phobia—extreme fears of negative evaluation, which is at the heart of cognitive models of social anxiety (e.g., Clark & Wells, 1995).

To date, many theorists contend that the distinction between social phobia and the more commonly experienced forms of shyness is a matter of degree rather than kind, with symptoms of social anxiety ranging along a continuum from mild and transient social unease to shyness to social phobia (see Heimberg & Becker, 2002). Thus, while social phobia and shyness have many similarities, symptoms of social phobia are more extreme across a variety of domains, including avoidance behaviors, chronicity, and extent of impairment (Turner, Beidel, & Townsley, 1990).

The issue of diagnosis becomes further complicated when one considers the relationship between social phobia and avoidant personality disorder. Given the striking similarities and high rates of comorbidity between these two disorders (as they were defined in DSM-IV, which mainly guided this research), some theorists believe that there is not a "distinct symptomatic delineation" between them (see Reich, 2001, p. 157). Furthermore, unlike persons with "generalized" social phobia (as defined in DSM-IV), individuals with more circumscribed social fears (e.g., public speaking, writing in front of other people) comprise a heterogeneous group defined as having "discrete," "limited," "nongeneralized," or "specific" forms of social phobia, depending on the researcher or clinician (Heimberg & Becker, 2002). Note, however, that there does not appear to be strong evidence for the notion that there are meaningful subtypes of social phobia with distinct symptom profiles (for reviews, see Heimberg, Holt, Schneier, Spitzer, & Liebowitz, 1993; Rapee, 1995), and DSM-5 now specifies if the social fear is restricted to performing or speaking in public, but no longer emphasizes other subgroups and has deleted the "generalized" specifier.

The subjective anxiety experienced by individuals with social phobia is often extremely impairing and distressing, as are the physical sensations typically tied to social anxiety (e.g., "palpitations, tremors, sweating, gastrointestinal discomfort, diarrhea, muscle tension, blushing"; American Psychiatric Association, 2000, p. 451). Avoidance is also particularly problematic. For instance, a student who fears appearing inarticulate or stupid may avoid raising a question during class; a teenager who fears being rejected may never risk asking someone on a date; a middle-aged man who fears that others will notice his hands shaking or voice trembling may avoid giving presentations at work. In some cases, this avoidance behavior can even lead to employment or financial difficulties (e.g., when individuals pass up promotions at work because the new position would involve increased social interactions).

Alcohol problems within the context of social anxiety are also quite high, because many individuals with social phobia report that they drink to help them minimize anxiety when interacting socially (e.g., Holle, Heimberg, Sweet, & Holt, 1995). While estimates regarding the link between social phobia and alcohol abuse and/or dependence vary considerably, Amies, Gelder, and Shaw (1983) found that alcohol was "taken in excess" by approximately 20% of patients with social phobia in their sample (see also the section on comorbidity below). The presence of social phobia may also increase the probability of suicide attempts among individuals who suffer from other psychiatric disorders (Weissman et al., 1996), and individuals with social phobia have lower quality-of-life ratings compared to individuals without a mental illness (Safren, Heimberg, Brown, & Holle, 1997) .

Specific Phobia

"Specific phobias" are defined by disproportionate and persistent fear toward a particular object or situation that typically lasts at least 6 months to qualify for a diagnosis (see American Psychiatric Association, 2013). Unlike less intense, subclinical fears, a specific phobia must almost always evoke an extreme and immediate fear reaction. Furthermore, the phobic target must be avoided or endured with severe distress, and result in some impairment in functioning. Interestingly, while DSM-IV required adults to recognize their fear was unreasonable or excessive, this requirement was deleted in DSM-5 because of the tendency by many phobic individuals to have exaggerated perceptions of the danger in phobic situations. Note that we focus in this chapter on panic and phobias among adults, but given the relatively high prevalence of phobias in children, the interested reader is encouraged to see excellent summaries of fear and phobias in children and adolescents (e.g., Ollendick, King, & Muris, 2002).

The overlap in criteria and feared situations for panic disorder, agoraphobia, social phobia, and specific phobias can make their differential diagnosis a challenge. More generally, determining whether a fear target constitutes a specific phobia or another anxiety problem is sometimes difficult. For example, a fear of dirt can reflect either obsessive–compulsive disorder for a person with contamination obsessions or be part of a specific phobia. Similarly, fear of a particular situation may be tied to a traumatic event in the context of posttraumatic stress disorder or reflect a more circumscribed specific phobia. Distinguishing among these possibilities involves a functional analysis that includes a careful assessment of the triggers and feared consequences associated with encountering the feared object or situation.

In theory, a phobia can be directed toward almost any target, and identifying some of the more esoteric phobias, often by their Greek or Latin names, can be an entertaining party game (e.g., "apeirophobia," a fear of infinity). Notwithstanding, in clinical practice a smaller set of phobias tend to be represented, and these have been organized into subtypes in recent DSM versions. The subtype delineations were based in part on differences across the phobias in typical ages of onset, comorbidity patterns, physiological responses, and gender prevalence (e.g., Craske & Sipsas, 1992). For instance, the "animal" (e.g., snakes, spiders) and "natural environment" (e.g., water, heights, storms) types were so grouped because phobias within each type tend to co-occur. The "blood–injection–injury" fears were made a subtype in part because they have a unique physiological profile that includes a tendency to faint. The "situational" (e.g., enclosed places, airplanes, elevators) type was separated in part due to the need to clarify the boundary between these specific fears and agoraphobia, given some similarities in their presentation and feared settings (see Horwath, Lish, Johnson, Hornig, & Weissman, 1993). Finally, an "other" type is listed in the DSM to reflect those fears not subsumed within one of the previously mentioned subtypes. While these types have some heuristic value for research and communication purposes, the utility of using subtype specifiers as part of the diagnostic label has been questioned (see Antony & Barlow, 2002). Indeed, factor analyses have not consistently supported the groupings (e.g., Landy & Gaupp, 1971), and it can be difficult to classify some fears because of potential overlap across subtypes.

As with panic disorder and the other phobias reviewed in this chapter, specific phobias are associated with a strong physiological response, characterized by increased heart rate and skin conductance. In fact, a panic attack is a common reaction for persons with specific phobias upon encountering their feared object/situation (Antony, 1994). While increased arousal is common across various types of specific phobias, blood–injection–injury phobia has a unique, additional component to its physiological response. In particular, Page (1994) noted a diphasic response that initially involves the usual increase in arousal in which heart rate and blood pressure rise, but in blood–injection–injury phobia this is followed by a sudden decrease in heart rate and blood pressure. This diphasic pattern can lead to fainting, which occurs commonly in blood–injection–injury phobias but not in other phobias (e.g., 70% of those with blood phobia and 56% with injection phobia reported a history of fainting; Öst, 1992). This diphasic response has led to specialized treatment techniques to manage the potential for fainting.

Specific phobias are also characterized by a pattern of biased information processing (akin to that seen in panic disorder and the other phobias) that favors fear-relevant stimuli. Despite some inconsistent results, the general pattern of findings indicates that individuals with specific phobias selectively attend to fear-relevant information (e.g., van den Hout, Tenney, Huygens, & de Jong, 1997) and interpret ambiguous information in a threatening manner (e.g., de Jong & Muris, 2002). Support for the presence of memory biases (preferential recall or recognition of phobic material) has been far more mixed (see Coles & Heimberg, 2002), though there is considerable evidence that phobic individuals have automatic associations in memory linking their phobic target with fear at a level outside conscious control (e.g., Teachman & Woody, 2003). There is also some indication that individuals with phobic symptoms may actually see their environment as more threatening at a perceptual level, in addition to thinking it is more dangerous. For instance, Teachman, Stefanucci, Clerkin, Cody, and Proffitt (2008) found that persons with high acrophobia symptoms (height fear) had a visual perception bias in which they saw a balcony as higher than did persons with low height fear.

One of the interesting characteristics of certain specific phobias, such as spider, snake, and blood–injury–injection fears, is that patients often feel a strong disgust reaction to their feared object (see review in Cisler, Olatunji, & Lohr, 2009). It is not yet known whether disgust plays a special role in the etiology or maintenance of these specific phobias (see Woody & Teachman, 2000), or whether disgust is just an epiphenomenon of the fear response (Thorpe & Salkovskis, 1998). However, the association between disgust sensitivity and specific fears cannot be accounted for by their shared relationship with neuroticism (Mulkens, de Jong, & Merckelbach, 1996) or trait anxiety (Matchett & Davey, 1991). This suggests that disgust is not simply tied to specific phobias as a general indicator of negative affect. One theory (which requires more empirical validation), known as the "disease avoidance model," is that disgust serves an adaptive function, in that it promotes avoidance, which helps to prevent the transmission of disease (Davey, 1992). The avoidance of disgust elicitors to prevent disease may function similarly to the avoidance in panic disorder of bodily sensations to prevent physical illness; both cases involve an oversensitive "false alarm" system that exaggerates the presence of danger.

The combination of distress (be it fear and/or disgust), physiological arousal, biased information processing, and avoidance behavior likely contributes to the impairment associated with specific phobias. Avoidance appears to be especially problematic, because it can result in limited functioning in social, recreational, and work situations (see Rowa, McCabe, & Antony, 2006), and persons with blood–injection–injury fears often do not adhere to recommended medical regimens (Mollema, Snoek, Ader, Heine, & van der Ploeg, 2001). At the same time, the impairment associated with specific phobias has more often been described as moderate rather than severe (e.g., Becker et al., 2007), in part because it is often possible to avoid encountering one's feared situation/object effectively because of the circumscribed nature of the fear. For instance, organizing one's life to avoid seeing a snake is far easier than trying to avoid all social performance situations or triggers of bodily sensations (as might be desired in social anxiety or panic disorder, respectively). Thus, it is not surprising that specific phobias are often thought to be less impairing than other anxiety disorders (though this is by no means always true), and it is not unusual for people to meet all of the diagnostic criteria for a specific phobia except for the impairment in functioning requirement (e.g., Romano, Tremblay, Vitaro, Zoccolillo, & Pagani, 2001).

Clinical Implications

The typical symptoms associated with anxiety disorders can be manifested in one or more responses systems: behavioral, physiological, expressive emotion, and/or cognitive. We deal with some of the clinical implications associated with each of these domains, considering the behavioral (e.g., avoidance of therapy), physiological (e.g., difficulty tolerating physiological reactions), expressive emotion (e.g., dysregulation of multiple emotions), and cognitive (e.g., beliefs about not feeling in control, selective processing of threatening information) features of anxiety. One considerable challenge in assessing and treating anxiety difficulties is that these different response systems are often not closely aligned and may not change in tandem (see Lang, Cuthbert, & Bradley, 1998), a process termed "desynchrony" or "uncoupling." Thus, it is important to consider multiple outcome markers to determine the success of therapy, because there is no one *true* measure of fear or anxiety. Analogously, evaluating other markers of impairment in functioning, such as quality of relationships and work life, is critical.

Avoidance of Therapy Itself

Reducing the avoidance of cues associated with panic and phobic targets is typically a key focus in therapy, but avoidance symptoms also have other important treatment implications. In particular, individuals who use avoidance as a coping strategy, albeit a maladaptive one, to reduce their anxiety in the short term also may sometimes desire to avoid treatment and therapy homework, especially if exposure to fear cues is involved in therapy. This may be particularly true in a group treatment context, where it can be slightly more challenging to permit total flexibility for each individual to set the pace for his or her exposures. Thus, building a strong therapeutic alliance is essential to help patients become willing to face their fears, and enhancing motivation for treatment may be needed to reduce patients' ambivalence about making changes in their lives, or even about being in treatment (motivational interviewing approaches can be very helpful in this regard; see Miller & Rollnick, 2002). This, of course, would be in conjunction with careful monitoring of patients' avoidance, as well as successful exposure practice between sessions.

Physiological Reactions

A salient characteristic of anxiety disorders is the increased activation of the sympathetic nervous system. Thus, in addition to the subjective feeling of anxiety and the associated behavioral manifestations, there are physiological symptoms such as rapid breathing, increased heart rate, and sweating. These reactions are involuntary and contribute to the feeling of not being in control—a point we return to later. At times, patients are encouraged to tolerate these physiological sensations to learn that they are not actually dangerous, so that the sensations become less frightening; at other times, the patients may want to reduce the arousal.

As a means of helping patients reduce their physiological reaction, it can be helpful in some cases to teach them how to use relaxation as a coping skill. This can be accomplished by various methods, most of which involve learning to differentiate between feelings of tension and relaxation, and to use the tension as a signal for reducing their arousal. Using external cues to remind patients to apply the relaxation response can be helpful. Thus, anxious patients can learn to use recurrent situational cues as reminders to relax, such as putting the key in the ignition of the car or sitting down in front of one's computer. Another example is a patient who tended to have panic attacks at restaurants, and was able to use the placement of the napkin on her lap as a cue to relax. She was successful in reducing the physiological arousal that was the precursor to panic, and soon she jokingly referred to this as "the magic napkin."

Dysregulation of Multiple Emotions

In some respects, the term "anxiety disorders" is somewhat limiting. While it is certainly true that fear, panic, and anxiety are central emotional states in these disorders, they are not the only forms of affect that become dysregulated or that may require therapeutic attention. For instance, as noted earlier, patients with certain specific phobias often feel a strong disgust reaction to their feared object (see Olatunji & McKay, 2009). Yet the extent to which it is important to reduce disgust (as well as fear) in treatment remains an open empirical question. While there is some evidence that disgust related to spiders is reduced following successful exposure therapy (e.g., de Jong, Andrea, & Muris, 1997), there is also some indication that disgust may be slower than fear to decline during exposure (e.g., Olatunji, Forsyth, & Cherian, 2007).

Social phobia is often characterized by feelings of shame and embarrassment, and it is not uncommon for people with panic disorder or phobias to feel intense sadness in response to their anxiety disorder symptoms. Along these lines, it is helpful to consider possible interactions between different emotional presentations and traditional gender expectations (e.g., women expressing sadness about their inability to manage their anxiety, and men expressing anger when they feel threatened), though more research is needed to determine the empirical support for these possible gender differences in the treatment context.

Finally, in panic disorder, it is not unusual to see anger as a central aspect of the presentation (Moscovitch, McCabe, Antony, Rocca, & Swinson, 2008; though the tie between anger and depression in these cases needs to be considered). Indeed, even though the relevance of anger in panic disorder has only recently been reported in the research literature, we have found that anger—and the lack of self-assertiveness that is frequently antecedent to this—is fairly common. Notably, the early clinical literature (e.g., Chambless & Goldstein, 1982) reported this frequent presence of anger and the eventual need for assertiveness training. In the case of a panic patient with whom we were unable to simulate panic sensations during the session by means of hyperventilation, we inadvertently triggered a panic attack when he discussed his relationship with his brother—with whom he had been in conflict. After the panic symptoms had subsided, he reluctantly acknowledged that he was indeed angry at his brother. However, he was raised with a strict religious background and was told at a young age that being angry meant that "the devil was in him." Given that he was fearful of feeling or expressing anger, he was first encouraged to acknowledge that he was "frustrated" with his brother, after which he agreed that he was "upset." With further encouragement, he allowed that perhaps he was "annoyed," and finally that he was "angry." Thus, desensitization to his concerns about anger became an integral part of the treatment of his panic disorder, as did work on increasing his assertiveness toward his brother.

Not Feeling "in Control"

The belief that the world is somehow unpredictable and uncontrollable is central to many anxiety difficulties (Barlow, 2002). Furthermore, one of the clinical hallmarks of panic disorder is that the patient feels "out of control" when panic symptoms arise. In this regard, it is important to frame the therapy intervention as a means by which patients can learn to *manage* their anxiety, so that they no longer feel they are at the mercy of anxiety symptoms and do not find them as threatening. Along these lines, in treatment we aim to reduce the unhelpful belief that the patient is totally "out of control" and cannot cope when anxious (e.g., by teaching patients that control is really a continuum, despite the popular but misleading terminology of being "in" vs. "out" of control). At the same time, we normalize the experience of anxiety and seek to reduce the belief that all anxiety needs to be controlled. Using a coping skills approach to treatment, it is often helpful to tell patients that our goal is not to eliminate all anxiety symptoms, but to help them learn to manage their anxiety by becoming less frightened of anxiety symptoms and their reaction to these symptoms. By understanding that they can tolerate some anxiety and still function, patients actually tend to become less anxious and feel less need always to control their internal (e.g., anxiety symptoms) and external (e.g., rigid behavior) environments.

Selective Processing of Threatening Information

We have noted that one of the factors associated with phobias and social anxiety is selective processing of threatening information. Although we wholeheartedly endorse exposure as an invaluable method of intervention, there are times when anxiety reduction can be greatly aided by cognitive techniques as well. Certainly, cognitive restructuring (i.e., explicitly altering thoughts and beliefs that fuel anxiety) is a core intervention for many anxiety problems. What we would like to add here, however, is the possibility that a relatively simple refocus of attention and shift of disorder-relevant automatic associations or negative interpretations can also prove to be clinically valuable. A growing body of research indicates that it is possible experimentally to manipulate or "retrain" cognitive biases, including biased attention and interpretation, in order to influence subsequent anxiety symptoms (e.g., in social anxiety: Amir, Weber, Beard, Bomyea, & Taylor, 2008; see review in Hertel & Mathews, 2011).

Limitations of the DSM

It is also important for clinicians to go beyond global diagnostic categories, such as "social phobia," to assess adequately and treat patients' presenting problems. Specific, idiographic targets of intervention need to be identified (e.g., delineating public speaking concerns or dating fears is more informative than "social phobia"). Identification of symptoms alone is insufficient, however. A broad biopsychosocial evaluation is critical to learn the strengths and weaknesses, and the challenging realities within which some of our patients live.

While improvements in the DSM have clearly been made since it was first published in 1952, it continues to have its shortcomings—particularly for the practicing clinician. The changes have not only helped to bring the classification system more closely in line with the disorders' phenomenology but they also present some challenges in differential diagnosis. For instance, the fact that panic attacks can occur across multiple anxiety problems beyond panic disorder can make it difficult to differentiate whether panic attacks occur in the context of panic disorder (with or without agoraphobia), social phobia, or specific phobia. Imagine a person who regularly has panic attacks while driving; it is possible this person has panic disorder because he fears the consequences of the attack (e.g., that he might faint while driving and cause an accident). Alternatively, it is plausible that this person has a specific driving phobia and has panic attacks tied to his general fears about driving and having an accident. To distinguish among these options, it is helpful to assess whether the attacks also occur in other situations (e.g., when he is not driving), as well as the specific fear triggers and perceived consequences tied to the attacks. Thought experiments in which a patient tries to isolate a given symptom can be helpful in this regard. Consider a patient who has panic attacks when asked to speak in public, and the challenge of determining whether panic disorder and/or social phobia diagnoses are warranted. Asking the patient how extensively she would still fear public speaking if she could take a magic pill and know that she would not have a panic attack while giving a speech to her coworkers can be useful to determine whether the fears are tied to panic attacks per se, or to fears of negative evaluation. Alternatively, asking how much she would still fear public speaking if there were a risk of having a panic attack but she could take a magic pill, causing her coworkers to think she did a great job, can help to rule in or out fears about the consequences of panic. Thus, *focus* of the fear is important (fear of fainting, bodily sensations, etc., vs. fear of being ridiculed, appearing stupid, etc.). Not surprisingly, making these fine distinctions in practice can be challenging, especially given that it is quite possible for the patient in this example to have both panic disorder and social phobia.

Another clinical issue stems from the fact that the social anxiety category is quite heterogeneous, including anxiety in interpersonal interactions, anxiety in public speaking situations, fear of using public bathrooms, and anxiety experienced when signing one's name in public. Moreover, patients who are socially anxious may vary in their social skills, such that behavioral skills training may be appropriate for some but not others (see Rapee & Spence, 2004). Researchers have also found that many gay men who appear to be "socially anxious" are responding appropriately to realistic fears of rejection (Pachankis & Goldfried, 2006); hence, their anxiety may not necessarily be considered unwarranted or maladaptive.

In writing about panic and agoraphobia some years ago, Goldstein and Chambless (1978) made an important distinction that was not reflected in DSM-IV-TR. Although the symptoms of panic and agoraphobia may be the same, for some the onset may have been focal and situational (e.g., an adverse reaction to a drug), whereas for others it may be related to a more general problematic life pattern (e.g., having conflictual relationships with others). The former they labeled as being "simple" and the latter, as "complex." In the treatment of a complex panic disorder, it is not unusual to have symptom reduction followed by a clinical focus on relationships with others. In a sense, the symptoms of a complex panic disorder may be viewed as a signal that something is not working in the patient's life.

Impairment in Functioning: Love and Work

Given the disruption to relationships caused by avoidance behavior that is characteristic of panic disorder and phobias, and the consequent dependence on loved ones, it is not unusual for families to need some help renegotiating their roles when a patient starts making progress in treatment and is able to function more independently. While this is usually a very exciting step, it is not always easy for family members to change long-standing patterns of who are the "strong" or "helper" members of the household. Thus, even with significant progress in achieving anxiety symptom reduction, it is important to evaluate how these life changes influence other aspects of a person's functioning, including possible impairment in work and interpersonal relationships. Monitoring and therapeutically addressing impairment in functioning may well decrease the risk for relapse, even when treatment may have successfully addressed the anxiety symptoms associated with the panic and phobia.

We should also emphasize that family members can either assist or interfere with therapeutic progress. For example, researchers found that spousal assistance in the treatment of agoraphobia helped to facilitate the reduction of avoidance behavior (Barlow, O'Brien, & Last, 1984). Serving as a therapeutic aide, the agoraphobic's partner can encourage graduated exposure to feared situations. Sometimes, however, such "assistance" can undercut the therapist's best efforts. One of us (M. G.) worked with a woman suffering from panic and agoraphobia, whose husband not only encouraged her to cope with panic by holding her breath but also discouraged her from traveling! The best efforts of the therapist, unfortunately, were no match for this very dominating husband.

COURSE

The conclusions one draws about the typical course and outcomes for persons with panic and phobic disorders depends in large part one's focus on the statistics.

Evidence tied to the natural course of these disorders leads to a pessimistic view about their chronic nature, whereas evidence that highlights the tremendous strides in treating these disorders presents a more optimistic picture. At the same time, there is considerable variability in outcomes across disorders, even using similar treatment approaches (e.g., as described below, medication is far more helpful for panic disorder than it is for specific phobias, whereas exposure-based therapies have impressive outcomes for both specific phobias and panic disorder, with more moderate success rates for treating social phobia).

Panic Disorder and Agoraphobia

The frequency of panic attacks may wax and wane over time quite dramatically (e.g., a person may have daily attacks for a couple weeks, then far more irregularly spaced attacks over a period of months), though these fluctuations do not seem to occur randomly. The presence of life stressors appears to be a predictor of both the initial onset of panic and its intensity over time (see Craske, Miller, Rotunda, & Barlow, 1990). Interestingly, stressors that are tied to either interpersonal difficulties or physical well-being (e.g., scary experiences with drugs) are particularly potent risk factors.

Although the course of panic disorder and agoraphobia may show considerable fluctuations over time, it is difficult to escape the conclusion that the disorders are chronic and disabling. For instance, Yonkers et al. (1998) found that the remission rate for panic disorder (with or without agoraphobia) was only 39% at a 5-year follow-up evaluation. This rate was similar for men and women, though interestingly the rate of recurrence was higher for women (82%) than for men (51%). Unfortunately, even among patients who attain remission, relapse is not unusual (see Keller et al., 1994). With a naturalistic follow-up period of 4 to 6 years posttreatment, 30% of patients from a "specialized"/tertiary care setting were labeled as well (mostly asymptomatic), 40–50% were defined as improved but symptomatic, and the remaining 20–30% had stable or slightly worsened symptoms (Katschnig, Amering, Stolk, & Ballenger, 1996; Roy-Byrne & Cowley, 1995). Thus, while most people showed some improvement in this study, residual symptoms were the norm, and relapse was not unusual.

Coinciding with this somewhat discouraging data are the impressive data on treatment outcome, particularly for cognitive-behavioral therapy (CBT) and pharmacotherapy. For instance, a meta-analysis for treatment outcomes for panic disorder (with or without agoraphobia) found that CBTs produced the highest mean effect sizes (ES = 0.68), relative to pharmacological treatment (ES = 0.47; Gould, Otto, & Pollack, 1995), with both treatments showing clear efficacy relative to a variety of control conditions. Note that the term "effect size" refers to the magnitude of a given finding, with higher numbers indicating a larger effect.

CBT can take many forms but typically includes a combination of psychoeducation, exposure therapy, cognitive restructuring, and relapse prevention (see the widely used manual by Barlow & Craske, 2006). Initially, patients are given psychoeducation about the nature of anxiety and panic, and the "fear of fear" cycle (the idea that reacting in catastrophic ways to benign physical sensations makes those sensations more intense and fuels panic attacks). Exposures focus on reducing avoidance behaviors to both internal and external panic cues. The exposure assignments typically involve reentering feared situations (e.g., crowds), while learning to tolerate the anxiety without trying to escape or avoid, as well as interoceptive exposure exercises, in which patients repeatedly expose themselves to their feared bodily sensations to learn that they can cope with these feelings, and that their anxiety habituates as the feared consequences do not occur. During cognitive restructuring, patients are taught to identify and challenge their maladaptive beliefs about the consequences of anxiety and their ability to tolerate bodily sensations. Also, in some panic treatment protocols, patients are taught diaphragmatic breathing and/or progressive muscle relaxation to encourage a more relaxed resting state.

The typical length of a CBT panic control treatment protocol, as used in randomized clinical trials, is 10–15 weekly sessions; however, there is evidence that positive outcomes can be achieved in much shorter time periods (e.g., six sessions: Clark et al., 1999; 2 intensive days: Evans, Holt & Oei, 1991). Efficacy has also been found for the administration of CBT by means of a palm-held computer (Newman, Kenardy, Herman, & Taylor, 1997). Both individual and group treatments have demonstrated efficacy and are reasonable choices, though outcomes may be slightly enhanced with individual therapy (see review in Craske & Barlow, 2008). Exposure-based therapy for agoraphobia also appears to work well in a group format (Lidren et al., 1994). In addition to the initial positive outcomes immediately posttreatment (e.g., 82% response rate based on the Panic Disorder Severity Scale among patents completing CBT in Shear, Houck, Greeno, & Masters, 2001), the available data suggest long-lasting benefits following CBT (e.g., based on 1-year follow-up data; see review by Furukawa, Watanabe, & Churchill, 2006), though residual symptoms are certainly not unusual. Furthermore, CBT appears to be a helpful treatment for patients who have not responded to a prior medication treatment (Otto, Pollack, Penava, & Zucker, 1999). For more information on empirically supported therapies for panic disorder, see Division 12's Website on Research-Supported Psychological Treatments (2008): *www.psychology.sunysb.edu/eklonsky-/ division12/index.html.*

There is also good evidence for the efficacy of medication to manage panic disorder (see summary of pharmacotherapy evidence and guidelines; American Psychiatric Association, 2009). Four classes of medication have demonstrated efficacy: Selective serotonin reuptake inhibitors (SSRIs), serotonin–norepinephrine reuptake inhibitors (SNRIs), tricyclic antidepressants (TCAs), and benzodiazepines. Although they are relatively comparable in their efficacy, their side effect profiles, risk of dependence, and quality of evidence bases vary considerably. Typically, SSRIs and SNRIs are recommended as a first-line medication treatment, because they do not lead to the serious cardiovascular and anticholinergic side effects linked with TCAs, or the high rate of addiction that occurs with benzodiazepines. In fact, there is considerable evidence for long-term negative outcomes with chronic use of high-potency benzodiazepines (see Otto, Pollack, & Sabatino, 1996). Thus, benzodi-azepine use may be most helpful as part of a short-term addition to one of the other antidepressants to help control symptoms while the antidepressant has a chance to take effect (Pollack et al., 2003). Even then, the challenge of tolerating the symptoms that often accompany the subsequent discontinuation of benzodiazepines needs to be weighed against the value of the rapid symptom relief they can provide. Fortunately, results for the many trials with SSRIs indicate that there are effec-tive, less addictive medication options available (e.g., Shear et al. [2001] found a 93% response rate based on the Panic Disorder Severity Scale among patents completing an imipramine trial).

More patients receive medication than CBT as a treatment for panic disorder and agoraphobia, in part because treatment is often sought in primary care set-tings (where medication is the norm), and in part because CBT is not yet offered in many health care settings despite its established efficacy (see Craske & Barlow, 2008). Any discussion of treatment outcomes for panic disorder and agoraphobia must also consider the typical short- and long-term response of patients receiving a combination of psychotherapy and pharmacotherapy, given how frequently this occurs. There are still some open questions about when outcomes may be enhanced by combining or sequencing medication and CBT. However, it is clear that combin-ing the treatments is often not necessary and can even be detrimental, despite the seemingly intuitive appeal of using two efficacious approaches. For instance, in a large, multisite clinical trial, Barlow, Gorman, Shear, and Woods (2000) found that CBT alone, medication alone, and the combination of medication and CBT were equally effective, both during and immediately after treatment for panic disorder and agoraphobia (but see de Beurs, van Balkom, Lange, Koele, & van Dyck [1995] for contradictory findings). Following medication discontinuation, however, the com-bination treatment condition had worse outcomes than the CBT-alone condition, suggesting that medication (and its subsequent withdrawal) can interfere with the application of CBT principles in the long term. The evidence does not seem to sug-gest that adding CBT to a medication treatment has the same negative impact. For example, adding even single components of CBT to the medication management offered for patients with panic disorder in a primary care setting led to improved outcomes posttreatment and 1 year later (Craske et al., 2005).

The choice to use CBT, medication, or their combination thus depends on the patient's wishes, past treatment history, and so on. However, it is important to high-light that treatment of panic disorder and agoraphobia is one of the field's success stories in terms of positive outcomes in mental health care. As described earlier, not all classes of medications are equal when long-term outcomes are taken into consideration, and caution should be used when combining treatments, as this may be unnecessary and unhelpful in the long run. At the same time, it is nice to have multiple efficacious options from which to choose when offering treatment. This is especially valuable given that not all patients respond to their first treatment trial. As noted earlier, CBT may be a useful second-line treatment for medication nonresponders (Otto et al., 1999). Similarly, for patients who do not respond to CBT, trying a subsequent medication trial (e.g., paroxetine, as used in Kampman, Keijsers, Hoogduin, & Hendriks, 2002) can be helpful, as opposed to just continuing CBT. Thus, sequencing treatments for people who do not respond to an initial CBT or medication trial may be a useful way to think about enhancing outcomes with multiple treatment modalities rather than simply combining treatments right away. The issue of using single or combined treatments is also important from a cost-cutting perspective given the tremendous financial burden posed by care for anxiety disorders (e.g., Markowitz et al., 1989). Notably, there is some indication that CBT may be more cost-effective than medication, based on total disability costs, work days missed, health care use, and so on (Heuzenroeder et al., 2004). Nonetheless, as noted earlier, because patients with panic disorder often seek out help at primary care facilities, the clinical reality is that they often come for CBT once they are already taking medication.

While CBT and medication approaches are the primary evidence-based options for treating panic disorder and agoraphobia, there is also some initial evidence that a panic-focused, psychodynamic, twice-weekly, 12-week psychotherapy may also be helpful for treating panic disorder (Milrod et al., 2007). This treatment focuses on confronting the emotional significance attached to panic symptoms, based on the idea that patients are avoidant in part because of difficulty separating from central attachment figures. Also significant is that this intervention explores the role that anger plays in panic attacks, a critical issue, as we noted earlier. It will be important to gather further evidence about the efficacy of this approach and its active components. Finally, it is notable that this therapy is still panic-focused and time-limited, and should not be confused with more general supportive psychotherapies that have not been found to be as efficacious as standard panic treatments (Shear et al., 2001).

There is thus both good and bad news when one examines the course and treatment outcomes for panic disorder and agoraphobia. Studies of the longitudinal course and relatively high relapse rates over time point to the need to develop better long-term management strategies for the disorders, while the impressive CBT and medication efficacy data suggest high treatment response rates. In reconciling these different pictures, a number of factors need to be considered. First, outcomes vary for persons with substantial comorbidity relative to those with relatively "cleaner" presentations of panic disorder. For instance, co-occurring depression is associated with a worse course of illness (e.g., Bruce et al., 2005; Tyrer, Seivewright, & Johnson, 2004), and there is mixed evidence regarding the impact of co-occurring personality disorders (Massion et al., 2002). Second, many people are simply not receiving treatment, or they are receiving substandard care, which may help explain the discrepant results for the negative, naturalistic course relative to the more positive outcomes for the CBT and medication trials. Finally, panic disorder is undertreated in both primary care (Stein et al., 2004) and mental health care settings (Bruce et al., 2003), with few people receiving CBT or evidence-based medication types and doses (see Goisman, Warshaw, & Keller, 1999). Thus, while panic disorder and ago-raphobia *can* be treated quite effectively, the field has a long way to go to make this ideal a reality.

Social Phobia

Social phobia tends to be a fairly chronic disorder with relatively low rates of recov-ery and high rates of recurrence when left untreated. Estimates for the naturalis-tic course of social phobia vary widely depending on methodological differences across studies. For instance, retrospective cross-sectional studies have found that social phobia persists anywhere between 19 and 30 years in community samples, with recovery rates ranging from 27 to 52% (e.g., see Kessler, Stein, & Berglund, 1998). In a prospective study, Bruce et al. (2005) found that individuals with social phobia had only a 37% chance of achieving recovery over the course of 12 years (defined as being virtually asymptomatic for at least 2 months). Of those patients with social phobia who did recover, there was also a 39% chance of a recurrence of social phobia. Similarly, Vriends and colleagues (2007) found that while 64% of young German women diagnosed with social phobia had *partially* recovered over a 1.5-year period, only 36% had achieved a full recovery (defined as fulfilling no DSM-IV criteria at follow-up). Taken together, research suggests that social phobia is an insidious, often unremitting disorder when untreated.

Fortunately, there are a variety of successful psychological interventions avail-able for treating social phobia, including CBT and cognitive-behavioral group ther-apy (CBGT). Research generally suggests that combining both cognitive and expo-sure techniques is recommended (Mattick, Peters, & Clarke, 1989). Indeed, while CBT and CBGT can take many forms (incorporating relaxation techniques, social skills training, etc.), treatment typically consists of both cognitive restructuring to evaluate beliefs that fuel social anxiety concerns, such as fears of negative evalua-tion, and exposure exercises to help patients learn to tolerate anxiety and feel more comfortable interacting socially. For instance, cognitive restructuring may target the belief that one will humiliate him- or herself by performing "inadequately." Meanwhile, exposures generally focus on encouraging patients gradually to confront and try to remain in socially threatening situations. This is achieved through the creation of individually tailored fear hierarchies, which begin with mildly anxiety-provoking situations and end with the situations that are most feared. When developing hierarchies, it is important to remember that avoidance associated with social phobia can take many forms, including not fully engaging with a given situation (e.g., through excessive use of alcohol), or refusing to enter a situation in the first place.

CBTs for social phobia are demonstrably effective; however, estimates vary con-siderably in terms of *how* effective. For instance, in one meta-analysis, Feske and Chambless (1995) concluded that patients showed "substantial improvement" on measures of social phobia as a result of CBT, including improvement on cognitive and mood/anxiety symptoms. However, estimates of clinically significant change or "high endstate functioning" ranged enormously from 22 to 95% (p. 714). Meanwhile, in a review of five meta-analyses evaluating CBT techniques (exposure only; cognitive restructuring only; cognitive restructuring and exposure; social skills training; applied relaxation), Rodebaugh, Holaway, and Heimberg (2004) concluded that each of the CBT interventions revealed moderate to large ES when comparing post-treatment to a wait-list control condition, as well as moderate to large within-group effects from pre- to posttreatment. For more information on empirically supported treatments for social phobia, see Division 12's website on Research-Supported Psychological Treatments (2008: *www.psychology.sunysb.edu/eklonsky-/division12/index.html*), in addition to one of the many meta-analyses (e.g., Fedoroff & Taylor, 2001).

A variety of pharmacological agents have also been used to treat social phobia. For instance, Gould, Buckminster, Pollack, Otto, and Yap (1997) conducted a meta-analysis to evaluate both CBT and pharmacological treatments for social phobia. Results indicated that the mean ES across CBT interventions (ES = 0.74) and pharmacological treatments (ES = 0.62) were significantly different from zero, although they did not differ from one another. In another meta-analysis evaluating pharmacological treatments for social phobia, Blanco et al. (2003) found that phenelzine (a monoamine oxidase inhibitor [MAOI]) led to the largest symptom improvements in social anxiety symptoms (ES = 1.02), but it did not produce significantly better outcomes than other medications included in the investigation (e.g., clonazepam, ES = 0.97; SSRIs, ES = 0.65). Given the problematic side effects tied of MAOIs (e.g., risk of hypertension) and benzodiazepines (e.g., physical dependence), medications such as the SSRIs may provide a better first-line pharmacological treatment option for social phobia (Rodebaugh et al., 2004). Indeed, the only drugs currently indicated for treating social phobia by the FDA are paroxetine and sertraline (both SSRIs), and venlafaxine (XR version only, an SNRI; Drug Reference for FDA Approved Psychiatric Drugs 2008: *www.neurotransmitter.net/drug_reference.html*).

To date, there is not a clear answer to whether pharmacological or psychotherapeutic interventions are preferable for treating social phobia. Some studies have demonstrated that pharmacotherapies may be more effective than CBT in the short-term (Fedoroff & Taylor, 2001), and that the effects of medication on social anxiety may occur more rapidly (Heimberg et al., 1998). In contrast, there is also evidence that the coping skills learned during CBT may help patients better maintain their treatment gains in the long term (Liebowitz et al., 1999). Finally, some research indicates no clear differences in the effectiveness of medication and CBT techniques (Gould et al., 1997). Thus, any treatment decisions will likely need to be made on a case-by-case basis, ideally in consultation with both a psychiatrist and a psychologist.

There are also insufficient data to determine whether combined psychological and pharmacological treatments for social phobia are more (or less) effective than either treatment in isolation (Gould et al., 1997). For example, there is some evidence that the combination of pharmacotherapy (e.g., sertraline) and exposure interventions may lead to quicker symptom change (see discussion in Blomhoff et al., 2001); however, in the long term, the effects of medication may actually interfere with the efficacy of exposures (Haug et al., 2003). On the other hand, Davidson et al. (2004) found that CBT combined with medication was not more effective at treatment termination than either treatment in isolation, but all active treatments were significantly more effective than a placebo. Some studies have even found that outcomes for combined CBT and medications did not differ in effectiveness from a placebo (Clark & Agras, 1991; Falloon, Lloyd, & Harpin, 1981). In light of the minimal and inconsistent evidence regarding the effectiveness of combined treatments, Turk, Heimberg, and Hope (2001) recommended that patients with social phobia stabilize their medication regimens prior to starting therapy and refrain from adjusting or changing their medications during treatment.

Finally, there is promising initial evidence for experimental anxiety reduction interventions designed directly to "retrain" cognitive processing biases away from threatening cues. For example, Amir and colleagues (2008) found that socially anxious participants trained to attend away from threat-relevant social information experienced decreased social anxiety as assessed by an independent rater. Similarly, Murphy, Hirsch, Mathews, Smith, and Clark (2007) demonstrated that it is possible experimentally to manipulate catastrophic misinterpretations and reduce social anxiety symptoms, even with one brief session of training.

This research is still in its preliminary stages, but these experimental interventions raise a number of intriguing theoretical and clinical implications. For instance, in line with cognitive models, this research suggests that cognitive processing biases are not only significantly correlated with symptoms of social anxiety but they may also be *causally* related. Additionally, because state anxiety is typically not directly influenced by the training procedures, these studies question the belief that it is necessary to activate subjective fear or anxiety directly in order to change elements of the fear network (see Foa & Kozak, 1986). Furthermore, these paradigms challenge the notion that verbal mediation is essential in order to influence cognition and behavior (see Beck & Clark, 1997).

Specific Phobia

Data speaking to the naturalistic course of specific phobias are relatively sparse, but the general impression is that the disorder in adults tends to be quite stable and enduring without treatment (Becker et al., 2007), although there is variability across phobia subtypes (Depla, ten Have, van Balkom, & de Graaf, 2008). Children with specific phobias, on the other hand, often grow out of their fears (see Starcevic, 2005). For instance, Agras, Chapin, and Oliveau (1972) found that the vast majority of patients under age 20 with specific phobias reported improvement in their fear at a 5-year follow-up assessment. In contrast, fewer than half of adult patients reported improvement.

The picture is quite different when one examines treatment outcome. While individuals with specific phobias rarely present for treatment (Antony, 2000), the success rate for exposure-based treatments is very high (e.g., a recent meta-analysis indicated that the average person receiving treatment was better off than approximately 85% of nontreated persons; Wolitzky-Taylor, Horowitz, Powers, & Telch, 2008). As previously discussed, one reason for this discrepancy between rates of treatment seeking and treatment outcome may be that treatment seems less critical given the relative ease with which many patients can avoid their feared stimuli (see Antony & Barlow, 2002).

It is unfortunate that more people do not seek treatment given that improvement can occur rapidly. In fact, there is evidence that a single session of exposure therapy is effective to treat spider phobia (e.g., Öst, Ferebee, & Furmark, 1997). For specific phobias in general, multi-session (vs. single-session) treatments tend to achieve slightly more favorable results (see Wolitzky-Taylor et al., 2008), but even the multisession treatments are often brief (e.g., three to eight sessions). Furthermore, the gains made in treatment tend to be maintained for at least 1 year, though more studies with longer follow-up periods are necessary (Choy, Fyer, & Lipsitz, 2007).

"Exposure therapies" refer to a class of behavioral approaches that are all based on exposing phobic persons to the stimuli that frighten them. The goal is to provide usually avoidant persons an opportunity to learn that they can tolerate the fear, which will come down on its own without avoiding or escaping it, and that feared outcomes (e.g., that a snake will lunge, lightning will strike, the person will lose all control) often do not come true or are not as awful as imagined. The choice of situations to encounter usually follows an individually tailored fear hierarchy that starts with situations that are mildly anxiety-provoking and builds up to extremely feared situations (though in "flooding" therapy, exposure starts with a very anxiety-provoking stimulus).

Numerous variants of exposure therapy have also been examined, and while many have been found to work effectively, research suggests more favorable outcomes for *in vivo* exposure (which involves actually confronting the feared stimuli) than for other approaches (e.g., systematic desensitization, in which fear-evoking images and thoughts or actual phobic stimuli are paired with relaxation or another response that is incompatible with fear; Choy et al., 2007). Actual contact with feared stimuli also seems to outperform other modes of exposure, such as imaginal or virtual reality exposure (which uses an immersive computer program to generate a phobic situation, e.g., a plane experiencing turbulence). Interestingly, this difference is evident at posttreatment, but *in vivo* exposure's advantage disappears at follow-up, seemingly because those receiving the less direct exposure therapies continue to improve after treatment ends (Wolitzky-Taylor et al., 2008). Another interesting (and effective) variant on standard exposure therapy involves adding applied muscle tension to *in vivo* exposure for the treatment of blood–injection–injury phobia (e.g., Öst, Fellenius, & Sterner, 1991). By adding exercises to manipulate muscle tension, patients are able to address the decreases in blood pressure that can lead to fainting with this phobia. Currently, there is some debate about whether the effectiveness of exposure therapies varies substantially across phobia subtypes (e.g., a qualitative review [Choy et al., 2007] reached different conclusions than a meta-analysis [Wolitzky-Taylor et al., 2008]).

A significant challenge with exposure therapies, especially *in vivo* exposure, concerns fairly high dropout rates and discomfort with the treatment because of the fear associated with trying exposures (Choy et al., 2007). Thus, other treatment options have also been examined, though far less extensively than exposure therapies, and there are some open questions about whether benefits from these non-exposure treatments reflect nonspecific treatment effects (due to attention, general support, etc.; see Wolitzky-Taylor et al., 2008). Notwithstanding, cognitive therapies, presented either alone or as an augmentation to exposure therapies, have received some support, though there is considerable heterogeneity in findings across studies and phobias types (Wolitzky-Taylor et al., 2008). Choy et al. (2007) interpret the available data to suggest cognitive therapy may be especially helpful for the treatment of claustrophobia (e.g., Öst, Alm, Brandberg, & Breitholtz, 2001); however, reasons for the discrepant findings across phobia subtypes are unclear.

A controversial therapy approach, eye movement desensitization and reprocessing (EMDR) therapy, adds movements (that typically involve shifting the eyes back and forth in line with the therapist's fingers) to an exposure-based therapy. EMDR appears to perform less well than traditional exposure therapies when large group designs are used (e.g., Muris, Merckelbach, Holdrinet, & Sijsenaar, 1998), and there is debate about whether adding eye movements to the treatment is essentially just an elaboration of imaginal exposure (see Lohr, Tolin, & Lilienfeld, 1998). Thus, this treatment is not currently recommended as a first-line therapeutic approach for specific phobias (see the American Psychological Association's Division 12 website on Research-Supported Psychological Treatments: *www.psychology.sunysb.edu/eklonsky-/division12/index.html*).

Finally, the evidence for medication treatment of specific phobias (e.g., use of benzodiazepines or beta-blockers, used either alone or in combination with exposure interventions) has not suggested that anti-anxiety medications consistently add much to treatment outcomes (beyond temporarily making a particular anxiety-provoking encounter, such as a plane flight, easier to endure; see Choy et al., 2007). It should be noted, however, that pharmacological treatments have not been as widely investigated for specific phobias as they have been for other anxiety disorders. One interesting possible exception to this conclusion about medications concerns D-cycloserine, which is a partial agonist at the *N*-methyl-D-aspartate (NMDA) receptor site. This medication is not designed to reduce fear or the phobia directly; instead, it appears to enhance the pace of exposure therapy by stimulating the amygdala and influencing how readily fear responses are unlearned. While it is too early to determine the ultimate potential for this medication to enhance treatment of specific phobias, initial evidence (e.g., examining D-cycloserine–enhanced virtual reality exposure for fear of heights; Ressler et al., 2004) has been promising (see Davis, Myers, Ressler, & Rothbaum, 2005).

Clinical Implications

As reviewed earlier, there is a large and helpful literature evaluating the efficacy of various treatments for panic and phobias. At the same time, this literature leaves open many questions about how to best implement these interventions and what to do when the first-line recommended treatment does not achieve maximal results. Among the clinical implications that follow from this research review are the importance of the therapeutic alliance and clinician's experience, the need to make exposure therapy more appealing to the patient, and the use of general principles of change associated with the treatment of anxiety disorders.

Importance of the Therapeutic Alliance and Experience

We can legitimately give patients good reason to be hopeful about exposure therapy; the challenge is to get them to try it in the first place and to recognize that tolerating anxiety and exposing themselves to the feared situation, object, or event do not impose any realistic danger. It is here that the therapeutic alliance is most important, in that there needs to be a strong bond between therapist and patient, and both need to be in agreement on the goals and methods of change (Goldfried & Davila, 2005; Newman, Stiles, Janeck, & Woody, 2005). There is no doubt that exposure can effectively reduce avoidance and anxiety—provided that the patient remains in treatment and agrees to engage in the therapeutic procedures. The therapy relationship can increase the likelihood that this will happen.

As we indicated earlier, framing the therapy as a means of teaching coping skills—where patients learn to manage and tolerate their anxiety—is particularly important. There is also some evidence that the experience level of the therapist can play an important role (though this has not been a consistent finding). Huppert et al. (2001) found that in using a standard protocol for the treatment of panic disorder, more experienced therapists were more successful, even though less experienced therapists were not rated as adhering less to, or being less competent in administering, the treatment. It is not clear whether the difference was a function of the alliance or the use of more general clinical skills in dealing with issues during the course of treatment.

Making Exposure Therapy More Appealing

In addition to making use of the therapeutic relationship as a means of having patients agree to expose themselves to that which is likely to cause anxiety, the judicial use of hierarchically graded situations to provide gradual exposure may make starting the exposure process easier for some patients to contemplate. Moreover, the use of relaxation as a coping skill can help patients to reduce their anxiety and obtain a sense of control. In this regard, however, it is important to note that the literature indicates that some patients (e.g., panic disorder, generalized anxiety disorder) experience a paradoxical *increase* in anxiety as a consequence of relaxation.

Lilienfeld (2007), who has reviewed some of the literature in this area, has even questioned whether relaxation training is potentially harmful in treating some patients with panic disorder. The phenomenon of relaxation-provoked anxiety in some patients has long been noted in the practice of behavior therapy (e.g., Goldfried & Davison, 1976), and there are indeed ways the skilled clinician can deal with it. Patients who are likely to fear losing control should be forewarned that the sensations they may experience are not signs that they are losing control, but that they are in fact *learning to manage* their sensations of anxiety (see Goldfried & Davison, 1976).

When utilizing relaxation techniques, it is also important to stress that the use of relaxation should not be confused with the inability to tolerate anxiety—an idea that clearly runs counter to the goals of exposure. Accordingly, one of the ways we introduce relaxation exercises in treatment for panic disorder is by noting that relaxation can help to reduce one's resting level of anxiety, making panic and intense anxiety reactions less likely in the first place. This gives patients more options when confronting feared situations and stimuli, namely, the option of whether they want to enhance a given exposure by fully tolerating anxiety symptoms or use relaxation techniques to decrease anxiety.

Being Familiar with Principles of Change

In addition to ensuring that clinical interventions are informed by the findings of basic research on anxiety and randomized clinical trials, therapists can enhance their clinical effectiveness by being familiar with general therapeutic principles of change (Castonguay & Beutler, 2005). Woody and Ollendick (2006) have extrapolated from the research literature a number of principles that can guide practicing therapists in implementing techniques for the treatment of anxiety disorders. Although space limitations prevent us from enumerating all of them, they include general guidelines such as fostering cognitive change (e.g., challenging misconceptions by reevaluating evidence for a given belief), increasing behavioral skills for coping with anxiety and reducing avoidance, and repeatedly using emotionally evocative procedures.

EPIDEMIOLOGY

Examining the prevalence rates for panic disorder and phobias highlights not only how common these problems are but also the fascinating differences in prevalence when comparing rates as a function of gender, age, race, ethnicity and nationality.

Panic Disorder and Agoraphobia

Lifetime prevalence estimates for panic disorder, with or without agoraphobia, range from 1.5 to 3.5%, with 1-year prevalence rate estimates between 1 and 2% (American Psychiatric Association, 1994). The presence of agoraphobia without panic is less common, with approximately a 1.3% lifetime prevalence, and a 0.8% 1-year prevalence (Kessler et al., 2005).

The panic disorder median age of onset is 24 years of age (Burke, Burke, Regier, & Rae, 1990), though some data suggest a bimodal distribution, with peak ages of onset at 15–24 years, then at 45–54 years (Eaton, Kessler, Wittchen, & Magee, 1994). The onset of panic disorder and agoraphobia appears to be less common in prepubescent children (Kearney, Albano, Eisen, Allan, & Barlow, 1997), with estimates of 0.5–1% in general pediatric populations (e.g., Essau, Conradt, & Petermann, 2000). Puberty seems to be an important predictor of panic attacks (even beyond age; Hayward et al., 1992), and many adolescents do experience panic attacks (e.g., King, Gullone, Tonge, & Ollendick, 1993).

In general, panic disorder and agoraphobia appear to be less pervasive in elderly populations (Flint, 1994), but there are not yet sufficient data to draw firm conclusions. Also, there is some debate about the validity of using DSM criteria with older adults that have been validated primarily in younger adult populations, especially given concerns about high rates of medical comorbidity in older populations in which the medical treatment may mask anxiety symptoms (see Palmer, Jeste, & Sheikh, 1997). While panic disorder in older adults typically reflects a preexisting condition (Flint, 1994), a later age of onset certainly does occur. New onset in older adulthood may be related to stressful life events, such as illness or injury, other medical or psychiatric disorders, or emerging dementia (see van Balkom et al., 2000).

Large gender differences in panic disorder and agoraphobia have been consistently reported (approximately 2:1 more women than men: see Kessler et al., 2006), even cross-culturally (Wittchen, Essau, Von Zerssen, Krieg, & Zaudig, 1992). The source of the gender differences is not entirely clear, though some have proposed that sex-based biological differences play a role (see Craske, 2003). Gender roles that indicate it is more acceptable for women to avoid (and for men to turn to substance abuse to self-medicate when they are emotionally dysregulated) may also be contributing factors (see Kushner, Abrams, & Borchardt, 2000). Notwithstanding the gender gap in prevalence, the general course, phenomenology, and treatment response do not vary strongly for men and women, except that women are more likely to have severe agoraphobia (e.g., Cameron & Hill, 1989).

The data are somewhat mixed with respect to prevalence differences based on ethnic or racial subgroups. Some data suggest that African Americans (compared to European Americans) have a higher lifetime prevalence of agoraphobia but not of panic disorder (Regier et al., 1984), and the National Comorbidity Survey Replication study found a lower risk of panic disorder among Hispanic (vs. non-Hispanic) whites in younger cohorts (less than 43 years old; Breslau et al., 2006). However, other population-based studies have not found differences in panic disorder and agoraphobia prevalence among African Americans, Hispanic Americans, and European American groups (see review by Neal & Turner, 1991). Notably, there may be some ethnic group differences in the presentation of panic disorder and agoraphobia. For instance, African Americans may have a later age of onset and more frequently use coping strategies tied to "counting one's blessings" or religiosity than European Americans (Smith, Friedman, & Nevid, 1999). African Americans with panic disorder and agoraphobia also show stronger associations with hypertension (e.g., Bell, Hildreth, Jenkins, & Carter, 1988) and are more likely to experience panic-like isolated sleep paralysis than European Americans or other groups with panic disorder and agoraphobia (Bell et al., 1984).

Epidemiological data across numerous countries suggest comparable lifetime prevalence, age of onset, and gender differences for panic disorder (Weissman et al., 1997), indicating considerable consistency in the cross-cultural presentation of panic. At the same time, there are some interesting cross-cultural differences in the experience of panic attacks. For instance, in some Hispanic populations, *ataques de nervios* is relatively common, sharing many symptoms of DSM-defined panic attacks, but the attacks include crying and uncontrollable shouting as common features as well (see Lewis-Fernandez et al., 2002). Khmer refugees in the United States also experience *kyol geo,* sometimes called "wind overload," which includes common panic symptoms and fear of orthostatic dizziness (dizziness upon standing; Hinton, Hinton, Pham, Chau, & Tran, 2003).

Social Phobia

Approximately 7–13% of individuals in Western societies have social phobia at some point in their lifetime (Furmark, 2002). For instance, the National Comorbidity Survey Replication Study of DSM-IV disorders found that social phobia has a lifetime prevalence rate of 12.1%, making it one of the most common disorders (Kessler et al., 2005). According to this study, the social phobia median age of onset is 13 years, which is consistent with other research indicating that social phobia typically develops at a fairly young age, usually prior to age 18 (Rapee, 1995). The age of onset for generalized social phobia in particular may be especially early (Wittchen, Stein, & Kessler, 1999).

While social phobia remains a common disorder in later life, the incidence appears to be lower in older than in younger cohorts. For example, research investigating Canadian older adults (defined as age 55 and over) found that the lifetime prevalence rate for social phobia in later life was only 4.9% (Cairney et al., 2007). Given the trend for greater lifetime prevalence rates of social phobia among younger (as opposed to older) cohorts, some researchers have suggested that social phobia may become an even more significant mental health concern in the future (Rapee & Spence, 2004). Without longitudinal epidemiology studies, however, this claim cannot be substantiated.

Similar to many anxiety disorders, social phobia appears to be more prevalent in women than men in the general population (Kessler et al., 1994). Interestingly, the sexes are more equally distributed among treatment-seeking populations (Chapman, Mannuzza, & Fyer, 1995), leading some researchers to speculate that having social phobia as a man may be relatively more difficult in certain societies (e.g., because of the impairment it can cause in work situations in societies where men tend to be more often in leadership positions that require public speaking; Rapee, 1995). At the same time, research suggests that among treatment-seeking populations, there are not many meaningful gender differences in severity of social phobia symptoms, including prior treatment history, comorbidity with other anxiety or affective disorders, and duration of social fears (Turk et al., 1998).

When evaluating the epidemiological profile of social phobia, it is also critical to incorporate cultural considerations. For instance, prevalence rates for social phobia in Southeast Asian countries (Korea and Taiwan) tend to be much lower than prevalence rates in Western countries (see Furmark, 2002). One explanation for this discrepancy is that the expression of social phobia may differ cross-culturally. For example, *taijin kyofusho*, a disorder characterized by the fear of embarrassing or causing offense to others, is categorized in DSM-5 as a "culture-related diagnostic issue," in spite of sharing some overlap with social phobia. Given the continuous nature of social anxiety symptoms, it is also plausible that the threshold for receiving a diagnosis of social phobia differs across cultures, even though symptom profiles are the same (Rapee & Spence, 2004). Finally, it is possible that social interactions may be more "scripted" or regulated in certain cultures, thereby leading to different rates of social phobia.

Specific Phobia

Although there is considerable variability in estimates across studies, the lifetime prevalence of specific phobias in two large epidemiological studies was approximately 11% (Eaton, Dryman, & Weissman, 1991; Kessler et al., 1994). Subclinical fears are also extremely common with the majority of the population reporting a significant fear (Birchall, 1996). The most frequent phobias in adult samples tend to focus on animals or heights (e.g., Becker et al., 2007), though, again, there is some inconsistency across studies.

Collapsing across different types of specific phobias (animal, situational, etc.), the mean age of onset is 15–16 years old (e.g., Magee, Eaton, Wittchen, McGonagle, & Kessler, 1996), with considerable differences observed across phobia subtypes. For instance, while animal and blood–injection–injury phobias often begin in childhood, situational and height phobias are more likely to emerge in adolescence or adulthood. There are also interesting age differences in overall prevalence rates of specific phobias. Prevalence seems to peak between 25 and 54 years of age (when specific phobias affect around 8–9% of samples), while lower rates are observed among both younger (ages 18–24) and older (age 55+) adults (Bland, Orn, & Newman, 1988).

As with the other anxiety disorders reviewed in this chapter, specific phobias are consistently found to be more prevalent among women (e.g., Curtis, Magee, Eaton, Wittchen, & Kessler, 1998), especially for fears of animals, lightning, enclosed places, and darkness (Fredrikson, Annas, Fischer, & Wik, 1996). Gender differences for phobias of heights, dentists, and flying tend to be lower (see Rowa et al., 2006). There are many possible reasons for the higher phobia prevalence among females, including some intriguing evidence that men tend to underreport their fear relative to women (see Pierce & Kirkpatrick, 1992). Also, more women are apt to seek treatment for specific phobias, so the gender gap is especially pronounced in treatment-seeking samples (see Antony & Barlow, 1997).

Research examining variation in the prevalence of specific phobias across diverse cultural, national, and ethnic groups is lacking, but the available studies suggest some interesting differences. For instance, while similar content of fears has been observed among African and European American children (Neal, Lilly, & Zakis, 1993), the overall prevalence rate of specific phobias among African American adults seems to be higher (Brown, Eaton, & Sussman, 1990). There is also some evidence for higher rates of specific phobias among Mexican Americans born in the United States, compared to both Mexican Americans born in Mexico and non-Hispanic whites born in the United States (Karno, Golding, Burnam, & Hough, 1989). Karno and colleagues suggest this difference may be partly due to a tendency for less distressed individuals to migrate. Not surprisingly, given variability in cultural norms, taboos, and so forth, across countries, there is also variability in phobia prevalence rates. In one striking example concerning a comparison between India and the United Kingdom, whereas phobias of animals, darkness, and bad weather were more common in India, other (in some cases, non-specific) phobias, such as agoraphobia and social phobia, were more common in the United Kingdom (Chambers, Yeragani, & Keshavan, 1986). The evidence to date also does not suggest that education level, socioeconomic status or employment is related to the prevalence of specific phobias (Costello, 1982).

Clinical Implications

The epidemiological findings reviewed earlier clearly indicate that the prevalence of anxiety disorders varies as a function of race, ethnicity, and other factors. Sharing a common diagnostic label is only the starting point in deciding on a treatment plan; cultural and diversity issues need to be carefully considered.

Cultural and Diversity Issues in Assessment and Treatment

In treating any anxiety disorder, it is essential to consider the sociocultural context of patients, such as their ethnic identity, age, gender expectations/roles, sexual orientation, and acculturation. These factors should be considered throughout case conceptualization, because they will likely play a role in symptom presentation, assessment, and treatment planning. For example, patients may have specific cultural beliefs that panic attacks reflect a punishment from God or an angry spirit. Indeed, there exist some disconcerting examples in which the failure to take into account the unique experiences and beliefs of certain minority groups has resulted in diagnostic bias and inappropriate treatment. Paradis, Friedman, Lazar, Grubea, and Kesselman (1992) found this to be the case in an outpatient clinic for black patients with panic disorder who had emigrated from the West Indies. The belief system of such patients often includes the practice of voodoo, resulting in an atypical description of symptoms. The authors provide an example of a young woman from Guyana, who came to the clinic describing the typical symptoms of panic that followed a breakup with a boyfriend (e.g., rapid heartbeat, dizziness). In addition to describing the traditional symptoms of panic, she added: "I feel like I'm going to die. . . . I worry it's not natural . . . not natural causes, evil like someone put a curse on me. . . . I'm afraid people might look at me and ridicule me because of how I look, people might talk about me" (Paradis et al., 1992. p. 63). The clinician who evaluated her gave her the diagnosis "schizophrenia, chronic paranoid type," with the following justification: "The patient's bizarre delusion of an evil spirit inside her body, persecutory delusions of her boyfriend plotting against her, her paranoid delusions of people thinking she is ugly and laughing at her all speak for the diagnosis of schizophrenia, although the onset of delusions at age 33, her normal affect, and the absence of formal thought disorder are inconsistent with the classical presentation of schizophrenia" (p. 64).

Misdiagnoses of social anxiety among gay men similarly fail to take into account the cultural and epidemiological context of the individuals. With the continued presence of verbal and physical harassment of sexual minorities in our society, there are legitimate reasons that such individuals may be concerned about the opinion and reaction of others. It should be noted, however, that individual differences exist within this group, and not all gay men are as sensitive to the reaction of others. For example, it has been found that less social anxiety among gay men is related to the extent to which these men feel comfortable being gay. Moreover, less socially anxious gay men are more likely to be "out" and have their sexual orientation supported by a parent (e.g., Pachankis, Goldfried, & Ramrattan, 2008).

Finally, when treating older adults, age may be an important consideration throughout case conceptualization. For instance, somatic complaints may mask anxiety problems among elderly patients with late-onset anxiety. Some older adults choose to describe their symptoms of anxiety as problems with sleep, for example, because this may be perceived as a less stigmatizing way of describing their experiences (Morin, Savard, & Blais, 2000). Older adults may also be particularly reactive to certain types of anxiety-provoking triggers, such as threats to physical health (Teachman & Gordon, 2009).

COMORBIDITY

Comorbidity among the anxiety disorders is the norm rather than the exception. Interestingly, however, the disorders are by no means uniform with respect to the likelihood or types of co-occurring psychological and medical disorders; thus, we evaluate each disorder in turn.

Panic Disorder and Agoraphobia

Comorbidity among individuals with panic disorder and agoraphobia is standard. For instance, Brown et al. (2001) found that 60% of persons with panic had an additional psychiatric disorder. As noted, rates of agoraphobia are very high, with approximately 20–50% of persons diagnosed with panic disorder in community samples also meeting criteria for agoraphobia, and even higher rates have been observed in clinical settings (Weissman et al., 1997). Comorbidity with other anxiety disorders is also quite common, including comorbidity with generalized anxiety disorder, as well as social and specific phobias (each occurring in around 15–16% of individuals with panic disorder: Brown et al., 2001). Fortunately, initial evidence indicates that some symptoms of anxiety disorders (that are not directly targeted in panic disorder treatment) will be reduced following medication and psychotherapy for panic, suggesting generalization of treatment effects.

Mood disorders, both unipolar and bipolar, also frequently co-occur with panic and agoraphobia (Simon et al., 2004). For instance, among individuals with panic disorder, with or without agoraphobia, the lifetime prevalence of major depression is 35–40% (Kessler et al., 2006). Notably, in two-thirds of cases, depression onset either follows or coincides with the onset of panic disorder (vs. preceding panic; Kessler et al., 1998). Critically, this additional diagnosis of a mood disorder is associated with a worse course for panic, including increased impairment and hospitalizations (Roy-Byrne et al., 2000). Although data are limited, there is some indication that depressive symptoms may improve spontaneously following CBT for panic (Tsao, Mystkowski, Zucker, & Craske, 2005).

Substance use also complicates the presentation of panic disorder; with around 20% of patients with panic disorder meeting criteria at some point for either alcohol or other substance abuse (Sansone, Griffiths, & Sansone, 2005). In one study, approximately half of those with comorbid panic and substance use disorders developed the panic difficulties prior to the onset of substance use, and 23% indicated that alcohol or drugs were used to help reduce anxiety symptoms (Bolton, Cox, Clara, & Sareen, 2006). Dual-diagnosis patients can be especially challenging to treat because of the numerous ways that substance abuse interferes with treatment participation, and there are many open questions about whether integrated or sequential treatment is recommended (see American Psychiatric Association, 2009).

Rates for comorbid personality disorders can also be extremely high, with estimates of 40–50% of persons with panic disorder also meeting criteria for at least one personality disorder (e.g., Grant et al., 2005; Mavissakalian, 1990), typically avoidant, obsessive–compulsive, or dependent personality disorder (Reich & Troughton, 1988). This comorbidity has the potential to interfere with treatment when the clinician must contend with pervasive and entrenched personality problems.

Complications may be particularly likely if personality difficulties interact with the aims of exposure-based therapy (e.g., building trust and a strong alliance with the therapist among individuals with borderline personality disorder, or encouraging confrontation of fears among persons with avoidant personality disorder).

In addition to these high rates of comorbid psychiatric disorders, medical comorbidity is also a significant issue with panic disorder. Many symptoms of panic attacks share features with the presentation of other, nonpsychiatric medical illnesses, such as myocardial infarction, diabetes, arrhythmia, mitral valve prolapse, hypoglycemia, irritable bowel syndrome, asthma, and chronic obstructive pulmonary disease. This apparent overlap likely contributes to the tendency of people with panic disorder to believe they are experiencing a serious medical illness (Ratcliffe, MacLeod, & Sensky, 2006) and their consequent frequent trips to the emergency room during panic attacks (see Klerman, Weissman, Ouellette, Johnson, & Greenwald, 1991). While panic attacks themselves are not a sign of a serious medical illness, individuals with panic disorder, compared to the general population, do have higher reported prevalence of hypertension, angina, and other cardiac problems; ulcer disease; and thyroid disease, among other illnesses (Rogers et al., 1994).

Social Phobia

As previously mentioned, there are high rates of comorbidity between social phobia and avoidant personality disorder, with the frequency of avoidant personality disorder among patients with social phobia ranging from 25 to 89% across a series of studies (median = 52.5%; see Heimberg & Becker, 2002). While estimates vary widely, there also appears to be a high rate of comorbidity between social phobia and both depression and alcohol abuse and/or dependence. In fact, according to the National Comorbidity Survey, 41.4% of individuals who met criteria for social phobia had a coexisting affective disorder (37% had major depressive disorder; Magee et al., 1996). Meanwhile, 11% of individuals with social phobia met criteria for alcohol abuse, and 24% met criteria for alcohol dependence (Magee et al., 1996; note, DSM-5 no longer delineates substance abuse from dependence). Studies have also revealed high rates of comorbidity between social phobia and other anxiety and mood disorders. Indeed, the National Comorbidity Survey found that a striking 81% of individuals with social phobia qualified for another disorder (Magee et al., 1996). It is also notable that when social phobia is comorbid with another psychological disorder, individuals typically report that social phobia occurred first (Wittchen et al., 1999). However, this may be an artifact of the early age of onset for social phobia, as opposed to indicating a causal developmental relationship.

Specific Phobia

Data from the National Comorbidity Survey suggest that specific phobias often co-occur with other specific phobias; in fact, only 24.4% of individuals diagnosed with specific phobia had a single specific phobia (Curtis et al., 1998) and many individuals had more than three phobias. At the same time, other studies have found multiple specific phobias to be relatively rare (e.g., in a Swedish sample, only 18.1% of patients with specific phobias had multiple phobias; Fredrikson et al., 1996), leaving open questions about how measurement issues and cohort effects may be influencing results.

Severity of the phobia appears related to comorbidity in interesting ways. Individuals who have multiple specific phobias are also likely to have another anxiety disorder (Curtis et al., 1998), but the specific phobia in these cases is usually less severe than the other disorder(s). When specific phobia is the most severe and impairing disorder (i.e., is the principal diagnosis), it is less likely to be associated with other disorders. For instance, Brown et al. (2001) found that only 34% of patients with a principal diagnosis of specific phobia met criteria for any other clinical disorder (usually another anxiety or mood disorder when comorbidity was present).

Clinical Implications

Responding to Co-Occurring Symptoms of Physical Illness

It is common for patients with panic disorder to label their physical symptoms as a heart attack. Although this is usually a mislabeling, there nonetheless exists a somewhat higher prevalence of cardiac problems in patients with panic disorder than in the general population. It is therefore important to help patients distinguish between signs of a heart attack and those of a panic attack, and, when relevant, to encourage them to get a full medical examination to determine the presence of a complicating medical condition. When co-occurring medical illnesses are present in the context of CBT for panic, some creativity is often required to adjust exposure exercises so that patients can still meet the goal of eliciting fear and panic sensations while being careful of medically relevant limitations (e.g., hyperventilation exercises can be modified for patients with asthma, so they still get the feeling of shortness of breath).

Alternate Ways to View Comorbidity

As our conceptualization of psychological problems has been shaped over the years by the ascendancy of the DSM, our thinking has changed, so that we understand clinical problems in terms of their diagnostic category. No longer "problems in living," what we see clinically are "disorders." Along with this shift, our understanding of multiple problems is viewed in terms of "comorbidity" rather than the potential functional relationship between problematic emotions, behaviors, and cognitions. The labeling of comorbidity of anxiety and depression in many individuals is quite typical, but unfortunately does not provide the practicing therapist with guidelines for how to proceed. On the other hand, if one thinks in terms of the functional rela-tionship between anxiety and depression, it is not at all unusual to see functioning impaired because of anxiety and behavioral avoidance, resulting in patients feeling helpless and hopeless about being able to cope with the demands of their lives. For example, patients might receive a diagnosis of both social phobia and depression due to the fact that they are impaired in both their social and occupational lives by behavioral avoidance, and this failure to function competently leads to depression. Practicing therapists know this to be the case, and it is important for research to focus more on this important clinical issue.

Notably, by focusing on principles of change (e.g., reducing avoidance of dis-tressing situations), rather than diagnoses, it becomes easier to tackle multiple problem areas simultaneously. Notwithstanding, it is often necessary to prioritize targets of therapy, because not every problem can be addressed at once. When comorbidity occurs, we generally think about prioritizing or ordering the foci of treatment based on multiple considerations. For instance, is improvement in one domain likely to generalize to other areas of functioning (e.g., will reduced fears of flying likely alleviate depressive symptoms)? What domain does the patient feel is most important to target first? Is one domain versus another (e.g., fear of future panic vs. anhedonia in depression) more clearly contributing to impairments in functioning or life crises? Where are we most likely to effect positive change? Answering these questions is often challenging and may involve some trial and error.

Some research also indicates that the treatment of an anxiety disorder is less successful if there is a comorbid personality disorder (see discussion in American Psychiatric Association, 2009), although the data here are somewhat mixed. Regard-less, a clinically more useful way to conceptualize this phenomenon parallels the distinction noted earlier between simple and complex panic disorder. Goldstein and Chambless (1978) characterize individuals on the simple end of the continuum as those whose initial panic attack may have been the result of a specific adverse drug experience, whereas a more complex case would involve a person with a maladap-tive interpersonal style. Here, too, thinking along the lines of functional analysis has important implications for intervention. Considering common vulnerability factors that can account for multiple problem manifestations can be helpful in this situation. For instance, recognizing the role of a common underlying personality style, such as neuroticism, can help make sense of a complex symptom presentation given evidence from hierarchical models of psychopathology that suggest neuroti-cism is common to a range of depressive and anxiety disorders (see Watson et al., 1995). Similarly, experiencing numerous stressful life circumstances (difficulties with finances, work, the legal system, etc.) can enhance vulnerability to a broad range of disorders. At times, we need to teach problem-solving approaches to help patients manage some of their difficult life circumstances, before they are able to work on other presenting clinical symptoms.

ETIOLOGY

As with most (if not all) psychological disorders, a multitude of factors contribute to the onset of panic disorder and phobias. Thus, isolating the "cause" of a disorder is rarely a realistic goal. Instead, we can talk to patients about the levels of vulnerability and causal factors that may interact to lead to the expression of a specific problem. Barlow (2002) outlines a model of triple vulnerabilities. The first, a general biological vulnerability, makes an individual more susceptible to becoming anxious. This first level interacts with a second, general psychological vulnerability, which focuses on a sense that the environment is uncontrollable and unpredictable. The combination of these two broad vulnerabilities can lead an individual to become extremely fearful in situations that are not objectively dangerous (termed "false alarms"). The third level constitutes specific psychological vulnerabilities that lead to the expression of an identifiable anxiety disorder as a function of an individual's particular learning experiences about what aspects of the environment are threatening. For instance, learning that evaluation by others can be dangerous may lead to social phobia, and learning that heights are hazardous may result in a specific phobia, whereas learning to fear changes in bodily sensations may manifest as panic disorder. Given the considerable overlap in etiological models, we highlight the common vulnerabilities for panic disorder and phobias in this section. However, we also provide examples of the unique ways in which these vulnerability factors manifest across the specific disorders.

General Biological Vulnerabilities

There is considerable empirical support for each of these levels of vulnerability. At the biological level, family and genetic studies point to the conclusion that there is a broad genetic basis to anxiety and related areas of emotion dysregulation (e.g., depression). For example, first-degree relatives of samples with anxiety disorders have higher rates of anxiety difficulties than the relatives of nonanxious control samples (e.g., Weissman, 1993). Similarly, the children of parents with anxiety disorders have been observed to have more than nine times greater risk of having a psychiatric disorder than the children of nonanxious control parents (see Turner, Beidel, & Costello, 1987; see replication in Beidel & Turner, 1997). More specifically, the children of parents with panic disorder tend to be more anxious than the children of nonanxious control parents (e.g., Sylvester, Hyde, & Reichler, 1988). These children also tend to be more depressed, pointing to the general nature of the vulnerability (though some anxiety disorders may have a more disorder-specific transmission, such as specific phobias; Page & Martin, 1998). Along these lines, genetic factors appear to play a moderate but meaningful role in the development of social phobia, explaining approximately 30–50% of the variance in the disorder (Kendler, Karkowski, & Prescott, 1999). However, it is less clear whether these genetic factors are specific to the development of social phobia, as opposed to the development of mental health problems more broadly (Kimbrel, 2008). Finally, twin studies, which help to minimize potential confounds between genetic and nongenetic influences, also support the heritability of a general anxiety proneness. For instance, there are higher concordance rates of anxiety disorders in monozygotic (34%) than in dizygotic (17%) twins (Torgersen, 1983). Critically, the evidence to date does not point to a specific anxiety gene; instead, there appear to be relatively weak contributions from an array of genes (Plomin, DeFries, McClearn, & Rutter, 1997). It is also important to highlight that many of the studies on biological vulnerabilities do not guarantee that the finding of higher rates of anxiety disorders among family members is due purely to genetic factors, as opposed to other influences, such as social learning experiences.

Temperamental vulnerabilities tied to anxiety (Clark, Watson, & Mineka, 1994) also seem to play a role in setting the stage for later expression of an anxiety problem. For example, behavioral inhibition, "a temperamental trait observed in infants and young children characterized by behavioral withdrawal, decreased approach behavior, increased vigilance, and increased arousal in response to novel and unfamiliar situations" (Kimbrel, 2008, p. 594), has been found to predict later anxiety disorders. Persons with a stable pattern of high behavioral inhibition over a 5- to 6-year period were more likely to develop an anxiety disorder, especially a phobia (Hirshfeld et al., 1992), and behavioral inhibition at age 8 was linked to increased risk for anxiety and depressive disorders at ages 16–21 (Goodwin, Fergusson, & Horwood, 2004). Behavioral inhibition has received considerable attention as an early risk factor within the context of social phobia. For example, Schwartz, Snidman, and Kagan (1999) found that 61% of children who received a diagnosis of social phobia had been previously classified as behaviorally inhibited (compared to 27% of children previously classified as uninhibited).

Numerous other biomarkers have also been linked to heightened risk for anxiety disorders, though the strength of the evidence varies considerably across markers. For instance, an imbalance of the neurotransmitter serotonin has often been proposed as a factor in the etiology of anxiety pathology (e.g., in panic disorder; Stein & Hugo, 2004), but this proposal is based mostly on the effective treatment response of anxiety to SSRIs rather than on prospective evidence. Other proposed neuropsychiatric contributions, derived in part from animal models, include differences in the anatomy of the amygdala and hippocampus, and altered stress responses with respect to cortisol levels and the hypothalamic–pituitary–adrenal axis (see review by Uhde & Singareddy, 2002).

There is also considerable evidence that certain biological triggers make panic attacks more likely, and there is a rich tradition of eliciting panic attacks in the laboratory by altering respiration in vulnerable individuals (e.g., through inducing hyperventilation or inhaling CO_2; see Barlow, 2002, Chapter 5). This has led to the suggestion that individuals who are particularly sensitive to increased levels of CO_2 may be at greater risk of developing panic attacks, an idea known as the false-suffocation alarm theory (Klein, 1993), though this hypothesis has received only mixed empirical support (see Barlow, 2002). Notably, the likelihood of cueing a panic attack through a biochemical or respiration challenge depends in part on other biological vulnerabilities (e.g., higher baseline heart rate; Liebowitz et al., 1985). Furthermore, the occurrence of panic attacks following a biological challenge is heavily influenced by other psychological vulnerabilities, such as greater baseline subjective distress (e.g., Coplan et al., 1998) and whether the challenge activates perceptions of loss of control (e.g., Zvolensky, Eifert, Lejuez, & McNeil, 1999), which brings us to the second level of vulnerabilities.

General Psychological Vulnerabilities

Interacting with general biological vulnerabilities is a set of broad psychological vulnerabilities that set the individual up to see the world as an uncontrollable and unpredictable place. This focus on the importance of perceived and actual control is based partly on extensive evidence from animal models that show having minimal control over the environment during early development can lead to chronic difficulties with anxiety (e.g., work with rhesus monkeys; Suomi, 2000). In humans, an attributional style reflecting a sense that outcomes are uncontrollable, either in general or because of personal limitations, also seems to be a risk factor (see Luten, Ralph, & Mineka, 1997). Interestingly, this cognitive style may be more common in girls, which may contribute to the oft-cited gender differences in anxiety disorder prevalence rates. Nolen-Hoeksema and Girgus (1994) propose that this gender disparity may be due to higher rates of negative life events during childhood and adolescence among girls, and more experiences that suggest one's behavior has limited impact on the environment. Other evidence that early learning experiences about controllability and predictability are important follow from the finding that parenting styles promoting a sense of control by being contingently responsive yet not overprotective (i.e., permitting exploration) seem to protect against the development of anxiety problems (see Chorpita & Barlow, 1998). It is important to note that most of the evidence in humans linking uncontrollability with anxiety is correlational, because of the ethical barriers to manipulating children's environments to enhance uncontrollability.

In addition to early learning experiences that focus on uncontrollability, stressful life events more generally seem to enhance vulnerability. These events appear to serve as triggers for various forms of psychopathology, and seem most closely implicated in anxiety pathology if the events are either threatening (e.g., involvement in an accident) or uncontrollable in some way (e.g., Eley & Stevenson, 2000). For instance, patients with panic disorder reported a higher number of salient life events, especially those that seemed out of their control, in the 12 months before onset of panic, relative to the same time period for control participants (Faravelli & Pallanti, 1989).

The interpretation of an event as negative and stressful is, of course, highly dependent on how individuals process that event, and there is extensive evidence that anxious individuals selectively process threatening information (see Mathews & MacLeod, 2005). These cognitive biases are thought to maintain anxiety and dysfunctional avoidance behaviors by keeping threatening cues salient to the vulnerable person. This general pattern can be seen across disorders, with a focus on preferential processing of information that is considered most threatening for a given disorder. For instance, the general tendency among anxious samples to interpret ambiguous situations as threatening is to focus on (mis)interpretations of bodily sensations in panic disorder. Specifically, the cognitive model of panic attacks was developed in part from observations of pharmacological and neurochemical studies of agents that promoted panic attacks, but only in select individuals—those who tended to interpret the bodily sensations induced by the agents in a disastrous way (Clark, 1986). This led Clark to suggest that panic attacks occur because certain bodily sensations are misinterpreted as indicating a catastrophe, such as a heart attack or loss of control. In social phobia, cognitive processing biases and related emotional responses in social situations are thought to reinforce the idea that social or performance situations are threatening, and that negative evaluation is likely (Clark & Wells, 1995; Rapee & Heimberg, 1997). When conversing with acquaintances at a party, for instance, individuals with social phobia may notice the one person who does not smile at something they have said and interpret this as evidence that they are dull or uninteresting.

In addition to the abundant data indicating that selective information processing is associated with anxiety disorders (see review by Mathews & MacLeod, 2005), there is also some evidence that these information-processing biases enhance vulnerability to react more negatively to subsequent challenging life events (e.g., MacLeod & Hagan, 1992). Similarly, "anxiety sensitivity" (the belief that anxiety symptoms are themselves scary) and explicit threat appraisals have been found to predict the onset of anxiety disorder symptoms (e.g., Schmidt, Lerew, & Jackson, 1997).

Specific Psychological Vulnerabilities

The combination of general biological and psychological vulnerabilities is thought to enhance anxiety proneness, while an individual's particular learning experiences are expected to predict whether or not a specific type of anxiety disorder is expressed. For instance, the emergence of panic disorder would be especially likely if the dangers of somatic symptoms and illnesses were emphasized and reinforced during childhood (see Barlow, 2002). Meanwhile, "sensitizing social experiences," such as being excessively teased, are thought potentially to increase the risk for developing generalized social phobia (Kimbrel, 2008).

There is also considerable evidence that conditioning experiences can be central to the onset of phobias (see Öst, 1987), and stories of a traumatic dog bite leading to a dog phobia are not unusual. Furthermore, Mowrer's (1947) influential two-factor theory includes both classical and operant conditioning mechanisms—specifically, fear becomes a classically conditioned response to a previously neutral stimulus through a negative conditioning event, then avoidance and escape behaviors are operantly reinforced because of their (temporary) anxiety-reducing qualities. However, classical conditioning models are not able to explain all the varied ways that fear acquisition can occur (i.e., lots of people who experience dog bites do not go on to develop a phobia and many, if not most, people with phobias did not experience a bad bite). Thus, Rachman (1977, 1990) has suggested multiple pathways to acquire specific fears. In addition to classical conditioning, a person may vicariously learn via modeling (e.g., watching someone else be bitten by a dog), or simply through the transmission of information that a given situation is dangerous (e.g., reading about plane crashes; see also Mineka & Zinbarg, 2006).

An additional challenge in explaining the development of fear and phobias concerns the unequal distribution of fears in the population (e.g., particularly high rates of snake and spider phobias relative to other animal phobias, despite fewer stories of snake bites than dog bites). This has led to the suggestion that we are predisposed to acquire some fears very readily because it was adaptive to be fearful of certain objects or situations in our evolutionary past. This idea, termed "biological preparedness theory" (Seligman, 1971), has some support from nonhuman primate studies (e.g., monkeys are more likely to exhibit fear when observing another monkey showing fear to a snake than to a rabbit; Cook & Mineka, 1989), though the broader status of preparedness theory remains controversial (see Davey, 1995; McNally, 1987).

Linked to early learning experiences, social skills and behaviors also feature prominently in many etiological models of social phobia. For example, Rapee and Spence (2004) draw a distinction between poor social skills and "interrupted social performance," which they define as "the interference of appropriate social behavior due to heightened anxiety" (p. 758). According to Rapee and Spence, interrupted social performance likely plays a larger role in the maintenance (vs. development) of social anxiety. At extreme levels, however, interrupted social performance may also interfere with one's ability to obtain and nurture meaningful friendships, which in turn could contribute to the development of social phobia.

Regardless of the method by which a given learning experience occurs, it seems clear at this point that it is the interaction of a range of general and specific biological and psychological vulnerabilities that can explain why a given person develops an anxiety problem. Even in the primate studies, the likelihood of fear conditioning is dependent in part on the monkeys' prior experience. For instance, fear conditioning is less likely if the monkeys have previously observed nonfearful behavior in response to the potential fear stimulus (Mineka & Cook, 1986). Thus, updated learning models (e.g., Mineka & Zinbarg, 2006; see also Armfield, 2006) tend to be more comprehensive and reflect the likely interaction of biological, cultural, and environmental vulnerabilities, as well as particular stressors that can influence the impact of a given learning experience.

Clinical Implications

Here, we consider the question of connecting etiology to treatment, and the diversity of developmental pathways for a given anxiety disorder.

Connecting Etiology to Treatment

When behavioral approaches to treatment were first introduced in the late 1950s, it was proposed that knowledge of etiology was not needed in deciding upon a treatment plan. It was assumed that problematic behavior—especially anxiety—was learned, and what the patient needed were new learning experiences. Consequently, intervention procedures were developed that focused on the current life situation, and not the past. Although contemporary CBT continues to emphasize the here and now, a focus on etiology can have important therapeutic benefits, especially in discussing the ongoing contributions to current fears from early life experiences. Take the example of socially phobic individuals who were frequently berated by others for being shy or not appearing socially skilled. While their anxiety may be partially a function of a biological vulnerability, a psychoeducational intervention could potentially allow them to reattribute one of the "causes" of their problem to something other than themselves.

Diverse Developmental Pathways for a Given Disorder

Given that the DSM classification system is topographical and does not assess the function associated with the symptoms for a given disorder, it can include within a single category clinical problems that have different developmental pathways. Thus, one individual who is anxious in social situations may have adequate social skills but nevertheless be overly concerned about the negative reaction of others. Meanwhile, another individual may have serious deficiencies in their social skills, so his or her concern about the negative reaction of others would consequently be much more realistic.

The etiological factors underlying panic can be highly idiosyncratic. For example, one of us (M. G.) worked with an actress whose panic disorder caused her considerable anxiety prior to stage performances. In conducting an assessment of the trigger for her initial panic attack, the therapist inquired whether she had recently undergone any surgical procedures that might have been stressful. The actress indicated that she indeed had a "tummy tuck" shortly before her initial panic attack. As the therapy progressed and as abdominal breathing was introduced as one of the interventions, the patient indicated that she already knew how to do this, and had used this successfully throughout her career. However, when she was asked to demonstrate her abdominal breathing ability, it was apparent that she was not doing it properly; indeed, the tummy tuck interfered with her ability to engage in abdominal breathing, likely enhancing her anxiety and setting her up to panic when she practiced this technique before going on stage.

CONCLUSION: LINKS BETWEEN PSYCHOPATHOLOGY RESEARCH AND TREATMENT

Our goal in this chapter has been to summarize the basic and applied research on panic disorder and phobias, and to extrapolate clinical implications from these findings to aid therapists in developing their case formulations and treatment plans. In our review of the research literature on the treatment of panic disorder and agoraphobia, social phobia, and specific phobias, our focus has been primarily on the cognitive-behavioral techniques that are demonstrably efficacious. However, we have not neglected the very critical role of the therapeutic relationship, as well as the importance of an agreement between therapist and patient on the goals for treatment, and an agreement about the specific intervention procedures. What we also hope to make clear is that although specific techniques have been used in the treatment of anxiety disorders, it is important not to fall into the trap of thinking that one size fits all. Practicing clinicians have always known this to be the case, but it appears that the research literature needs to focus more on this concept. For instance, research focused on cultural considerations, treatment effectiveness in real-world settings, and therapeutic outcomes for patients with dual diagnoses is sorely needed.

Although there are specific procedures for particular clinical problems, it is also important for the clinician to keep in mind the overriding principles of change that may be reflected in the specific procedures. Among these are (1) a positive expectation that therapy will help, and the presence of sufficient motivation to participate; (2) an optimal therapeutic alliance; (3) doing what is necessary to help patients to become better aware of what they are doing and not doing, and how that contributes to their life problems and symptoms; (4) corrective experiences (e.g., via exposure) that encourage new learning and result in altered emotions and behavior, followed by changes in expectations that encourage further corrective experiences; and (5) reevaluation of biased thinking (Goldfried & Davila, 2005; see also Moses & Barlow, 2006).

Human behavior is far too varied and complex to be understood by any given therapeutic model or procedure. If we think in terms of general principles of change, we can then begin to investigate the parameters associated with their efficacy and effectiveness for different patients. In pursing such an evidenced-based approach, we can begin to build a body of knowledge that rather than being restricted by any single theoretical orientation is empirically based.

A final point we would like to make is that while this chapter is structured to derive clinical implications from research findings, the clinical situation should also be thought of as the context of discovery, whereby therapists' clinical observations provide invaluable directions for hypothesis generation and future research. In order to have a meaningful interaction between research and practice, the bridge needs to go both ways. After a drug has been approved by the U.S. Food and Drug Administration (FDA) following randomized clinical trials, practitioners have the opportunity to provide feedback to the FDA on the use of the drug in clinical practice. The Society of Clinical Psychology, Division 12 of the American Psychological Association, is now establishing such a mechanism, providing a two-way bridge between research findings on empirically supported treatments and therapy experiences that use these treatments in practice.

REFERENCES

Agras, W. S., Chapin, H. M., & Oliveau, D. C. (1972). The natural history of phobias: Course and prognosis. *Archives of General Psychiatry, 26*, 315–317.

Alonso, J., Angermeyer, M. C., Bernert, S., Bruffaerts, R., Brugha, T. S., Bryson, H., et al. (2004). Sampling and methods of the European Study of the Epidemiology of Mental Disorders (ESEMeD) project. *Acta Psychiatrica Scandinavica, 109*(Suppl. 420), 8–20.

American Psychiatric Association. (1994). *Diagnostic and statistical manual of mental disorders* (4th ed.). Washington, DC: Author.

American Psychiatric Association. (2000). *Diagnostic and statistical manual of mental disorders* (4th ed., text rev.). Washington, DC: Author.

American Psychiatric Association. (2009). Practice guidelines for the treatment of patients with panic disorder (2nd ed.). *American Journal of Psychiatry, 166*(1), 1–68.

American Psychiatric Association. (2013). *Diagnostic and statistical manual of mental disorders* (5th ed.). Arlington, VA: Author.

Amies, P. L., Gelder, M. G., & Shaw, P. M. (1983). Social phobia: A comparative clinical study. *British Journal of Psychiatry, 142*, 174–179.

Amir, N., Weber, G., Beard, C., Bomyea, J., & Taylor, C. T. (2008). The effect of a single session attention modification program on response to a public speaking challenge in socially anxious individuals. *Journal of Abnormal Psychology, 117*, 860–868.

Antony, M. M. (1994). *Heterogeneity among specific phobias types in DSM-IV.* Unpublished doctoral dissertation, State University of New York at Albany.

Antony, M. M. (2000). [Frequency of specific phobia referrals in an anxiety disorders clinic]. Unpublished raw data, Anxiety Treatment and Research Centre, Hamilton, Ontario, Canada.

Antony, M. M., & Barlow, D. H. (1997). Social and specific phobias. In A. Tasman, J. Kay, & J. A. Lieberman (Eds.), *Psychiatry* (pp. 1037–1059). Philadelphia: Saunders.

Antony, M. M., & Barlow, D. H. (2002). Specific phobias. In D. H. Barlow (Ed.), *Anxiety and its disorders: The nature and treatment of anxiety and panic* (pp. 380–417). New York: Guilford Press.

Armfield, J. M. (2006). Cognitive vulnerability: A model of the etiology of fear. *Clinical Psychology Review, 26*(6), 746–768.

Barlow, D. H. (1988). *Anxiety and its disorders: The nature and treatment of anxiety and panic* (1st ed.). New York: Guilford Press.

Barlow, D. H. (2002). *Anxiety and its disorders: The nature and treatment of anxiety and panic* (2nd ed.). New York: Guilford Press.

Barlow, D. H., & Craske, M. G. (2006). *Mastery of your panic and anxiety: Client workbook* (4th ed.). New York: Oxford University Press.

Barlow, D. H., Gorman, J. M., Shear, M. K., & Woods, S. W. (2000). Cognitive-behavioral therapy, imipramine, or their combination for panic disorder: A randomized controlled trial. *Journal of the American Medical Association, 283*(19), 2529–2536.

Barlow, D. H., O'Brien, G. T., & Last, C. A. (1984). Couples treatment of agoraphobia. *Behavior Therapy, 15,* 41–58.

Beck, A. T., & Clark, D. A. (1997). An information processing model of anxiety: Automatic and strategic processes. *Behaviour Research and Therapy, 35*(1), 49–58.

Becker, E. S., Rinck, M., Veneta, T., Kause, P., Goodwin, R., Neumer, S., et al. (2007). Epidemiology of specific phobia subtypes: Findings from the Dresden Mental Health Study. *European Psychiatry 22*(2), 69–74.

Beidel, D. C., & Turner, S. M. (1997). At risk for anxiety: I. Psychopathology in the offspring of anxious parents. *Journal of American Academy of Child and Adolescent Psychiatry 36,* 918–924.

Bell, C. C., Hildreth, C. J., Jenkins, E. J., & Carter, C. (1988). The relationship of isolated sleep paralysis and panic disorder to hypertension. *Journal of the National Medical Association, 80,* 289–294.

Bell, C. C., Shakoor, B., Thompson, B., Dew, D., Hughley, E., Mays, R., et al. (1984). Prevalence of isolated sleep paralysis in black subjects. *Journal of the National Medical Association, 76,* 501–508.

Birchall, H. M. (1996). Just how common are common fears? *Anxiety, 2,* 303–304.

Blanco, C., Schneier, F. R., Schmidt, A., Blanco-Jerez, C. R., Marshall, R. D., Sánchez-Lacay, A., et al. (2003). Pharmacological treatment of social anxiety disorder: A meta-analysis. *Depression and Anxiety, 18*(1), 29–40.

Bland, R. C., Orn, H., & Newman, S. C. (1988). Lifetime prevalence of psychiatric disorders in Edmonton. *Acta Psychiatrica Scandinavica, 77,* 24–32.

Blomhoff, S., Haug, T. T., Hellstrøm, K., Holme, I., Humble, M., Madsbu, H. P., et al. (2001). Randomised controlled general practice trial of sertraline, exposure therapy and combined treatment in generalised social phobia. *British Journal of Psychiatry, 179,* 23–30.

Bolton, J., Cox, B., Clara, I., & Sareen, J. (2006). Use of alcohol and drugs to self-medicate anxiety disorders in a nationally representative sample. *Journal of Nervous and Mental Disease, 194,* 818–825.

Breslau, J., Aguilar-Gaxiola, S., Kendler, K. S., Su, M., Williams, D., & Kessler, R. C. (2006). Specifying race–ethnic differences in risk for psychiatric disorder in a USA national sample. *Psychological Medicine, 36,* 57–68.

Brown, T. A., & Barlow, D. H. (2009). A proposal for a dimensional classification system based on the shared features of the DSM-IV anxiety and mood disorders: Implications for assessment and treatment. *Psychological Assessment, 21,* 256–271.

Brown, T. A., Campbell, L. A., Lehman, C. L., Grisham, J. R., & Mancill, R. B. (2001). Current and lifetime comorbidity of the DSM-IV anxiety and mood disorders in a large clinical sample. *Journal of Abnormal Psychology, 110,* 585–599.

Brown, D. R., Eaton, W., & Sussman, L. (1990). Racial differences in the prevalence of phobic disorders. *Journal of Nervous and Mental Disease, 178*(7), 434–441.

Bruce, S. E., Vasile, R. G., Goisman, R. M., Salzman, C., Spencer, M., Machan, J. T., et al. (2003). Are benzodiazepines still the medication of choice for patients with panic disorder with or without agoraphobia? *American Journal of Psychiatry, 160,* 1432–1438.

Bruce, S. E., Yonkers, K. A., Otto, M. W., Eisen, J. L., Weisberg, R. B., Pagano, M., et al. (2005). Influence of psychiatric comorbidity on recovery and recurrence in generalized anxiety disorder, social phobia, and panic disorder: A 12–year prospective study. *American Journal of Psychiatry, 162,* 1179–1187.

Burke, K. C., Burke, J. D., Jr., Regier, D. A., & Rae, D. S. (1990). Age at onset of selected mental disorders in five community populations. *Archives of General Psychiatry, 47*(6), 511–518.

Cairney, J., McCabe, L., Veldhuizen, S., Corna, L. M., Streiner, D., & Herrmann, N. (2007). Epidemiology of social phobia in later life. *American Journal of Geriatric Psychiatry, 15*(3), 224–233.

Cameron, O. G., & Hill, E. M. (1989). Women and anxiety. *Psychiatric Clinics of North America, 12,* 175–186.

Cannon, W. B. (1929). *Bodily changes in pain, hunger, fear and rage* (2nd ed.). New York: Appleton–Century–Crofts.

Castonguay, L. G., & Beutler, L. E. (Eds.). (2005). *Principles of therapeutic change that work.* New York: Oxford University Press.

Chambers, J., Yeragani, V. K., & Keshavan, M. S. (1986). Phobias in India and the United Kingdom: A trans-cultural study. *Acta Psychiatrica Scandinavica, 74*(4), 388–391.

Chambless, D. L., & Goldstein, A. J. (Eds.). (1982). *Agoraphobia: Multiple perspectives on theory and treatment.* New York: Wiley.

Chapman, T. F., Mannuzza, S., & Fyer, A. J. (1995). Epidemiology and family studies of social phobia. In R. G. Heimberg, M. R. Liebowitz, D. A. Hope, & F. R. Schneier (Eds.), *Social phobia: Diagnosis, assessment, and treatment* (pp. 21–40). New York: Guilford Press.

Chorpita, B. F., & Barlow, D. H. (1998). The development of anxiety: The role of control in the early environment. *Psychological Bulletin, 124*(1), 3–21.

Choy, Y., Fyer, A. J., & Lipsitz, J. D. (2007). Treatment of specific phobia in adults. *Clinical Psychology Review, 27,* 266–286.

Cisler, J. M., Olatunji, B. O., & Lohr, J. M. (2009). Disgust, fear, and the anxiety disorders: A critical review. *Clinical Psychology Review 29*(1), 34–46.

Clark, D. B., & Agras, W. S. (1991). The assessment and treatment of performance anxiety in musicians. *American Journal of Psychiatry, 148*(5), 598–605.

Clark, D. M. (1986). A cognitive approach to panic. *Behaviour Research and Therapy, 24,* 461–470.

Clark, D. M., Salkovskis, P. M., Hackman, A., Wells, A., Ludgate, J., & Gelder, M. (1999). Brief cognitive therapy for panic disorder: A randomized controlled trial. *Journal of Consulting and Clinical Psychology, 67,* 583–589.

Clark, D. M., & Wells, A. (1995). A cognitive model of social phobia. In R. Heimberg, M. Liebowitz, D. A. Hope, & F. R. Schneier (Eds.), *Social phobia: Diagnosis, assessment and treatment* (pp. 69–93). New York: Guilford Press.

Clark, L. A., Watson, D., & Mineka, S. (1994). Temperament, personality, and the mood and anxiety disorders. *Journal of Abnormal Psychology, 103,* 103–116.

Coles, M. E., & Heimberg, R. G. (2002). Memory bias in the anxiety disorders: Current status. *Clinical Psychology Review, 22,* 587–627.

Cook, M., & Mineka, S. (1989). Observational conditioning of fear to fear-relevant versus fear-irrelevant stimuli in rhesus monkeys. *Journal of Abnormal Psychology, 98,* 448–459.

Coplan, J. D., Goetz, R., Klein, D. F., Papp, L. A., Fyer, A. J., Liebowitz, M. R., et al. (1998). Plasma cortisol concentrations preceding lactate-induced panic: Psychological, biochemical, and physiological correlates. *Archives of General Psychiatry, 55,* 130–136.

Costello, C. G. (1982). Fears and phobias in women: A community study. *Journal of Abnormal Psychology, 91,* 280–286.

Craske, M. G. (2003). *Origins of phobias and anxiety disorders: Why more women than men?* (BRAT Series in Clinical Psychology). Oxford, UK: Elsevier.

Craske, M. G., & Barlow, D. H. (2008). Panic disorder and agoraphobia. In D. H. Barlow (Ed.), *Clinical handbook of psychological disorders* (pp. 1–64). New York: Guilford Press.

Craske, M. G., Golinelli, D., Stein, M. B., Roy-Byrne, P., Bystritsky, A., & Sherbourne, C. (2005). Does the addition of cognitive behavioral therapy improve panic disorder treatment outcome relative to medication alone in the primary-care setting? *Psychological Medicine, 35*(11), 1645–1654.

Craske, M. G., Lang, A. J., Mystkowski, J. L, Zucker, B. G., Bystritsky, A., & Yan-go, F. (2002). Does nocturnal panic represent a more severe form of panic disorder? *Journal of Nervous and Mental Disease, 190*(9), 611–618.

Craske, M. G., Miller, P. P., Rotunda, R., & Barlow, D. H. (1990). A descriptive report of features of initial unexpected panic attacks in minimal and extensive avoiders. *Behaviour Research and Therapy, 28*(5), 395–400.

Craske, M. G., & Sipsas, A. (1992). Animal phobias versus claustrophobias: Exteroceptive versus interoceptive cues. *Behaviour Research and Therapy, 30*(6), 569–581.

Curtis, G. C., Magee, W. J., Eaton, W. W., Wittchen, H. U., & Kessler, R. C. (1998). Specific fears and phobias: Epidemiology and classification. *British Journal of Psychiatry, 173,* 212–217.

Davey, G. C. L. (1992). Classical conditioning and the acquisition of human fears and phobias: A review and synthesis of the literature. *Advances in Behaviour Research and Therapy, 14,* 29–66.

Davey, G. C. L. (1995). Preparedness and phobias: Specific evolved associations or a generalized expectancy bias? *Behavioral and Brain Sciences, 18,* 289–325.

Davidson, J. R. T., Foa, E. B., Huppert, J. D., Keefe, F. J., Franklin, M. E., Compton, J. S., et al. (2004). Fluoxetine, comprehensive cognitive behavioral therapy, and placebo in generalized social phobia. *Archives of General Psychiatry, 61*(10), 1005–1013.

Davis, M., Myers, K. M., Ressler, K. J., & Rothbaum, B. O. (2005). Facilitation of Extinction of Conditioned Fear by D-Cycloserine: Implications for Psychotherapy. *Current Directions in Psychological Science, 14*(4), 214–219.

de Beurs, D., van Balkom, A. J. L. M., Lange, A., Koele, P., & van Dyck, R. (1995). Treatment of panic disorder with agoraphobia: Comparison of fluvoxamine, placebo, and psychological panic management combined with exposure and of exposure in vivo alone. *American Journal of Psychiatry, 152*(5), 683–691.

de Jong, P. J., Andrea, H., & Muris, P. (1997). Spider phobia in children: Disgust and fear before and after treatment. *Behaviour Research and Therapy, 35*(6), 559–562.

de Jong, P. J., & Muris, P. (2002). Spider phobia: Interaction of disgust and perceived likelihood of involuntary physical contact. *Journal of Anxiety Disorders, 16,* 51–65.

Depla, M. F. I. A., ten Have, M. L., van Balkom, A. J. L. M., & de Graaf, R. (2008). Specific fears and phobias in the general population: Results from the Netherlands mental health survey and incidence study (NEMESIS). *Social Psychiatry and Psychiatric Epidemiology, 43*(3), 200–208.

Drug Reference for FDA Approved Psychiatric Drugs. (2008). Retrieved April, 2009, from *www. neurotransmitter.net/drug_reference.html.*

Eaton, W. W., Dryman, A., & Weissman, M. M. (1991). Panic and phobia. In L. N. Robin & D. A. Regier (Eds.), *Psychiatric disorders in America* (pp. 155–179). New York: Free Press.

Eaton, W. W., Kessler, R. C., Wittchen, H. U., & Magee, W. J. (1994). Panic and panic disorder in the United States. *American Journal of Psychiatry, 151*(3), 413–420.

Eley, T. C., & Stevenson, J. (2000). Specific life events and chronic experiences differentially associated with depression and anxiety in young twins. *Journal of Abnormal Child Psychology, 28,* 383–394.

Essau, C. A., Conradt, J., & Petermann, F. (2000). Frequency, comorbidity, and psychosocial impairment of anxiety disorders in German adolescents. *Journal of Anxiety Disorders, 14,* 263–279.

Evans, L., Holt, C., & Oei, T. P. S. (1991). Long term follow-up of agoraphobics treated by brief intensive group cognitive behaviour therapy. *Australian and New Zealand Journal of Psychiatry, 25,* 343–349.

Falloon, I. R. H., Lloyd, G. G., & Harpin, R. E. (1981). The treatment of social phobia: Real-life rehearsal with non-professional therapists. *Journal of Nervous and Mental Disease, 169,* 180–184.

Faravelli, C., & Pallanti, S. (1989). Recent life events and panic disorder. *American Journal of Psychiatry, 146*(5), 622–626.

Federoff, I. C., & Taylor, S. (2001). Psychological and pharmacological treatments of social phobia: A meta-analysis. *Journal of Clinical Psychopharmacology, 21,* 311–324.

Feske, U., & Chambless, D. L. (1995). Cognitive behavioral versus exposure only treatment for social phobia: A meta-analysis. *Behavior Therapy, 26,* 695–720.

Flint, A. J. (1994). Epidemiology and comorbidity of anxiety disorders in the elderly. *American Journal of Psychiatry, 151*(5), 640–649.

Foa, E. B., & Kozak, M. J. (1986). Emotional processing of fear: Exposure to corrective information. *Psychological Bulletin, 99*(1), 20–35.

Fredrikson, M., Annas, P., Fischer, H., & Wik, G. (1996). Gender and age differences in the prevalence of specific fears and phobias. *Behaviour Research and Therapy, 34*(1), 33–39.

Furmark, T. (2002). Social phobia: Overview of community surveys. *Acta Psychiatrica Scandinavica, 105*(2), 84–93.

Furukawa, T. A., Watanabe, N., & Churchill, R. (2006). Psychotherapy plus antidepressant for panic disorder with or without agoraphobia: systematic review. *British Journal of Psychiatry, 188,* 305–312.

Goisman, R. M., Warshaw, M. G., & Keller, M. B. (1999). Psychosocial treatment prescriptions for generalized anxiety disorder, panic disorder, and social phobia, 1991–1996. *American Journal of Psychiatry, 156*(11), 1819–1821.

Goldfried, M. R., & Davila, J. (2005). The role of relationship and technique in therapeutic change. *Psychotherapy: Theory, Research, Practice and Training, 42,* 421–430.

Goldfried, M. R., & Davison, G. C. (1976). *Clinical behavior therapy.* New York: Holt, Rinehart & Winston.

Goldfried, M. R., Padawer, W., & Robins, C. (1984). Social anxiety and the semantic structure of heterosocial interactions. *Journal of Abnormal Psychology, 93,* 87–97.

Goldstein, A. J., & Chambless, D. L. (1978). A reanalysis of agoraphobia. *Behavior Therapy, 9,* 47–59.

Goldstein, A. J., & Chambless, D. L. (Eds.). (1982). *Agoraphobia.* New York: Wiley.

Goodwin, R. D., Fergusson, D. M., & Horwood, L. J. (2004). Childhood abuse and familial violence and the risk of panic attacks and panic disorder in young adulthood. *Psychological Medicine, 35,* 881–890.

Gould, R. A., Buckminster, S., Pollack, M. H., Otto, M. W., & Yap, L. (1997). Cognitive-behavioral and pharmacological treatment for social phobia: A meta-analysis. *Clinical Psychology: Science and Practice, 4*(4), 291–306.

Gould, R. A., Otto, M. W., & Pollack, M. H. (1995). A meta-analysis of treatment outcome for panic disorder. *Clinical Psychology Review, 15*(8), 819–844.

Grant, B. F., Hasin, D. S., Stinson, F. S., Dawson, D. A., Chou, S. P., Ruan, W. J., et al. (2005). Co-occurrence of 12–month mood and anxiety disorders and personality disorders in the US: Results from the national epidemiologic survey on alcohol and related conditions. *Journal of Psychiatric Research, 39*(1), 1–9.

Gray, J. A., & McNaughton, N. (1996). The neuropsychology of anxiety: Reprise. In D. A. Hope (Ed.), *Nebraska Symposium on Motivation, 1995: Perspectives on anxiety, panic, and fear* (pp. 61–134). Lincoln: University of Nebraska Press.

Harris, E. C., & Barraclough, B. (1997). Suicide as an outcome for mental disorders: A meta-analysis. *British Journal of Psychiatry, 170*(3), 205–228.

Haug, T. T., Blomhoff, S., Hellstrom, K., Holme, I., Humble, M., Madsbu, H. P., et al. (2003). Exposure therapy and sertraline in social phobia: 1–year follow-up of a randomised controlled trial. *British Journal of Psychiatry, 182,* 312–318.

Hayward, C., Killen, J. D., Hammer, L. D., & Litt, I. F., Wilson, D. M., Simmonds, B., et al. (1992). Pubertal stage and panic attack history in sixth- and seventh-grade girls. *American Journal of Psychiatry, 149*(9), 1239–1243.

Heimberg, R. G., & Becker, R. E. (2002). *Cognitive-behavioral group therapy for social phobia: Basic mechanisms and clinical strategies*. New York: Guilford Press.

Heimberg, R. G., Holt, C. S., Schneier, F. R., Spitzer, R. L., & Liebowitz, M. R. (1993). The issue of subtypes in the diagnosis of social phobia. *Journal of Anxiety Disorders, 7*(3), 249–269.

Heimberg, R. G., Liebowitz, M. R., Hope, D. A., Schneier, F. R., Holt, C. S., Welkowitz, L., et al. (1998). Cognitive-behavioral group therapy versus phenelzine in social phobia: 12-week outcome. *Archives of General Psychiatry, 55*, 1133–1141.

Heimberg, R. G., Sweet, R. A., & Holt, C. S. (1995). Alcohol and caffeine use by social phobics: An initial inquiry into drinking patterns and behavior. *Behaviour Research and Therapy, 33*(5), 561–566.

Hertel, P. T., & Mathews, A. (2011). Cognitive bias modification: Past perspectives, current findings, and future applications. *Perspectives on Psychological Science, 6*(6) 521–536.

Heuzenroeder, L., Donnelly, M., Haby, M. M., Mihalopoulos, C., Rossell, R., Carter, R., et al. (2004). Cost-effectiveness of psychological a pharmacological interventions for generalized anxiety disorder and panic disorder. *Australian and New Zealand Journal of Psychiatry, 38*(8), 602–612.

Hinton, D., Hinton, S., Pham, T., Chau, H., & Tran, M. (2003). "Hit by the wind" and temperature-shift panic among Vietnamese refugees. *Transcultural Psychiatry, 40*, 342–376.

Hirshfeld, D. R., Rosenbaum, J. F., Biederman, J., Bolduc, E. A., Faraone, S. V., Snidman, N., et al. (1992). Stable behavioral inhibition and its association with anxiety disorder. *Journal of the American Academy of Child and Adolescent Psychiatry, 31*, 103–111.

Holle, C., Heimberg, R. G., Sweet, R. A., & Holt, C. S. (1995). Alcohol and caffeine use by social phobics: An initial inquiry into drinking patterns and behavior. *Behaviour Research and Therapy, 33*, 561–566.

Horwath, E., Lish, J. D., Johnson, J., Hornig, C. D., & Weissman, M. M. (1993). Agoraphobia without panic: Clinical reappraisal of an epidemiologic finding. *American Journal of Psychiatry, 150*(10), 1496–1501.

Huppert, J. D., Bufka, L. F., Barlow, D. H., Gorman, J. M., Shear, M. K., & Woods, S. W. (2001). Therapists, therapist variables, and cognitive-behavioral therapy outcome in a multicenter trial for panic disorder. *Journal of Consulting and Clinical Psychology, 69*, 747–755.

Kampman, M., Keijsers, G. P. L., Hoogduin, C. A. L., & Hendriks, G.-J. (2002). A randomized, double-blind, placebo controlled study of the effects of adjunctive paroxetine in panic disorder patients unsuccessfully treated with cognitive-behavioral therapy alone. *Journal of Clinical Psychiatry, 63*(9), 772–777.

Karno, M., Golding, J. M., Burnam, M. A., & Hough, R. L. (1989). Anxiety disorders among Mexican Americans and non-Hispanic Whites in Los Angeles. *Journal of Nervous and Mental Disease, 177*(4), 202–209.

Katschnig, H., Amering, M., Stolk, J. M., & Ballenger, J. C. (1996). Predictors of quality of life in a long-term followup study in panic disorder patients after a clinical drug trial. *Psychopharmacology Bulletin, 32*, 149–155.

Kearney, C. A., Albano, A. M., Eisen, A. R., Atlan, W. D., & Barlow, D. H. (1997). The phenomenology of panic disorder in youngsters: An empirical study of a clinical sample. *Journal of Anxiety Disorders, 11*(1), 49–62.

Keller, M. B., Yonkers, K. A., Warshaw, M. G., Pratt, L. A., Gollan, J. K., Massion, A. O., et al. (1994). Remission and relapse in subjects with panic disorder and panic with agoraphobia: A prospective short interval naturalistic follow-up. *Journal of Nervous and Mental Disease, 182*(5), 290–296.

Kendler, K. S., Karkowski, L. M., & Prescott, C. A. (1999). Fears and phobias: Reliability and heritability. *Psychological Medicine, 29*, 539–553.

Kessler, R. C., Berglund, P., Demler, O., Jin, R., Merikangas, K. R., & Walters, E. E. (2005). Lifetime prevalence and age-of-onset distributions of DSM-IV disorders in the National Comorbidity Survey Replication. *Archives of General Psychiatry, 62*(6), 593–602.

Kessler, R. C., Chiu, W. T., Jin, R., Ruscio, A. M., Shear, K., & Walters, E. E. (2006). The epidemiology of panic attacks, panic disorder, and agoraphobia in the National Comorbidity Survey Replication. *Archives of General Psychiatry, 63*, 415–424.

Kessler, R. C., McGonagle, K. A., Zhao, S., Nelson, C. B., Hughes, M., Eshleman, S., et al. (1994). Lifetime and 12-month prevalence of DSM-III-R psychiatric disorders in the United States: Results from the National Comorbidity Survey. *Archives of General Psychiatry, 51*, 8–19.

Kessler, R. C., Stein, M. B., & Berglund, P. (1998). Social phobia subtypes in the National Comorbidity Survey. *American Journal of Psychiatry, 155*(5), 613–619.

Kimbrel, N. A. (2008). A model of the development and maintenance of generalized social phobia. *Clinical Psychology Review, 28*, 592–612.

King, N. J., Gullone, E., Tonge, B. J., & Ollendick, T. M. (1993). Self-reports of panic attacks and manifest anxiety in adolescents. *Behaviour Research and Therapy, 31*, 111–116.

Klein, D. F. (1993). False suffocation alarms, spontaneous panics, and related conditions: An integrative hypothesis. *Archives of General Psychiatry, 50*, 306–317.

Klerman, G. L., Weissman, M. M., Ouellette, R., Johnson, J., & Greenwald, S. (1991). Panic attacks in the community: Social morbidity and health care utilization. *Journal of the American Medical Association, 265*, 742–746.

Kushner, M. G., Abrams, K., & Borchardt, C. (2000). The relationship between anxiety disorders and alcohol use disorders: A review of major perspectives and findings. *Clinical Psychology Review, 20*(2), 149–171.

Landau, R. J. (1980). The role of semantic schemata in phobic word interpretation. *Cognitive Therapy and Research, 4*, 427–434.

Landy, F. J., & Gaupp, L. A. (1971). A factor analysis of the Fear Survey Schedule–III. *Behaviour Research and Therapy, 9*(2), 89–93.

Lang, P. J. (1985). The cognitive physiology of emotion: Fear and anxiety. In A. H. Tuma & J. D. Maser (Eds.), *Anxiety and the anxiety disorders* (pp. 131–170). Hillsdale, NJ: Erlbaum.

Lang, P. J., Cuthbert, B. N., & Bradley, M. M. (1998). Measuring emotion in therapy: Imagery, activation, and feeling. *Behavior Therapy*, 655–674.

Lewis-Fernandez, R., Guarnaccia, P. J., Martinez, I. E., Salman, E., Schmidt, A., & Liebowitz, M. (2002). Comparative phenomenology of *ataques de nervios*, panic attacks, and panic disorder. *Culture, Medicine and Psychiatry, 26*, 199–223.

Lidren, D. M., Watkins, P. L., Gould, R. A., Clum, G. A., Asterino, M., & Tulloch, H. L. (1994). A comparison of bibliotherapy and group therapy in the treatment of panic disorder. *Journal of Consulting and Clinical Psychology, 62*, 865–869.

Liebowitz, M., Gorman, J., Fyer, A., Levitt, M., Dillon, D., Levy, G., et al. (1985). Lactate provocation of panic attacks: Clinical and behavioral findings. *Archives of General Psychiatry, 41*, 764–770.

Liebowitz, M. R., Heimberg, R. G., Schneier, F. R., Hope, D. A., Davies, S., Holt, C. S., et al. (1999). Cognitive-behavioral group therapy versus phenelzine in social phobia: Long-term outcome. *Depression and Anxiety, 10*, 89–98.

Lilienfeld, S. O. (2007). Psychological treatments that cause harm. *Perspectives on Psychological Science, 2*, 53–70.

Lohr, J. M., Tolin, D. F., & Lilienfield, S. O. (1998). Efficacy of eye movement desensitization and reprocessing: Implications for behavior therapy. *Behavior Therapy, 29*(1), 123–156.

Luten, A., Ralph, J. A., & Mineka, S. (1997). Pessimistic attributional style: Is it specific to depression versus anxiety versus negative affect? *Behaviour Research and Therapy, 35*(8), 703–719.

MacLeod, C., & Hagan, R. (1992). Individual differences in the selective processing of threatening information, and emotional responses to a stressful life event. *Behaviour Research and Therapy, 30,* 151–161.

Magee, W. J., Eaton, W. W., Wittchen, H., McGonagle, K. A., & Kessler, R. C. (1996). Agoraphobia, simple phobia, and social phobia in the National Comorbidity Survey. *Archives of General Psychiatry, 53,* 159–168.

Markowitz, J. S., Weissman, M. M., Ouellette, R., Lish, J. D., & Klerman, G. L. (1989). Quality of life in panic disorder. *Archives of General Psychiatry, 46,* 984–992.

Massion, A. O., Dyck, I. R., Shea, M. T., Phillips, K. A., Warshaw, M. G., & Keller, M. B. (2002). Personality disorders and time to remission in generalized anxiety disorder, social phobia, and panic disorder. *Archives of General Psychiatry, 59,* 434–440.

Matchett, G., & Davey, G. C. L. (1991). A test of a disease avoidance model of animal phobias. *Behaviour Research and Therapy, 29,* 91–94.

Mathews, A., & MacLeod, C. (2005). Cognitive vulnerability to emotional disorders. *Annual Review of Clinical Psychology, 1,* 167–195.

Mattick, R. P., Peters, L., & Clarke, J. C. (1989). Exposure and cognitive restructuring of social phobia: A controlled study. *Behavior Therapy, 20*(1), 3–23.

Mavissakalian, M. (1990). The relationship between panic disorder/agoraphobia and personality disorders. *Psychiatric Clinics of North America, 13,* 661–684.

McNally, R. J. (1987). Preparedness and phobias: A review. *Psychological Bulletin, 101,* 283–303.

Miller, W., & Rollnick, S. (2002). *Motivational interviewing: Preparing people for change* (2nd ed.). New York: Guilford Press.

Milrod, B., Leon, A. C., Busch, F., Rudden, M., Schwalberg, M., Clarkin, J., et al. (2007). A randomized controlled clinical trial of psychoanalytic psychotherapy for panic disorder. *American Journal of Psychiatry, 164*(2), 265–272.

Mineka, S., & Cook, M. (1986). Immunization against the observational conditioning of snake fear in rhesus monkeys. *Journal of Abnormal Psychology, 95,* 307–318.

Mineka, S., & Zinbarg, R. (2006). A contemporary learning theory perspective on the etiology of anxiety disorders: It's not what you thought it was. *American Psychologist, 61*(1), 10–26.

Mollema, E. D., Snoek, F. J., Ader, H. J., Heine, R. J., & van der Ploeg, H. M. (2001). Insulin-treated diabetes patients with fear of self-injecting or fear of self-testing: Psychological comorbidity and general well-being. *Journal of Psychosomatic Research, 51,* 665–672.

Moran, C. C. (1986). Depersonalization and agoraphobia associated with marijuana use. *British Journal of Medical Psychology, 59*(2), 187–196.

Morin, C. M., Savard, J., & Blais, F. (2000). Cognitive therapy of late-life insomnia. In K. Lichstein & C. M. Morin (Eds.), *Treatment of late-life insomnia* (pp. 207–230). Oakland, CA: Sage.

Moscovitch, D. A., McCabe, R. E., Antony, M. M., Rocca, L., & Swinson, R. P. (2008). Anger experience and expression across the anxiety disorders. *Depression and Anxiety, 25*(2), 107–113.

Moses, E. B., & Barlow, D. H. (2006). A new unified treatment approach for emotional disorders based on emotion science. *Current Directions in Psychological Science, 15,* 146–150.

Mowrer, O. H. (1947). On the dual nature of learning: A reinterpretation of "conditioning" and "problem solving. " *Harvard Educational Review, 17,* 102–148.

Mulkens, S. A. N., de Jong, P. J., & Merckelbach, H. (1996). Disgust and spider phobia. *Journal of Abnormal Psychology, 105*(3), 464–468.

Muris, P., Merckelbach, H., Holdrinet, I., & Sijsenaar, M. (1998). Treating phobic children: Effects of EMDR versus exposure. *Journal of Consulting and Clinical Psychology, 66*(1), 193–198.

Murphy, R., Hirsch, C., Mathews, A., Smith, K., & Clark, D. M. (2007). Facilitating a benign interpretation bias in a high socially anxious population. *Behaviour Research and Therapy, 45,* 1517–1529.

Neal, A. M., Lilly, R. S., & Zakis, S. (1993). What are African American children afraid of?: A preliminary study. *Journal of Anxiety Disorders, 7*(2), 129–139.

Neal, A. M., & Turner, S. M. (1991). Anxiety disorders research with African Americans: Current status. *Psychological Bulletin, 109*, 400–410.

Newman, M. G., Kenardy, J., Herman, S., & Taylor, C. B. (1997). Comparison of palmtop-computer-assisted brief cognitive-behavioral treatment to cognitive-behavioral treatment for panic disorder. *Journal of Consulting and Clinical Psychology, 65*, 178–183.

Newman, M. G., & Stiles, W. B., Janeck, A., & Woody, S. R. (2005). Techniques factors in treating anxiety disorders. In L. G. Castonguay, & L. E. Beutler (Eds.), *Principles of therapeutic change that work* (pp. 187–200). New York: Oxford University Press.

Nolen-Hoeksema, S., & Girgus, J. S. (1994). The emergence of gender differences in depression during adolescence. *Psychological Bulletin, 115*, 424–443.

Olatunji, B. O., Forsyth, J. P., & Cherian, A. (2007). Evaluative conditioning of disgust: A sticky form of relational learning that is resistant to extinction. *Journal of Anxiety Disorders, 21*, 820–834.

Olatunji, B. O., & McKay, D. (2009). *Disorders of disgust: Assessment, theory, and treatment.* Washington, DC: American Psychological Association.

Ollendick, T. H., King, N. J., & Muris, P. (2002). Fears and phobias in children: Phenomenology, epidemiology, and aetiology. *Child and Adolescent Mental Health, 7*(3), 98–106.

Öst, L. G. (1987). Age of onset in different phobias. *Journal of Abnormal Psychology, 96*(3), 233–229.

Öst, L. G. (1992). Blood and injection phobia: Background and cognitive, physiological, and behavioral variables. *Journal of Abnormal Psychology, 101*(1), 68–74.

Öst, L. G., Alm, T., Brandberg, M., & Breitholtz, E. (2001). One vs five sessions of exposure and five sessions of cognitive therapy in the treatment of claustrophobia. *Behaviour Research and Therapy, 39*(2), 167–183.

Öst, L. G., Fellenius, J., & Sterner, U. (1991). Applied tension, exposure *in vivo*, and tension-only in the treatment of blood phobia. *Behaviour Research and Therapy, 29*(6), 561–574.

Öst, L. G., Ferebee, I., & Furmark, T. (1997). One-session group therapy of spider phobia: Direct versus indirect treatments. *Behaviour Research and Therapy, 35*(8), 721–732.

Otto, M. W., Pollack, M. H., Penava, S. J., & Zucker, B. G. (1999). Group cognitive-behavior therapy for patients failing to respond to pharmacotherapy for panic disorder: A clinical case series. *Behaviour Research and Therapy, 37*, 763–770.

Otto, M. W., Pollack, M. H., & Sabatino, S. A. (1996). Maintenance of remission following cognitive behavior therapy for panic disorder: Possible deleterious effects of concurrent medication treatment. *Behavior Therapy, 27*, 473–482.

Pachankis, J. E., & Goldfried, M. R. (2006). Social anxiety in young gay men. *Journal of Anxiety Disorders, 20*, 996–1015.

Pachankis, J. E., Goldfried, M. R., & Ramrattan, M. E. (2008). Extension of the rejection sensitivity construct to the interpersonal functioning of gay men. *Journal of Consulting and Clinical Psychology, 76*, 306–317.

Page, A. C. (1994). Blood–injury phobia. *Clinical Psychology Review, 14*(5), 443–461.

Page, A. C., & Martin, N. G. (1998). Testing a genetic structure of blood–injury–injection fears. *American Journal of Medical Genetics, 81*, 377–384.

Palmer, B. W., Jeste, D. V., & Sheikh, J. I. (1997). Anxiety disorders in the elderly: DSM-IV and other barriers to diagnosis and treatment. *Journal of Affective Disorders, 46*, 183–190.

Paradis, C. M., Friedman, S., Lazar, R. M., Grubea, J., & Kesselman, M. (1992). Use of a structured interview to diagnosis anxiety disorders in a minority population. *Hospital and Community Psychiatry, 43*, 61–64.

Pierce, K. A., & Kirkpatrick, D. R. (1992). Do men lie on fear surveys? *Behaviour Research and Therapy, 30*(4), 415–418.

Plomin, R., DeFries, J. C., McClearn, G. E., & Rutter, M. (1997). *Behavioral genetics: A primer* (3rd ed.). New York: Freeman.

Pollack, M. H., Simon, N. M., Worthington, J. J., Doyle, A. L., Peters, P., Toshkov, F., et al. (2003). Combined paroxetine and clonazepam treatment strategies compared to paroxetine mono-therapy for panic disorder. *Journal of Psychopharmacology, 17,* 276–282.

Rachman. S. J. (1977). The conditioning theory of fear acquisition: A critical examination. *Behaviour Research and Therapy, 14,* 125–131.

Rachman, S. J. (1990). *Fear and courage* (2nd ed.). New York: Freeman.

Rachman, S. J. (1994). The overprediction of fear: A review. *Behaviour Research and Therapy, 32,* 683–690.

Rapee, R. M. (1995). Descriptive psychopathology of social phobia. In R. G. Heimberg, M. R. Liebowitz, D. A. Hope, & F. R. Schneier (Eds.), *Social phobia: Diagnosis, assessment, and treatment* (pp. 41–66). New York: Guilford Press.

Rapee, R. M., & Heimberg, R. G. (1997). A cognitive-behavioral model of anxiety in social phobia. *Behaviour Research and Therapy, 35,* 741–756.

Rapee, R. M., & Lim, L. (1992). Discrepancy between self- and observer ratings of performance in social phobics. *Journal of Abnormal Psychology, 101*(4), 728–731.

Rapee, R. M., & Spence, S. H. (2004). The etiology of social phobia: Empirical evidence and an initial model. *Clinical Psychology Review, 24,* 737–767.

Ratcliffe, D., MacLeod, A., & Sensky, T. (2006). Anxiety in patients who have had a myocardial infarction: The maintaining role of perceived physical sensations and causal attributions. *Behavioural and Cognitive Psychotherapy, 34*(2), 201–217.

Regier, D. A., Myers, J. K., Kramer, M., Robins, L. N., Blazer, D. G., Hough, R. L., et al. (1984). The NIMH Epidemiologic Catchment Area program: Historical context, major objectives, and study population characteristics. *Archives of General Psychiatry, 41,* 934–941.

Reich, J. (2001). The relationship of social phobia to avoidant personality disorder. In S. G. Hofmann & P. M. DiBartolo (Eds.), *From social anxiety to social phobia: Multiple perspectives* (pp. 148–161). Boston: Allyn & Bacon.

Reich, J., & Troughton, E. (1988). Frequency of DSM-III personality disorders in patients with panic disorder: Comparison with psychiatric and normal control subjects. *Psychiatry Research, 26,* 89–100.

Ressler, K. J., Rothbaum, B. O., Tannenbaum, L., Anderson, P., Graap, K., Zimand, E., et al. (2004). Cognitive enhancers as adjuncts to psychotherapy: Use of D-cycloserine in phobic individuals to facilitate extinction of fear. *Archives of General Psychiatry, 61*(11), 1136–1144.

Rodebaugh, T. L., Holaway, R. M., & Heimberg, R. G. (2004). The treatment of social anxiety disorder. *Clinical Psychology Review, 24,* 883–908.

Rogers, M., White, K., Warshaw, M., Yonkers, K., Rodriguez-Villa, F., Chang, G., et al. (1994). Prevalence of medical illness in patients with anxiety disorders. *International Journal of Psychiatry in Medicine, 24*(1), 83–96.

Romano, E., Tremblay, R. E., Vitaro, F., Zoccolillo, M., & Pagani, L. (2001). Prevalence of psychiatric diagnoses and the role of perceived impairment: findings from an adolescent community sample. *Journal of Child Psychology and Psychiatry and Allied Disciplines, 42*(4), 451–461.

Rowa, K., McCabe, R. I., & Antony, M. M. (2006). Specific phobias. In F. Andrasik (Ed.), *Comprehensive handbook of personality and psychopathology: Vol. 2. Adult psychopathology* (pp. 154–168). Hoboken, NJ: Wiley.

Roy-Byrne, P. P., & Cowley, D. S. (1995). Course and outcome in panic disorder: A review of recent follow-up studies. *Anxiety, 1,* 150–160.

Roy-Byrne, P. P., Stang, P., Wittchen, H. U., Ustun, B., Walters, E. E., & Kessler, R. C. (2000). Lifetime panic-depression comorbidity in the National Comorbidity Survey: Association with symptoms, impairment, course and help-seeking. *British Journal of Psychiatry, 176,* 229–235.

Safren, S. A., Heimberg, R. G., Brown, E. J., & Holle, C. (1997). Quality of life in social phobia. *Depression and Anxiety, 4,* 126–133.

Sansone, R. A., Griffith, K. A., & Sansone, L. A. (2005). Panic disorder, alcohol and substance abuse, and benzodiazepine prescription primary care companion. *Journal of Clinical Psychiatry, 7*(5), 246–248.

Schmidt, N. B., Lerew, D. R., & Jackson, R. J. (1997). The role of anxiety sensitivity in the pathogenesis of panic: Prospective evaluation of spontaneous panic attacks during acute stress. *Journal of Abnormal Psychology, 106*(3), 355–364.

Schwartz, C. E., Snidman, N., & Kagan, J. (1999). Adolescent social anxiety as an outcome of inhibited temperment in childhood. *Journal of the American Academy of Child and Adolescent Psychiatry, 38*(8), 1008–1015.

Seligman, M. E. P. (1971). Phobias and preparedness. *Behavior Therapy, 2,* 307–320.

Shear, M. K., Houck, P., Greeno, C., & Masters, S. (2001). Emotion-focused psychotherapy for patients with panic disorder. *American Journal of Psychiatry, 158*(12), 1993–1998.

Simon, N. M., Otto, M. W., Wisniewski, S. R., Fossey, M., Sagduyu, K., Frank, E., et al. (2004). Anxiety disorder comorbidity in bipolar disorder patients: Data from the first 500 participants in the Systematic Treatment Enhancement Program for Bipolar Disorder (STEP-BD). *American Journal of Psychiatry, 161,* 2222–2229.

Smith, L. C., Friedman, S., & Nevid, J. (1999). Clinical and sociocultural differences in African Americans and European American patients with panic disorder and agoraphobia. *Journal of Nervous and Mental Disease, 187,* 549–561.

Starcevic, V. (2005). *Anxiety disorders in adults: A clinical guide* (pp. 191–215). New York: Oxford University Press.

Stein, D. J., & Hugo, F. (2002). Neuropsychiatric aspects of anxiety disorders. In S. C. Yudofsky & R. E. Hales (Eds.), *The American Psychiatric Publishing textbook of neuropsychiatry and clinical neurosciences* (pp. 1049–1068). Washington, DC: American Psychiatric Publishing.

Stein, M. B., Sherbourne, C. D., Craske, M. G., Means-Christensen, A., Bystritsky, A., Katon, W., et al. (2004). Quality of care for primary care patients with anxiety disorders. *American Journal of Psychiatry, 161,* 2230–2237.

Stopa, L., & Clark, D. M. (1993). Cognitive processes in social phobia. *Behaviour Research* Therapy, *31*(3), 255–267.

Suomi, S. J. (2000). A biobehavioral perspective on developmental psychopathology. In A. J. Sameroff, M. Lewis, & S. M. Miller (Eds.), *Handbook of developmental psychopathology* (pp. 237–256). New York: Kluwer Academic/Plenum.

Sylvester, C. E., Hyde, T. S., & Reichler, R. J. (1988). Clinical psychopathology among children of adults with panic disorder. In D. L. Dunner, E. S. Gershon, & J. E. Barrett (Eds.), *Relatives at risk for mental disorders* (pp. 87–102). New York: Raven Press.

Teachman, B. A., & Gordon, T. G. (2009). Age differences in anxious responding: Older and calmer, unless the trigger is physical. *Psychology and Aging, 24,* 703–714.

Teachman, B. A., Stefanucci, J. K., Clerkin, E. M., Cody, M. W., & Proffitt, D. R. (2008). A new mode of fear expression: Perceptual bias in height fear. *Emotion, 8,* 296–301.

Teachman, B. A., & Woody, S. (2003). Automatic processing among individuals with spider phobia: Change in implicit fear associations following treatment. *Journal of Abnormal Psychology, 112,* 100–109.

Thorpe, S. J., & Salkovskis, P. M. (1998). Studies on the role of disgust in the acquisition and maintenance of specific phobias. *Behaviour Research and Therapy, 36*(9), 877–893.

Torgersen, S. (1983). Genetic factors in anxiety disorders. *Archives of General Psychiatry, 40*(10), 1085–1089.

Trower, P., Bryant, B., & Argyle, M. (1978). *Social skills and mental health*. London: Methuen.

Tsao, J. C. I., Mystkowski, J. L., Zucker, B. G., & Craske, M. G. (2005). Impact of cognitive-behavioral therapy for panic disorder on comorbidity: A controlled investigation. *Behaviour Research and Therapy, 43*, 959–970.

Turk, C. L., Heimberg, R. G., & Hope, D. A. (2001). Social anxiety disorder. In D. H. Barlow (Ed.), *Clinical handbook of psychological disorders: A step-by-step treatment manual* (3rd ed., pp. 114–153). New York: Guilford Press.

Turk, C. L., Heimberg, R. G., Orsillo, S. M., Holt, C. S., Gitow, A., Street, L. L., et al. (1998). An investigation of gender differences in social phobia. *Journal of Anxiety Disorders, 12*, 209–223.

Turner, S. M., Beidel, D. C., & Costello, A. (1987). Psychopathology in the offspring of anxiety disorders parents. *Journal of Consulting and Clinical Psychology, 55*, 229–235.

Turner, S. M., Beidel, D. C., & Townsley, R. M. (1990). Social phobia: Relationship to shyness. *Behaviour Research and Therapy, 28*(6), 497–505.

Tyrer, P., Seivewright, H., & Johnson, T. (2004). The Nottingham Study of Neurotic Disorder: Predictors of 12-year outcome of dysthymic, panic and generalized anxiety disorder. *Psychological Medicine, 34*, 1385–1394.

Uhde, T. W., & Singareddy, R. (2002). Biological research in anxiety disorders. In J. J. López-Ibor, W. Gaebel, M. Maj, & N. Sartorius (Eds.), *Psychiatry as a neuroscience* (pp. 237–285). New York: Wiley.

van Balkom, A. J., Beekman, A. T., de Beurs, E., Deeg, D. J., van Dyck, R., & van Tilburg, W. (2000). Comorbidity of the anxiety disorders in a community-based older population in The Netherlands. *Acta Psychiatrica Scandinavica, 101*, 37–45.

van den Hout, M., Tenney, N., Huygens, K., & de Jong, P. (1997). Preconscious processing bias in specific phobia. *Behaviour Research and Therapy, 35*(1), 29–34.

Vriends, N., Becker, E. S., Meyer, A., Williams, S. L., Lutz, R., & Margraf, J. (2007). Recovery from social phobia in the community and its predictors: Data from a longitudinal epidemiological study. *Journal of Anxiety Disorders, 21*, 320–337.

Wallace, S. T., & Alden, L. E. (1997). Social phobia and positive social events: The price of success. *Journal of Abnormal Psychology, 106*(3), 416–424.

Watson, D., Clark, L. A., Weber, K., Assenheimer, J. S., Strauss, M. E., & McCormick, R. A. (1995). Testing a tripartite model: II. Exploring the symptom structure of anxiety and depression in student, adult, and patient samples. *Journal of Abnormal Psychology, 104*, 15–25.

Watts, F. N., McKenna, F. P., Sharrock, R., & Trezise, L. (1986). Colour naming of phobia-related words. *British Journal of Psychology, 77*, 97–108.

Website on Research-Supported Psychological Treatments. (2008). Society of Clinical Psychology, American Psychological Association, Division 12. Retrieved April, 2009, from *www.psychology.sunysb.edu/eklonsky-/division12/index.html*.

Weissman, M. M. (1993). Family genetic studies of panic disorder. *Journal of Psychiatric Research, 27*(Suppl.), 69–78.

Weissman, M. M., Bland, R. C., Canino, G. J., Faravelli, C., Greenwald, S., Hwu, H. G., et al. (1997). The cross-national epidemiology of panic disorder. *Archives of General Psychiatry, 54*(4), 305–309.

Weissman, M. M., Bland, R. C., Canino, G. J., Greenwald, S., Lee, C.-K., Newman, S. C., et al. (1996). The cross-national epidemiology of social phobia: A preliminary report. *International Clinical Psychopharmacology, 11*, 9–14.

Weissman, M. M., Klerman, G. L., Markowitz, J. S., & Ouellette, R. (1989). Suicidal ideation and suicide attempts in panic disorder and attacks. *New England Journal of Medicine 321*(18), 1209–1214.

Williams, J. M. G., Watts, F. N., MacLeod, C., & Mathews, A. (1997). *Cognitive psychology and emotional disorders* (2nd ed.). Chichester, UK: Wiley.

Wittchen, H. U., & Essau, C. A. (1991). The epidemiology of panic attacks, panic disorder, and agoraphobia. In J. R. Walker, G. R. Norton, & C. A. Ross (Eds.), *Panic disorder and agoraphobia: A comprehensive guide for the practitioner* (pp. 103–149). Belmont, CA: Thomson Brooks/Cole.

Wittchen, H. U., Essau, C. A., Von Zerssen, D., Krieg, J. C., & Zaudig, M. (1992). Lifetime and six-month prevalence of mental disorders in the Munich Follow-Up Study. *European Archives of Psychiatry and Clinical Neuroscience, 241*(4), 247–258.

Wittchen, H. U., Stein, M. B., & Kessler, R. C. (1999). Social fears and social phobia in a community sample of adolescents and young adults: Prevalence, risk factors and co-morbidity. *Psychological Medicine, 29*, 309–323.

Wolitzky-Taylor, K. B., Horowitz, J. D., Powers, M. P., & Telch, M. J. (2008). Psychological approaches in the treatment of specific phobias: A meta-analysis. *Clinical Psychology Review, 28*(6), 1021–1037.

Woody, S. R., & Ollendick, T. H. (2006). Technique factors in treating anxiety disorders. In L. G. Castonguay & L. E. Beutler (Eds.), *Principles of therapeutic change that work* (pp. 167–200). New York: Oxford University Press.

Woody, S., & Teachman, B. A. (2000). Intersection of disgust and fear: Normative and pathological views. *Clinical Psychology: Science and Practice, 7*, 291–311.

Yonkers, K. A., Zlotnick, C., Allsworth, J., Warshaw, M., Shea, T., & Keller, M. B. (1998). Is the course of panic disorder the same in men and women? *American Journal of Psychiatry, 155*, 596–602.

Zvolensky, M. J., Eifert, G. H., Lejuez, C. W., & McNeil, D. W. (1999). The effects offset control over 20% carbon dioxide–enriched air on anxious responding. *Journal of Abnormal Psychology, 108*, 624–632.

CHAPTER 5

Obsessive–Compulsive Disorder

Jonathan S. Abramowitz
Lynne Siqueland

Our goal in this chapter is to outline and discuss the psychopathology of obsessive–compulsive disorder (OCD), especially as it guides implementation of treatment of this often baffling disorder.

TYPICAL SYMPTOMS

OCD is characterized by two main symptoms: obsessions and compulsions (American Psychiatric Association, 2013). "Obsessions" are unwanted thoughts, ideas, images, or impulses that are experienced as repugnant, threatening, obscene, blasphemous, nonsensical, or all of these. The content of obsessions is highly individualized and shaped by the thinker's personal experiences, although the general themes of obsessions can be organized into several general categories: contamination, responsibility for harm, violence, sex, religion, and the need for order or exactness (e.g., Abramowitz et al., 2010; McKay et al., 2004). Most people with OCD evince multiple obsessional themes and forms, and the form and content of these may shift over time. Table 5.1 provides examples of common obsessions. Obsessions often evoke intense distress and impairment that result from avoidance of related situations. For example, someone with obsessions about hurting or killing family members (e.g., spouse, child) may avoid loved ones and experience depressive symptoms as a result.

Three characteristics set clinical obsessions apart from other types of repetitive thinking (e.g., worries, daydreams). First, obsessions are experienced as *unwanted* or *uncontrollable,* in that they *intrude* into consciousness (often triggered by something in the environment). Second, while personally relevant, the content of obsessions is

TABLE 5.1. Common Obsessions

Category	Examples
Contamination	• Concerns about getting AIDS from touching a bathroom door knob • Fear of getting cancer from using lawn fertilizer • Fear that "germs" will spread to others and make them ill • Fear of getting sick from touching dirty laundry
Responsibility for harm	• Thought that you've hit someone with your car without realizing • Doubts about whether the door is locked or the oven is turned off • Doubts about whether you dropped pills on the floor and a child thought they were candy and ate them
Symmetry/order	• The need to have the environment "balanced" on the left and right sides • Thoughts that a parent will die if the books aren't arranged in alphabetical order
Sexual	• Impulses to kiss one's boss • Thoughts of having sex with children or family members • Doubts regarding whether one is homosexual or heterosexual
Violence/aggression	• Impulses to harm loved ones • Thoughts of injuring a vulnerable person (small child or elderly)
Religious	• Blasphemous images of Jesus with an erection on the cross • Doubts about whether one is "faithful enough"

incongruent with the individual's belief system and is not the type of thought one would normally expect him- or herself to have. Third, obsessions are *resisted*; that is, they are accompanied by the sense that they must be "dealt with," neutralized, or altogether avoided. The motivation to resist is activated by the fear that if action is not taken, disastrous consequences may occur.

Compulsive rituals are the most noticeable feature of OCD and, in many instances, account for the most functional impairment. The DSM specifies that "compulsions" are motivated and intentional, in contrast to mechanical or robotic repetitive behaviors, as observed in disorders such as Tourette's. Moreover, compulsions are performed in response to obsessions and to reduce obsession-related distress. This is in contrast to repetitive behaviors in addictive or impulse control disorders (e.g., "sexual addiction," trichotillomania), which are carried out because they may produce pleasure or gratification. Examples of the most common compulsive rituals include washing and cleaning, checking and seeking reassurance, ordering and arranging, repeating routine behaviors (e.g., stepping through a doorway, flicking a light switch, getting up from a chair), and counting. Specific examples of common rituals are listed in Table 5.2.

In most instances, it is clear how compulsive rituals are intended to reduce obsessional anxiety about particular feared consequences—for example, compulsively checking the door locks to reduce fears of a break-in, or hand washing rituals

TABLE 5.2. Common Compulsive Rituals

Category	Examples
Decontamination	• Handwashing for 15 minutes at a time • Ritualized showering routines, including washing the shower itself • Wiping down mail and groceries before bringing them into the house • Demanding that others wash before touching items in the house
Checking	• Locks, windows, appliances, paperwork • That others are safe • Asking repeated questions of others to gain assurances
Repeating	• Going up and down the stairs several times until an unwanted thought is dismissed • Getting dressed and undressed over and over, until it feels "just right"
Mental rituals	• Repeating prayers, words, or phrases to oneself to neutralize unwanted thoughts • Mentally reviewing what one said or did (reassurance)

intended to remove contaminants and prevent disease. In some cases, patients perform rituals simply to reduce a general sense of anxiety or to achieve a feeling of "completeness." Compulsive rituals can also be overt behaviors or covert mental acts aimed at preventing a negative outcome. Examples of common mental rituals include repetition of special phrases, prayers, or numbers in a specific manner, and ritualistically going over (mentally reviewing, analyzing) one's behavior or conversations to reassure oneself that one has not made egregious mistakes or said anything offensive.

In addition to compulsive rituals, many people with OCD use various overt and covert strategies that do not meet DSM criteria for compulsions (i.e., they are not stereotyped or repeated according to rigid rules) to control, remove, or prevent their obsessions (Freeston & Ladouceur, 1997; Ladouceur et al., 2000). Examples include overanalyzing the meaning of obsessional thoughts, rational self-talk (i.e., to convince oneself of the unimportance of the obsession), reassurance seeking, replacing the obsessional thought with a "safe" thought, performing a brief behavioral act (e.g., putting one's hand in one's pockets to prevent losing control), distraction, and thought suppression (Ladouceur et al., 2000). Because these strategies may be covert and automatic, the individual may not even recognize them as part of OCD. Thus, the assessment should include examples to help the individual identify neutralization.

Avoidance is also present to some degree in most individuals with OCD, and is intended to prevent exposure to situations that provoke obsessional thoughts and urges to ritualize. Sometimes the aim of avoidance is to prevent specific feared consequences, such as illness or harm. Other times, avoidance is used to prevent obsessional thoughts, such as avoiding public stairways because they evoke obsessions of impulsively pushing people down the steps.

Insight

Although most people with OCD view their obsessions and rituals as more or less senseless, the degree of insight into the irrationality of symptoms varies from person to person, and even within patients across time. Whereas some individuals readily acknowledge the senselessness of their symptoms, others remain convinced that their obsessional fears will come true, and that their rituals and avoidance patterns serve to prevent disaster. An individual's degree of insight may also vary between his or her obsessions. For example, she may recognize her obsessive thoughts about contamination as irrational, yet believe her harming obsessions have a basis in reality. As we discuss later in this chapter, the level of a patient's insight can have implications for treatment response.

Clinical Implications

The essential features of OCD are unwanted anxiety-provoking thoughts (obsessions) and deliberate anxiety-reducing behaviors that can be overt or covert and take a variety of forms. Thus, the clinician should keep in mind that obsessions and rituals (including avoidance and neutralizing) are *functionally related*—the compulsive ritual is an attempt to reduce obsessional distress. For example, the obsession that one has mistakenly hit a pedestrian while driving would *increase* anxiety and lead to the urge compulsively to check (ritual) or ask for assurances to *reduce* this anxiety. It is therefore not surprising that certain types of obsessions and rituals co-occur in the following patterns: (1) Obsessions about responsibility for harm and mistakes are associated with checking rituals; (2) symmetry obsessions occur along with ordering and counting rituals; (3) contamination obsessions co-occur with washing and cleaning rituals; and (4) religious, sexual, and violent obsessions often trigger mental rituals and reassurance seeking (e.g., McKay et al., 2004).

With respect to assessment, it is important for the clinician to understand the content and triggers of obsessional thoughts, as well as the feared consequences predicted to result from the obsessions. As well, information about the compulsive rituals and avoidance strategies must be collected, including the individual's rationale for deploying each type of ritual (e.g., Abramowitz et al., 2010); that is, how does the ritual reduce anxiety or prevent feared negative consequences? The effectiveness of psychological treatments for OCD hinge on the clinician (and patient) having a good understanding of the patient's symptoms in this way. Finally, it is important to determine the individual's insight into the senselessness of his or her symptoms, since poor insight is associated with attenuated treatment response (e.g., Foa, Abramowitz, Franklin, & Kozak, 1999).

CLASSIFICATION

Dimensions of OCD

Studies on the structure of OCD symptoms consistently identify *symptom dimensions* that comprise certain obsessions and compulsions (Abramowitz et al., 2010; for a review see McKay et al., 2004). The most commonly detected dimensions are (1) harming (aggressive obsessions and checking rituals), (2) contamination (contamination obsessions and decontamination rituals), (3) symmetry (obsessions about order or neatness and arranging rituals), (4) unacceptable immoral or violent thoughts with mental rituals and neutralization, and (5) hoarding symptoms. These symptom dimensions overlap in individuals with OCD, such that someone might have both contamination and harming symptoms. In addition, some sufferers undergo changes in their symptom picture over time, for example, shifting from unacceptable thoughts to symmetry concerns. With respect to the hoarding dimension, recent research has raised doubts about whether this is actually a symptom of OCD, since individuals with OCD who report hoarding symptoms have a clinical profile distinct from those who do not hoard (e.g., Abramowitz, Wheaton, & Storch, 2008). This is not to say that some people with OCD also have hoarding symptoms, but that hoarding itself does not appear to be a symptom of OCD. Each of these symptom dimensions also has implications for the psychological treatment of OCD because the use (and effectiveness) of specific treatment techniques depends in part on the patient's symptom presentation, which we discuss in the section on treatment in this chapter.

Obsessive–Compulsive Spectrum Disorders

Seeming overlaps between the symptoms of OCD and those of other psychological disorders (e.g., impulse control disorders) have prompted the proposal of an "OCD spectrum" that includes various conditions involving "obsessional" thinking and repetitive or "compulsive" behaviors (Hollander, Friedberg, Wasserman, Yeh, & Iyengar, 2005). The boundaries of such a spectrum (and its very existence), however, are the subject of debate (Abramowitz & Deacon, 2005). Table 5.3 lists the three categories of disorders currently included in the proposed spectrum.

The main conceptual problem with the OCD spectrum notion as displayed in Table 5.3 is that the symptoms of most of the proposed spectrum disorders do not show the same functional relationship as is present in OCD; that is, whereas OCD involves obsessional thinking that provokes anxiety and avoidance, or ritualistic behavior that reduces anxiety, such phenomena are not present in most of the proposed spectrum conditions. Impulse control disorders, for example, involve no obsessional fear, and the repetitive behaviors are not performed to reduce anxiety or distress. In fact, impulsive behaviors are associated with pleasure seeking. Similarly, anorexia and bulimia do not involve overt fears of disastrous consequences, as is observed in OCD, and these are differentiated from OCD by the presence of

TABLE 5.3. Putative Obsessive–Compulsive Spectrum Disorders

Impulse control disorders	Appearance/bodily sensations	Neurological disorders characterized by repetitive behaviors
Intermittent explosive disorder	Body dysmorphic disorder	Autism
Pyromania	Hypochondriasis	Asperger syndrome
Kleptomania	Depersonalization disorder	Tourette syndrome
Pathological gambling	Anorexia nervosa	Sydenham's chorea
Trichotillomania	Bulimia nervosa	
Paraphilias and nonparaphilic compulsive sexual behavior		
Impulsive and aggressive personality disorders such as borderline, narcissistic, and antisocial personality disorders		

body image distortion (although some have advocated that hypochondriasis and body dysmorphic disorder might be related to OCD; Abramowitz & Deacon, 2005). Finally, the repetitive (or perseverative) behaviors found in neurological disorders are not aimed at reducing distress but are instead more or less automatized and pointless motoric behaviors. There are also no obsessions present in these neurological conditions. Thus, although the disorders in the putative OCD spectrum bear some superficial resemblance to OCD—all involve repetitive thinking or behaviors—when one more closely examines the function of these behaviors, the similarities seem to fall away, with the possible exception of hypochondriasis and body dysmorphic disorder, as discussed in the section that follows.

Differentiating OCD from Similar Disorders

Hypochondriasis and Body Dysmorphic Disorder

Hypochondriasis (HC) is a somatoform disorder characterized by a preoccupation with fears of having a serious disease (e.g., cancer). The intrusive health-related preoccupations in HC have been compared to obsessional thoughts or fears in OCD, and the repetitive attempts to seek reassurance in HC, to compulsive checking rituals (e.g., Fallon, Javitch, Hollander, & Liebowitz, 1991). Body dysmorphic disorder (BDD) involves excessive preoccupation with an imagined defect in appearance (e.g., "My nose is too large"). The thoughts of unsightliness occur in the absence of any noticeable physical defect, are often resisted, and lead to significant anxiety about how the person appears to others. In this way, preoccupations in BDD are functionally similar to obsessions in OCD. To circumvent anticipated embarrassment, individuals with BDD may avoid certain social situations or engage in behaviors aimed to reduce distress or the visibility of their imagined defect, including excessive checking in mirrors, grooming, and hiding the perceived defect (e.g., with large sunglasses or a hat). Because HC and BDD involve anxiety-provoking preoccupations and excessive behaviors aimed at reducing this anxiety, these problems might be related to OCD. In clinically distinguishing these somatoform disorders from OCD, it is important to assess the full range of obsessions and compulsions, and determine whether any health and appearance concerns occur along with other more quintessential types of obsessions and compulsions. If this is the case, OCD is the proper diagnosis. If the person appears singly obsessed with appearance or health concerns, somatoform disorder is likely the correct diagnosis.

Generalized Anxiety Disorder

The main features of generalized anxiety disorder (GAD) are chronic worry and tension that are unfounded or more severe than would be expected in most people. Because of their intense worrying, people with GAD often suffer from insomnia and other physical symptoms, including fatigue, headaches, irritability, and hot flashes. Worries in GAD can be intrusive, unwanted, repetitive, and highly distressing to the individual; thus, it is common for such symptoms to be mistaken for obsessions. Yet whereas the content of worries in GAD is focused on real-life circumstances such as finances, social and family relationships, work, and school performance, obsessional content in OCD does not typically concern everyday problems. Worries also tend to involve exclusively verbal content, whereas obsessions are often experienced as images and impulses, along with thoughts and doubts. Worry content often shifts from one topic to another over time, whereas the focus of obsessions is typically stable. Some individuals with GAD show ritual-like reassurance-seeking and checking behavior (e.g., calling one's spouse repeatedly if one is late getting home); however, these behaviors are more specific to worry content and do not neutralize anxiety in same way that compulsive rituals neutralize obsessions. Thus, the presence of "obsessions" that pertain to everyday circumstances indicates the presence of GAD rather than OCD.

Obsessive–Compulsive Personality Disorder

The main features of obsessive–compulsive personality disorder (OCPD) are an enduring pattern of perfectionism, rigidity, stubbornness, and orderliness that interferes with task completion; preoccupation with rules, organization, and schedules, so that the point of activities is lost; overconscientiousness and inflexibility regarding ethical or moral issues (not accounted for by normal cultural or religious values); and excessive devotion to work and productivity to the exclusion of friendships or leisure time (American Psychiatric Association, 2013). Although some of these characteristics are informally referred to as "compulsive" and might be found among individuals with OCD, there are important differences in the function of these symptoms. In OCD, perfectionistic behavior is provoked by fear and is resisted; the person wishes he or she did not feel compelled to behave this way. In contrast, people with OCPD do not have obsessional fears and instead perceive their "compulsive" traits as useful, agreeable, and consistent with their worldview. Thus, when individuals do not resist their behavior patterns and are often resistant to the suggestion of adapting a less rigid lifestyle, OCPD is the likely diagnosis rather than OCD.

Schizophrenia and Delusional Disorders

It is important to distinguish schizophrenia and delusional disorders from OCD, since these conditions possess superficial similarities that have led some to speculate a relationship among them (e.g., Enright, 1996). For instance, these other conditions may involve bizarre thoughts (i.e., "delusions") and behavior. Yet unlike in OCD, most people with schizophrenia and other psychotic disorders do not resist their bizarre, intrusive, thoughts, and the thoughts do not produce anxiety or urges to neutralize. Rather, the bizarre ideation might be believed or even defended as reasonable (i.e., as in delusions). Other differences are that repetitive behaviors in schizophrenia (e.g., undifferentiated or catatonic subtypes) and other psychotic disorders are pointless motor behaviors rather than responses to obsessional anxiety. Nevertheless, patients with OCD are sometimes misdiagnosed as having delusions or psychotic thinking by those who are not knowledgeable about the nature of OCD, especially when the OCD is characterized by bizarre obsessions (e.g., fear of making a pact with the devil, intrusions about murdering loved ones, fears of turning into someone else). Therefore, the unwanted nature of the thoughts and the anxiety response; in concert with the presence of avoidance and compulsions (overt and covert), must be carefully assessed, as these features differentiate psychotic symptoms from those of OCD.

COURSE AND ASSOCIATED FEATURES

OCD is a chronic condition with a very low rate of spontaneous remission. Left untreated, symptoms fluctuate, with worsening during periods of increased life stress. In a 40-year follow-up study of 144 individuals with OCD (Skoog & Skoog, 1999), 83% of this cohort had improved, and 48% no longer met diagnostic criteria for OCD; although about half of the nonclinical individuals reported some residual symptoms. Thus, although OCD symptoms are likely to improve with treatment, full recovery is the exception rather than the rule. The clinical implications of this fact are discussed in the section on treatment.

Having OCD is associated with impaired social and role functioning, troubled romantic and family relationships, diminished academic performance, unemployment, comorbid psychological disorders, sleep and sexual problems, and increased receipt of disability income (Koran, 2000). Despite the fact that severe OCD can lead to functional impairment, people with OCD do not differ substantially from the general U.S. population in terms of the rates of alcohol abuse, suicide, or marriage. Relatives of patients with OCD also suffer, since symptoms often result in restricted access to certain rooms, involvement of others in compulsive rituals, and difficulty in enjoying life (e.g., the inability to enjoy a family vacation because of the sufferer's obsessions and rituals; Black, Gaffney, Schlosser, & Gabel, 1998). A diagnosis of OCD is also related to increased (non-mental health) medical utilization.

Clinical Implications

Accordingly, at the beginning and end of treatment, therapists should assess for associated features of OCD such as mood and other anxiety disorders, interpersonal functioning, academic and occupational performance, general quality of life, and physiological indices such as sleep and sexual functioning. Assessment of these variables before beginning treatment helps the therapist plan for therapy that addresses, as comprehensively as possible, the clinical problems frequently associated with OCD. The same assessment at the end of treatment might also help therapists prepare patients who might be at greater risk for relapse, especially since some of the associated features, such as poor family functioning and mood disturbance, are associated with greater OCD symptom severity.

EPIDEMIOLOGY

Prevalence and Onset

Once considered a rare condition, OCD is known to affect from 2 to 3% of the adult population across the world (Weissman et al., 1994). The disorder is slightly more common among females than males. OCD onset is in childhood or adolescence, typically begins by the age of 25, and only rarely after age 50 (Rasmussen & Tsuang, 1986). The mean age of onset tends to be earlier in males (about 21 years of age) than in females (22 to 24 years; Lensi et al., 1996).

Although most individuals with OCD do not identify clear-cut precipitants to symptom onset, stressful or traumatic events and experiences may play a role for some patients (Gershuny, Baer, Radomsky, Wilson, & Jenike, 2003). Symptoms also occur at higher than expected rates among childbearing women (Abramowitz, Schwartz, Moore, & Luenzmann, 2003). Moreover, the content of obsessional thoughts and rituals is clearly influenced by environmental and sociological factors, as evidenced by the predominance of obsessions concerning timely issues. For example, the highly prevalent contamination obsessions relating to gonorrhea in the 1970s have largely been replaced by fears of acquiring AIDS since the mid-1980s. Similarly, individuals with religious obsessions show concerns related to their specific religion (e.g., Jewish patients afraid of violating the dietary laws associated with that religion).

COMORBIDITY

Individuals with OCD are at an increased risk for additional forms of psychopathology, with depressive disorders among the most commonly co-occurring difficulties. The lifetime prevalence of major depressive disorder (MDD) among patients with OCD ranges from 12.4 to 60.3% cross-nationally (mean = 29%; Weissman et al. (1994) and, for the most part, OCD predates MDD, suggesting that depressive symptoms usually occur in response to the distress and impairment associated with OCD. Depressive symptoms also seem to be more strongly related to the severity of obsessions than to compulsions (Ricciardi & McNally, 1995). Also, coexisting depressive symptoms are especially predictive of poor quality of life for those suffering with OCD.

OCD may also be accompanied by additional anxiety disorders (e.g., Weissman et al., 1994), with social phobia, panic disorder, and GAD being the most commonly reported (Nestadt et al., 2001). Estimates of comorbidity between OCD and personality disorders vary widely (from 8.7 to 87.5%), yet those personality disorders belonging to the anxious cluster (e.g., obsessive–compulsive, avoidant) are more common than those of other clusters (e.g., Crino & Andrews, 1996; Steketee, Eisen, Dyck, Warshaw, & Rasmussen, 1999). Clinical implications of comorbid conditions, especially the impact of mood and personality disorders, are presented later in the chapter.

ETIOLOGY

Biological Models

The Serotonin Hypothesis

The serotonin hypothesis was the leading neurochemical theory of OCD. It proposed that obsessions and compulsions arise from abnormalities in the serotonin neurotransmitter system, specifically a hypersensitivity of the postsynaptic serotonergic receptors (Zohar & Insel, 1987). The most consistent findings in support of this model came from the pharmacotherapy literature, which suggests that selective serotonin reuptake inhibitors (SSRIs; e.g., fluoxetine) are more effective than medications with other mechanisms of action (e.g., norepineherine inhibitors) in reducing OCD symptoms. Studies of biological markers—such as blood and cerebrospinal fluid levels of serotonin metabolites—largely do not support a relationship between serotonin and OCD (e.g., Insel, Mueller, Alterman, Linnoila, & Murphy, 1985). As a result of these findings, contemporary biological theorists have all but abandoned the serotonin hypothesis of OCD.

Structural Models

Structural models hypothesize that OCD symptoms are caused by neuroanatomical abnormalities in localized brain regions, specifically the orbitofrontal–subcortical circuits (Saxena, Bota, & Brody, 2001), which are thought to connect regions of the brain responsible for the initiation of behaviors implemented with little conscious awareness. These models were derived from neuroimaging studies comparing brain function between people with and without OCD (for a review, see Whiteside, Port, & Abramowitz, 2004). Although findings vary across studies, a meta-analysis of 10 positron emission tomographic (PET) and single-proton emission computed tomographic (SPECT) studies found that relative to healthy individuals, those with OCD evidence more activity in the orbital gyrus and the head of the caudate nucleus (Whiteside et al., 2004).

Limitations of Biological Models

There are important limitations of biological models of OCD. First, there is little correspondence between the patterns of symptoms that patients report and the biological mechanisms proposed to account for them; that is, there is no sufficient explanation for how neurotransmitter or neuroanatomical abnormalities translate into obsessions and compulsions, but not into other psychological symptoms such as panic attacks or eating disorder symptoms (e.g., body image disturbance). Second, biological models are unable to explain the fact that OCD symptoms concern some themes (e.g., fears of harming vulnerable individuals), but not others (e.g., fears of harming those who could defend themselves). Also, why do some people experience contamination-related obsessions, whereas others have intrusive sexual obsessions? Finally, existing serotonin and neuroimaging studies are correlational in design and therefore do not provide evidence that biological abnormalities *cause* OCD symptoms.

Psychological Models

Learning Theory

Behavioral (learning and conditioning) models of OCD were based on Mowrer's (1960) two-stage theory of fear acquisition and maintenance. Obsessional fears were thought to be acquired (Stage 1: classical conditioning) as a result of traumatic conditioning experiences in which a previously neutral stimulus (the conditioned stimulus, or CS) was paired with an aversive stimulus (the unconditioned stimulus, or UCS; e.g., a traumatic experience), so that the CS comes to elicit a conditioned fear response (CR). As a result of this associative learning process, specific situations (e.g., using a public bathroom), objects (e.g., door knobs), and thoughts, images, doubts, or impulses (e.g., incestuous images) that pose no objective threat may come to evoke obsessional fear. Stage 2 of the model (operant conditioning) proposes that avoidance behaviors and compulsive rituals become habitual, because they reduce obsessional anxiety immediately (i.e., negative reinforcement). By the 1980s, however, limitations of learning models had become apparent. Specifically, many people with OCD did not describe the types of classical conditioning experiences that were thought to lead to obsessions. Thus, additional models were sought to explain obsessional thinking.

Information-Processing Deficit Models

Theorists trying to understand the role of cognition in OCD proposed that obsessions and compulsions were caused by abnormally functioning executive processes, such as memory. Compulsive checking, for example, might develop as a consequence of *not being able to remember* whether one has locked the door, turned off the oven, or unplugged the iron. Despite its face validity, however, little evidence of overall memory deficit among individuals with OCD was found. As a result, theorists proposed that individuals with OCD have memory problems *only where their obsessional fears are concerned*. This would explain, for example, why a patient who fears house fires might spend hours rechecking the stove and oven, yet have no urges to check door locks. The few studies that have examined this selective memory hypothesis, however, suggest just the opposite: Patients appear to have a selectively *better* memory for OCD-related information relative to non-OCD-relevant stimuli (e.g., Radomsky, Rachman, & Hammond, 2001).

Although information-processing deficit models of OCD have intuitive appeal, they have very limited empirical support. Additionally, they do not explain the heterogeneity of OCD symptoms (e.g., why some have religious obsessions, while others have contamination fears), and cannot account for the fact that mild memory "problems" are present in many disorders (e.g., panic disorder, social phobia, posttraumatic stress disorder, and bulimia nervosa; Taylor, Thordarson, & Sochting, 2002). Thus, the question remains as to why such deficits would give rise to *OCD* instead of one of these other disorders. Thus, if dysfunctional information processing plays any causal role in OCD, it is most likely to be a nonspecific vulnerability factor, as opposed to a specific cause.

Cognitive-Behavioral Models

Most theorists and researchers now apply Beck's (1976) cognitive specificity theory of emotion to understanding the development and persistence of OCD. This model proposes that emotional distress—such as anxiety and fear—arises not from negative or threatening situations and stimuli themselves, but from how one *interprets* or *appraises* such stimuli. Accordingly, obsessional fears are thought to arise from inaccurate beliefs about the importance of intrusive thoughts. Indeed, unpleasant mental intrusions (i.e., thoughts, images, and impulses that intrude into consciousness) are a normal and universal experience for people with and without OCD (Rachman

& de Silva, 1978). Rachman (1997) and Salkovskis (1996) have proposed that these mental intrusions develop into clinical obsessions when they are *misappraised* as overly significant, threatening, harmful, or as posing a threat for which the individual is personally responsible.

A number of similar cognitive-behavioral theories have been proposed, each emphasizing a slightly different type of belief or appraisal of intrusive thoughts. Salkovskis (1996), for example, emphasized inflated responsibility as a key cognitive bias in OCD. Rachman (1997) emphasized the overimportance of thoughts. Clark (2004) emphasized the need to control intrusive thoughts as the main dysfunctional belief. A comprehensive model that incorporates all of these types of beliefs and appraisals is that developed by the Obsessive Compulsive Cognitions Working Group (e.g., Frost & Steketee, 2002), which identified six domains of dysfunctional beliefs that play a role in OCD, as described in Table 5.4.

To illustrate, consider an intrusive unwanted image of murdering a loved one. Most people would regard such a thought as "mental noise" (i.e., having no harm-related implications). Such a senseless intrusion, however, might develop into a clinical obsession if the person appraises it as having serious consequences, for example, "Thoughts like this mean I am a dangerous person." Such appraisals evoke anxiety and motivate the person to try to suppress or remove the unwanted intrusion and the anxiety using compulsive rituals or other neutralizing strategies, and to attempt to avoid reminders of the thought (e.g., by locking up all the knives in the house), so that worries about dreadful outcomes may be kept to a minimum.

Salkovskis (1996) proposed that compulsive rituals and avoidance develop into strong patterns because they seem to work immediately (albeit temporarily)

TABLE 5.4. Domains of Dysfunctional Beliefs Associated with OCD as Identified by the Obsessive–Compulsive Cognitions Working Group

Belief domain	Description
Excessive responsibility	Belief that one has the special power to cause and/or the duty to prevent negative outcomes.
Overimportance of thoughts	Belief that the mere presence of a thought indicates that the thought is significant. For example, the belief that the thought has ethical or moral ramifications, or that thinking the thought increases the probability of the corresponding behavior or event.
Need to control thoughts	Belief that complete control over one's thoughts is both necessary and possible.
Overestimation of threat	Belief that negative events are especially likely and would be especially awful.
Perfectionism	Belief that mistakes and imperfection are intolerable.
Intolerance for uncertainty	Belief that it is necessary and possible to be completely certain that negative outcomes will not occur.

to reduce distress and remove the unwanted obsessional thought, and are therefore negatively reinforced. Such behaviors, however, also prevent the person from discovering that the feared outcome (e.g., acting on a senseless intrusive thought) is highly unlikely in the first place. Thus, the mistaken interpretation of the thought persists and the obsessional fear is maintained.

Treatment approaches derived from the biological and psychological models are reviewed in the following section on treatment outcome.

TREATMENT OUTCOME

Behavioral and cognitive-behavioral models hold the greatest promise for understanding and treating OCD symptoms. The cognitive-behavioral approach, in particular, is empirically supported (e.g., Abramowitz, Khander, Nelson, Deacon, & Rygwall, 2006, Abramowitz, Nelson, Rygwall, & Khander, 2007) and provides a logically consistent treatment approach. In particular, from this perspective, successful treatment for OCD must (1) correct maladaptive beliefs and appraisals that lead normal intrusive thoughts to escalate into obsessional fear and (2) terminate avoidance and compulsive rituals that prevent the correction of these maladaptive beliefs. Two approaches have been developed for these purposes: (a) exposure and response prevention (ERP), and (b) cognitive therapy. This section provides a concise description of these interventions, which can be used on their own or in tandem to reduce OCD symptoms. Detailed guidelines for their use are available in various treatment manuals (e.g., Abramowitz, 2006; Kozak & Foa, 1997; Wilhelm & Steketee, 2006).

Exposure and Response Prevention

Exposure therapy comprises a set of psychological treatment procedures designed to help individuals confront stimuli that provoke obsessional fear, but that objectively pose a low risk of harm. Exposure for OCD can occur in the form of repeated encounters with the actual feared situations (situational exposure) and imaginal confrontation with the feared disastrous consequences of confronting these situations (imaginal exposure). For example, an individual with obsessional thoughts of harming children might for situational exposure be asked to go to playgrounds and schools where there are small children. He might also practice imaginal exposure to images of harming chidren. A patient with fears of contamination from disabled persons might for situational exposure shake hands with a visually or hearing-impaired individual. For imaginal exposure, she would then confront thoughts of losing her vision or hearing as a result of the encounter. During exposure tasks individuals experience temporary increases in anxiety, which naturally subside—a process called *habituation*. With each repetition of the exposure task, habituation occurs more rapidly.

The response prevention component of treatment entails refraining from compulsive rituals and other strategies that serve as an escape from obsessional fear. Response prevention helps to prolong exposure and facilitate the long-term habituation of obsessional anxiety. In the earlier examples, the first patient might practice refraining from any strategies he typically uses to reassure himself that he won't act on his thoughts of harming children. The second patient would be instructed to refrain from decontamination rituals such as washing.

Most ERP treatment manuals (e.g., Abramowitz et al., 2006; Kozak & Foa, 1997) recommend that ERP be conducted over the course of 12–20 sessions. The initial few sessions include a thorough assessment of obsessions, compulsive rituals, avoidance strategies, and anticipated consequences of confronting feared situations. This information is used to plan the specific ERP exercises that will be pursued. The therapist also never physically restrains the individual from performing rituals; rather, he or she helps the person to resist these behaviors. Exposure exercises progress gradually using a hierarchy—a list of feared situations and thoughts arranged from the least to the most anxiety provoking. Beginning exposure with less anxiety-evoking tasks increases the likelihood that the patient will learn to manage distress and fosters confidence in the treatment. At the end of each treatment session, the therapist instructs the patient to continue exposure for several hours and in different environmental contexts, without the therapist.

Numerous studies involving thousands of individuals with OCD affirm that ERP is an effective treatment for this condition. Randomized controlled trials (RCTs) show the superiority of ERP over placebo treatments such as progressive muscle relaxation training (e.g., Fals-Stewart, Marks, & Schafer, 1993), anxiety management training (Lindsay, Crino, & Andrews, 1997), and pill placebo (Foa et al., 2005). RCTs also show that ERP is more effective than the antidepressant clomipramine, believed to be the most effective form of pharmacotherapy for OCD (Foa et al., 2005). Although patients receiving ERP typically show a 50–60% reduction in their OCD symptoms, some residual symptoms usually remain even posttreatment (Abramowitz, 1998).

Cognitive Therapy

Cognitive therapy typically begins with the therapist presenting a rationale for treatment that incorporates the notion that intrusive obsessional thoughts are normal experiences rather than indicative of anything threatening or important. He or she also explains how misinterpreting unwanted mental intrusions as very significant leads to anxiety, obsessional preoccupation, and avoidance and compulsive rituals that unwittingly maintain the obsessional preoccupation and anxiety. Next, a set of verbal techniques helps patients challenge and correct their erroneous beliefs and appraisals, such as didactic presentation of educational material (e.g., information about the rates of distressing thoughts in the general population) and Socratic dialogue aimed at helping patients recognize faulty interpretations. "Behavioral experiments," in which patients enter and observe situations that exemplify their fears, also facilitate the collection of information that allows individuals to revise their judgments about the degree of risk associated with their obsessions.

Some specific cognitive therapy techniques used in the treatment of OCD are as follows: For a patient who overestimates personal responsibility, the "pie technique" (Clark, 2004) involves the patient giving an initial estimate of the percentage of responsibility that would be attributable to him or her if a feared consequence were to occur. The patient then generates a list of the parties (other than him- or herself) who would also have some responsibility for the feared consequence. They then draw a pie chart, each slice of which represents one of the responsible parties identified. Next, the patient labels all parties' slices according to their percentage of responsibility and labels his or her own slice last. By the exercise's end, it is generally clear to patients that the majority of the responsibility for the feared event would not be their own.

For patients with difficulty discriminating between unwanted obsessional thoughts and actions, the "cognitive continuum" technique involves rating how immoral they perceive themselves to be for having the intrusive obsessional thoughts. Next, patients rate the morality level of other individuals who have committed acts of varying degrees of immorality (e.g., a serial rapist, abusive parents). Then, patients rerate themselves and reevaluate how immoral they are for simply experiencing intrusive thoughts.

Compared to ERP, fewer studies have examined the efficacy of cognitive therapy. Clinical observations suggest, however, that using cognitive techniques along with ERP enhances the effects of ERP. For example, during exposure, patients often need to be persuaded that confronting feared situations and images will be beneficial for them. This typically requires discussion of fear-related beliefs and assumptions (e.g., about the importance of senseless intrusive thoughts). Thus, cognitive interventions can be used to "tenderize" distorted cognitions that underlie obsessional fears, thereby setting the table for individuals to engage in and get the most out of ERP.

Hypothesized Mechanisms of Change in Psychological Treatments

A cognitive mechanism is proposed to account for how ERP modifies obsessional anxiety and compulsive urges. Specifically, Foa and Kozak (1986) hypothesized that repeated and prolonged exposure to feared stimuli, in the absence of rituals and avoidance behavior, correct the catastrophic overestimates of danger that underlie obsessional anxiety and fear. These authors point to three requirements for successful outcome with ERP. First, physiological arousal and subjective fear must be evoked during exposure. Second, the fear responses must gradually diminish during the exposure session in the absence of compulsive rituals (within-session habituation). Third, the initial fear response at the beginning of each exposure session should decline across sessions (between-session habituation).

Pharmacotherapy

SSRI medication is the most widely used pharmacological treatment for OCD. The specific agents in this class of drugs include fluoxetine, paroxetine, sertraline, citalopram, and fluvoxamine. Clomipramine, a tricyclic medication that also possesses serotonergic properties, is also used in the treatment of OCD. On average, relative to placebo, SSRIs produce a 20–40% reduction in obsessions and compulsions (Rauch & Jenike, 1998). The major strengths of a pharmacological approach to treating OCD include the convenience and the little effort required on the individual's part. Limitations include the relatively modest improvement and likelihood of residual symptoms, high rate of nonresponse (40–60% of patients do not show any favorable response), and the prospect of unpleasant side effects (which can often be stabilized by adjusting the dose). Moreover, once SSRIs are terminated, OCD symptoms typically return rapidly (Pato, Zohar-Kadouch, Zohar, & Murphy, 1988).

CLINICAL IMPLICATIONS
OF BASIC RESEARCH FOR TREATMENT

Various aspects of the psychopathology of OCD have direct treatment implications and can be used to establish informal guidelines regarding the use of ERP, cognitive therapy, and medication, or their combination. We discuss these implications in this section.

Poor Insight

Research consistently demonstrates that relative to individuals who recognize their obsessions and compulsions as illogical and senseless, those with poor insight into senselessness of their symptoms show attenuated response to both ERP and pharmacotherapy (e.g., Foa et al., 1999). It appears that patients with poor insight have difficulty consolidating information that is inconsistent with their obsessional fears; thus, their beliefs and expectations of danger are not modified with repeated exposure to obsessional cues. Moreover, because of their extreme fear, these patients might not engage in ERP tasks as well as do those with good insight. As a result, they do not gain opportunities to correct strongly held inaccurate beliefs and appraisals. The reason that poor insight hinders response to medication is not well understood, yet the fact that both of these treatments are attenuated by poor insight suggests that augmentation strategies are necessary. In the case of psychological treatment, some authors suggest the use of cognitive therapy to help with verbally changing beliefs and appraisals rather than using exposure alone (Salkovskis & Westbrook, 1989).

Severe Depression

Between 25 and 50% of patients with OCD suffer from comorbid depressive disorders (Abramowitz, 2004), and studies that have examined the effects of depressive symptoms on the outcome of ERP have revealed that relative to mildly and moderately depressed patients with OCD, those with severe depression—and indeed a diagnosis of MDD—have attenuated outcomes with ERP. Perhaps because of their high emotional activity, severely depressed individuals fail to undergo a reduction in anxiety/distress (i.e., habituation) that normally occurs following extended exposure to feared stimuli. Thus, depressed patients with OCD may not learn how to feel comfortable in the presence of obsessionally feared situations. Motivational difficulties, which often accompany depression, may also account for poor treatment outcome; that is, patients may not adhere to instructions to face their fears and resist urges to ritualize if they are extremely depressed and unmotivated to help themselves. Some research points to the use of antidepressant medication to help depressed patients benefit from ERP (e.g., Simpson & Liebowitz, 2005). Other authors have proposed that the use of cognitive therapy for both OCD and depression may enhance outcome for this group of patients (Abramowitz, 2004).

Personality Disorders

The presence of certain personality traits and personality disorders is known to hinder response to ERP and medication for OCD (Steketee, Chambless, & Tran, 2001). OCPD and histrionic personality disorder traits, for example, might interfere with developing rapport and adherence to ERP instructions. If, however, a good therapeutic relationship can be developed, ERP can be successful despite these traits. Clinicians should also consider that some patients with dramatic traits gain reinforcement for their OCD symptoms. In such circumstances, psychological treatment approaches are unlikely to succeed, because patients do not perceive themselves as gaining rewards for their efforts to reduce obsessions and rituals. Individuals with personality traits in the odd cluster (e.g., schizotypal personality disorder) present a challenge for clinicians, because such patients have a reduced ability to profit from corrective information obtained during exposure or cognitive interventions.

OCD Symptom Presentation

As described earlier in this chapter, the symptoms of OCD vary considerably. Below are some specific treatment implications for particular presentations of this clinical disorder.

Contamination Concerns

Contamination obsessions and decontamination rituals respond well to ERP involving planned exposure to sources of contamination, contaminated objects, or "dirty" environments. Response prevention can pose a challenge, especially if the patient fears situations such as using the bathroom, which will be confronted multiple times per day. Ideally, response prevention should include no washing at all, although exceptions for bathroom use and before meals can be made initially (until such items are confronted for exposure). If the patient is reluctant to end all washing, a limited amount of ritualizing may be permitted per day, with gradual reductions over time. It is important for the therapist to attend closely to the actual washing methods, which may be lengthy, detailed, or completed according to a set of "rules."

Order and Symmetry Concerns

This symptom dimension often responds well to ERP, which emphasizes the response prevention component, because rather than specific obsessions, there may be only anxiety about "not feeling right" unless rituals are carried out. Exposure may involve deliberately leaving things "not just right"—pictures hung crookedly, books arranged in a haphazard manner, doors left open, and so forth—in which case the urge to complete the associated ordering or arranging rituals is resisted. The focus is on tolerating the anxiety and "not just right" feelings, and finding out they diminish with time, even without performing compulsive rituals.

Responsibility Obsessions and Checking Rituals

Responsibility obsessions often require the use of both situational exposure to feared situations and imaginal exposure to feared consequences. For example, a women afraid of hitting pedestrians while she is driving, and who checks the roadside for bodies, might perform situational exposure to driving in areas with high pedestrian traffic (e.g., parking lots) and subsequently imagine that she hit someone but didn't realize it. Instead of acting on her urges to return to the parking lot to check, she would be helped to use response prevention to remain exposed to her uncertainty and learn that her obsessional anxiety eventually subsides. Cognitive therapy might also be used directly to address dysfunctional guilt and inflated perceptions of responsibility.

Mental Rituals

It has long been thought that mental rituals, which are often accompanied by disturbing obsessional thoughts about violence (e.g., images of stabbing loved ones), sex (e.g., doubts about whether one is becoming gay), and religion (e.g., blasphemous ideas), are the most difficult presentation of OCD to manage with psychological treatments. In addition to the typical anxiety and fear of acting on intrusive thoughts that seem senseless, individuals with these types of symptoms often become concerned that their obsessions reflect their true nature (e.g., "Why would I be thinking about this if I didn't really feel this way?"). An important goal for the clinician is to assess carefully rituals and other strategies used to respond to such obsessions, and to avoid falling into the trap of labeling such individuals as "pure obsessional" even if no rituals can be observed. Most likely, the patient is using covert (mental) rituals and brief neutralizing strategies in response to his or her obsessions. Mental rituals can take many forms, such as replacing a "bad" thought with a "good" one, mentally blocking a "bad" thought by imagining an X through it, saying a prayer, repeating magic words or phrases to oneself ("God keep them safe"), or mentally reviewing one's behavior.

Exposure therapy involves confronting stimuli that trigger obsessional thoughts (e.g., places of worship, knives), as well as imaginal confrontation with the obsession itself, and the feared consequences of not ritualizing (e.g., thoughts and images of molesting children). Imaginal exposure tasks usually involve first writing scripts of the patient's obsessional fears that incorporate varying amounts of detail to modulate anxiety (e.g., "I have a thought about my grandmother dying, but I don't say a prayer for her. As a result, she dies, it is all my fault, and my family abandons me"). The patient is then helped to record and listen to the scenario, or simply to read it, repeatedly until habituation occurs (i.e., the scene becomes "boring" or does not provoke anxiety). In addition, the patient is helped to refrain from rituals that would artificially reduce the obsession and the resulting anxiety.

Engaging Patients, Motivation, and Collaboration

Most psychological therapies require engaging patients and motivating them for treatment but it is especially true in treatment of OCD when trying to convince patients to stay with anxiety-provoking thoughts, take risks, and not engage in behaviors that they usually believe are essential for their own well-being or survival, or to protect their loved ones. One thing that would surprise most clinicians who do not work in a cognitive-behavioral format is how much education alone can help with engagement and motivation. Clearly, this interacts with relationship variables. Patients often say to clinicians familiar with OCD, "I really get this" or "I know what I am talking about." This knowledge increases the therapist's credibility and increases hope that recovery is possible.

Especially with OCD that can appear so "crazy" in terms of both thoughts and behaviors, it is comforting that there is some explanation about how patients get stuck and why. Fortunately, education about how OCD works both teaches the patient about the problem and leads directly to how to treat it. Education is essential before any treatment can begin. Therapists who talk to patients about the fact that they have a low tolerance for uncertainty and respond more negatively to that uncertainty or intrusive thoughts resonates with patients. Also framing why rituals start and continue—rituals continued because they work in the short run by decreasing anxiety—teaches patients why they feel better right after they do their rituals because it relieves anxiety. Also telling patients that everyone would do some rituals if they felt it was only way to keep their family safe or protected from unending anxiety expresses empathy. Indeed, rituals may seem like a small price to pay if they were the only way and they worked.

However, the cruel trick of OCD is that performing the ritual makes the thoughts come more frequently and the ritual feel more necessary. The short-term relief is traded for longer-term loss of freedom and interference with living. The other lie of OCD is that the intense distress the patient experiences after the obsession continues on—that day, that night, or longer, if the ritual is not performed. CBT therapists talk to patients about retraining their brains to respond differently to the error message or danger warning, and to break the cycle between the ritual and relief. While education is not enough, therapists who use it are continually reminded of how important it can be. This might be especially true of OCD, because so little about it seems to make sense, and patients know they are not only doing "crazy" things but also how difficult it is to stop.

One important aspect of motivation is discussing the loss of freedom and time, and ascertaining what the patient is missing because of OCD. They may lose time for favored activities, sleep, enjoying a meal, being able to touch or hug a family member, travel, and so forth. Each person is different, but it is important for each person to have a reason to start this effective but difficult treatment, and it has to be their own motivation. Motivational interviewing, formal or informal, can be extremely helpful to discuss the reasons whether to change or not. It is important to be clear that one expects to be ambivalent and afraid. It is also crucial to talk to the patient about what he or she believes about the obsessions when in a state of calm versus an OCD crisis moment. The therapist sets the tone of a collaborative venture in discussing, planning, and designing treatment goals. Patients are told that they are in charge of the pace and content of their exposures, since they cannot and will not be forced to do anything. However, the therapist will be using his or her knowledge to guide treatment, to recommend and select goals, and to push patients past their comfort zone. Indeed, patients need to understand that if they do not feel anxiety, the treatment is not working. The goal is to start with manageable levels of anxiety and easier tasks, and build competence and confidence, session by session.

While education is very important, clinical experience suggests that patients only begin to believe in the treatment of OCD and hope for recovery when they do something different relative to their OCD. What patients with OCD need, in other words, are corrective experiences, particularly about the nature of anxiety and their ability to tolerate it. In contrast, patients with OCD can be experts at engaging therapists in endless discussions and questions about their fears and obsessions. A more supportive, exploratory "talk-oriented" therapy can get kidnapped by OCD, with therapists' spending months of sessions reassuring, answering questions, endlessly reviewing past events, or trying to be logical about OCD. While the treatment of other anxiety disorders may benefit from supportive therapy or logical analysis of thought styles or patterns, OCD rarely does, and it often worsens due to the increased ritualizing in therapy. Indeed, what is helpful is to perform early exposures with the therapist in the office, or in the situation, so that the patient can understand and experience what exposure is like, and see how to address issues that arise and to modify plans to be most useful and successful.

While the goal of the treatment of OCD is to eliminate rituals, there are a number of ways to address this other than full-scale elimination. This is where the protocol-limited research programs and independent clinical work may diverge. Often after the education component is completed, the patient who is not ready to begin exposure may be "deemed inappropriate for the treatment program." Some research-based programs require full adherence to a planned limitation of rituals (e.g., a week of no washing or limited showering); however, only some patients can do this, and other options are available for the private practice clinician. Actually the patients who agree readily to treatment and jump in are often the easiest to treat. It is important to tell patients that while it may be more difficult and anxiety provoking to try to eliminate rituals (e.g., washing only before meals or after going to the bathroom), they will get faster relief. While the former may be preferable, a more gradual approach is workable and more patients may be able to comply. Indeed, both of us have treated "research rejects" who became actively involved in treatment and had very good outcomes.

For all OCD symptom types, there are ways to delay or modify rituals. Many patients are more willing to consider these as first steps to delay a ritual (e.g., delay checking for 20 minutes). The other option is to pick one period of day to be OCD free (e.g., "From 9:00–12:00 P.M., I won't rearrange things in my kitchen"). Also a patient can work to reduce the frequency of the ritual (limit reassurance questions to 10 rather than usual 30 per day). Finally a patient can "do OCD wrong" (e.g., use two squirts of soap instead of four, or do their full OCD prayer ritual, but in a different order). A certain number of sessions can be devoted to establishing a therapeutic relationship and providing information, learning anxiety management skills, or discussing problematic relationships, but CBT therapists are clear that this is not *treating* the OCD. Therapists of other orientations might not take the same approach. The only way to do CBT is to face feared situations and to eliminate rituals. In other words, a CBT therapist might distinguish between providing therapy and treating OCD. Behavioral treatment of OCD cannot involve just talking; it has to include doing. Rather than being asked, "What can't you do?" the patient is often asked, "What can you do?" Doing nothing is not an option. Any small step can provide an opening.

An important component of retraining the brain is not to break the ritual, then sit around waiting for anxiety to recede or white knuckling it through. Patients need to have a plan about what to do with themselves while anxiety resets, either to go about their lives or to engage in desired activity. All of these components of treatment—education, defining the motivation, and collaboration—are essential for all therapeutic approaches to be successful. These components are a basis for a good therapeutic alliance, along with the empathy and regular feedback that have been found to be associated with good outcomes for empirically supported treatments across multiple disorders. These relationship qualities are likely to be especially essential when treatment of OCD requires clients to take risks in facing fears, and to trust the process and the therapist to do so. Compliance, an additional treatment variable with in-session and out-of-session tasks, is crucial to the success of OCD treatment and likely is far more important than in the treatment of other anxiety disorders or other disorders overall.

Implications of Client Variables for Treatment Planning

As in the predictors of outcome for other anxiety disorders, severity of disorder, comorbidity with other psychological disorders, and overvalued ideation of OCD thoughts are predictors of poorer outcome in OCD treatment. It may be that these patients show slower progress, need more sessions, set more modest goals, and demonstrate more modest outcomes. However, clinically we have found with OCD that severity may interact with motivation, such that if the OCD is very distressing or interfering, patients are motivated to reclaim their lives or "not want to continue like this anymore." Very serious depression or substance use may require alternative psychosocial and/or medication treatments before the person has enough energy and focus to engage in the challenging work of ERP. Overvalued ideation may require more cognitive therapy before ERP can begin. Finally, demographic variables have not been strong predictors of response to treatments for anxiety.

Group Therapy

A few studies have examined the effectiveness of group treatment (ERP and cognitive therapy) for OCD (McLean et al., 2001). One strength of a group approach is that patients can get support and understanding, and learn that they do not suffer alone. Education about OCD can be delivered in a didactic format, since the general cognitive-behavioral model of OCD applies to patients across symptom dimensions. However, the symptom heterogeneity in OCD also limits this approach. Specifically, different patients in the group may require individual ERP plans that cannot practically be implemented in group format, or even within a group therapy room. Still, patients may experience vicarious learning by watching others engage and manage feared situations, and help their cohorts to challenge mistaken beliefs. Patients can also provide support and encouragement to each other. There are also consumer-led support groups that supplement professional treatment or help with relapse prevention.

Partner or Family Involvement in Symptoms

Individuals with OCD who live with a partner (e.g., spouse) or relatives often involve these other people in obsessions, avoidance, and compulsive rituals. For example, a man with contamination obsessions required that his family take showers with a specific type of soap before coming into his bedroom. In a less direct manner, OCD can affect friends and coworkers. People interacting with individuals with OCD often comply with requests to follow rituals, provide reassurance, and engage in avoidance strategies to keep their loved ones from experiencing anxiety. Because such accommodation is akin to the OCD sufferer performing rituals by him- or herself, it must be targeted in treatment, and the extent to which others can be helped to cut down on such behavior is a predictor of more successful treatment outcome. Additional suggestions for treating OCD in the context of family accommodation can be found in Abramowitz (2006). In a more global manner, low levels of social support or, in contrast, high levels of hostility and criticism are negative predictors of outcome and influence relapse across multiple disorders, including anxiety disorders. Therefore, interventions that increase social support and decrease negative social interactions are likely to impact treatment outcome. These interventions need to be "responsive." Some families that are very supportive have low levels of OCD accommodation. Other family work is crucial for treatment success to address impediments that are clearly present and impactful.

Relapse Prevention

For the majority of people with OCD, treatment produces noticeable improvement in symptoms; but residual obsessional fears, avoidance, and compulsive urges usually remain (Abramowitz, 1998). In addition, these residual symptoms are likely to wax and wane over time, often becoming more intense during periods of stress (e.g., relationship difficulties, job loss). Thus, any improvement attained during treatment should be carefully monitored to ensure that temporary lapses do not turn into full-blown relapses. Relapse prevention programs for OCD using ERP and cognitive therapy have been developed and tested (e.g., Hiss, Foa, & Kozak, 1994), and can be used as a way to taper off of treatment.

An important part of preventing relapse is recognizing that obsessions and compulsions may be inevitable. Thus, the patient should not be surprised or frightened by such symptoms when they occur. Cognitive therapy techniques can be used to modify any maladaptive beliefs about the recurrence of symptoms (e.g., "It's my fault that I'm slipping," "I'll be back to how I was before treatment"). Psychoeducation helps patients understand that OCD is usually a chronic problem, that they should expect symptom exacerbation during times of life stress, and that they should interpret symptoms within this framework and use the skills they have learned during treatment to manage these residual problems. Relapse prevention also teaches patients to recognize when new or different obsessions and compulsions arise, and how to view these as similar to symptoms that may already have been addressed. Indeed, rapid application of ERP techniques can prevent symptoms from escalating or interfering with functioning.

Other Treatment Approaches

While a wealth of research evidence supports the use of ERP, pharmacotherapy, and to a lesser extent, cognitive approaches, other forms of psychotherapy have not been evaluated for OCD. Unfortunately, at times, therapists who do not use these empirically supported approaches end up inadvertently reinforcing OCD symptoms. For example, therapists who repeatedly try to provide reassurance to patients with obsessional doubts—instead of helping them face their anxiety and learn to manage obsessional uncertainty and doubt—are helping the patient ritualize by reassurance-seeking. Others try to "help" patients overcome obsessions by trying to stop these thoughts (e.g., by snapping a rubber band on their arm when an obsession comes to mind) rather than confronting them therapeutically to learn that they are not dangerous. This "thought stopping" technique, however, is akin to mental rituals such as thought suppression, which, as we have discussed, do not work in the long run (i.e., obsessions return, especially when the person tries to dismiss them). Finally, the first inclination of many therapists when they see anxious and fearful individuals may be to try to soothe them, perhaps by teaching them relaxation strategies or biofeedback. Unfortunately, however, this approach is the opposite of exposure therapy, in which the person is helped to go *toward* anxiety in order to learn that it is a temporary feeling, that, although unpleasant, is not dangerous. Approaches such as these are not consistent with the conceptual models of OCD described earlier; therefore, they are not likely to provide patients with long-term relief from obsessions and compulsions.

Additional Approaches under Investigation

Acceptance and commitment therapy (ACT) and mindfulness-based approaches have been tested for OCD, assessed as both adjunctive treatments and alternative treatments, especially for those patients who absolutely refuse ERP (e.g., Whittal, 2009). Interestingly, if patients could be taught to view thoughts as thoughts and nothing more and would therefore not be compelled to act in response to them, these approaches might work similarly to ERP. In a different approach, patients might not begin to engage in rituals, might face anxiety differently, and might change their emotional reactions and relationship to OCD thoughts and feelings. If ACT or mindfulness approaches were utilized, the experience might also mean finding out that bad things do not happen, and that anxiety passes or is manageable.

SUMMARY AND CONCLUSION

OCD is a severe and functionally impairing condition with a heterogeneous presentation. Even the most experienced clinicians find themselves at once astounded and baffled by the complexity of the psychopathology, the rich patterns of anxiety-provoking thoughts and anxiety-reducing behaviors, and the severity of the impairment that occur in OCD. Although a definitive cause has not been established, various biological and psychological models have been proposed. Yet, as with many psychological disorders, more is understood about the *symptoms* of OCD than about its etiology. Fortunately, understanding the symptoms—specifically, that obsessional thoughts provoke anxiety and compulsive rituals are performed to reduce anxiety—has led to tremendous breakthroughs in treatment. Exposure, response prevention, and cognitive therapy are all effective strategies for reducing symptoms, although each comes with its own barriers to success. Although many patients achieve excellent outcomes that were unheard of before the 1960s, residual symptoms are still the norm. The field has, however, begun to identify factors that may reliably predict poorer response, such as poor insight into the senselessness of obsessional fears, severe depression, and family hostility.

Still, important topics require further study. For example, patient readiness programs would ensure a lower refusal or premature dropout rate. Treatments that teach partners (and other family members) effectively how to assist with a loved one's ERP would also prove beneficial given the high prevalence of relational problems and symptom accommodation in families of patients with OCD. From the clinical perspective, providing successful treatment for OCD can be one of the greatest challenges a therapist may experience. Yet the fact that most patients show at least some response to contemporary cognitive and behavioral techniques makes working with this patient population highly rewarding.

REFERENCES

Abramowitz, J. S. (1998). Does cognitive-behavioral therapy cure obsessive–compulsive disorder?: A meta-analytic evaluation of clinical significance. *Behavior Therapy, 29*, 339–355.

Abramowitz, J. S. (2004). Treatment of obsessive–compulsive disorder in patients with comorbid major depression. *Journal of Clinical Psychology: In Session, 60*, 1133–1141.

Abramowitz, J. S. (2006). *Understanding and treating obsessive–compulsive disorder: A cognitive-behavioral approach.* Mahwah, NJ: Erlbaum.

Abramowitz, J. S., & Deacon, B. J. (2005). The OC spectrum: A closer look at the arguments and the data. In J. Abramowitz & A. C. Houts (Eds.), *Concepts and controversies in obsessive–compulsive disorder* (pp. 141–149). New York: Springer.

Abramowitz, J. S., Deacon, B., Olatunji, B., Wheaton, M. G., Berman, N., Losardo, D., et al. (2010). Assessment of obsessive–compulsive symptom dimensions: Development and evaluation of the Dimensional Obsessive–Compulsive Scale. *Psychological Assessment, 22*, 180–198.

Abramowitz, J. S., Khandher, M., Nelson, C., Deacon, B. J., & Rygwall, R. (2006). The role of cognitive factors in the pathogenesis of obsessive–compulsive symptoms: A prospective study. *Behaviour Research and Therapy, 44,* 1361–1374.

Abramowitz, J. S., Nelson, C., Rygwall, R., & Khandher, M. (2007). The cognitive mediation of obsessive–compulsive symptoms: A longitudinal study. *Journal of Anxiety Disorders, 21,* 91–104.

Abramowitz, J. S., Schwartz, S. A., Moore, K. M., & Luenzmann, K. R. (2003). Obsessive–compulsive symptoms in pregnancy and the puerperium: A review of the literature. *Journal of Anxiety Disorders, 17,* 461–478.

Abramowitz, J. S., Wheaton, M., G., & Storch, E. A. (2008). The status of hoarding as a symptom of obsessive–compulsive disorder. *Behaviour Research and Therapy, 46,* 1026–1033.

American Psychiatric Association. (2013). *Diagnostic and statistical manual of mental disorders* (5th ed.). Arlington, VA: Author.

Beck, A. T. (1976). *Cognitive therapy of the emotional disorders.* New York: International Universities Press.

Black, D. W., Gaffney, G., Schlosser, S., & Gabel, J. (1998). The impact of obsessive–compulsive disorder on the family: Preliminary findings. *Journal of Nervous and Mental Disease, 186,* 440–442.

Clark, D. A. (2004). *Cognitive-behavioral therapy for OCD.* New York: Guilford Press.

Crino, R. D., & Andrews, G. (1996). Personality disorder in obsessive compulsive disorder: A controlled study. *Journal of Psychiatric Research, 30,* 29–38.

Enright, S. (1996). Obsessive–compulsive disorder: Anxiety disorder or schizotype? In R. Rapee (Ed.), *Current controversies in the anxiety disorders* (pp. 161–190). New York: Guilford Press.

Fallon, B. A., Javitch, J. A., Hollander, E., & Liebowiz, M. R. (1991). Hypochondriasis and obsessive–compulsive disorder: Overlaps in diagnosis and treatment. *Journal of Clinical Psychiatry, 52,* 457–460.

Fals-Stewart, W., Marks, A. P., & Schafer, J. (1993). A comparison of behavioral group therapy and individual behavior therapy in treating obsessive–compulsive disorder. *Journal of Nervous and Mental Disease, 181,* 189–193.

Foa, E. B., Abramowitz, J. S., Franklin, M. E., & Kozak, M. J. (1999). Feared consequences, fixity of belief and treatment outcome in obsessive–compulsive disorder. *Behavior Therapy, 30,* 717–724.

Foa, E. B., & Kozak, M. (1986). Emotional processing of fear: exposure to corrective information. *Psychological Bulletin, 99,* 20–35.

Foa, E. B., Liebowitz, M. R., Kozak, M. J., Davies, S., Campeas, R., Franklin, M. E., et al. (2005). Randomized, placebo-controlled trial of exposure and ritual prevention, clomipramine, and their combination in the treatment of obsessive–compulsive disorder. *American Journal of Psychiatry, 162,* 151–161.

Freeston, M. H., & Ladouceur, R. (1997). What do patients do with their obsessive thoughts? *Behaviour Research and Therapy, 35,* 335–348.

Frost, R. O., & Steketee, S. (2002). *Cognitive approaches to obsessions and compulsions: Theory, assessment, and treatment.* Oxford, UK: Elsevier.

Gershuny, B. S., Baer, L., Radomsky, A. S., Wilson, K. A., & Jenike, M. A. (2003). Connections among symptoms of obsessive–compulsive disorder and posttraumatic stress disorder: A case series. *Behaviour Research and Therapy, 41,* 1029–1041.

Hiss, H., Foa, E. B., & Kozak, M. J. (1994). Relapse prevention program for treatment of obsessive–compulsive disorder. *Journal of Consulting and Clinical Psychology, 62,* 801–808.

Hollander, E., Friedberg, J., Wasserman, S., Yeh, C.-C., & Iyengar, R. (2005). The case for the OCD spectrum. In J. Abramowitz & A. C. Houts (Eds.), *Concepts and controversies in obsessive–compulsive disorder* (pp. 95–118). New York: Springer.

Insel, T. R., Mueller, E. A., Alterman, I., Linnoila, M., & Murphy, D. L. (1985). Obsessive–compulsive disorder and serotonin: Is there a connection? *Biological Psychiatry, 20,* 1174–1188.

Koran, L. M. (2000). Quality of life in obsessive–compulsive disorder. *Psychiatric Clinics of North America, 23,* 509–517.

Kozak, M. J., & Foa, E. B. (1997). *Mastery of obsessive–compulsive disorder: Therapist manual.* San Antonio, TX: Psychological Corp.

Ladouceur, R., Freeston, M. H., Rheaume, J., Dugas, M. J., Gagnon, F., Thibodeau, N., et al. (2000). Strategies used with intrusive thoughts: A comparison of OCD patients with anxious and community controls. *Journal of Abnormal Psychology, 109,* 179–187.

Lensi, F., Cassano, G. B., Correddu, G., Ravagli, S., Kunovac, J. L., & Akiskal, H. S. (1996). Obsessive–compulsive disorder. Familial–developmental history, symptomatology, comorbidity and course with special reference to gender-related differences. *British Journal of Psychiatry, 169,* 101–107.

Lindsay, M., Crino, R., & Andrews, G. (1997). Controlled trial of exposure and response prevention in obsessive–compulsive disorder. *British Journal of Psychiatry, 171,* 135–139.

McKay, D., Abramowitz, J. S., Calamari, J. E., Kyrios, M., Radomsky, A. S., Sookman, D., et al. (2004). A critical evaluation of obsessive–compulsive disorder subtypes: Symptoms versus mechanisms. *Clinical Psychology Review, 24,* 283–313.

McLean, P. D., Whittal, M. L., Thordarson, D. S., Taylor, S., Sochting, I., Koch, W. J., et al. (2001). Cognitive versus behavior therapy in the group treatment of obsessive–compulsive disorder. *Journal of Consulting and Clinical Psychology, 69,* 205–214.

Mowrer, O. (1960). *Learning theory and behavior.* New York: Wiley.

Nestadt, G., Samuels, J., Riddle, M. A., Liang, K.-Y., Bienvenu, O. J., Hoehn-Saric, R., et al. (2001). The relationship between obsessive–compulsive disorder and anxiety and affective disorders: Results from the Johns Hopkins OCD Family Study. *Psychological Medicine, 31,* 481–487.

Pato, M. T., Zohar-Kadouch, R., Zohar, J., & Murphy, D. L. (1988). Return of symptoms after discontinuation of clomipramine in patients with obsessive–compulsive disorder. *American Journal of Psychiatry, 145,* 1521–1525.

Rachman, S. (1997). A cognitive theory of obsessions. *Behaviour Research and Therapy, 35,* 793–802.

Rachman, S., & de Silva, P. (1978). Abnormal and normal obsessions. *Behaviour Research and Therapy, 16,* 233–248.

Radomsky, A. S., Rachman, S., & Hammond, D. (2001). Memory bias, confidence and responsibility in compulsive checking. *Behaviour Research and Therapy, 39,* 813–822.

Rasmussen, S. A., & Tsuang, M. T. (1986). Clinical characteristics and family history in DSM-III obsessive–compulsive disorder. *American Journal of Psychiatry, 143,* 317–322.

Rauch, S., & Jenike, M. (1998). Pharmacological treatment of obsessive compulsive disorder. In P. E. Nathan & J. M. Gorman (Eds.), *A guide to treatments that work.* London: Oxford University Press.

Ricciardi, J. N., & McNally, R. J. (1995). Depressed mood is related to obsessions but not compulsions in obsessive–compulsive disorder. *Journal of Anxiety Disorders, 9,* 249–256.

Salkovskis, P. (1996). Cognitive-behavioral approaches to the understanding of obsessional problems. In R. Rapee (Ed.), *Current controversies in the anxiety disorders* (pp. 103–133). New York: Guilford Press.

Salkovskis, P. M., & Westbrook, H. M. (1989). Cognitive therapy of obsessive–compulsive disorder: Treating treatment failures. *Behavioural Psychotherapy, 13,* 243–255.

Saxena, S., Bota, R. G., & Brody, A. L. (2001). Brain–behavior relationships in obsessive–compulsive disorder. *Seminars in Clinical Neuropsychiatry, 6,* 82–101.

Simpson, H., & Liebowitz, M. (2005). Combining pharmacotherapy and cognitive behavioral therapy in the treatment of OCD. In J. Abramowitz & A. Houts (Eds.), *Concepts and controversies in OCD* (pp. 359–376). New York: Springer Science.

Skoog, G., & Skoog, I. (1999). A 40-year follow-up of patients with obsessive–compulsive disorder. *Archives of General Psychiatry, 56,* 121–127.

Steketee, G. S., Chambless, D. L., & Tran, G. Q. (2001). Effects of Axis I and II comorbidity on behavior therapy outcome for obsessive–compulsive disorder and agoraphobia. *Comprehensive Psychiatry, 42,* 76–86.

Steketee, G., Eisen, J., Dyck, I., Warshaw, M., & Rasmussen, S. (1999). Predictors of course in obsessive–compulsive disorder. *Psychiatry Research, 89,* 229–238.

Taylor, S., Thordarson, D., & Sochting, I. (2002). Obsessive–compulsive disorder. In M. Antony & D. H. Barlow (Eds.), *Handbook of assessment and treatment planning for psychological disorders* (pp. 182–214). New York: Guilford Press.

Weissman, M. M., Bland, R. C., Canino, G. J., Greenwald, S., Hwu, H.-G., Kyoon Lee, C., et al. (1994). The cross national epidemiology of obsessive compulsive disorder. *Journal of Clinical Psychiatry, 55,* 5–10.

Whittal, M. (2009). Special section: Cognitive and behavioral practice comes of age. *Cognitive and Behavioral Practice, 16*(1), 161–175.

Whiteside, S. P., Port, J. D., & Abramowitz, J. S. (2004). A metaanalysis of functional neuroimaging in obsessive–compulsive disorder. *Psychiatry Research: Neuroimaging, 132,* 69–79.

Wilhelm, S., & Steketee, G. (2006). *Cognitive therapy for obsessive–compulsive disorder: A guide for professionals.* Oakland CA: New Harbinger.

Zohar, J., & Insel, T. R. (1987). Obsessive–compulsive disorder: Psychobiological approaches to diagnosis, treatment, and pathophysiology. *Biological Psychiatry, 22,* 667–687.

CHAPTER 6

Posttraumatic Stress Disorder

Richard A. Bryant
Terence M. Keane

The adverse psychological effects of being exposed to a traumatic event have been documented for many years. Earlier conceptualizations of traumatic stress typically regarded these reactions as transient responses that would normally abate shortly after trauma exposure. In the first edition of the DSM (American Psychiatric Association, 1952), traumatic stress reactions were classified as acute posttrauma responses under gross stress reaction, and longer lasting reactions were subsumed under the anxiety or depressive neuroses. A major change occurred in DSM-III (American Psychiatric Association, 1980), in which the diagnosis of posttraumatic stress disorder (PTSD) was formally introduced. This formal recognition of the syndrome was partly influenced by the need to understand and meet the needs of veterans returning from Vietnam with PTSD reactions.

TYPICAL SYMPTOMS

PTSD describes severe and persistent stress reactions after exposure to a traumatic event. In the DSM-5 (American Psychiatric Association, 2013), Cluster A involves exposure to a life-threatening event either directly, through witnessing the event, or indirectly by learning about the event. PTSD comprises four additional symptom clusters to include: intrusive symptoms (Cluster B), avoidance symptoms (Cluster C), negative alterations in mood and cognitions (Cluster D), and alterations in arousal and reactivity (Cluster E). Examples for the intrusive symptoms of Cluster B are intrusive, distressing memories of the traumatic event; recurrent, distressing dreams/nightmares; flashbacks that recapitulate the event in a dissociative manner; intense distress when exposed to reminders of the traumatic experience;

and marked physiological reactions (panic-like) to reminders or cues. Criterion C includes avoidance of stimuli that are reminiscent of the traumatic event, but it can also include avoidance of thoughts or feelings associated with that event, as well as avoidance of external reminders.

Criterion D represents a new component of the PTSD diagnosis in that it separates avoidance from other emotional facets of the condition. Negative alterations in cognitions and mood include the following components: the inability to remember an important aspect of the event; persistent and exaggerated negative beliefs about oneself, the world, or others; persistent distorted blame of self or others for the occurrence of the event; persistent negative emotional state; markedly diminished interest in activities; feelings of detachment or estrangement; and difficulty experiencing positive emotions or feelings.

Acute stress disorder (ASD), a new diagnosis in DSM-IV, was introduced for two primary reasons: to describe acute stress reactions that occur in the initial month after trauma exposure, and to identify trauma survivors who are high risk for developing subsequent PTSD (Harvey & Bryant, 2002). A major rationale for the introduction of this diagnosis was because PTSD can only be diagnosed at least 1 month following trauma, and there was a diagnostic gap in the initial month of trauma. The lack of a formal diagnosis to describe posttraumatic stress in the initial month potentially limited some trauma survivors to having ready access to mental health services and, in this sense, a formal diagnosis was intended to alleviate this potential barrier to care. In DSM-5, the stressor criterion (Criterion A) for acute stress disorder was changed from DSM-IV. The criterion now requires, as with PTSD, being explicit as to whether the qualifying traumatic events were experienced directly, witnessed, or experienced indirectly. Also the DSM-IV Criterion A2 regarding the subjective reaction to the traumatic event (e.g., "the person's response involved intense fear, helplessness, or horror") was eliminated. Based on evidence that acute posttraumatic reactions are very heterogeneous and that DSM-IV's emphasis on dissociative symptoms is too restrictive, individuals may meet diagnostic criteria in DSM-5 for acute stress disorder if they report any 9 of 14 listed symptoms in these categories: intrusion, negative mood, dissociation, avoidance, and arousal.

A diagnosis of ASD requires that the individual has at least three of the following: (1) subjective sense of numbing or detachment, (2) reduced awareness of one's surroundings, (3) derealization, (4) depersonalization, or (5) dissociative amnesia. DSM-IV stated that these dissociative responses can occur either at the time of the trauma or in the month after trauma exposure. The emphasis on dissociative symptoms can be traced back to the work of Janet (1907), which suggested that people who are overwhelmed by traumatic experiences may attempt to reduce the emotional pain of the trauma by restricting awareness of the traumatic experience. He proposed that although this splitting of traumatic memories from awareness led to some reduction in distress, there was a loss of mental functioning, because mental resources were not available for other processes. It has subsequently been proposed that dissociating from awareness trauma memories and emotions in the immediate aftermath of trauma impedes processing of these reactions and thereby leads to subsequent PTSD. Support for the inclusion of dissociative symptoms in the ASD diagnosis to predict subsequent PTSD came from evidence demonstrating an association between "peritraumatic dissociation" (i.e., dissociation occurring in the immediate aftermath of a traumatic experience) and subsequent levels of PTSD, a finding that has been replicated across numerous longitudinal studies (Murray, Ehlers, & Mayou, 2002).

COURSE

There is strong evidence that most people who are recently exposed to a traumatic experience commonly report posttraumatic stress reactions in the initial weeks after trauma. Despite the prevalence of acute stress reactions, the majority of these stress responses are transient (Bryant, 2003). For example, whereas 94% of rape victims displayed sufficient PTSD symptoms 2 weeks posttrauma to meet criteria (excluding the 1-month time requirement), 11 weeks later this rate dropped to 47% (Rothbaum, Foa, Riggs, Murdock, & Walsh, 1992). In another study, 70% of women and 50% of men were diagnosed with PTSD at an average of 19 days after an assault; the rate of PTSD at 4-month follow-up dropped to 21% for women and zero for men (Riggs, Rothbaum, & Foa, 1995). Similar patterns have been observed following motor vehicle accidents (Blanchard, Hickling, Barton, & Taylor, 1996), the New York terrorist attacks (Galea et al., 2003), and the 2004 tsumani (van Griensven et al., 2006).

Despite a general trend for people to adapt after trauma, it is also important to note that there are different trajectories from acute reactions to chronic PTSD. The main exemplar of a different trajectory is delayed-onset PTSD. Delayed onset is an uncommon response in civilian populations, although there is some evidence that it is more common in military contexts (for a review, see Andrews, Brewin, Philpott, & Stewart, 2007). Although the mechanisms underpinning delayed-onset PTSD are not well understood, several explanations have been offered. These include the implementation of numbing responses that inhibit expression of distress (Horowitz & Solomon, 1975), preoccupation with more immediate needs (e.g., pain, surgery) that distract attention from one's symptoms (Andreasen, 2004), the increase of stressors in the posttrauma period that compound the initial stress response (Bryant & Harvey, 2002), or rising demands on cognitive resources that are required to manage emotional responses and which then lead to increased distress (Grossman, Levin, Katzen, & Lechner, 2004). There is evidence that it represents subsyndromal levels of PTSD that accumulate over time, potentially as a function of increasing posttraumatic stress; that is, prospective evidence indicates that cases described as delayed onset actually display elevated levels of posttraumatic stress in the initial period after the trauma (Andrews et al., 2007). Interesting evidence on this issue emerged in a recent study on the trajectory of adaptation after Hurricane Katrina, which found that rates of PTSD actually increased over time following Hurricane

Katrina (Kessler et al., 2008). It is possible that the lengthy periods of relocation, lack of housing, and loss of basic infrastructures resulted in increased psychological strain, which led to rising rates of PTSD. Delayed-onset PTSD appears to be more common in military settings than in civilian contexts, with accumulating evidence from military populations that soldiers do not appear to have PTSD immediately after deployment but do develop the disorder months later (Andrews et al., 2007). One possibility is that the relief of leaving the immediate context of threat and the attention given to soldiers in the immediate postdeployment environment result in a period of minimal posttraumatic stress; however as time passes they are increasingly aware of the negative aftereffects of their trauma.

CLASSIFICATION

Posttraumatic Stress Disorder

In the discussions preceding DSM-5, considerable attention had been devoted to the classification of PTSD, in terms of both where it belongs in the broader spectrum of psychiatric disorders and its own definition. One important decision was to reclassify PTSD in a new category of trauma-related and stressor-related disorders (rather than with the anxiety disorders, where it appeared in DSM-IV). Recent debate has focused on the possibility of identifying a subset of anxiety disorders termed "fear circuitry disorders" that arise after a traumatic/stressful event. Some experts proposed that this category would include PTSD, panic disorder/agoraphobia, social anxiety disorder, and specific phobia (Andrews, Charney, Sirovatka, & Regier, 2009). Although there is some evidence that aversive or traumatic experiences do precede onset of panic disorder (Manfro et al., 1996) and social phobia (McCabe, Antony, Summerfeldt, Liss, & Swinson, 2003), other evidence suggests a different pattern (Rapee, Litwin, & Barlow, 1990). There is also increasing evidence that a range of other disorders do develop after trauma exposure. Depression is a commonly observed psychological disorder in survivors of traumatic events, along with various anxiety disorders (Norris, Friedman, & Watson, 2002). After the Oklahoma City Bombing, 22% of people suffered depression, 7% suffered panic disorder, 4% had generalized anxiety disorder, 9% had alcohol use disorder, and 2% had drug use disorder; overall, 30% of people had a psychiatric disorder other than PTSD (North et al., 1999). In another study of over 1,000 traumatic injury survivors, depression was the most common disorder (16%), followed by generalized anxiety disorder (11%), agoraphobia (9%), and PTSD (9%) (Bryant, Creamer, O'Donnell, Silove, Clark, & McFarlane, 2010). These patterns highlight that PTSD is not the only condition that can develop following trauma. However, the evidence that these other disorders are not distinctive to the aftermath of trauma is not consistent with their being part of a fear circuitry category. Another challenge is that the fear circuitry construct does not give adequate attention to other emotions associated with PTSD, including sadness, grief, anger, guilt, and shame (Friedman, Resick, Bryant & Brewin, 2011).

One line of research supporting the fear circuitry category comes from neu-roimaging research. The prevailing model of fear circuitry posits that these disor-ders are characterized by impaired medial prefrontal cortex activation, which leads to excessive amygdala response, and this network is responsible for fear reactivity (Charney, 2003) . Across an increasing body of evidence in which researchers con-ducted neuroimaging studies across the relevant disorders, there is evidence that whereas fear circuitry disorders tend to be characterized by excessive amygdala reactivity, and to a lesser extent impaired regulation of that response by the medial prefrontal cortex (e.g., Shin & Liberzon, 2010), different neural networks appear to be involved in nonfear circuitry anxiety disorders (e.g., Rauch et al., 2007).

DSM-5 suggests several important changes based upon key findings in the literature. The subjective response to the trauma at the time of the event is now eliminated (A2). Second avoidance is redefined and includes only active avoidance of thoughts, feelings, and situations associated with the traumatic event. This is in deference to the many factor-analytic studies suggesting PTSD is composed of four factors: intrusive thoughts; active avoidance; numbing/passive avoidance; and arousal symptoms (King, Leskin, King, & Weathers, 1998). These studies have found that emotional numbing and social withdrawal are distinct from more active avoidance strategies. The latter symptoms will be included in a separate cluster that also involves negative alterations in cognitions and mood, which also includes negative appraisals about oneself and one's future, and persistent negative emo-tional states, including anger, guilt, or shame. This addition is included because of the overwhelming evidence that PTSD can be characterized by catastrophic cogni-tive interpretations of the experience (Ehlers & Clark, 2000), and by a range of emo-tional responses beyond fear and anxiety (Brewin, Andrews, & Valentine, 2000). The arousal cluster is retained, with several minor modifications; aggressive behav-ior and self-destructive/reckless behavior are included.

Acute Stress Disorder

Since its introduction, the ASD diagnosis has been widely criticized for several rea-sons. In terms of describing acute posttraumatic stress, approaches that focus on fear responses alone may neglect other psychological reactions (Isserlin, Zerach, & Solomon, 2008). In contrast to ASD, the construct of acute stress reactions described in the *International Classification of Diseases* (ICD; World Health Organization, 1995) conceptualizes acute stress reaction as a transient reaction that can be evident immediately after the traumatic event and usually resolves within 2–3 days after trauma exposure. The ICD description of acute stress reaction includes dissociative (daze, stupor, amnesia), anxiety (tachycardia, sweating, flushing), anger, or depres-sive reactions, which may have more utility for clinicians than the more focused ASD criteria (Isserlin et al., 2008) . This approach presumes that the initial period after trauma exposure may result in a rather amorphous state of distress that can include many emotional responses that cannot be readily classified into different responses (Yitzhaki, Solomon, & Kotler, 1991).

A secondary goal of the ASD diagnosis is to discriminate between recent trauma survivors who are experiencing transient stress reactions and those who are suffering reactions that will persist into long-term PTSD. A large number of prospective studies have assessed trauma survivors for ASD in the initial month after trauma and subsequently assessed for PTSD months or years later (for a review, see Bryant, 2011). Across these studies, at least half of trauma survivors with ASD subsequently meet criteria for PTSD. In contrast, the majority of survivors who eventually developed PTSD did not initially meet ASD criteria. This pattern suggests that if a major goal of ASD is to predict who will subsequently develop PTSD, it is failing to identify half of those who will meet criteria for PTSD at some later time.

DSM-5 reformulates the construct of ASD in a way that its basis isn't solely as a state that predicts PTSD. Evidence in the past 15 years suggests that ASD does not seem to be able to identify the majority of people who develop PTSD upon exposure to a traumatic event (Bryant, Friedman, Spiegel, Ursano, & Strain, 2011). For the current edition of the DSM, the goal is to describe severe acute stress reactions that may or may not be transient responses but might nonetheless benefit from mental health interventions. The ASD definition now requires that the patient satisfy a minimum of nine out of a total fourteen potential symptoms in recognition that ASD presentations are heterogeneous.

ASSOCIATED CLINICAL FEATURES

There is much evidence that PTSD is linked to a wide range of other mental health and psychosocial problems, both of which contribute to impaired functioning and also compound the PTSD itself. PTSD has been linked to a large range of impairment indicators. In the large-scale National Vietnam Veterans Readjustment Study, those with PTSD had lower levels of impairment in terms of employment, marital difficulties, divorce rates, poor self-reported health, and higher utilization of medical services (Zatzick et al., 1997). It appears that avoidance and numbing are the PTSD symptoms that most contribute to impairment (Shea, Vujanovic, Mansfield, Sevin, & Liu, 2010). There is convergent evidence that trauma exposure is linked to a range of poor physical health outcomes, and it appears that this effect can be largely attributed to PTSD (Friedman & Schnurr, 1995). Several mechanisms have been proposed for this relationship, including biological (e.g., increased cardiovascular reactivity, altered hypothalamic–pituitary–adrenal [HPA] activity), behavioral (e.g., increased substance use, smoking), and psychological (e.g., chronic depression, hostility) factors that may impair health (Friedman & McEwen, 2004). PTSD is also linked to impaired sleep function (Neylan et al., 1998); not only do nightmares and hyperarousal lead to sleep disturbance, but also sleep disturbance immediately prior to trauma exposure enhances risk for PTSD (Bryant, Creamer, O'Donnell, Silove, & McFarlane, 2010). PTSD also is associated with interpersonal, marital, and sexual dysfunction. For example, individuals with PTSD are more likely to have diminished sexual drive and erectile dysfunction (Anticevic & Britvic, 2008), social withdrawal, and interpersonal conflict (MacDonald, Chamberlain, Long, & Flett, 1999). Finally, it is important to note that suicide risk is increased with PTSD; for example, large-scale studies of veterans of the Vietnam (Bullman & Kang, 1996) and Iraq (Kang & Bullman, 2008) wars who display posttraumatic stress tend to have higher rates of suicidal risk than other veterans. This pattern has led the Institute of Medicine (2007) conclude that suicide risk is heightened in the initial years following deployment. The issue of suicide risk in PTSD is particularly relevant because of the elevated rates of suicidality in other mental disorders (e.g., depression) that are highly comorbid with PTSD (Zivin et al., 2007).

EPIDEMIOLOGY

Population studies have shown that many people in the community have been exposed to traumatic stressors. The U.S. National Comorbidity Survey indicated that 61% of randomly sampled adults reported exposure to a traumatic stressor (Kessler, Sonnega, Hughes, & Nelson, 1995). A study of adults living in Detroit found that 90% reported exposure to a traumatic stressor (Breslau, Davis, Andreski, & Peterson, 1991). Despite the frequency of exposure to potentially traumatizing events, relatively few people actually develop PTSD. For example, the National Comorbidity Survey found that only 20.4% of the women and 8.2% of the men ever developed PTSD (Kessler et al., 1995). Similarly, the Detroit study found that only 13% of the women and 6.2% of the men had developed PTSD (Breslau et al., 1991). These studies indicate that the normative response following trauma exposure is to adapt to the experience and to not develop PTSD. Although men are more likely than women to be exposed to trauma, women have at least a twofold risk of developing PTSD compared to men (Breslau, Davis, Peterson, & Schultz, 1997). There is a tendency for more severe traumas to result in more severe PTSD. There is evidence that interpersonal violence leads more to PTSD than does impersonal trauma; for example, whereas 55% of rape victims develop PTSD, only 7.5% of accident victims do so. Meta-analytic studies of international research highlight how torture results in markedly higher rates of PTSD than other forms of trauma (Thomas et al., 2008).

Prevalence rates are not the same everywhere. Across countries and cultural settings there is marked variability in the occurrence of PTSD. Comparing these studies is difficult because of methodological differences, different patterns in trauma exposure, variability in access to health care, and cultural distinctiveness in definition of posttraumatic symptoms. Accordingly, to address the role of ethnicity in PTSD, it is important to consider ethnic variation in similar settings, with exposure to comparable traumatic events. In this context, there are different prevalence rates across ethnic groupings. For example, in the wake of the September 11, 2001, terrorist attack in New York, Hispanics, blacks, and other minority ethnicities were more likely than whites to develop PTSD (Adams & Boscarino, 2005; DiGrande et al., 2008). In addition to civilian samples, there is also evidence in military samples that Hispanics are particularly at risk of PTSD development (Schlenger et al., 1992).

It is difficult to identify the reason for this pattern; it may be attributable to lower socioeconomic status and associated resource availability to manage trauma, racial discrimination, or cultural differences in expressing and coping with adversity (Ruef, Litz, & Schlenger, 2000).

COMORBIDITY

There is overwhelming evidence that PTSD is more often associated with other psychiatric disorders than occurring as the sole diagnosis. Lifetime comorbidity prevalence rates with PTSD have been reported in at least two-thirds of cases (Kessler Sonnega, et al., 1995). The major overlap is between PTSD and other disorders: depression, other anxiety disorders, and substance abuse. Although it is possible that a degree of comorbidity may be attributed to overlapping symptoms between PTSD and both depressive and anxiety disorders, several studies have confirmed that there is marked comorbidity with these disorders and PTSD, even when controlling for this overlap. There is also considerable comorbidity with personality disorders. PTSD has frequently been shown to be comorbid with borderline personality disorder, which arguably is not surprising, as there is often a significant trauma history in the profile of those with borderline personality disorder. There is also significant overlap between PTSD and antisocial personality disorder (Sareen, Stein, Cox, & Hassard, 2004); it has been suggested that the antisocial tendencies may precede the PTSD, and that dangerous behaviors may predispose the person to suffer traumatic events.

Two major mechanisms have been proposed to explain these high rates of comorbidity. One pathway may involves people developing a psychiatric disorder, which predisposes people to experiencing trauma and associated PTSD. The other pathway is the primary onset of PTSD, which leads to simultaneous or subsequent comorbid disorders. It appears that a significant proportion of comorbid cases reflect the development of PTSD after the initial onset of another disorder (Breslau et al., 1997). It appears that anxiety disorders and substance use disorders are particularly influential in increasing risk for trauma exposure and PTSD (e.g., Stein et al., 2002). There is also strong evidence that much comorbidity develops following PTSD onset, implying that PTSD can increase the likelihood of developing distinct disorders (Perkonigg, Kessler, Storz, & Wittchen, 2000). One important consequence of PTSD is increased substance use, which has been conceptualized as a form of self-medication and can lead to marked long-term dysfunction in the context of chronic PTSD (McFarlane, 1998).

TREATMENT

Chronic PTSD

The treatment of choice for chronic PTSD is trauma-focused psychotherapy. Comprehensive treatment based on systematic reviews of the evidence including guidelines from the U.K. National Institute for Clinical Excellence (2005), the U.S. Department of Veterans Affairs (U.S. Department of Defense, 2004), the U.S. Institute of Medicine (2007), the Australian National Health and Medical Research Council (Australian Centre for Posttraumatic Mental Health, 2007a), and the International Society of Traumatic Stress Studies (Foa, Keane, Friedman, & Cohen, 2009), have reached this conclusion. A similar conclusion has been drawn from major meta-analyses (Bradley, Greene, Russ, Dutra, & Westen, 2005). Importantly, trauma-focused psychotherapy has been shown to be efficacious across different trauma-exposed populations, including survivors of traumatic injury and assault (Bryant, Moulds, et al., 2008), sexual assault (Foa, Rothbaum, Riggs, & Murdock, 1991), combat (Schnurr et al., 2003), terrorist attacks (Duffy, Gillespie, & Clark, 2007), and child sexual abuse (McDonagh et al., 2005).

The major form of trauma-focused psychotherapy, cognitive-behavioral therapy (CBT), usually commences with psychoeducation about the trauma responses, then focuses on three major strategies: anxiety management, exposure, and cognitive restructuring. In psychoeducation the patient is informed about common symptoms following a traumatic event and the way in which the core symptoms will be treated during the course of therapy. Anxiety management techniques aim to reduce anxiety through a range of techniques that may include breathing retraining, relaxation skills, and self-talk. Exposure therapy usually involves both imaginal and *in vivo* exposure. Imaginal exposure typically requires patients to imagine their traumatic experience vividly for prolonged periods, usually for at least 30 minutes. The therapist asks patients to provide a narrative of their traumatic experience in a way that emphasizes all relevant details, including sensory cues and affective responses. *In vivo* exposure involves graded exposure to feared stimuli, in which patients are asked to remain in close proximity to mildly fearful reminders of the trauma, then repeat this exercise with increasingly fearful situations until they feel comfortable with most reminders of their experience. Exposure may be therapeutic because of habituation of anxiety, integration of corrective information, knowledge that the trauma is a discrete event that is no longer threatening, and self-mastery through management of exposure (Rothbaum & Schwartz, 2002). Cognitive restructuring involves teaching patients to identify and evaluate the evidence for negative automatic thoughts, as well as helping them to evaluate their beliefs about the trauma, the self, the world, and the future. In most controlled trials, CBT programs usually require eight to 12 sessions conducted on an individual basis.

The majority of studies indicate that treatments incorporating prolonged exposure either to trauma memories or situations that remind the individual of trauma are beneficial. There is some debate over the relative contributions of different CBT components. Several studies suggest that exposure and cognitive restructuring provide comparable treatment gains, and others indicate that combining cognitive restructuring with exposure does not provide additive effects above beyond exposure alone (Foa et al., 2005). There is limited evidence that the addition of cognitive restructuring may enhance the effect of exposure (Bryant, Moulds, Guthrie,

Dang, & Nixon, 2003). The overall finding that other CBT components do not markedly enhance exposure suggests that exposure is a critical ingredient in facilitating recovery from PTSD (Cahill, Rothbaum, Resick, & Follette, 2009). Because exposure typically includes a form of cognitive reframing in which the therapist discusses the mastery of exposure to trauma reminders, it seems that the change mechanisms involved in both exposure and cognitive restructuring may overlap. In summary, the largest body of evidence supports the use of exposure-based CBT that typically employs exposure to trauma memories and feared situations that result in a sense of safety or mastery over those stimuli.

A variant of CBT is eye movement desensitization and reprocessing (EMDR). This treatment differs from CBT insofar as it requires patients to focus their attention on a traumatic memory, while simultaneously visually tracking the therapist's finger as it is moved across their visual field, then to engage in restructuring of the memory (Shapiro, 1995). The patient is asked to identify more adaptive or positive thoughts related to the memory or traumatic experience, and to again track the therapist's fingers. EMDR often also includes other coping techniques, such as relaxation skills or positive visualization. Although the specific mechanisms by which eye movements are purported to enhance treatment gains are not well specified, moving one's eyes after engaging the trauma memory is intended to facilitate information processing (Shapiro & Maxfield, 2002).

Across a series of controlled trials, EMDR has been shown to be an effective treatment for PTSD relative to wait-list and to perform comparably to standard CBT. Accordingly, it is recommended, along with CBT, as a frontline treatment in a number of recent treatment guidelines (Australian Centre for Posttraumatic Mental Health, 2007b; National Institute of Clinical Excellence, 2005). In evaluating EMDR, however, it is important to note that eye movements are not pivotal in the treatment effects of EMDR (Australian Centre for Posttraumatic Mental Health, 2007b). This conclusion is supported by evidence from studies that manipulated eye movement, in addition to other strategies, and found that the eye movements themselves were not important in relieving the symptoms relative to the other components of EMDR (Foley & Spates, 1995). Additionally, the Australian National Health and Medical Research council (NHMRC) guidelines concluded that EMDR was as efficacious as CBT only when EMDR also included *in vivo* exposure (Australian Centre for Posttraumatic Mental Health, 2007b).

Another variant of trauma-focused therapy, cognitive processing therapy (CPT), was developed as a form of cognitive therapy to address the specific cognitive responses of survivors of rape (Resick & Schnicke, 1993). In CPT, attention is focused on reframing unrealistic beliefs about safety, trust, control, esteem, and intimacy; CPT also engages trauma memories by requiring the patient to write detailed accounts of the trauma and relating these accounts to the therapist. Randomized controlled CPT trials have reported strong effects of CPT relative to a wait list (Chard, 2005). Furthermore, a recent trial that compared (1) full CPT, (2) the writing component, and (3) the cognitive component found that the writing component did not provide any additive gain over the cognitive element (Resick et al., 2008).

There has been concern that CBT techniques may not be appropriate for patients with more complex PTSD. "Complex PTSD" describes cases of PTSD (often secondary to childhood abuse) in which the patient has marked difficulties with emotion regulation, which may manifest in strong mood swings, difficulty stabilizing emotional reactions, impulsive behaviors, self-harm, and difficulties with interpersonal relationships (Cloitre, Miranda, Stovall-McClough, & Han, 2005). On the premise that patients with emotion regulation deficits may have difficulty managing the emotional demands of exposure-based therapy, attempts have been made to prepare these patients for CBT by teaching them skills to regulate emotions. These skills involve distress tolerance, labeling emotions, and emotion management. Two randomized trials have now demonstrated that this modified form of CBT is efficacious in treating complex PTSD, and there is evidence that it is more effective than standard CBT for patients with complex PTSD (Cloitre et al., 2010). Considering that people who suffer more severe traumatic exposures, and often endure prolonged childhood trauma, can have difficulty regulating emotions, this approach appears to augment the efficacy of CBT.

Cognitive-Behavioral Therapy for Children

Compared to studies of adults, relatively less attention has been given to treatment of childhood PTSD. In general terms, children appear to experience PTSD as often as adults, although there have been proposals that symptom manifestation may be marginally different in children (e.g., Salmon & Bryant, 2002). Treatment programs for children often modify CBT by integrating strategies that teach regulation of affect or behavior, including parents in treatment, adapting treatment delivery to the developmental stage of the child, and placing strong emphasis on rapport factors between therapist and patient (Cohen, Mannarino, Deblinger, & Berliner, 2009). Consistent with the adult literature, available trials support the conclusion that trauma-focused psychotherapy is the treatment of choice for childhood PTSD.

Global Early Interventions

A major debate that has persisted over recent years concerns the merits of intervening shortly after a traumatic event potentially to prevent PTSD. For many years psychological debriefing has been the most common approach immediately after trauma exposure, and critical incident stress debriefing (CISD) was arguably the most common variant of this approach (Mitchell, 1983). In the original iteration of this strategy, a debriefing session that typically occurred within 48 hours of the trauma involved education about trauma reactions; required participants to describe what occurred and their cognitive, emotional, and physical responses to the event; and provided suggestions for stress reduction (Mitchell & Everly, 1996). Although difficult to assess because of the many uncontrollable factors that exist in a post-disaster setting, a series of studies have compared trauma survivors who received CISD and those who did not receive the intervention (Rose, Brewin, Andrews, & Kirk, 1999). Systematic reviews of these studies indicate that people who receive CISD did not have better outcomes than those who do not (Rose, Bisson, & Wessely, 2001). Furthermore, some tentative evidence indicates that very distressed people who receive debriefing immediately after a trauma may subsequently have worse PTSD symptoms than those who do not receive debriefing (Hobbs, Mayou, Harrison, & Worlock, 1996). It has been suggested that requiring people to ventilate their emotions within days of trauma exposure may hasten arousal and strengthen their trauma memories, which may impede natural recovery (McNally, Bryant, & Ehlers, 2003). In the wake of this evidence, the field has moved toward recognition that single-session interventions after trauma may not be sufficient to avert subsequent PTSD. At present the most common alternative to debriefing is psychological first aid (PFA; Young, 2006), which attempts to assist adaptation by ensuring that patients' needs are met, facilitating problem solving, reducing acute arousal, and accessing social supports. PFA attempts to enhance coping skills in the immediate aftermath of a disaster *without* causing undue distress by directing the survivor to revisit the traumatic experience. Importantly, PFA has not yet been tested, and one obstacle to evaluation is that PFA does not have clearly stated goals or outcomes, and is not a standardized intervention that is amenable to controlled evaluation. Whereas CISD explicitly attempts to reduce subsequent PTSD, PFA assists coping rather than serving a secondary prevention role (for full details of PFA, see *www.ncptsd.va.gov/ncmain/ncdocs/manuals/nc_manual_psyfirstaid.html*).

Targeted Early Interventions

In contrast to interventions provided to all trauma survivors shortly after exposure, there has also been a focus on interventions for survivors who are deemed to be at high risk for developing PTSD. The focus of most of these studies has been on trauma survivors who display ASD in the first month after trauma exposure, because of evidence that these individuals are more likely than other survivors to develop chronic PTSD (Bryant, 2003). Attempts at secondary prevention have typically modified standard CBT approaches by abridging them to five or six sessions. The common factor across interventions for ASD/acute PTSD is that their trauma-focused exposure approach that involves imaginal or *in vivo* exposure. Across a series of controlled trials, there is now convergent evidence that exposure-based CBT provided within a month of trauma exposure prevents PTSD in the majority of cases relative to nondirective counseling (Bryant, Mastrodomenico, et al., 2008). These treatment gains have been shown to maintain up to four years after treatment (Bryant et al., 2006). Additionally, providing CBT to trauma survivors with acute PTSD in the initial months after trauma exposure results in reduced levels of PTSD at subsequent time points (Ehlers et al., 2003). Overall, the evidence indicates that exposure-based therapies are indicated for early intervention with people with ASD/acute PTSD.

PRINCIPLES OF CHANGE

This review has highlighted the heterogeneity of PTSD. The potential variability and complexity of PTSD highlights how clinicians need to be cognizant of the various techniques from evidence-supported research that can be administered to posttraumatic presentations. Table 6.1 presents a summary of principles and related strategies that can be applied to the variety of PTSD presentations. It is apparent that a range of evidence-based interventions is available to the clinician to address the array of presentations that frequently exist with PTSD. The sequence in which one implements these strategies is usually determined by several factors. As always, with any clinical intervention, any presentation that poses a risk for a patient (e.g.,

TABLE 6.1. Principles of Change and Treatment Choices

Principle	Treatment strategy
Understanding of trauma reactions	Psychoeducation and normalization of symptoms
Enhancing distress tolerance	Emotion regulation skills training (breathing retraining, emotion labeling, mindfulness)
Extinction learning of trauma memory	Prolonged imaginal exposure
Extinction of situational reminders	*In vivo* exposure
Modifying maladaptive appraisals of the trauma or one's response	Cognitive restructuring
Managing harmful substance use	Initially provide exposure to reduce source of self-medication. Give medication and implement behavioral control and motivational interviewing to address substance abuse
Reducing sleep disturbance	Address nightmares through imaginal exposure and, if necessary, implement a sleep hygiene regimen to reduce sleep-incompatible behaviors
Reducing rumination on trauma or one's response	Prolonged exposure to minimize ruminative response, motivational interviewing to understand the impact of rumination, and distraction or mindfulness to manage rumination
Managing anger	Motivational interviews concerning the benefits and costs of anger, cognitive restructuring of beliefs driving anger, and mindfulness practice to reduce anger-related thoughts
Addressing comorbid depression	Prolonged exposure to reduce PTSD symptoms, cognitive restructuring to address self-esteem and hopelessness beliefs, and event scheduling to increase positive activities

self-harm, reckless behavior) needs to be addressed first. It is for this reason that programs targeting patients with complex PTSD who may be engaging in harmful behaviors typically commence with skills to assist emotion tolerance (Cloitre, Koenen, Cohen, & Han, 2002). Having ensured the safety of the patient, the next principle is to sequence those strategies that lead to generalized improvement. In the context of PTSD, it is often understood that many of the related problems, including depression, sleep disturbance, or substance use, may be exacerbated by the symptoms of PTSD. In fact, these related problems often diminish following successful treatment of the PTSD; accordingly, treatment should focus on exposure and cognitive restructuring strategies, with the expectation that reduction of trauma-related distress will generalize to improvements in other domains. If residual problems remain, then specific techniques can be applied to these remaining problems (e.g., sleep hygiene).

ETIOLOGY

Biological Theories of PTSD

Biological models of PTSD have predominantly focused on fear conditioning concepts to explain the genesis and maintenance of PTSD (Milad, Rauch, Pitman, & Quirk, 2006). Fear conditioning models posit that when a traumatic event (unconditioned stimulus) occurs, people typically respond with fear (unconditioned response). It is argued that the strong fear elicited by the trauma will lead to strong associative conditioning between the fear and the events surrounding the trauma. As reminders of the trauma occur (conditioned stimuli), people then respond with fear reactions (conditioned response). It is postulated that release of stress neurochemicals (including norepinephrine and epinephrine) in the context of the traumatic experience results in very strong conditioning and overconsolidation of trauma memories (Rauch, Shin, & Phelps, 2006). This model proposes that successful recovery from trauma involves extinction learning, in which repeated exposure to trauma reminders or memories results in new learning that these reminders no longer signal threat (Davis & Myers, 2002).

In support of these proposals, there is evidence that people who eventually develop PTSD display elevated resting heart rates (Shalev et al., 1998) and respiration rates (Bryant, Creamer, O'Donnell, Silove, & McFarlane, 2008) in the initial days after trauma. There have been reports that other indices of elevated arousal in the immediate posttrauma phase are associated with subsequent PTSD, such as lower gamma-aminobutyric acid (GABA) levels (Vaiva et al., 2006). Psychophysiological studies have also explored the responses of individuals with PTSD, using their own recollections of the trauma as the eliciting stimulus. Paradigms that have employed script-driven imagery in which trauma survivors with PTSD listen to accounts of their traumatic experience consistently find larger psychophysiological responses, including heart rate, skin conductance, and facial electromyogram (EMG), than responses of individuals with a similar trauma history without PTSD (Pitman, Orr, Forgue, de Jong, & Claiborn, 1987).

Biological models propose that PTSD occurs when the amygdala is hyper-responsive to fear-related stimuli, and there is a concomitant lack of "top-down" inhibition from the medial prefrontal cortex (MPFC; Rauch et al., 2006). There is reduced MPFC recruitment in PTSD during fear processing, particularly in rostral anterior cingulate cortex (Shin et al., 2005). There is also some evidence for increased amygdala response to fear stimuli in PTSD (e.g., Armony, Corbo, Clement, & Brunet, 2005), although this evidence is mixed (Lanius, Bluhm, Lanius, & Pain, 2006). It is worth noting that trauma-focused therapy is conceptualized as a form of extinction learning, in which conditioned fear responses are inhibited by learning of new, safe associations (Rothbaum & Davis, 2003). In this context, it is interesting to note that the same neural networks implicated in extinction learning are also involved in successful CBT. The neural mechanisms implicated in extinction learning (i.e., MPFC–amygdala network) have been shown to predict positive response to CBT in patients with PTSD in both functional (Bryant, Felmingham, Kemp, et al., 2008) and structural (Bryant, Felmingham, Whitford, et al., 2008) magnetic resonance imaging (MRI). Furthermore, as patients with PTSD successfully respond to CBT, they are better able to recruit the MPFC during fear processing (Felmingham et al., 2007).

Cognitive Models of PTSD

Cognitive models of PTSD posit that the development and maintenance of PTSD rely heavily on two processes: (1) maladaptive appraisals of the trauma and its aftermath, and (2) disturbances in autobiographical memory (Ehlers & Clark, 2000). These models posit that trauma memories are encoded in a fragmented manner because of the elevated arousal that occurs at the time of trauma. It is proposed that the disorganized nature of these memories precludes a coherent narrative, and this can impede adaptive processing of the experience and limit the extent to which the traumatic experience can be placed in the context of other nontraumatic memories the person may retrieve. It is also proposed that the manner in which people appraise the traumatic event, their responses to it, and their environment after the trauma are pivotal in terms of perpetuating their sense of threat or sense of vulnerability.

There is a great body of evidence supporting this model. Individuals with PTSD have an attentional bias to threat stimuli (McNally, Kaspi, Riemann, & Zeitlin, 1990), are deficient in recalling specific positive memories (McNally, Lasko, Macklin, & Pitman, 1995), and engage in maladaptive thoughts about how they responded to the trauma or to future negative events that may happen to them (Warda & Bryant, 1998). Catastrophic appraisals about the experience shortly after the trauma are also strongly predictive of subsequent PTSD (Ehlers, Mayou, & Bryant, 1998).

RISK FACTORS

The robust finding that only a minority of trauma survivors develop PTSD raises the issue about variables that increase risk for PTSD development. In terms of pre-existing risk factors, prior psychological disturbance, family history of psychological disorders, abusive childhoods, and female gender are predictive of PTSD development (Brewin et al., 2000). In terms of factors associated with the trauma, a major predictor of PTSD is the nature of the traumatic event itself. The more one is exposed to threat and to grotesque or distressing events, the more likely one is to develop PTSD (Brewin et al., 2000). Although PTSD can develop in response to a wide range of traumatic events, there is strong evidence of a dosage relationship between severity of trauma and PTSD development (March, 1993). As noted earlier in the discussion of ASD, there is considerable evidence that peritraumatic responses can predict subsequent PTSD. Symptom severity, including dissociation, reexperiencing, avoidance, and arousal, several weeks after exposure can be predictive of subsequent PTSD. Consistent with cognitive models, there is evidence that catastrophic appraisals of the stressor and of one's reactions to the stressor influence whether chronic PTSD develops (Ehlers, Mayou, et al., 1998). In relation to posttrauma factors, there is evidence that self-reported levels of low social support and the presence of ongoing stressors are important predictors of PTSD (Brewin et al., 2000).

Most of the literature on risk factors for PTSD has been limited by inferring risk on the basis of data collected retrospectively after trauma exposure; this data can be confounded by mood biases in retrospective reports. In more recent years researchers have focused on populations with high risk for trauma exposure, assessed these people prior to trauma exposure, with subsequent follow-up after trauma exposure. Using medical records from military sources, there is evidence that precombat school problems and lower arithmetic aptitude predict PTSD in military personnel (Pitman, Orr, Lowenhagen, Macklin, & Altman, 1991). Personality variables measured before deployment to war zones, such as hypochondriasis, diagnosis of psychopathic deviate, paranoia, and femininity on the Minnesota Multiphasic Personality Inventory (MMPI), are predictive of PTSD (Schnurr, Friedman, & Rosenberg, 1993). Lower predeployment intelligence test scores predict PTSD in men who subsequently enter combat zones (Macklin et al., 1998). There is also evidence that the tendency to engage in catastrophic thinking before trauma exposure predicts subsequent PTSD in firefighters (Bryant & Guthrie, 2005, 2007).

Twin studies indicate the role of genetic contribution given the increased prevalence of PTSD in monozygotic compared to dizygotic twins (True et al., 1993). It is important to note, however, that the genetic influences on PTSD are common to other (frequently comorbid with PTSD) disorders, including depression, other anxiety disorders, and substance use (Koenen et al., 2008). Using MRI to study monozygotic co-twins, Gilbertson et al. (2002) found that Vietnam veterans with PTSD were characterized by smaller hippocampi than those without PTSD, but that the co-twins of veterans with PTSD (but had not served in Vietnam) had hippocampi that were just as small. These findings suggest that small hippocampal volume may constitute a vulnerability factor for PTSD among people exposed to trauma. There is initial evidence that genetic differences may influence the development of PTSD. Initial evidence implicates a functional polymorphism in the promoter region of the human serotonin transporter gene (*SLC6A4*). The short allele (5-HTTLPR S) reduces serotonergic expression and uptake by nearly 50% (Lesch et al., 1996). Healthy individuals with one or two copies of the short allele of the serotonin transporter (5-HTT) polymorphism have higher rates of neuroticism and harm avoidance (Steptoe, Gibson, Hamer, & Wardle, 2007), greater conditioned startle responses (Lonsdorf et al., 2009), increased amygdala activity in response to fearful and angry faces (Hariri et al., 2002), and more startle responses following stressful events (Armbruster et al., 2009). There is a greater incidence of 5-HTTLPR S in subjects with PTSD (Lee et al., 2005) relative to controls, and the 5-HTTLPR S coupled with low social support increases the risk of PTSD (Kilpatrick et al., 2007).

There is also evidence that people's capacity for conditioning may be a risk factor for PTSD development. One study compared startle responses in pairs of Vietnam combat veterans and their non-combat-exposed monozygotic twins (Orr et al., 2003). This study found evidence of more slowly habituating skin conductance to startle responses in veterans with PTSD and their non-combat-exposed co-twins compared to veterans without PTSD and their non-combat-exposed co-twins. This finding suggests that more slowly habituating skin conductance responses to startle stimuli may represent a pretrauma vulnerability factor for PTSD. A prospective study of newly recruited firefighters found that skin conductance and eyeblink EMG startle responses before trauma exposure in a cohort of trainees predicted acute stress reactions after subsequent trauma exposure (Guthrie & Bryant, 2005). Other studies have found that impaired extinction learning prior to trauma exposure is predictive of subsequent posttraumatic stress in firefighters and paramedics (Guthrie & Bryant, 2006).

CLINICAL IMPLICATIONS

The preceding review of treatment evidence and proposed mechanisms underpinning development and maintenance of PTSD should guide the clinician in treatment planning. One of the first decisions is whether a patient is appropriate for exposure-based therapy. Although it is the treatment of choice, some patients may not be able to manage it appropriately for several reasons. Patients who are potentially psychotic, severely suicidal, or substance dependent may be better managed with medication or supportive therapy, until these conditions are adequately controlled. There is some evidence that patients who are prone to ruminating about their condition (Ehlers, Clark, et al., 1998) or whose predominant response to the trauma memory is anger (Jaycox & Foa, 1996) may not be as responsive to exposure, and may benefit from more cognitively oriented approaches prior to exposure. It is also crucial to determine whether the patient is ready to allocate sufficient resources to therapy. It is common in the posttraumatic period, especially in the acute phase, for the trauma survivor to be challenged with a range of environmental and personal demands, including pain, surgery, legal processes, housing disturbance, or ongoing threat. In these circumstances, it is appropriate to question whether patients can focus appropriately on therapy when they are attempting to manage the demands of their environment.

One also needs to be cognizant of the frequent comorbidity with PTSD, and consider sequencing treatment components or adjusting treatment delivery to accommodate this. For example, substance use is often a result of PTSD and will abate once the PTSD symptoms have been addressed; in other cases, however, chronic substance use may be so entrenched and habitual that it needs to be specifically targeted, and in cases when one suspects that exposure may exacerbate substance use, it is wise to manage the abuse prior to exposure. Any condition that may undermine extinction learning during exposure should be managed prior to exposure. As we noted earlier, there is already strong evidence that teaching emotion regulation skills leads to better response with exposure therapy in patients who have deficits in emotion regulation (Cloitre et al., 2010). It is common for patients with PTSD to present with panic attacks, and these usually subside during the course of exposure. In the case of patients who have panic disorder, the clinician who wants to reduce the likelihood of full panic attacks in the course of exposure can conduct interoceptive exposure prior to exposure. Another common comorbidity is traumatic brain injury. These cases pose a challenge for exposure, because they typically involve some degree of amnesia of the event that triggered the disorder. In mild traumatic brain injury, there are usually islands of memory that allow exposure to be administered in the normal manner (Bryant, Moulds, Guthrie, & Nixon, 2003). In more severe cases of brain injury, when there is often no discursive memory of the trauma, patients often experience psychological or physiological distress in response to reminders of the trauma, without actually recalling the event (Bryant, Marosszeky, Crooks, & Gurka, 2000). In these cases it is more useful to focus on *in vivo* rather than imaginal exposure, because situational factors tend to be the major triggers of fear.

PTSD is also associated with a number of debilitating clinical features that should be systematically assessed, such as employment problems, health difficulties, marital and interpersonal problems, sleep and sexual dysfunction, as well as suicidal risk. In order to respond most effectively to clients' needs and to reduce possible interference to therapy, some of these issues may need to be addressed before and/or during exposure-based therapy. These issues should also be assessed at the end of successful exposure-based treatment to determine whether additional interventions are necessary to improve clients' health and functioning.

CONCLUSION

Much has been learned about human response to psychological trauma since the introduction of the PTSD diagnosis. In the wake of large-scale natural and man-made disasters, and the continuing effects of war, research continues to shed light on the biological, cognitive, and social factors that influence the different trajectories of response to trauma. The evidence emerging from these studies continues to shape policy and practice to enhance the ways we attempt to prevent, assess, and treat PTSD. There is no doubt that traumatic experiences will continue to affect people at a very frequent rate, and it is critical that we constantly adopt scientific approaches to help people respond to these events in ways that enhance adaptation.

REFERENCES

Adams, R. E., & Boscarino, J. A. (2005). Differences in mental health outcomes among whites, African Americans, and Hispanics following a community disaster. *Psychiatry: Interpersonal and Biological Processes, 68*(3), 250–265.

American Psychiatric Association. (1952). *Diagnostic and statistical manual of mental disorders.* Washington, DC: Author.

American Psychiatric Association. (1980). *Diagnostic and statistical manual of mental disorders* (3rd ed.). Washington, DC: Author.

American Psychiatric Association. (2013). *Diagnostic and statistical manual of mental disorders* (5th ed.). Arlington, VA: Author.

Andreasen, N. C. (2004). Acute and delayed posttraumatic stress disorder: A history and some issues. *American Journal of Psychiatry, 161*(8), 1321–1323.

Andrews, B., Brewin, C. R., Philpott, R., & Stewart, L. (2007). Delayed-onset posttraumatic stress disorder: A systematic review of the evidence. *American Journal of Psychiatry, 164*(9), 1319–1326.

Andrews, G., Charney, D. S., Sirovatka, P. J., & Regier, D. A. (Eds.). (2009). *Stress-induced and fear circuitry disorders: Refining the research agenda for DSM-V.* Arlington, VA: American Psychiatric Association.

Anticevic, V., & Britvic, D. (2008). Sexual functioning in war veterans with posttraumatic stress disorder. *Croatian Medicine Journal, 49*(4), 499–505.

Armbruster, D., Moser, D. A., Strobel, A., Hensch, T., Kirschbaum, C., Lesch, K. P., et al. (2009). Serotonin transporter gene variation and stressful life events impact processing of fear and anxiety. *International Journal of Neuropsychopharmacology, 12*(3), 393–401.

Armony, J. L., Corbo, V., Clement, M. H., & Brunet, A. (2005). Amygdala response in patients with acute PTSD to masked and unmasked emotional facial expressions. *American Journal of Psychiatry, 162*(10), 1961–1963.

Australian Centre for Posttraumatic Mental Health. (2007a). *Australian guidelines for the treatment of adults with acute stress disorder and posttraumatic stress disorder.* Melbourne: Author.

Australian Centre for Posttraumatic Mental Health. (2007b). *Australian guidelines for the treatment of adults with acute stress disorder and posttraumatic stress disorder: Practitioner guide.* Melbourne: Author.

Blanchard, E. B., Hickling, E. J., Barton, K. A., & Taylor, A. E. (1996). One-year prospective follow-up of motor vehicle accident victims. *Behaviour Research and Therapy, 34*(10), 775–786.

Bradley, R., Greene, J., Russ, E., Dutra, L., & Westen, D. (2005). A multidimensional meta-analysis of psychotherapy for PTSD. *American Journal of Psychiatry, 162*(2), 214–227.

Breslau, N., Davis, G. C., Andreski, P., & Peterson, E. (1991). Traumatic events and post-traumatic stress disorder in an urban population of young adults. *Archives of General Psychiatry, 48,* 216–222.

Breslau, N., Davis, G. C., Peterson, E. L., & Schultz, L. R. (1997). Psychiatric sequelae of posttraumatic stress disorder in women. *Archives of General Psychiatry, 54*(1), 81–87.

Brewin, C. R., Andrews, B., & Valentine, J. D. (2000). Meta-analysis of risk factors for posttraumatic stress disorder in trauma-exposed adults. *Journal of Consulting and Clinical Psychology, 68*(5), 748–766.

Bryant, R. A. (2003). Early predictors of posttraumatic stress disorder. *Biological Psychiatry, 53*(9), 789–795.

Bryant, R. A. (2011). Acute stress disorder as a predictor of posttraumatic stress disorder: A systematic review. *Journal of Clinical Psychiatry, 72,* 233–239.

Bryant, R. A., Creamer, M., O'Donnell, M., Silove, D., Clark, C. R., & McFarlane, A. C. (2010). The psychiatric sequelae of traumatic injury. *American Journal of Psychiatry, 167,* 312–320.

Bryant, R. A., Creamer, M., O'Donnell, M., Silove, D., & McFarlane, A. C. (2008). A multisite study of initial respiration rate and heart rate as predictors of posttraumatic stress disorder. *Journal of Clinical Psychiatry, 69*(11), 1694–1701.

Bryant, R. A., Creamer, M., O'Donnell, M., Silove, D., & McFarlane, A. C. (2010). Sleep disturbance immediately prior to trauma predicts subsequent psychiatric disorder. *Sleep, 33*(1), 69–74.

Bryant, R. A., Felmingham, K., Kemp, A., Das, P., Hughes, G., Peduto, A., et al. (2008). Amygdala and ventral anterior cingulate activation predicts treatment response to cognitive behaviour therapy for post-traumatic stress disorder. *Psychological Medicine, 38*(4), 555–561.

Bryant, R. A., Felmingham, K., Whitford, T. J., Kemp, A., Hughes, G., Peduto, A., et al. (2008). Rostral anterior cingulate volume predicts treatment response to cognitive-behavioural therapy for posttraumatic stress disorder. *Journal of Psychiatry and Neuroscience, 33*(2), 142–146.

Bryant, R. A., Friedman, M. J., Spiegel, D., Ursano, R., & Strain, J. (2011). A review of acute stress disorder in DSM-5. *Depression and Anxiety, 28*(9), 802–817.

Bryant, R. A., & Guthrie, R. M. (2005). Maladaptive appraisals as a risk factor for posttraumatic stress: A study of trainee firefighters. *Psychological Science, 16*(10), 749–752.

Bryant, R. A., & Guthrie, R. M. (2007). Maladaptive self-appraisals before trauma exposure predict posttraumatic stress disorder. *Journal of Consulting and Clinical Psychology, 75*(5), 812–815.

Bryant, R. A., & Harvey, A. G. (2002). Delayed-onset posttraumatic stress disorder: A prospective evaluation. *Australian and New Zealand Journal of Psychiatry, 36*(2), 205–209.

Bryant, R. A., Marosszeky, J. E., Crooks, J., & Gurka, J. A. (2000). Posttraumatic stress disorder after severe traumatic brain injury. *American Journal of Psychiatry, 157*(4), 629–631.

Bryant, R. A., Mastrodomenico, J., Felmingham, K. L., Hopwood, S., Kenny, L., Kandris, E., et al. (2008). Treatment of acute stress disorder: A randomized controlled trial. *Archives of General Psychiatry, 65*(6), 659–667.

Bryant, R. A., Moulds, M. L., Guthrie, R. M., Dang, S. T., Mastrodomenico, J., Nixon, R. D., et al. (2008). A randomized controlled trial of exposure therapy and cognitive restructuring for posttraumatic stress disorder. *Journal of Consulting and Clinical Psychology, 76*(4), 695–703.

Bryant, R. A., Moulds, M. L., Guthrie, R. M., Dang, S. T., & Nixon, R. D. (2003). Imaginal exposure alone and imaginal exposure with cognitive restructuring in treatment of posttraumatic stress disorder. *Journal of Consulting and Clinical Psychology, 71*(4), 706–712.

Bryant, R. A., Moulds, M., Guthrie, R., & Nixon, R. D. (2003). Treating acute stress disorder following mild traumatic brain injury. *American Journal of Psychiatry, 160*(3), 585–587.

Bryant, R. A., Moulds, M. L., Nixon, R. D. V., Mastrodomenico, J., Felmingham, K., & Hopwood, S. (2006). Hypnotherapy and cognitive behaviour therapy of acute stress disorder: A 3–year follow-up. *Behaviour Research and Therapy, 44*(9), 1331–1335.

Bullman, T. A., & Kang, H. K. (1996). The risk of suicide among wounded Vietnam veterans. *American Journal of Public Health, 86*(5), 662–667.

Cahill, S. P., Rothbaum, B. O., Resick, P. A., & Follette, V. M. (2009). Cognitive-behavioral therapy for adults. In E. B. Foa, T. M. Keane, M. J. Freidman, & J. A. Cohen (Eds.), *Effective treatments for PTSD: Practice guidelines from the International Society of Traumatic Stress Studies* (pp. 139–222). New York: Guilford Press.

Chard, K. M. (2005). An evaluation of cognitive processing therapy for the treatment of post-traumatic stress disorder related to childhood sexual abuse. *Journal of Consulting and Clinical Psychology, 73*(5), 965–971.

Charney, D. S. (2003). Neuroanatomical circuits modulating fear and anxiety behaviors. *Acta Psychiatrica Scandinavica, 108*, 38–50.

Cloitre, M., Koenen, K. C., Cohen, L. R., & Han, H. (2002). Skills training in affective and inter-personal regulation followed by exposure: A phase-based treatment for PTSD related to childhood abuse. *Journal of Consulting and Clinical Psychology, 70*(5), 1067–1074.

Cloitre, M., Miranda, R., Stovall-McClough, K. C., & Han, H. (2005). Beyond PTSD: Emotion regu-lation and interpersonal problems as predictors of functional impairment in survivors of childhood abuse. *Behavior Therapy, 36*(2), 119–124.

Cloitre, M., Stovall-McClough, K. C., Nooner, K., Zorbas, P., Cherry, S., Jackson, C. L., et al. (2010). Treatment for PTSD related to childhood abuse: A randomized controlled trial. *American Journal of Psychiatry, 167*(8), 915–924.

Cohen, J. A., Mannarino, A. P., Deblinger, E., & Berliner, L. (2009). Cognitive-behavioral therapy for children and adolscents. In E. B. Foa, T. M. Keane, M. J. Friedman, & J. A. Cohen (Eds.), *Effective treatments for PTSD: Practice guidelines from the International Society of Traumatic Stress Studies* (pp. 223–244). New York: Guilford Press.

DiGrande, L., Perrin, M. A., Thorpe, L. E., Thalji, L., Murphy, J., Wu, D., et al. (2008). Posttraumatic stress symptoms, PTSD, and risk factors among lower Manhattan residents 2–3 years after the September 11, 2001 terrorist attacks. *Journal of Traumatic Stress, 21*(3), 264–273.

Duffy, M., Gillespie, K., & Clark, D. M. (2007). Post-traumatic stress disorder in the context of terrorism and other civil conflict in Northern Ireland: Randomised controlled trial. *British Medical Journal, 334*(7604), 1147.

Ehlers, A., & Clark, D. M. (2000). A cognitive model of posttraumatic stress disorder. *Behaviour Research and Therapy, 38*(4), 319–345.

Ehlers, A., Clark, D. M., Dunmore, E., Jaycox, L., Meadows, E., & Foa, E. B. (1998). Predicting response to exposure treatment in PTSD: The role of mental defeat and alienation. *Journal of Traumatic Stress, 11*(3), 457–471.

Ehlers, A., Clark, D. M., Hackmann, A., McManus, F., Fennell, M., Herbert, C., et al. (2003). A randomized controlled trial of cognitive therapy, a self-help booklet, and repeated assess-ments as early interventions for posttraumatic stress disorder. *Archives of General Psychiatry, 60*(10), 1024–1032.

Ehlers, A., Mayou, R. A., & Bryant, B. (1998). Psychological predictors of chronic posttraumatic stress disorder after motor vehicle accidents. *Journal of Abnormal Psychology, 107*(3), 508–519.

Felmingham, K., Kemp, A., Williams, L., Das, P., Hughes, G., Peduto, A., et al. (2007). Changes in anterior cingulate and amygdala after cognitive behavior therapy of posttraumatic stress disorder. *Psychological Science, 18*(2), 127–129.

Foa, E. B., Hembree, E. A., Cahill, S. P., Rauch, S. A. M., Riggs, D. S., Feeny, N. C., et al. (2005). Ran-domized trial of prolonged exposure for posttraumatic stress disorder with and without cognitive restructuring: Outcome at academic and community clinics. *Journal of Consulting and Clinical Psychology, 73*(5), 953–964.

Foa, E. B., Keane, T. M., Friedman, M. J., & Cohen, J. A. (Eds.). (2009). *Effective treatments for PTSD: Practice guidelines from the International Society of Traumatic Stress Studies* (2nd ed.). New York: Guilford Press.

Foa, E. B., Rothbaum, B. O., Riggs, D. S., & Murdock, T. B. (1991). Treatment of posttraumatic stress disorder in rape victims: A comparison between cognitive-behavioral procedures and counseling. *Journal of Consulting and Clinical Psychology, 59*(5), 715–723.

Foley, T., & Spates, C. R. (1995). Eye movement desensitization of public-speaking anxiety: A partial dismantling. *Journal of Behavior Therapy and Experimental Psychiatry, 26*(4), 321–329.

Friedman, M. J., & McEwen, B. S. (2004). Posttraumatic stress disorder, allostatic load, and medical illness. In P. P. Schnurr & B. L. Green (Eds.), *Trauma and health: Physical health consequences of exposure to extreme stress* (pp. 157–188). Washington, DC: American Psychological Association.

Friedman, M. J., Resick, P. A., Bryant, R. A., & Brewin, C. R. (2011). Considering PTSD for DSM-V. *Depression and Anxiety, 28*, 750–769.

Friedman, M. J., & Schnurr, P. P. (1995). The relationship between trauma, post-traumatic stress disorder, and physical health. In M. Friedman, D. Charney, & A. Y. Deutch (Eds.), *Neurobiological and clinical consequences of stress: From adaptation to PTSD*. Philadelphia: Raven.

Galea, S., Vlahov, D., Resnick, H., Ahern, J., Susser, E., Gold, J., et al. (2003). Trends of probable post-traumatic stress disorder in New York City after the September 11 terrorist attacks. *American Journal of Epidemiology, 158*(6), 514–524.

Gilbertson, M. W., Shenton, M. E., Ciszewski, A., Kasai, K., Lasko, N. B., Orr, S. P., et al. (2002). Smaller hippocampal volume predicts pathological vulnerability to psychological trauma. *Nature Neuroscience, 5*, 1242–1247.

Grossman, A. B., Levin, B. E., Katzen, H. L., & Lechner, S. (2004). PTSD symptoms and onset of neurologic disease in elderly trauma survivors. *Journal of Clinical and Experimental Neuropsychology, 26*, 698–705.

Guthrie, R. M., & Bryant, R. A. (2005). Auditory startle response in firefighters before and after trauma exposure. *American Journal of Psychiatry, 162*(2), 283–290.

Guthrie, R. M., & Bryant, R. A. (2006). Extinction learning before trauma and subsequent posttraumatic stress. *Psychosomatic Medicine, 68*(2), 307–311.

Hariri, A. H., Mattay, V., Tessitore, A., Kolachana, B., Fera, F., & Goldman D. (2002). Serotonin transporter genetic variation and the response of the human amygdala. *Scence, 297*, 400–403.

Harvey, A. G., & Bryant, R. A. (2002). Acute stress disorder: A synthesis and critique. *Psychological Bulletin, 128*(6), 886–902.

Hobbs, M., Mayou, R., Harrison, B., & Worlock, P. (1996). A randomised controlled trial of psychological debriefing for victims of road traffic accidents. *British Medical Journal, 313*(7070), 1438–1439.

Horowitz, M. J., & Solomon, G. F. (1975). A prediction of delayed stress response syndromes in Vietnam veterans. *Journal of Social Issues, 31*, 67–80.

Institute of Medicine. (2007). *Treatment of posttraumatic stress disorder: An assessment of the evidence.* Washington, DC: Author.

Isserlin, L., Zerach, G., & Solomon, Z. (2008). Acute stress responses: A review and synthesis of ASD, ASR, and CSR. *American Journal of Orthopsychiatry, 78*(4), 423–429.

Janet, P. (1907). *The major symptoms of hysteria.* New York: Macmillian.

Jaycox, L. H., & Foa, E. B. (1996). Obstacles in implementing exposure therapy for PTSD: Case discussions and practical solutions. *Clinical Psychology and Psychotherapy, 3*, 176–184.

Kang, H. K., & Bullman, T. A. (2008). Risk of suicide among US veterans after returning from the Iraq or Afghanistan war zones. *Journal of the American Medical Association, 300*(6), 652–653.

Kessler, R. C., Galea, S., Gruber, M. J., Sampson, N. A., Ursano, R. J., & Wessely, S. (2008). Trends in mental illness and suicidality after Hurricane Katrina. *Molecular Psychiatry, 13*(4), 374–384.

Kessler, R. C., Sonnega, A., Hughes, M., & Nelson, C. B. (1995). Posttraumatic stress disorder in the National Comorbidity Survey. *Archives of General Psychiatry, 52*, 1048–1060.

Kilpatrick, D. G., Koenen, K. C., Ruggiero, K. J., Acierno, R., Galea, S., Resnick, H. S., et al. (2007). The serotonin transporter genotype and social support and moderation of posttraumatic stress disorder and depression in hurricane-exposed adults. *American Journal of Psychiatry, 164*(11), 1693–1699.

King, D. W., Leskin, G. A., King, L. A., & Weathers, F. W. (1998). Confirmatory factor analysis of the clinician-administered PTSD Scale: Evidence for the dimensionality of posttraumatic stress disorder. *Psychological Assessment, 10*(2), 90–96.

Koenen, K. C., Fu, Q. J., Ertel, K., Lyons, M. J., Eisen, S. A., True, W. R., et al. (2008). Common genetic liability to major depression and posttraumatic stress disorder in men. *Journal of Affective Disorders, 105*(1–3), 109–115.

Lanius, R. A., Bluhm, R., Lanius, U., & Pain, C. (2006). A review of neuroimaging studies in PTSD: Heterogeneity of response to symptom provocation. *Journal of Psychiatric Research, 40*(8), 709–729.

Lee, H. J., Lee, M. S., Kang, R. H., Kim, H., Yim, S. D., Kee, B. S., et al. (2005). Influence of the serotonin transporter promoter gene polymorphism on susceptibility to posttraumatic stress disorder. *Depression and Anxiety, 21*(3), 135–139.

Lesch, K. P., Bengel, D., Heils, A., Sabol, S. Z., Greenberg, B. D., Petri, S., et al. (1996). Association of anxiety-related traits with a polymorphism in the serotonin transporter gene regulatory region. *Science, 274*, 1527–1531.

Lonsdorf, T. B., Weike, A. I., Nikamo, P., Schalling, M., Hamm, A. O., & Ohman, A. (2009). Genetic gating of human fear learning and extinction: Possible implications for gene–environment interaction in anxiety disorder. *Psychological Science, 20*(2), 198–206.

MacDonald, C., Chamberlain, K., Long, N., & Flett, R. (1999). Posttraumatic stress disorder and interpersonal functioning in Vietnam War veterans: A mediational model. *Journal of Traumatic Stress, 12*(4), 701–707.

Macklin, M. L., Metzger, L. J., Litz, B. T., McNally, R. J., Lasko, N. B., Orr, S. P., et al. (1998). Lower precombat intelligence is a risk factor for posttraumatic stress disorder. *Journal of Consulting and Clinical Psychology, 66*(2), 323–326.

Manfro, G. G., Otto, M. W., McArdle, E. T., Worthington, J. J., III, Rosenbaum, J. F., & Pollack, M. H. (1996). Relationship of antecedent stressful life events to childhood and family history of anxiety and the course of panic disorder. *Journal of Affective Disorders, 41*(2), 135–139.

March, J. S. (1993). The stressor criterion in DSM-IV post traumatic stress disorder. In J. R. T. Davidson & E. B. Foa (Eds.), *Posttraumatic stress disorder in review: Recent research and future development* (pp. 37–54). Washington, DC: American Psychiatric Press.

McCabe, R. E., Antony, M. M., Summerfeldt, L. J., Liss, A., & Swinson, R. P. (2003). Preliminary examination of the relationship between anxiety disorders in adults and self-reported history of teasing or bullying experiences. *Cognitive Behaviour Therapy, 32*(4), 187–193.

McDonagh, A., Friedman, M., McHugo, G., Ford, J., Sengupta, A., Mueser, K., et al. (2005). Randomized trial of cognitive-behavioral therapy for chronic posttraumatic stress disorder in adult female survivors of childhood sexual abuse. *Journal of Consulting and Clinical Psychology, 73*(3), 515–524.

McFarlane, A. C. (1998). Epidemiological evidence about the relationship between PTSD and alcohol abuse: The nature of the association. *Addictive Behaviors, 23*(6), 813–825.

McNally, R. J., Bryant, R. A., & Ehlers, A. (2003). Does early psychological intervention promote recovery from posttraumatic stress? *Psychological Science, 4*, 45–79.

McNally, R. J., Kaspi, S. P., Riemann, B. C., & Zeitlin, S. B. (1990). Selective processing of threat cues in posttraumatic stress disorder. *Journal of Abnormal Psychology, 99*(4), 398–402.

McNally, R. J., Lasko, N. B., Macklin, M. L., & Pitman, R. K. (1995). Autobiographical memory disturbance in combat-related posttraumatic stress disorder. *Behaviour Research and Therapy, 33*(6), 619–630.

Milad, M. R., Rauch, S. L., Pitman, R. K., & Quirk, G. J. (2006). Fear extinction in rats: Implications for human brain imaging and anxiety disorders. *Biological Psychology, 73*(1), 61–71.

Mitchell, J. T. (1983). When disaster strikes: The critical incident stress debriefing process. *Journal of Emergency Medical Services, 8*, 36–39.

Mitchell, J. T., & Everly, G., Jr. (1996). *Critical incident stress debriefing: An operations manual for the prevention of traumatic stress among emergency services and disaster workers* (Vol. 2). Ellicott City, MD: Chevron.

Murray, J., Ehlers, A., & Mayou, R. A. (2002). Dissociation and post-traumatic stress disorder: Two prospective studies of road traffic accident survivors. *British Journal of Psychiatry, 180,* 363–368.

National Institute of Clinical Excellence. (2005). *The management of PTSD in adults and children in primary and secondary care* (Vol. 26). Wiltshire, UK: Author.

Neylan, T. C., Marmar, C. R., Metzler, T. J., Weiss, D. S., Zatzick, D. F., Delucchi, K. L., et al. (1998). Sleep disturbances in the Vietnam generation: Findings from a nationally representative sample of male Vietnam veterans. *American Journal of Psychiatry, 155*(7), 929–933.

Norris, F. H., Friedman, M. J., & Watson, P. J. (2002). 60,000 disaster victims speak: Part I. An emirical review of the empirical literature, 1981–2001. *Psychiatry, 65,* 207–239.

North, C. S., Nixon, S. J., Shariat, S., Mallonee, S., McMillen, J. C., Spitznagel, E. L., et al. (1999). Psychiatric disorders among survivors of the Oklahoma City bombing. *Journal of the American Medical Association, 282*(8), 755–762.

Orr, S. P., Metzger, L. J., Laska, N. B., Macklin, M. L., Hu, F. B., Shalev, A. Y., et al. (2003). Physiologic responses to sudden, loud tones in monozygotic twins discordant for combat exposure: Association with posttraumatic stress disorder. *Archives in General Psychiatry, 60,* 283–288.

Perkonigg, A., Kessler, R. C., Storz, S., & Wittchen, H. U. (2000). Traumatic events and post-traumatic stress disorder in the community: Prevalence, risk factors and comorbidity. *Acta Psychiatrica Scandinavica, 101*(1), 46–59.

Pitman, R. K., Orr, S. P., Forgue, D. F., de Jong, J. T., & Claiborn, J. (1987). Psychophysiologic assessment of posttraumatic stress disorder imagery in Vietnam combat veterans. *Archives of General Psychiatry, 44*(11), 970–975.

Pitman, R. K., Orr, S. P., Lowenhagen, M. J., Macklin, M. L., & Altman, B. (1991). Pre-Vietnam contents of posttraumatic stress disorder veterans' service medical and personnel records. *Comprehensive Psychiatry, 32*(5), 416–422.

Rapee, R. M., Litwin, E. M., & Barlow, D. H. (1990). Impact of life events on subjects with panic disorder and on comparison subjects. *American Journal of Psychiatry, 147*(5), 640–644.

Rauch, S. L., Shin, L. M., & Phelps, E. A. (2006). Neurocircuitry models of posttraumatic stress disorder and extinction: Human neuroimaging research—past, present, and future. *Biological Psychiatry, 60*(4), 376–382.

Rauch, S. L., Wedig, M. M., Wright, C. I., Martis, B., McMullin, K. G., Shin, L. M., et al. (2007). Functional magnetic resonance imaging study of regional brain activation during implicit sequence learning in obsessive–compulsive disorder. *Biological Psychiatry, 61*(3), 330–336.

Resick, P. A., Galovski, T. E., Uhlmansiek, M. O, Scher, C. D., Clum, G. A., et al. (2008). A randomized clinical trial to dismantle components of cognitive processing therapy for posttraumatic stress disorder in female victims of interpersonal violence. *Journal of Consulting and Clinical Psychology, 76*(2), 243–258.

Resick, P. A., & Schnicke, M. K. (1993). *Cognitive processing therapy for sexual assault victims: A treatment manual.* Newbury Park, CA: Sage.

Riggs, D. S., Rothbaum, B. O., & Foa, E. B. (1995). A prospective examination of symptoms of posttraumatic stress disorder in victims of nonsexual assault. *Journal of Interpersonal Violence, 10*(2), 201–214.

Rose, S., Bisson, J., & Wessely, S. (2001). Psychological debriefing for preventing posttraumatic stress disorder (PTSD). *Cochrane Database of Systematic Reviews, 3,* CD000560.

Rose, S., Brewin, C. R., Andrews, B., & Kirk, M. (1999). A randomized controlled trial of individual psychological debriefing for victims of violent crime. *Psychological Medicine, 29*(4), 793–799.

Rothbaum, B. O., & Davis, M. (2003). Applying learning principles to the treatment of post-trauma reactions. *Annals of the New York Academy of Sciences, 1008,* 112–121.

Rothbaum, B. O., Foa, E. B., Riggs, D. S., Murdock, T., & Walsh, W. (1992). A prospective examination of post-traumatic stress disorder in rape victims. *Journal of Traumatic Stress, 5*(3), 455–475.

Rothbaum, B. O., & Schwartz, A. C. (2002). Exposure therapy for posttraumatic stress disorder. *American Journal of Psychotherapy, 56*(1), 59–75.

Ruef, A. M., Litz, B. T., & Schlenger, W. E. (2000). Hispanic ethnicity and risk for combat-related posttraumatic stress disorder. *Cultural Diversity and Ethnic Minority Psychology, 6*(3), 235–251.

Salmon, K., & Bryant, R. A. (2002). Posttraumatic stress disorder in children—the influence of developmental factors. *Clinical Psychology Review, 22*(2), 163–188.

Sareen, J., Stein, M. B., Cox, B. J., & Hassard, S. T. (2004). Understanding comorbidity of anxiety disorders with antisocial behavior—findings from two large community surveys. *Journal of Nervous and Mental Disease, 192*(3), 178–186.

Schlenger, W. E., Kulka, R. A., Fairbank, J. A., Hough, R. L., Jordan, B. K., Marmar, C. R., et al. (1992). The prevalence of post-traumatic stress disorder in the Vietnam generation: A multimethod, multisource assessment of psychiatric disorder. *Journal of Traumatic Stress, 5*(3), 333–363.

Schnurr, P. P., Friedman, M. J., Foy, D. W., Shea, M. T., Hsieh, F. Y., Lavori, P. W., et al. (2003). Randomized trial of trauma-focused group therapy for posttraumatic stress disorder: Results from a Department of Veterans Affairs Cooperative Study. *Archives of General Psychiatry, 60*(5), 481–489.

Schnurr, P. P., Friedman, M. J., & Rosenberg, S. D. (1993). Preliminary MMPI scores as predictors of combat related PTSD symptoms. *American Journal of Psychiatry, 150,* 479–483.

Shalev, A. Y., Sahar, T., Freedman, S., Peri, T., Glick, N., Brandes, D., et al. (1998). A prospective study of heart rate response following trauma and the subsequent development of posttraumatic stress disorder. *Archives of General Psychiatry, 55*(6), 553–559.

Shapiro, F. (1995). *Eye movement desensitization and reprocessing: Basic principles, protocols, and procedures.* New York: Guilford Press.

Shapiro, F., & Maxfield, L. (2002). Eye movement desensitization and reprocessing (EMDR): Information processing in the treatment of trauma. *Journal of Clinical Psychology, 58*(8), 933–946.

Shea, M. T., Vujanovic, A. A., Mansfield, A. K., Sevin, E., & Liu, F. (2010). Posttraumatic stress disorder symptoms and functional impairment among OEF and OIF National Guard and Reserve veterans. *Journal of Traumatic Stress, 23*(1), 100–107.

Shin, L. M., & Liberzon, I. (2010). The neurocircuitry of fear, stress, and anxiety disorders. *Neuropsychopharmacology, 35*(1), 169–191.

Shin, L. M., Wright, C. I., Cannistraro, P. A., Wedig, M. M., McMullin, K., Martis, B., et al. (2005). A functional magnetic resonance imaging study of amygdala and medial prefrontal cortex responses to overtly presented fearful faces in posttraumatic stress disorder. *Archives of General Psychiatry, 62*(3), 273–281.

Stein, M. B., Höfler, M., Perkonigg, A., Lieb, R., Pfister, H., Maercker, A., et al. (2002). Patterns of incidence and psychiatric risk factors for traumatic events. *International Journal of Methods in Psychiatric Research, 11*(4), 143–153.

Steptoe, A., Gibson, E. L., Hamer, M., & Wardle, J. (2007). Neuroendocrine and cardiovascular correlates of positive affect measured by ecological momentary assessment and by questionnaire. *Psychoneuroendocrinology, 32*(1), 56–64.

Thomas, P. A., Brackbill, R., Thalji, L., DiGrande, L., Campolucci, S., Thorpe, L., et al. (2008). Respiratory and other health effects reported in children exposed to the World Trade Center disaster of 11 September 2001. *Environmental Health Perspectives, 116*(10), 1383–1390.

True, W. R., Rice, J., Eisen, S. A., Heath, A. C., Goldberg, J., Lyons, M. J. et al. (1993). A twin study of genetic and environmental contributions to liability for posttraumatic stress symptoms. *Archives of General Psychiatry, 50,* 257–264.

U.S. Department of Defense. (2004). *Clinical practice guideline for the management of posttraumatic stress, version 1.0.* Washington, DC: Author.

Vaiva, G., Boss, V., Ducrocq, F., Fontaine, M., Devos, P., Brunet, A., et al. (2006). Relationship between posttrauma GABA plasma levels and PTSD at 1-year follow-up. *American Journal of Psychiatry, 163*(8), 1446–1448.

van Griensven, F., Chakkraband, M. L. S., Thienkrua, W., Pengjuntr, W., Cardozo, B. L., Tantipiwatanaskul, P., et al. (2006). Mental health problems among adults in tsunami-affected areas in southern Thailand. *Journal of the American Medical Association, 296*(5), 537–548.

Warda, G., & Bryant, R. A. (1998). Cognitive bias in acute stress disorder. *Behaviour Research and Therapy, 36*(12), 1177–1183.

World Health Organization. (1995). *The ICD-10 classification of mental and behavioural disorders: Clinical descriptions and diagnostic guidelines.* Geneva: World Health Organization.

Yitzhaki, T., Solomon, Z., & Kotler, M. (1991). The clinical picture of acute combat stress reaction among Israeli soldiers in the 1982 Lebanon war. *Military Medicine, 156*(4), 193–197.

Young, B. H. (2006). The immediate response to disaster: Guidelines for adult psychological first aid. In E. C. Ritchie, P. J. Watson, & M. J. Friedman (Eds.), *Interventions following mass violence and disasters: Strategies for mental health practice* (pp. 134–154). New York: Guilford Press.

Zatzick, D. F., Weiss, D. S., Marmar, C. R., Metzler, T. J., Wells, K., Golding, J. M., et al. (1997). Posttraumatic stress disorder and functioning and quality of life outcomes in female Vietnam veterans. *Military Medicine, 162*(10), 661–665.

Zivin, K., Kim, H. M., McCarthy, J. F., Austin, K. L., Hoggatt, K. J., Walters, H., et al. (2007). Suicide mortality among individuals receiving treatment for depression in the Veterans Affairs Health System: Associations with patient and treatment setting characteristics. *American Journal of Public Health, 97*(12), 2193–2198.

CHAPTER 7

Eating Disorders

Deborah R. Glasofer
Evelyn Attia
Kathleen M. Pike

This chapter presents an overview of the clinical features, risk factors, and treatment of three eating disorders: anorexia nervosa (AN), bulimia nervosa (BN), and binge-eating disorder (BED). Throughout the chapter, we highlight clinical implications that may arise in relation to the psychopathology characteristic of or commonly associated with eating disorders.

TYPICAL SYMPTOMS AND ASSOCIATED FEATURES

Anorexia Nervosa

AN is characterized by a failure to maintain a minimally acceptable weight (e.g., a body mass index [BMI] of less than 18.5 kg/m^2) and an intense fear of being or becoming fat. Low weight is accompanied by a distortion or disturbance in experience of body shape or weight, the overvaluing of body shape or weight on self-evaluation, or denial of the seriousness of current low weight (American Psychiatric Association, 2013). Females commonly experience an interruption in menstrual activity for at least 3 months. However, increasing evidence suggests that the presence or absence of amenorrhea does not meaningfully distinguish the clinical status of those who otherwise meet criteria for the AN diagnosis (Attia & Roberto, 2009). Individuals who are not regularly engaged in binge-eating or purging behaviors (e.g., self-induced vomiting, misuse of laxatives/diuretics) are diagnosed with AN, restricting subtype (AN-R; American Psychiatric Association, 2013). Those who are regularly engaging in binge-eating or purging behaviors while underweight meet criteria for AN, binge-eating/purging subtype (AN-B/P; American Psychiatric Association, 2013).

Psychological symptoms associated with AN include depression, distractibility, anxiety, insomnia, and increased obsessionality (Attia, 2010). These symptoms have also been observed in non-eating-disordered individuals undergoing an induced state of semistarvation and in the case of AN are often secondary to underweight status (Keys, Brozek, Henschel, Mickelsen, & Taylor, 1950). Medical complications of AN include cardiac abnormalities (e.g., bradycardia, hypotension), osteopenia or osteoporosis, and endocrine disturbances (Mehler, Birmingham, Crow, & Jahraus, 2010). Electrolyte imbalances may be present, including hypokalemia in individuals with vomiting or laxative use, and hyponatremia in those who ingest large amounts of water or other noncaloric beverages (Attia, 2010).

Anorexia nervosa is a serious psychiatric illness associated with increased morbidity and mortality (Steinhausen, 2002). In a meta-analysis of outcome studies, Steinhausen reported that, over the long-term, while approximately one-half of the individuals with AN achieve full recovery, approximately one-third remain partially symptomatic and approximately one-fifth remain chronically ill. Moreover, a recent longitudinal study of mortality using the National Death Index determined a crude mortality rate of 4.0% for individuals with AN seeking treatment in an outpatient setting (Crow et al., 2009). Overall, crude mortality rates reported in AN studies since 2004 range from 0 to 8%, with a cumulative mortality rate of 2.8% (Keel & Brown, 2010). Mortality estimates rise for patients with AN who require hospitalization, with as much as a sixfold increased mortality rate in comparison to the general population (Papadopoulos, Ekbom, Brandt, & Ekselius, 2009). Studies of mortality associated with AN indicate that the cause of death is equally likely, or in some studies more likely, to be suicide than to be medical problems resulting from complications associated with compromised nutritional status (Holm-Denoma et al., 2008).

In terms of comorbidity with other clinical disorders, high rates of depression, dysthymia, social phobia, generalized anxiety disorder, specific phobia, and obsessive–compulsive disorder (OCD) are commonly reported in clinical samples of adolescents and adults with AN (Herzog & Eddy, 2007). Individuals with AN report elevated lifetime alcohol use disorder (alcohol abuse or dependence) that typically begins after onset of AN; however, the rate of alcohol use disorder for individuals with AN-R is significantly lower than for individuals with AN-B/P, BN, or BED (Bulik et al., 2004).

AN is associated with certain personality traits, including perfectionism, obsessive–compulsiveness, neuroticism, negative emotionality, harm avoidance, low self-directedness, low cooperativeness, and avoidant personality disorder traits (Cassin & von Ranson, 2005). Individuals with restricting AN also report high levels of constraint and persistence and low levels of novelty seeking (von Ranson, 2008). However, it is important to note that these personality dimensions are not characteristic of all individuals with AN, and a wide range of personality types are represented among individuals with AN. Perhaps the most consistent and significant personality traits that appear to be premorbid to AN, enduring even after recovery from AN, are perfectionism and harm avoidance (Strober et al., 2006). In terms of personality disorders, studies indicate that the majority of individuals (77%) with chronic eating disorders meet criteria for at least one personality disorder (Ro, Martinsen, Hoffart, & Rosenvinge, 2005). Borderline personality disorder is more common among those who abuse laxatives (Tozzi et al., 2006), and presence of a personality disorder in early adulthood increases risk for onset of an eating disorder (Johnson, Cohen, Kasen, & Brook, 2006).

AN can also be associated with a range of social and interpersonal problems. Risk factors research indicates that significant interpersonal problems or stressors often occur in the year prior to onset of AN and cumulatively increase risk for AN (Pike et al., 2008). Individuals with AN often report social isolation and lack of pleasure in interpersonal relationships, and studies of sexual function and intimacy indicate that the majority of women with AN report dramatically decreased sexual interest and pleasure (Zemishlany & Weizman, 2008). Women with AN are also much less likely to be in a marital relationship or to report satisfaction in an intimate partnership than their peers without eating disorders (Raboch & Faltus, 1991). Relatedly, individuals with AN are likely to report lower rates of employment than non-eating-disordered peers given the all-consuming nature of the disorder. This is particularly true during the acute stages of the disorder; however, for individuals with long-standing AN and for those with significant comorbid associated psychopathology, employment continues to be a problem even following recovery (Hjern, Lindberg, & Lindblad, 2006).

These data suggest that for many individuals with AN, the impact of the disorder can be pervasive and long-lasting; however, it is important to note that most follow-up studies of AN have been conducted with individuals who have pursued intensive treatment and are therefore likely to represent a more severely ill subset of individuals with AN. Among those with AN who develop their eating disorder in adolescence, and for whom the disorder is not enduring, associated psychopathology and related problems in social and interpersonal functioning are accordingly more limited. Moreover, even for those with more longstanding AN, it is important to recognize that certain interpersonal problems and personality dimensions (and even disorders) are unstable over time and improve with recovery from AN. Thus, clinicians should be careful not to overinterpret personality disorders and interpersonal problems during the acute stage of AN, but rather should monitor an individual's clinical presentation, including these features, and address them as an integrated part of the clinical work. The more enduring interpersonal and personality problems will become self-evident over time and as the eating disorder resolves.

Bulimia Nervosa

Individuals meeting diagnostic criteria for BN engage in recurrent binge eating and inappropriate compensatory behavior over a 3-month period (American Psychiatric Association, 2013). By definition, an episode of binge eating involves eating an objectively large amount of food in a discrete period of time *and* simultaneously experiencing a sense of loss of control over eating. Similar to AN, BN is characterized by an overvaluing of body shape and weight on self-evaluation.

The medical complications associated with BN are primarily related to the deleterious effects of purging. The most common problems are erosion of dental enamel, swollen salivary glands, edema, electrolyte abnormalities (e.g., hypokalemia), and esophageal tears (Mehler et al., 2010). BN is also associated with disturbances in mood, with studies suggesting that 50–70% of patients with BN experience depression at some point during the illness (Crow & Brandenburg, 2010). Depressive symptoms endorsed by individuals with BN may include distress about binge-eating episodes (Roberto, Grilo, Masheb, & White, 2010), and depressive symptoms or negative affect may also be associated with the onset of aberrant eating (Smyth et al., 2007).

Given the lack of agreement on definitions of remission, recovery, and relapse in BN (Shapiro et al., 2007), the evaluation of outcome for this patient population remains problematic. A longitudinal study reported that approximately 75% of female college students diagnosed with BN by structured interview were in remission at 20-year follow-up (Keel & Klump, 2003). However, in an analysis of available data on treatment-seeking individuals with BN, Steinhausen and Weber (2009) found that approximately 45% of patients achieved full recovery, 27% showed improvement, and close to 23% remained chronically ill. In addition, 22.5% of those with BN cross over to another eating disorder category over time (Steinhausen & Weber, 2009). The most common crossover observed was from BN to eating disorder not otherwise specified (EDNOS), which may reflect partial remission of symptoms, followed by AN and, less commonly, BED (Steinhausen & Weber, 2009).

Crude mortality rates for individuals with BN are generally lower than what has been reported in AN (Papadopoulos et al., 2009). The highest mortality rate by far (3.9%) was reported by Crow and colleagues (2009). However, this estimate was based upon an outpatient sample with the BN category broadly defined to include individuals with a body mass index above 17.5 (i.e., a combination of individuals in normal weight range and those below a minimally medically acceptable weight). Steinhausen and Weber (2009), in a comprehensive analysis of data from 76 studies of patients with BN, estimated a more modest crude mortality rate of 0.32% in this patient population. This is consistent with the 0.40% cumulative mortality rate recently determined from studies of BN between 2004 and 2009 (Keel & Brown, 2010).

Similar to individuals with AN, individuals with BN report significant rates of comorbid psychiatric diagnoses. Among individuals with a lifetime history of

BN, mood and anxiety disorders are common. Reports of comorbid mood disorder range from approximately 33 to 75% for individuals with BN (Binford & Le Grange, 2005; Duncan et al., 2005; Fichter & Quadflieg, 2004; Kaye, Bulik, Thornton, Barbarich, & Masters, 2004). Recent studies suggest that the majority of individuals with BN also experience some form of anxiety disorder (68%), with the most common diagnoses being OCD, social phobia, and posttraumatic stress disorder (PTSD) (Binford & LeGrange, 2005; Fichter & Quadflieg, 2004; Kaye et al., 2004). Compared to people with AN, individuals with BN are more likely to report a lifetime history of an alcohol use disorder (46.1%); similar to AN, the majority of individuals with BN who develop an alcohol use disorder do so subsequent to the onset of their eating disorder (Bulik et al., 2004).

A high percentage of individuals with BN also meet criteria for comorbid personality disorders, with borderline personality disorder and avoidant personality disorder being most common, followed by obsessive–compulsive, paranoid, and dependent personality disorder (Ro et al., 2005). Studies also indicate that impulsivity and, more specifically, negative urgency is commonly associated with BN and significant in predicting treatment outcome (Fischer, Smith, & Cyders, 2008). Impulsiveness has been associated with poorer outcome and more frequent hospitalizations (von Ranson, 2008). Data suggest that suicide attempts are not uncommon among individuals with BN, with a recent study reporting that 26.9% of women with a lifetime history of BN have attempted suicide. However, the rate of completed suicides for individuals with BN is generally reported to be significantly lower than that for those with AN. Self-harm, including suicide attempts, is associated with borderline personality disorder, and given the high rate of comorbid borderline personality disorder associated with BN, it may be that this personality disorder is the significant factor that increases risk of such behaviors for individuals with BN (Forcano et al., 2009).

Given the high rates of comorbidity with other mental disorders, it is not surprising that individuals with BN report significant difficulties in interpersonal relationships, and data suggest that interpersonal problems are correlated with treatment outcome (Hartmann, Zeeck, & Barrett, 2010). However, in comparison to those with AN, individuals with BN are much more likely to be able to continue working and to be socially engaged in their peer communities, even while symptomatic.

Binge-Eating Disorder

BED is characterized by recurrent episodes of "binge eating" (i.e., the ingestion of a large amount of food, accompanied by a sense of loss of control) that occur in the absence of any compensatory behaviors (e.g., self-induced vomiting, laxative misuse, excessive exercise). The binge eating that occurs in BED must be recurrent, associated with significant emotional distress, and characterized by three or more of the following features: (1) eating more rapidly than normal, (2) eating until uncomfortably full, (3) eating in the absence of hunger, (4) eating alone because of embarrassment over the amount eating, and (5) feelings of disgust, depression, or guilt after overeating (American Psychiatric Association, 2013). While BED was previously considered a condition in need of further study under the umbrella category of EDNOS in DSM-IV (American Psychiatric Association, 1994), BED has become a formal diagnostic category in DSM-5 (American Psychiatric Association, 2013). Unlike AN and BN, BED has no diagnostic criterion specifying the cognitive feature of undue influence of body shape or weight on self-evaluation. Studies indicate, however, that individuals with BED do report more concern with their body shape and weight than do overweight (Eldredge et al., 1997; Grilo et al., 2008) and normal-weight (Eldredge & Agras, 1996) individuals without BED. The degree of overvaluation reported by patients with BED is similar to that reported by individuals with BN (Grilo, Masheb, & White, 2010). Moreover, data suggest that the undue influence of body shape and weight on self-evaluation may indicate a more severe variant of BED (Goldschmidt et al., 2010).

Individuals with BED are more likely than those without the disorder to be obese (Hudson, Hiripi, Pope, & Kessler, 2007), but they can also be distinguished reliably from non eating-disordered obese individuals (Wonderlich, Gordon, Mitchell, Crosby, & Engel, 2009). When compared to weight-matched individuals without BED, those with BED endorse significantly more eating disorder psychopathology and lower quality of life (Wonderlich et al., 2009). BED is associated with co-occurring medical problems such as diabetes (Johnson, Spitzer, & Williams, 2001); irritable bowel syndrome and fybromyalgia (Javaras et al., 2008); and psychological correlates, including the presence of depressive symptoms and low self-esteem (Hrabosky, Masheb, White, & Grilo, 2007). While a recent meta-analysis of BED studies from 2004 to 2009 reported the disorder to have a cumulative mortality rate of 0.5%, more data are needed from studies with longer follow-up periods to appreciate better any possible elevated mortality risk in this group (Keel & Brown, 2010).

Since BED's introduction into the nomenclature in 1994, there has been debate about whether regular binge eating in the absence of compensatory behavior represents a unique disorder or instead serves as an indicator of other psychological problems. However, there is now ample evidence that BED can be distinguished from other eating disorders and is associated with both heightened eating-disordered psychopathology and functional impairment (Wonderlich et al., 2009). Though longitudinal data are limited, the course of BED appears quite distinct from that of AN, and although BED shares core features with BN and crossover occurs between these two disorders, there are also clear differences in risk, course, and outcome. Individuals with BED who receive treatment are more likely to experience a reduction in symptoms and less likely to cross over into another eating disorder diagnostic group over time (Wonderlich et al., 2009).

BED is commonly associated with obesity in clinical samples, and compared to obese individuals without BED, individuals with BED show higher rates of mood disorders and personality disorders, with major depressive disorder being the most commonly reported comorbid psychiatric condition for BED (lifetime rate of

50–60%). (Wonderlich et al., 2009). In addition, alcohol abuse and dependence and anxiety disorders are also elevated in clinical samples (Grilo, 2002). The degree of associated psychopathology reported by individuals with BED appears to be associated with the eating disorder, not the degree of obesity (Dingemans, Bruna, & van Furth, 2002). In comparison to individuals with BN-purging subtype, individuals with BED tend to show fewer comorbid psychiatric symptoms (Tobin, Griffing, & Griffing, 1997); however, in comparison to individuals with nonpurging BN, individuals with BED show comparable levels of eating-related and associated psychopathology on average, but with much greater variance (Santonastaso, Ferrara, & Favaro, 1999). Similar to AN and BN, research on life events and interpersonal functioning suggests that interpersonal problems and work stresses are significant as potential precipitants of BED and can endure throughout the course of the disorder (Pike et al, 2006; Striegel-Moore et al., 2005).

EPIDEMIOLOGY

It is now widely recognized that eating disorders occur across culture, socioeconomic class and race (Becker, 2007; Soh, Touyz, & Surgenor, 2006). Much more research is necessary to more understand fully and explicate the rise of eating disorders in cultures around the globe, and the differential distribution of AN, BN, and BED; however, as discussed earlier, it is widely held that the distribution of eating disorders in a population reflects the confluence of biological, environmental, cultural, and psychological factors.

Anorexia Nervosa

AN, while a severe psychiatric illness, is also a relatively uncommon disorder. A review of epidemiological studies of eating disorders placed the average prevalence rate (total number of cases in the population) at 0.29%, with higher prevalence for subthreshold AN (Hoek & van Hoeken, 2003). A subsequent study, in which information was collected over 50 years in one region of the United States, yielded estimates of the incidence of AN (total number of new cases in the population over a specified period of time) to be 8 per 100,000 per year (Hoek, 2006). Overall, the average prevalence rate of AN among females is estimated to be 0.3% (Hoek, 2006). While limited research has evaluated the prevalence or clinical presentation of AN in men, best estimates indicate the disorder affects one-tenth as many males as females (Hoek & van Hoeken, 2003).

In the United States, recently pooled data from national epidemiological studies suggests the prevalence of AN to be similar among non-Latino whites, Latinos, Asians, and blacks (Marques et al., 2011). AN has also been described in non-Western cultures (Cummins, Simmons, & Zane, 2005; Eddy, Hennessey, & Thompson-Brenner, 2007; Pike & Mizushima, 2005). However, prevalence of the illness among culturally diverse groups has not yet been adequately determined and as a result, misclassification of cases may occur. One apparent cultural variation of AN, for example, is the absence of fat phobia among Asian and Indian individuals who otherwise meet diagnostic criteria for the disorder (Lee, Ho, & Hsu, 1993; Lee, 1994). False-positive results of eating disorder symptoms have been noted in the literature as well, for example, in South African youth who reported a preoccupation with food that was related to poverty, shortage of resources, and hunger rather than to an eating disorder (Le Grange, Luow, Breen, & Katzman, 2004). Increased focus upon phenomenological differences and culturally sensitive "idioms of distress" is clearly necessary to understand better and accurately classify these problems (Becker, 2007).

Incidence and prevalence rates of AN appear to have risen over the 20th century, but it is unclear whether more individuals are affected by the disease, or whether the increase instead reflects increased utilization of the health care system, improved diagnostics, or greater acceptability/feasibility of treatment (Grilo, 2006; Hoek, 2006). Estimates of incidence and prevalence of AN may be complicated by the illness's rarity and patient characteristics, including the secrecy and denial around symptoms that may interfere with accurate reporting (Grilo, 2006).

Bulimia Nervosa

Estimates of the prevalence of BN suggest that it is a slightly more common disorder than AN. Hoek and van Hoeken's (2003) epidemiological review described a 1.0% aggregated prevalence rate for BN (range: 0.0–4.5%), with higher rates for more broadly defined BN. The National Comorbidity Survey Replication study, based on surveys of a large, nationally representative, random sample of adults in the United States, yielded similar prevalence rates of 1.5 and 0.5% for females and males, respectively (Hudson et al., 2007). While disease frequency estimates of AN may be complicated by the disorder's rarity, the wide variation of prevalence estimates of BN may be attributed to changing definitions of the illness since its introduction in 1980 (Crow & Brandenburg, 2010). Moreover, given the secrecy and ease of hiding disordered behaviors in BN, incidence rates are generally considered to underestimate the true rate of illness (Grilo, 2006).

Nationally, recent research suggests that BN may be more prevalent among Latinos and blacks than non-Latino whites (Marques et al., 2011). Associated distress with bulimic symptoms may vary cross-culturally, with preliminary data suggesting binge eating as the best predictor of distress among whites, blacks, and Latinos, in contrast with vomiting as the most salient predictor of distress among Asians (Franko, Becker, Thomas, & Herzog, 2007). The cross-cultural variation in experience of this eating disorder supports the development of flexibility within the classification system that would promote cultural sensitivity and allow for phenomenologic distinctions (Becker, 2007).

Though the prevalence and incidence of BN has primarily been documented in North American and European cultures, the disorder has been described in a variety of non-Western cultures (Nobakht & Dezhkam, 2000; Pike & Mizushima, 2005). Unlike in AN, the transmission of Western ideals (e.g., thin beauty) and economic factors (e.g., an abundance of food available for binge eating) is thought to play an important role in the prevalence of BN in non-Western cultures (Keel & Klump, 2003).

Binge-Eating Disorder

BED is estimated to affect 3% of adults, based on the aforementioned National Comorbidity Survey Replication study (Hudson et al., 2007). In addition to being more common than either AN or BN, BED is associated with later age of onset and longer duration (Hudson et al., 2007; Striegel-Moore & Franko, 2003). This disorder is more commonly seen in men (2.5%) than other eating disorders, though available data indicate that full-syndrome BED is still at least 1.75 times more common in women (Hudson et al., 2007). Among obese individuals, prevalence estimates of BED range from 2 to 5% in community samples, and as high as 30% among individuals seeking bariatric surgery or alternative weight loss treatments (de Zwaan, 2001; Kalarchian et al., 2007). Relative to other eating disorders, BED is known to be more prevalent across a variety of racial and ethnic groups within North American samples (see Wonderlich et al., 2009).

ETIOLOGY

Given the long-standing recognition of eating disorders, it is notable that the empirical literature on the etiology of eating disorders is still quite limited. Although the field has a large body of correlational studies, prospective and experimental research designs that can identify directional and causational effects are few. Several case–control studies have been conducted to identify risk correlates of eating disorders (Fairburn et al., 1998; Karwautz et al., 2001; Striegel-Moore et al., 2005; Pike et al., 2008). These studies offer the advantage of examining actual clinical cases, and they advance the field by narrowing the number of potential risk factors for prospective study; however, they are also subject to potential reporting bias given that the data are gathered retrospectively from individuals with eating disorders. Thus, risk correlates identified in case–control studies need to be examined prospectively or experimentally before they can be described as true risk factors. On the flip side, the majority of the prospective and experimental studies of eating disturbance are limited by the fact that they do not examine true cases of individuals with eating disorders. These studies typically demonstrate risk for eating problems but not necessarily clinical eating disorders (for review, see Jacobi, Hayward, de Zwaan, Kraemer, & Agras, 2004).

In 1986, Striegel-Moore, Sliberstein, and Rodin posed the following set of heuristic questions to guide the study of the development of eating disorders: Why now? Why women? Why some women and not others? These questions reflect several important understandings of risk for eating disorders. First, eating disorders are a contemporary problem; prevalence rates have increased during the past century in Western cultures, and rates of eating psychopathology continue to increase across the globe (Becker, Thomas, & Pike, 2009). Second, gender is perhaps the most significant and unequivocal risk factor for eating disorders. Although males do present with eating disorders, adolescent and young adult females are at dramatically elevated risk, especially for AN and BN. And finally, the questions posed by Striegel-Moore and colleagues (1986) recognize that despite widespread sociocultural and environmental factors, only a small percentage of individuals actually develops significant eating disturbances, implying that individual risk factors are essential to understanding why some individuals develop eating psychopathology while others from the same environmental context do not.

Why Now?

At the broadest level, sociocultural factors set the general stage of risk. Socio-cultural studies of the development of eating disorders suggest a complex interplay between increased abundance in the food supply, increased sedentary lifestyles, and societal overvaluation of a thin beauty ideal (Brownell, 2010). The transformation to modern, industrialized societal structures is associated with dramatic increases in food supply, especially highly palatable, caloric foods, and equally dramatic decreases in energy expenditure in daily living. In addition, as societies modernize and industrialize, traditional gender roles are often put in flux. Economic, social, and political changes that characterize societies in transition bring not only tremendous opportunity but also instability in terms of role models and societal expectations. It has been argued that the actual dynamic of social transition increases risk for eating disorders at the broadest level, because such societal flux increases the developmental challenges of coming of age given the lack of role models and societal norms to guide the course (Katzman & Lee, 1997). In clinical practice, it is useful to assess a given patient's cultural context and potential role models better to understand maintaining and perpetuating factors.

Why Women?

In addition to biological vulnerabilities that likely predispose women to develop eating disorders, environmental factors associated with industrialization and modernization over the past century have profoundly impacted women's place in society. Across the globe, issues of women's roles and rights have been at the forefront of much societal change, and although this has ushered forth many positive changes in women's roles, a concomitant phenomenon has been the rise in societal overvaluation of a thin beauty ideal for women. Although the meaning of thinness may vary somewhat across cultures, it appears that young women coming of age are consistently the most vulnerable and targeted group. The confluence of these factors results in significant pressure conveyed by family, peers, and mass media to achieve an unrealistically thin beauty ideal within a social context that is associated with increased caloric consumption and reduced energy expenditure. To the extent that an individual internalizes the thin beauty ideal, the tension that ensues has been shown to be associated with increased body dissatisfaction and dieting, and prospective studies suggest that body dissatisfaction and dieting are significant risk factors for eating psychopathology, particularly bulimic symptomatology (Ogden & Mundray, 1998; Stice & Agras, 1998).

Why Some Women and Not Others?

Given the widespread societal values and pressures to achieve an unrealistically thin beauty ideal, it is notable that only a minority of individuals actually develops eating disorders. Exposure to particular life events, individual characteristics, and genetic differences and vulnerabilities have been examined in an attempt to identify why particular individuals are at increased risk for the development of eating disorders.

The genetics data suggest some biological heritability of risk for AN, BN, and BED; however, it is unclear what the genetic vulnerability is, whether it is the same across eating disorders, and the degree of variance accounted for by genetic factors in an etiological model (Commission on Adolescent Eating Disorders, 2005; Mazzeo, Slof-Op't Landt, van Furth, & Bulik, 2006). It appears that one biological component of risk centers on weight regulation. Individuals with AN appear to have a biology that can sustain extreme weight loss that the majority of the population could not tolerate. In contrast, it appears that individuals with BED and BN are much more likely to have a history of being overweight. There are likely other biological factors that contribute to risk; however, without the existence of specific biological or genetic markers, studies must identify variables that may further be explored in terms of both biological and environmental transmission.

In terms of the development of AN, no prospective and experimental studies exist to inform the discussion of risk factors. Several case–control studies suggest that the personal vulnerabilities of perfectionism and negative affectivity, family discord and high parental demands, and childhood physical and sexual abuse are potential risk correlates in the developmental history reported by individuals in treatment for AN (Fairburn, Cooper, Doll, & Welch, 1999; Karwautz et al., 2001; Pike et al., 2008). Interestingly, individuals with AN do not report a long history of weight and shape concerns; instead, the salience of these factors appears to be greatest in the year immediately preceding the onset of their eating psychopathology. In fact, it may be that dieting and weight concern are more accurately understood as prodromal correlates of AN rather than potential risk factors. The convergence of the data from these case–control studies is noteworthy; however, given that these studies all included individuals with relatively long-standing AN, it may be that the identified risk correlates are most accurately understood for a more severe and/or more chronic clinical condition. Based on the extant data, prospective studies that focus on the identified risk correlates would potentially advance the field in terms of understanding the interplay of variables that increase risk specifically for AN and more generally for clinical impairment and chronicity.

The mechanism of risk for many of these variables may be biological or environmental, or most likely a combination of biological vulnerabilities that interact with certain environmental exposures or triggers. For example, a majority of girls engage in dieting at some point during adolescence. In the case of AN, it may be that dieting and weight loss trigger a certain biological vulnerability among individuals who also have some anxious and perfectionistic traits, such that they would be able to lose and sustain significant weight loss when others could not.

In the case of BN, extant data converge to suggest that genetic vulnerability, childhood obesity, weight concern, negative body image and dieting, sexual abuse and adverse family factors (including parental obesity, parental mood or substance abuse disorder, and highly critical parenting), along with individual factors of social anxiety, negative affectivity, and low self-esteem, may contribute to increased risk (Fairburn et al., 1998; Jacobi et al., 2004; Stice, 2001). Also, although perfectionistic qualities appear to increase risk for AN, impulsivity and externalizing behaviors may be associated with increased risk for bulimic psychopathology (Stice, 2001).

BED shares with BN the common feature of binge eating at the core of the syndrome; thus, certain risk correlates also appear to be common across these disorders. In particular, childhood obesity, adverse family factors (including family discord, high parental demands, and parental history of mood and substance disorder), mood disorder and negative affectivity have been identified as risk correlates in case–control studies of BED (Fairburn et al., 1998; Striegel-Moore et al., 2005). It is likely that both biological and environmental factors contribute to increased risk for childhood obesity, which is often associated with teasing and body dissatisfaction as the individual matures. Many individuals with BED report that they engage in emotional binge eating due to mood disturbance, negative affectivity, and difficulties in affect regulation. Many also describe binge eating as result of dieting to lose weight due to the subjectively intolerable deprivation they experience when dieting. Both pathways reflect the interplay of biological, psychological, and experiential factors in increasing risk for BED.

As noted earlier, research designs exploring risk for eating disorders are limited by the fact that most of the data represent retrospective reports from individuals with eating disorders or prospective studies that assess risk for eating problems but not clinical eating disorders. Prospective studies that focus on high-risk groups and assess whether risk correlates represent true risk factors would greatly advance the field. Also, collateral reports from significant others would provide important additional information to solve the puzzle of risk for eating disorders. Moreover, it is important to note that many of the possible risk factors associated with eating disorders may be shared with other psychiatric disorders. For example, childhood abuse increases risk for not only eating disorders but also anxiety and mood disorder (Pope & Hudson, 1992; Jonas et al., 2011). Finally, it is essential to note that none of the risk correlates or risk factors are pathognomonically associated with any of the eating disorders. Unlike the presence of a certain cellular abnormality that indicates without a doubt the presence of a particular cancer, for example, the variables associated with eating disturbances represent increased risk but do not definitively determine the presence of an eating disorder.

MULTIVARIATE MODELS OF ONSET
AND MAINTENANCE OF EATING DISORDERS

Although many questions regarding risk factors in the development of eating disorders remain unanswered, it is widely recognized that these disorders are multidetermined, with both broad societal factors and individual environmental, psychological, and biological factors interacting to increase risk for eating disorders (Stice, 2001; Smolak & Murnen, 2001).

It is also widely acknowledged that the factors contributing to the onset of the disorder are not necessarily the factors that contribute to maintenance of the disorder. Cognitive-behavioral treatment (CBT) interventions across the spectrum of eating disorders emphasize this point (Fairburn, Marcus, & Wilson, 1993; Garner, Vitousek, & Pike, 1997; Pike, Carter, & Olmsted, 2010). These models maintain that certain variables very likely increase risk during a developmentally vulnerable period of time (e.g., overvaluation of shape and/or weight), and that other variables contribute to the persistence of the eating psychopathology (e.g., strict dietary rules or rigid eating behavior). Specific components of the eating disorders (e.g., severe weight loss, binge eating and purging) have significant biological, behavioral, and psychological effects that serve to complicate the clinical picture and perpetuate the disturbance. In fact, the evidence-based treatments for eating disorders largely focus on maintenance factors based on the tenet that addressing these issues first will result in the most significant and tangible clinical improvement initially. Other more long-standing issues, including factors that may have contributed to the development of the disorder (e.g., poor self-esteem, interpersonal stressors), will more readily be addressed once these maintenance behaviors have resolved to a sufficient degree. CBT maintains that addressing the current issues and bringing some resolution of symptoms will bring some immediate relief and increase the patient's sense of self-efficacy in achieving resolution of the eating disorder. Moreover, from a CBT perspective, resolution of the acute issues will bring clarity of vision in analyzing the more distal, developmental factors, because by the time individual presents for treatment, the eating disorder has often taken on a life of its own. As we discuss in more detail later in the chapter, CBT treatments that focus first on regaining control of eating behaviors and challenging what has become automatic in terms of maintenance of the eating disorder psychopathology have strong empirical support in the field.

CLINICAL IMPLICATIONS, TREATMENT PLANNING, AND EVIDENCE-BASED TREATMENT OF EATING DISORDERS

Anorexia Nervosa

Individuals with AN are unlikely to present with complaints about their change in weight or nutritional intake. They may be identified on routine medical assessment or may present for evaluation following concern expressed by family, friends, coworkers, or coaches. The evaluation of individuals with AN is challenging because of the thought content frequently associated with the illness, including a belief that one is fat or would become fat with weight gain, and a denial of the seriousness of the low weight state. Life events and psychological traits that were present before the onset of eating behavioral change are part of any comprehensive evaluation of an individual with an eating disorder, but the clinician should use caution in making any causal hypotheses regarding the development of the eating disorder, since little is known about factors that directly influence the development of these conditions. Evaluation should include detailed assessment of daily food and beverage intake, including quantities of the foods cited. Additionally, clinicians should assess weight history (including lifetime highest–lowest weights; time course of significant weight changes; and associated changes in menstrual status, if applicable), body image concerns, and exercise routines. Assessments should include direct questioning about purging behaviors, including vomiting, as well as the use of laxatives, diuretics, and diet pills in traditional pharmaceutical, as well as alternative or health supplement, preparations. Parallel history from family members may be necessary to confirm an eating disorder diagnosis. In younger patients, weight loss may not be present; rather, the diagnosis of AN may be made if expected goals for weight gain and growth are not met (Rosen, 2010). The evaluation of AN will likely include medical assessment, including vital signs such as heart rate, blood pressure, and temperature, in addition to height and weight. Low weight patients will frequently have changes consistent with a hypometabolic state, and both these findings and other physical signs, such as amenorrhea, can be useful indicators of the severity of illness. In fact, some patients are concerned enough about these changes that they are willing to consider engaging in weight restoration treatment. Even in the context of significant low weight, laboratory assessments may not identify abnormalities. Clinicians should not be reassured by these results, because total body levels of micronutrients and minerals may not be reflected in blood tests.

Case formulation in AN should include a narrative that helps the patient understand the emergence and perpetuation of illness symptoms. The narrative should include the patient's predisposing factors such as pre-illness anxiety or obsessionality, family history of an eating disorder, dieting behaviors, or activi- ties (e.g., athletics, dance or modeling) that may significantly reinforce leanness. Dietary changes, even those that the patient dismisses as distinct from the formal eating disorder, such as lists of disliked foods, recently acquired vegetarian prac- tices, and food allergies, should be considered as possible symptoms of the illness itself. Patients should be informed about the physical and psychological risks of malnutrition, including the development or intensification of distressing symptoms such as depression, anxiety, and social isolation. Basic principles of nutritional reha- bilitation should be reviewed, such as the fact that adolescents and young adults usually require 1,800–2,400 kcal (kilocalories) for weight maintenance, and that 3,500 kcal above maintenance requirements are necessary in order to gain 1 pound. Patients (and families) may have to hear this repeatedly in order to process the fact that nutritional plans will need to include 500–1,000 kcal/day above maintenance requirements in order for an individual to gain 1–2 pounds per week.

Treatment plans for individuals with AN need to emphasize weight restora- tion and normalization of eating behaviors. After evaluation of illness severity, available psychosocial supports, prior treatment history, and treatment availability, evaluations should conclude with recommendations for treatment type and set- ting. Patients, and their families, whenever possible, should participate in treatment planning. Most treatments include a team of clinicians with medical, psychologi- cal, and nutritional expertise. Target weight goals (and the rationale for these rec- ommendations) should be provided, along with explicit expectations about rate of weight gain and plans for weight monitoring. Clearly identified treatment goals are imperative, so that individuals with AN can receive appropriate levels of care dependent on their progress. Once a recommended weight has been achieved, goals can be reevaluated to incorporate weight maintenance. Psychoeducation about nor- mal fluctuations in weight and healthy weight *ranges* often is required. Ambivalence about various aspects of recovery and denial about the seriousness of the problem can be framed as symptomatic of the illness, and should be explicitly addressed at the onset of treatment and repeatedly as needed.

Clearly, treatment for AN can be both challenging and complicated, and the lack of clear empirical support for any single treatment approach may be a result of different factors, including several difficulties inherent to treating this clinical group (Attia, 2010). Associated features of AN, such as the ego-syntonic nature of the disorder (Vitousek, Watson, & Wilson, 1998) and the medical complications that can arise during treatment (Halmi et al., 2005), can have profound implications on patient motivation, compliance, and outcome. Patients with AN are also typically hesitant to participate in treatments with the goal of weight normalization, which impacts both recruitment and retention rates (Halmi et al., 2005). Treatment research in individuals with AN is complicated by their varying needs in terms of intensity of services (e.g., inpatient hospitalization, day treatment, outpatient treatment) and the tendency for patients to be withdrawn from outpatient treatment for a higher level of care (Bulik, Berkman, Brownley, Sedway, & Lohr, 2007). Additionally, the rarity of the illness makes it challenging to recruit adequate samples for rigorous study.

Overall, psychotherapeutic interventions for AN target either acute treatment for underweight (e.g., refeeding and normalization of weight) or the prevention of relapse to a low weight. The theoretical foundations and existing treatment efficacy data of family therapy and CBT for AN are described below. Novel approaches for treatment of this disorder are also briefly introduced.

Family Therapy

Preliminary evidence supports the use of family-based treatment of adolescents with AN, though only a handful of randomized controlled psychotherapy trials have been completed. One type of family therapy, called the Maudsley approach because of its origins at the Maudsley Hospital in England (Russell, Szmukler, Dare, & Eisler, 1987), stands out in particular from the existing empirical database as potentially promising.

The Maudsley approach assumes that normal adolescent development has been disturbed by the presence of the eating disorder; thus, parents' involvement in treatment is essential to the this therapeutic intervention (Lock, Le Grange, Agras, & Dare, 2001). Parents temporarily oversee the refeeding process, and once successful in this task, gradually return an age-appropriate degree of control and autonomy back to the patient. After eating and weight have normalized, treatment focuses on feelings underlying the disordered behaviors and the developmental issues that may have been ignored due to the illness. This treatment modality is best suited to individuals with AN who are younger than 18, who live at home with their families, and whose families are able and willing to set aside other issues in the service of treating the eating disorder (Lock et al., 2001). The entire household (e.g., parents, siblings, child care providers) is typically involved in the psychotherapy and must therefore be committed to the approach and involved in the day-to-day routines around meals.

Overall, this treatment appears to be a reasonable choice for young adolescents with AN who have a short duration of illness (Russell et al., 1987). Moreover, existing data suggest long-term benefit of a Maudsley family-based intervention (Eisler, et al., 1997; Eisler, Simic, Russell, & Dare, 2007). For example, a recent study of adolescents with AN receiving Maudsley treatment observed that 78% of patients no longer met criteria for an eating disorder at 36-month follow-up (Paulson-Karlsson, Engstrom, & Nevonen, 2009). In weighing the need for a high level of family commitment and involvement against the possible long-term benefits of Maudsley treatment, researchers have become particularly interested in identifying the essential elements of this approach. Studies comparing subtle variations of the Maudsley approach (Eisler et al., 2000; Lock, Agras, Bryson, & Kraemer, 2005) suggest that parental involvement may be the most salient feature of the treatment (Varchol & Cooper, 2009). Thus, careful consideration must be given by the evaluating clinician as to whether parents *and* patients can be adequately committed to this psycho-therapy. If not, alternative interventions should be considered.

Cognitive-Behavioral Therapy

CBT, pioneered by Aaron Beck (1976), has demonstrated efficacy for a wide range of psychiatric illnesses, including depression, anxiety disorders, substance abuse, and eating disorders (Nathan & Gorman, 2002; Wilson, Grilo, & Vitousek, 2007; Young, Weinberger, & Beck, 2001).

A central tenet of the CBT model of AN is that eating disorder symptoms are maintained by the interaction between cognitive disturbances (e.g., preoccupation with shape, weight, and eating) and behavioral disturbances (e.g., rigid dietary rules, overexercise, purging) that impact eating and weight control (Fairburn, 2008; Pike et al., 2010). Personality characteristics (e.g., perfectionism), stressors associated with mood changes, and underlying low self-esteem are theorized to contribute to the onset and perpetuation of the illness. The primary dysfunctional schema is one in which a high value is placed on control over eating, shape, and weight. This over-valuation, which is coupled with internalization about the importance of thinness in combating feelings of inadequacy, leads to the implementation of rigid dietary rules (Pike et al., 2010). The resulting extreme weight control behaviors engender a state of starvation, which in and of itself is known to exacerbate impairment in psy-chological functioning (low mood, increased preoccupation with food, etc.; Keys et al., 1950). In AN-B/P subtype, dietary restriction leads to episodes of bingeing and purging that result in a renewed resolve to limit caloric intake. The CBT model acknowledges that as an individual becomes more entrenched in AN, the cognitive and behavioral disturbances are increasingly self-perpetuating.

Though available data on CBT for AN are quite limited, there is some indica-tion that this approach may be of use preventing relapse in weight-restored patients (Carter et al., 2009; Pike, Walsh, Vitousek, Wilson, & Bauer, 2003). Studies compar-ing CBT to alternative approaches have consistently reported lower rates of prema-ture dropout (Pike et al., 2003) and significantly longer time to relapse (Carter et al., 2009) in weight-restored individuals receiving CBT.

This modality's efficacy in treating acute AN is considerably more ambiguous. In the first published case series of CBT for individuals with acute AN, Fairburn and Cooper reported that two patients did well, one showed some improvement, and two did not benefit from the intervention at all (Cooper & Fairburn, 1984). Overall, however, subsequent randomized controlled trials have found no differences in out-come for underweight patients receiving CBT compared to other treatments (Ball & Mitchell, 2004; Channon, DeSilva, Hemsley, & Pekins, 1989; McIntosh et al., 2005). However, studies of CBT for acute AN are limited by small study samples, shorter duration of treatment than recommended by CBT experts (Wilson et al., 2007), and high attrition rates. In fact, findings from two CBT studies cannot even be inter-preted, with the first noting a 100% dropout rate from the nutritional counseling comparison intervention (Serfaty, Turkington, Heap, Ledsham, & Jolley, 1999), and the second retaining less than 40% of patients across all groups (Halmi et al., 2005).

Thus, while there is no evidence that CBT for people with acute, low-weight AN offers a superior treatment in comparison to other approaches, existing studies in this subgroup are limited by methodological problems. Taken together, studies of CBT in weight-restored individuals with AN suggest that this may be a promising intervention for preventing relapse in an illness known to have an overall poor long-term prognosis (Steinhausen, 2002).

Additional Approaches

Given the limited evidence in support of any one psychotherapeutic intervention for AN, clinical researchers have begun adapting treatments originally studied in other patient populations, such as cognitive remediation therapy (CRT) and exposure therapy and response prevention (EX/RP), for use in individuals with AN.

Developed as an intervention for patients with impaired cognitive functioning due to brain lesions, CRT aims to identify, then strengthen impaired cognitive processes through repetitive cognitive and behavioral exercises (Tchanturia & Hambrook, 2010). The therapy is tailored to address areas of relative cognitive weakness, based upon neuropsychological assessment, neuroimaging findings, and studies comparing individuals with AN to healthy counterparts (e.g., Roberts, Tchanturia, Stahl, Southgate, & Treasure, 2007; Steinglass, Walsh, & Stern, 2006; Zastrow et al., 2009). Areas of impairment include "set shifting" (i.e., an inability to move easily back and forth between tasks or mental sets) or "cognitive flexibility" (to adapt behavior to changing demands in the environment), and "central coherence" (i.e., a difficulty in holistic information processing whereby details are integrated and put in a broader context). CRT sessions require patients to work on versions of different tasks to address inflexibility in thinking and overly detailed processing biases (for details, see Tchanturia & Hambrook, 2010). At present, only case series data on this approach have been published. Initial findings indicate that CRT yields improvement on neuropsychological measures in patients with AN (Tchanturia et al., 2008), but its utility in addressing disturbances in weight and eating behavior remains unknown.

In EX/RP for AN, disturbances in eating behavior are explicitly targeted. This cognitive-behavioral intervention, predicated upon patients' learning through experience that anticipated negative consequences do not occur when a fearful stimulus is approached, is the psychotherapy of choice for several anxiety disorders (Craske & Barlow, 2001; Foa & Franklin, 2001). In EX/RP for AN, the avoidance of food likely to produce weight gain is hypothesized to result from anxiety. Rigid dietary rules and ritualized eating behaviors (e.g., eating slowly, cutting food in small pieces) are conceptualized as strategies to avoid or minimize distress around eating (Steinglass et al., 2011). To promote experiential learning and habituation to anxiety, EX/RP for AN utilizes session time to put the patient in direct contact with feared foods and eating situations. This treatment is currently in early phases of development for use in patients with AN. While an initial study observed significantly increased caloric intake during a laboratory meal in patients with AN following a brief trial of EX/RP (Steinglass et al., 2007), further research is warranted to determine the overall acceptability and feasibility of this type of psychotherapy.

Bulimia Nervosa

While individuals with BN are more likely than individuals with AN to present with clear interest in symptom resolution, it is not unusual for those with BN to delay their presentation because of shame and reluctance to discuss symptoms with a clinician. All comprehensive psychological evaluations should include questions about eating, body shape, and weight concerns, and individuals who report concerns in these areas should be asked about binge-eating and purging behaviors. As with AN, assessment should include gathering information about typical overall eating pattern (and associated dietary rules) and binge episodes (e.g., amounts of food, type of food, time of day, context/triggers). Patients with BN may report an escalating pattern of binge and purge frequency. They may even have had an earlier period of restrictive food intake, and may have met full criteria for AN prior to the development of their BN symptoms. Younger patients may report less frequent episodes of binge eating or purging. Self-induced vomiting at any frequency should be identified as a problem, likely associated with an eating disorder, and should be addressed in the evaluation and treatment plan. Assessments for BN should include questions about social functioning, because patients with BN may eat secretively, or pair restrictive eating when alone with apparently "normal" eating with friends, accompanied by purging following a fuller meal. Patients should be made aware of the risks of frequent vomiting, including dental erosion and decay, and electrolyte instability associated with serious medical risks, such as cardiac arrhythmia or seizures. Individuals who abuse laxatives may develop significant difficulties with intestinal motility, as well as fluid and electrolyte abnormalities.

As previously mentioned, the symptoms of BN are often the source of great shame, and patients should be commended for speaking honestly with their clinicians about their symptoms and seeking help. Patients with BN require education about the cycle of thoughts and behaviors that frequently perpetuate the symptoms of illness and need support in order to break this cycle, introduce healthier eating behaviors, and manage the consequent anxiety about whether eating without purging can be accomplished without feared weight gain. Treatment planning should include education about effective treatments for BN, including psychotherapy and antidepressant medication. Regular evaluation of medical status should be required if patients with BN continue to be notably symptomatic as treatment progresses.

There has been great progress in the development and rigorous empirical study of several psychotherapies for BN in the past two decades. This body of research has identified substantial differences in the effectiveness of distinct psychotherapies, allowing for clearly delineated treatment guidelines (Grilo, 2006). In contrast to AN, the prognosis for patients with BN who receive adequate treatment is good. Approximately 50% of individuals with BN who receive manual-based CBT, for example, achieve either near or full remission of symptoms that appears to be maintained over time (Wilson et al., 2007). Given the robust empirical database of treatment research in BN, in 2004 the United Kingdom's National Institute for Health and Clinical Excellence (NICE) issued a detailed list of evidence-based treatment guidelines. CBT was designated as the treatment of choice for BN, marking the first NICE recommendation of a psychotherapy as a first-line treatment for any psychiatric disorder. Other recommended psychotherapeutic interventions for BN treatment included interpersonal psychotherapy (IPT) and guided self-help (GSH). These approaches are reviewed briefly below to familiarize clinicians with the range of evidence-based interventions available to them. Alternative treatments currently being adapted for study and use in this population, such as dialectical behavioral therapy (DBT) and family therapy, are also discussed.

Cognitive-Behavioral Therapy

The model underlying CBT for BN, similar to that for AN, strongly emphasizes the role of disturbances in cognitions and behaviors in maintaining bulimic symptoms. Again, the overvaluation of shape and weight is hypothesized to be a critical conduit to the implementation of rigid dietary rules. Dietary restriction predisposes individuals to experience binge-eating episodes, which are characterized by a loss of control over eating. Inappropriate compensatory behaviors, such as self-induced vomiting, laxative misuse, or overexercise, are relied upon to counteract the effects of binge eating. These weight control behaviors instead perpetuate binge eating, either by reducing negative affect about weight gain or disrupting normative satiety cues. Additionally, the binge–purge cycle causes distress and reinforces low self-esteem, increasing the likelihood of continued cognitive distortions about shape and weight, and subsequent dietary restriction (Fairburn, Marcus, et al., 1993). CBT targets behavioral disturbances characteristic of BN by prescribing a regular pattern of eating and providing problem-solving skills to cope with high-risk situations. Cognitive distortions are addressed via cognitive restructuring, with an aim of modifying problematic shape and weight concerns (Fairburn, Marcus, et al., 1993).

Randomized controlled trials of CBT for BN support its efficacy in helping patients achieve abstinence from or a decreased frequency of binge–purge behaviors. Consistent with the conceptual model on which the treatment is based, the reduction in dietary restraint achieved by CBT partly mediates the intervention's efficacy in eliminating binge eating and purging (Wilson, Fairburn, Agras, Walsh, & Kraemer, 2002). CBT has been demonstrated to be superior to other psychological treatments in the short term (Wilson et al., 2002) and to antidepressant medications (Wilson et al., 2007) for achieving abstinence from bulimic symptoms. Furthermore, the effects of CBT for BN are evident in improvements in not only binge eating and purging but also general psychopathology, including depressive symptoms, self-esteem, and social functioning (e.g., Chen et al., 2003).

Based upon extant data, although CBT is a first-line intervention for BN, improvements are still needed, because many patients remain at least marginally symptomatic following treatment (Wilson et al., 2007). Thus, a current challenge is for a cognitive behavioral intervention to demonstrate efficacy for a wider range of individuals with BN. To this end, Fairburn introduced an enhanced version of CBT (CBT-E), proposed to be "transdiagnostic," in that it focuses on commonalities among the eating disorders rather than differences (Fairburn, 2008). CBT-E aims to provide a more individualized form of treatment, with an emphasis on personalized treatment formulations. The core treatment is similar to that in the earlier manual by Fairburn, Marcus, and colleagues (1993), with two substantial changes. First, Fairburn (2008) offered a reformulated strategy and method for addressing dysfunctional thought processes regarding the overvaluation body shape and weight. Second, a treatment module has been added to tackle "mood intolerance" as a trigger of aberrant eating episodes. In addition, the core focus on eating disorder symptoms is supplemented by a flexible use of modules to address maintaining mechanisms theorized to perpetuate the illness, including low self-esteem, clinical perfectionism, and difficulties in interpersonal functioning. The first controlled trial of CBT-E for BN suggests that it may indeed be a more effective treatment for individuals with complex cases (Fairburn et al., 2009).

GUIDED SELF-HELP USING CBT

Despite the effectiveness of CBT in the treatment of BN, access to this modality of treatment remains quite limited (Wilson et al., 2007). Self-help programs using the principles and procedures of CBT were developed to overcome the barriers to treatment dissemination (e.g., adequate therapist training and supervision). In contrast to pure self-help, in which individuals are not provided with any direct feedback or assistance, GSH combines a self-help manual with a limited number of brief "therapy" sessions administered by health care providers with differing degrees of expertise and experience.

Studies of GSH vary widely in methodological quality and in where, how, and with whom the intervention was applied (Wilson et al., 2007). Comparisons of GSH to a wait list uniformly demonstrate that this approach is associated with a greater reduction of symptoms than no treatment (for a complete list, see Sysko & Walsh, 2008). Findings from randomized controlled trials of GSH compared to alternative treatment are more challenging to interpret (for a complete list, see Sysko & Walsh, 2008). Some studies do suggest that there are no differences in outcome between GSH and individual CBT for BN. However, it remains unclear whether they are equally effective interventions or whether the nonsignificant differences are due to methodological issues (e.g., lack of a unique reference treatment group, small sample size, characteristics of study participants; Sysko & Walsh, 2008). Thus, it remains uncertain whether GSH offers a specific benefit to individuals with BN over alternative interventions, or whether this modality is most appropriate to recommend when no other established treatment is available.

Interpersonal Psychotherapy

Originally developed as a short-term, structured psychotherapy for depression (Klerman, Weissman, Rounsaville, & Chevron, 1984), IPT has been adapted for BN by Fairburn and colleagues Fairburn, Jones, Peveler, Hope, and O'Connor (1993). In contrast to CBT, IPT for BN does not overtly focus on the modification of disturbed eating behaviors or overvaluation of shape and weight. Binge eating is theorized to occur as a response to interpersonal disturbances (e.g., social isolation) and consequent negative mood (Fairburn, Jones, et al., 1993). Thus, the primary emphasis of IPT is on helping patients identify and address current interpersonal problems that are hypothesized to maintain and perpetuate the eating disorder. Treatment goals typically evolve from the four domains of interpersonal problems, as outlined by Klerman et al. (1984)—grief, interpersonal role disputes, role transitions, and interpersonal deficits—and encourage mastery of current social roles, as well as adjustment to evolving interpersonal situations (Wilfley et al., 2002). Eating disorder symptoms are linked consistently back to their role in the perpetuation or maintenance of the patient's interpersonal domain of focus (Tanofsky-Kraff & Wilfley, 2010).

The NICE (2004) guidelines identify IPT as a treatment with some empirical support that might be considered an alternative to CBT. Overall, controlled trials of IPT for BN show this approach to be less effective than CBT in reducing bulimic symptoms by the end of the active phase of treatment (Agras, Walsh, Fairburn, Wilson, & Kraemer, 2000; Fairburn et al., 1991). Nevertheless, studies have shown that by follow-up time points, there is no significant difference between IPT and CBT, with individuals receiving either treatment experiencing a similar degree of improvement in bulimic symptoms (Agras et al., 2000; Fairburn, Jones, et al., 1993). Thus, there appear to be clear temporal differences in response to treatment, with IPT taking longer to achieve its effects than CBT (Fairburn, Jones, et al., 1993; Wilson et al., 2002). Proponents of IPT assert that if this psychotherapy is delivered in such a way that interpersonal problems are repeatedly linked to the maintenance of the eating disorder, response to treatment may occur more rapidly (Tanofsky-Kraff & Wilfley, 2010).

Additional Approaches

Given the need for psychological treatments to address a broader range of individuals with BN (Wilson et al., 2007), DBT and family-based therapy for BN have recently garnered increased attention.

DBT, developed to treat borderline personality disorder (Linehan, 1993), is an empirically supported treatment that focuses primarily on affect regulation and development of adaptive coping strategies and interpersonal skills. The skills taught in DBT, including mindfulness, distress tolerance, and emotional regulation, may be a particularly good match for the high levels of negative affect frequently experienced by patients with BN (Safer, Telch, & Agras, 2001a; Wilson et al., 2007). While findings from the first wait-list controlled trial suggest that DBT can yield a reduction of bulimic symptoms (Safer, Telch, & Agras, 2001b), rigorous studies comparing it to an active treatment have not yet been conducted.

The Maudsley form of family therapy, which has an evidence base for use in adolescents with AN, has also been adapted to meet the needs of younger patients with BN. Thus far, research suggests that family-based treatment is useful in reducing eating disorder symptoms in adolescents with BN (Le Grange, Crosby, Rathouz, & Leventhal, 2007), but it may not be any more effective than other approaches (Russell et al., 1987; Schmidt et al., 2007).

Beyond meeting the needs of a broader range of patients with BN, there has been a growing interest in telemedicine (e.g., Internet-based intervention) as a strategy to "reach" more individuals overall and to provide treatment in a cost-effective manner. The use of Internet-based CBT, for example, has shown promise in reaching and treating individuals with anxiety disorders (Andersson, 2009). Consistent with these findings, preliminary data support the usefulness of telemedicine CBT for BN in reducing the frequency of binge eating and purging compared to a wait-list control condition (Fernandez-Aranda et al., 2009) and to face-to-face CBT (Mitchell et al., 2008). More research is needed to address logistical considerations in delivering telemedicine and to identify possible long-term differences in outcome between this and other treatment modalities (Mitchell et al., 2008).

Binge-Eating Disorder

BED is the eating disorder with the highest prevalence rates, yet it may be the condition about which mental health clinicians know the least. Having been introduced into the diagnostic nomenclature as only a provisional diagnosis requiring further study in the DSM-IV (American Psychiatric Association, 1994), and given that individuals with BED often present at obesity clinics and other medical venues, many psychologists and other therapists have had limited exposure to BED compared to other eating disorder diagnoses. BED symptoms include significant distress to the affected individual, in terms of both the experience of loss of control associated with binge eating and associated psychological symptoms, such as depression and anxiety. Additionally, BED is present in many individuals who present for treatment for other, identified psychiatric disorders. Individuals with mood disorders, psychotic disorders, and anxiety disorders should be assessed for binge eating because of the prevalence of co-occurring BED in these clinical populations.

Treatment planning for BED requires patient education and participation. BED treatment is not synonymous with weight loss treatment, and treatments that effectively decrease bingeing episodes may not be associated with much or any weight loss. Psychotherapy for BED is often one of several treatment components that overweight or obese individuals with BED may want to consider in deciding to move toward healthy eating and weight.

In contrast to the treatments available for acute AN, but similar to findings in BN, multiple therapeutic modalities show promise in the amelioration of symptoms for BED. Overall, however, BED treatment research is still in its early stages. Initial studies came from the field of obesity, where mixed findings led to concern that behavioral weight loss interventions and calorically restrictive diets might be unsuitable for obese individuals endorsing features of eating disorders (Yanovski, 1993). For the many obese individuals with BED, there continues to be debate in the eating disorder and obesity fields as to whether weight status or eating disorder symptoms should be first-line treatment goals (Krysanksi & Ferraro, 2008). Given limited data supporting maintenance of significant weight loss following behavioral weight loss, targeting a reduction in binge eating initially may allow for a slow, modest weight loss following BED treatment (Krysanski & Ferraro, 2008). However, treatment research including long-term follow-up in this area is limited. Additionally, more studies comparing obese and nonobese individuals with BED are warranted to clarify the extent to which the eating disorder diagnosis offers clinically relevant information in relation to obesity (Wonderlich et al., 2009).

The clinical concerns of practitioners treating obese individuals with BED inspired research on psychological treatments adapted from the empirical database for BN, and more specifically on the use of CBT and IPT for patients with BED. Currently, CBT conducted individually or in group format enjoys the strongest empirical support and a designation as the treatment of choice for BED by the United Kingdom's NICE (2004). In considering the treatment needs of individuals with BED, however, it is important to bear in mind that these patients struggle across domains (e.g., binge eating; attitudinal features of eating disorders; general psychological symptoms and distress; and, at times, obesity with its associated health risks; Grilo, 2006). Specialized psychotherapies for BED including CBT and IPT are reviewed below.

Cognitive-Behavioral Therapy

To date, treatment studies evaluating CBT for BED have typically relied upon the manual developed by Fairburn, Marcus, and colleagues (1993) for the treatment of BN. The conceptual model, emphasizing disturbances in both thinking and behavior, has been largely retained. However, in this iteration of CBT, patients are encouraged to challenge negative cognitions related to having a larger body size and to develop structured, healthy eating patterns, with an emphasis on moderation of amounts and types of foods. Adjustments to the theoretical understanding of mechanisms maintaining the illness recognize key differences between the disorders, namely, the absence of inappropriate compensatory behaviors and more generally chaotic, less restrictive eating in BED compared to BN (Masheb & Grilo, 2000, 2006).

Overall, in controlled trials of CBT for BED, substantial reductions in binge eating, and general and eating-disordered psychopathology are evident posttreatment and sustained through follow-up (Peterson et al., 2001; Wilfley et al., 2002). Though CBT interventions do not reliably result in substantial or sustained weight loss (e.g., Wilson, Wilfley, Agras, & Bryson, 2010), the approach is generally associated with good treatment completion rates, reduction in binge-eating episodes in more than half of patients, and improvement in psychosocial functioning and mood (Wilson et al., 2007). CBT has also proven more effective than pharmacological treatments for BED as a stand-alone treatment (Grilo, Masheb, & Wilson, 2005) and as an adjunct to behavioral weight loss (BWL) treatment (Devlin et al., 2005). A recent meta-analysis of randomized controlled trials of BED treatments observed large effect sizes for cognitive-behavioral interventions (e.g., traditional psychotherapy, GSH), compared to medium effects of pharmacotherapy (primarily antidepressants), in the reduction of binge eating (Vocks et al., 2010).

While data clearly and consistently support the use of CBT for BED, little is known about how this intervention produces its effects. Some investigators have proposed that the current cognitive-behavioral model of BED, adapted from BN, may pay insufficient attention to low levels of dietary restraint, high negative affect, and eating in response to emotion characteristic of individuals with this particular eating disorder (Wilson, et al., 2007). As more is learned about the underlying mechanisms perpetuating this illness, cognitive-behavioral interventions will likely target even better the treatment of BED.

GUIDED SELF-HELP USING CBT

Similar to what we described for BN, self-help based on the CBT model of eating disorders has been studied extensively, primarily using the Fairburn (1995) manual. Several investigations have tested therapist-guided self-help (GSH) approaches, as well as pure self-help (for a complete list, see Sysko & Walsh, 2008); emerging data suggest some advantage of GSH over pure self-help in the treatment of BED (Grilo & Masheb, 2005; Loeb, Wilson, Gilbert, & Labouvie, 2000). In a recent study, 10 sessions of CBT-GSH delivered by beginning clinical psychology graduate students with limited therapy experience proved to be as effective in reducing BED symptoms as 20 sessions of IPT conducted by intensively trained and supervised doctoral-level clinical psychologists (Wilson et al., 2010), providing further support that GSH may be a viable, appropriate intervention with advantages in dissemination and cost-effectiveness.

Interpersonal Psychotherapy

IPT for BED, formulated by Wilfley and colleagues (2002), was based upon interpersonal treatment for depression (Klerman et al., 1984) and BN (Fairburn, Jones, et al.,

1993). Although connections are made throughout therapy between interpersonal events and binge eating, the treatment does not overtly address disturbances in eating behavior. Instead, consistent with IPT for BN, patients' work focuses on making changes in specifically identified problematic areas of interpersonal functioning. In adapting IPT for BED, Wilfley and colleagues (Wilfley, MacKenzie, Welch, Ayres, & Weissman, 2000; Wilfley et al., 2002) developed a group format of the treatment. In group IPT, patients are encouraged to use the group to decrease isolation, enable the formation of new relationships, and practice new communication skills. The group format, by definition, provides a unique environment for individuals with BED, who may keep eating behaviors hidden from others due to feelings of guilt and shame (Tanofsky-Kraff & Wilfley, 2010).

At present, NICE (2004) guidelines for BED have designated a grade of B to IPT, possibly because of the paucity of controlled treatment trials investigating this approach relative to the number of studies using CBT. Rigorous investigations of IPT uniformly demonstrate the treatment's significant effect on diminishing the frequency of binge eating, with recovery rates comparable to CBT delivered in group format or as part of a GSH intervention (Wilfley et al., 2002; Wilson et al., 2010). The equivalent effects of these two treatments for BED contrast substantially with findings observed in patients with BN (Agras et al., 2000), and may underscore the utility of an IPT approach in patients known to suffer across domains of functioning (Grilo, 2006). For example, in the largest controlled outcome study to date, Wilson and colleagues (2010) noted IPT to be superior to BWL in patients with low self-esteem at 2-year follow-up, and superior to CBT-GSH in patients with low self-esteem and high eating disorder psychopathology. Also in contrast to the literature on IPT for BN, the time course of most outcome measures with IPT is similar to that of CBT (Wilfley et al., 2002). Taken together, these findings provide preliminary evidence that IPT may in the future be recommended as a first-line treatment for a subset of individuals with BED.

Additional Approaches

Few studies have considered novel approaches in the treatment of BED. One investigation of DBT, a well-validated intervention for affect regulation (Linehan, 1993), compared to a wait list, observed that the active treatment led to a greater reduction of binge-eating frequency and eating-disordered psychopathology compared to no treatment (Telch, Agras, & Linehan, 2001). However, no currently available data compare DBT to a unique reference treatment for BED.

One published study compared a virtual reality therapy to address body image attitudes and psychonutritional groups in inpatients with BED (Riva, Bacchetta, Baruffi, & Molinari, 2002). Both treatment groups achieved abstinence from binge eating (likely attributable to the structure of the inpatient program), with those participating in virtual reality therapy reporting improved body satisfaction, weight self-efficacy, and motivation for change relative to the control group. These preliminary findings, in conjunction with data supporting the importance of overvaluation of body shape and weight as an associated feature of BED, indicate the need for future studies that incorporate interventions for body image disturbance into broader BED treatment.

MEDICATION USE

Anorexia Nervosa

Currently there is no clearly established role for medication use in the treatment of acute AN. Given the prevalence of AN symptoms that are commonly responsive to medication in other clinical populations (e.g., depression, anxiety, and obsessionality), none of the classes of medication (e.g., antidepressants, anxiolytics, appetite-enhancing drugs) examined in patients with AN in small randomized clinical trials (Hay & Claudino, 2012), found clear benefit of medication versus placebo in effecting weight gain or improvements in general or eating disorder psychopathology. Investigators have theorized that the consistent lack of medication response may result from physiological changes that accompany malnutrition. Generally, weight restoration is emphasized, as psychological symptoms such as depression improve significantly with weight restoration alone (Meehan, Loeb, Roberto, & Attia, 2006). Recently, however, preliminary evidence indicates that olanzapine, an atypical antipsychotic medication, may help patients achieve normal weight in a shortened time and decrease obsessional symptoms relative to placebo (Bissada, Tasca, Barber, & Bradwejn, 2008). This finding is in need of replication and further study. However, medication studies in this population have proven challenging due to patients' high dropout rates and overall reluctance to comply with study medication regimens (Halmi et al., 2005).

Several studies have also considered the utility of medication for relapse prevention in weight-restored patients with AN. Findings are mixed, with initial reports that fluoxetine might be helpful (Kaye et al., 2001; Strober, Freeman, DeAntonio, Lampert, & Diamond, 1997). In contrast, a recent large, controlled study observed fluoxetine to be no more beneficial than placebo in preventing relapse during the first year after hospitalization among patients receiving CBT (Walsh et al., 2006). However, once patients with AN have achieved and maintained normal weight for some time, a medication evaluation may be warranted to assess for persistent co-occurring psychopathological symptoms.

Bulimia Nervosa

Medication treatment for BN should be considered when an individual prefers a medication approach, in the case of poor or partial response to CBT, or when CBT is unavailable. Generally, medication trials in BN have demonstrated that a variety of medications (e.g., antidepressants, including selective serotonin reuptake inhibitors, serotonin–norepinephrine reuptake inhibitors, tricyclics, and monoamine oxidase inhibitors) are superior to placebo in reducing binge–purge behavior (Bacaltchuk & Hay, 2003; Shapiro et al., 2007). Fluoxetine is commonly tried first, as it is the only medication with a specific indication for the treatment of AN by the U.S. Food and Drug Administration (Broft, Berner, & Walsh, 2010). There are two primary concerns about pharmacotherapy for BN: (1) Data suggest that patients may experience a relapse in symptoms after discontinuing medication, and (2) although medication may help to reduce binge eating, it does not appear to decrease extreme dietary restriction, a core behavioral symptom of the illness (Craighead & Agras, 1991). Given these clinical concerns, psychotherapists are advised to work collaboratively with prescribing physicians to monitor bulimic symptoms if patients are using medication as part of their eating disorder treatment.

Binge-Eating Disorder

Most, but not all, controlled medication studies for BED have observed a significant advantage for medication versus placebo in the short-term reduction of binge eating (Reas & Grilo, 2008). Investigations have largely evaluated the efficacy of different antidepressants, an anticonvulsant (topiramate), and weight loss medications including orlistat and sibutramine. Overall, there does not appear to be substantial difference in the efficacy of these different agents relative to placebo in treating BED psychothopathology (Grilo, 2006). Fluoxetine has also been noted to be associated with improvement in depressive symptoms in the short term (Devlin et al., 2005) and at follow-up (Devlin, Goldfein, Petkova, Liu, & Walsh, 2007) for individuals with BED. Not surprisingly, the use of obesity medication has been observed to result in more clinically meaningful weight loss concomitant with a reduction in binge frequency (Wilfley et al., 2008). A comprehensive meta-analysis of BED pharmacotherapy studies also determined that orlistat (a weight loss medication) and topiramate (an anticonvulsant) offer enhanced weight loss as adjunctive treatment to CBT and BWL (Reas & Grilo, 2008). Thus, medication might be recommended as part of a multidisciplinary treatment approach for individuals with BED, particularly for those who are significantly overweight or suffering from additional psychological problems.

TREATMENT MOTIVATION

The issue of motivation for treatment is embedded in the previous discussion of treatment approaches for AN, BN, and BED. As described, individuals with AN most frequently do not self-present for treatment, and the ego-syntonic nature of the disorder is perhaps its most dramatic and particularly challenging clinical feature (comparable to individuals with substance abuse disorders). Because investment in an excessively low weight is core to AN, treatment interventions must address motivational issues from the start. One of the particularly salient components of the Maudsley family therapy approach is to engage parents to assist with and lead in the recovery process, until their child is in a healthier state, such that the child is aligned with and able to assume responsibility for recovery from the eating disorder. In the case of BN and BED, goals regarding weight loss may compete with recovery from the eating disorder. In recent years a significant amount of work has been devoted to understanding the role of motivation in treatment and articulating approaches for enhancing motivation (Miller & Rollnick, 2002). Specific applications to treat eating disorders have been articulated by Vitousek and colleagues (1998). Issues of motivation can arise at multiple points in treatment, and the long-term success of treatment ultimately depends on the patient's sense of ownership about the goals of treatment and commitment to the goals of recovery. Clinicians' creativity (e.g., finding meaningful metaphors as patients grapple with ambivalence) and flexibility (e.g., developing and operationalizing mutually agreed upon intermediate goals while working toward long-term goals) may contribute to enhanced therapeutic alliance and motivation for change with individuals with eating disorders.

THE PROCESS OF CHANGE
IN EVIDENCE-SUPPORTED TREATMENTS

There is increasing interest in the field of psychotherapy research in exploring treatment mechanisms and identifying factors that may contribute to behavioral change in the context of successful treatment. While Castonguay and Beutler (2005) have outlined participant factors, technique factors, and clinical relationship factors that should be considered in examining principles of therapeutic change associated with evidence supported treatments, very little has been written about such principles of change associated with treatments for eating disorders. Treatment elements relevant to CBT that may represent principles for change include the challenge of cognitive distortions regarding ideas about body shape and weight, as well as the reinforcement of structured eating and other healthy eating behaviors. Elements relevant to IPT and possibly reflective of principles of change associated with this treatment approach include encouragement of normal socialization, cessation of social isolation, development of communication skills to improve relationships and decrease eating in response to negative affect, and selection of environmental factors that are conducive to healthy choices regarding eating behavior. Elements relevant to the evidence-supported family-based treatment for AN include structured eating and changing the environment to make eating and weight gain more likely. Further study of these and other treatment factors would provide useful information about the mechanism of symptom improvement associated with some of the more effective available treatments.

Several investigators have examined variables that may predict treatment outcome or serve as mediators for change in treatment studies. Across studies of different treatments, early treatment response appears to predict both shorter and longer-term outcomes. Specifically, improvement in binge eating and purging during the first 4 weeks of CBT or IPT treatment (Agras et al., 2000), as well as during the first few weeks of antidepressant treatment (Sysko, Sha, Wang, Duan, & Walsh, 2010; Sysko & Walsh, 2006), predicts symptom remission at the end of treatment for individuals with BN. While it is unclear whether there is something inherently different (and more likely to remit) about the individuals who respond quickly to treatment, these findings suggest that treatment should emphasize behavioral change and that individuals who do not experience symptom resolution early in a treatment course may need a change in the intervention to achieve the targeted symptom resolution. Relatedly, in an analysis of variables thought possibly to mediate treatment response, Wilson et al. (2002) found that improvement in dietary restraint mediated improvement in binge-eating behavior in individuals with BN receiving either CBT or IPT in a randomized trial. This finding was surprising, as normalization of eating behaviors was a direct treatment focus in CBT and not IPT, yet normalization of restraint appeared to be a mediator of both therapeutic approaches, questioning whether the mechanisms of therapeutic effect for these two seemingly different treatments are really so different (Wilson et al., 2002). Additionally, among weight-restored individuals with AN, consumption of a diet higher in variety and caloric density predict likelihood of maintaining normal weight during the year following acute weight restoration. Taken together, these findings on predictors and mediators of outcome suggest, though somewhat indirectly, that normalizing eating behavior is central to better outcomes in eating disorder treatments.

TREATMENT INTENSITY

Available services for treating patients with eating disorders range from varying levels of outpatient care (e.g., weekly or biweekly psychotherapy, nutritional counseling, psychiatric care) to intensive outpatient programs (i.e., day treatment), residential programs, and inpatient programs. Because specialized programs are not available in all geographic regions, it can be difficult to access appropriate care for an individual with an eating disorder. Nonetheless, we present guidelines below for how clinicians might choose the most appropriate level of care based on patients' clinical status. When available, relevant data regarding treatment intensity are included.

Anorexia Nervosa

While the specific mechanism responsible for psychological changes in individuals with AN remains uncertain, the improved nutritional state that accompanies refeeding is presumed to enable better cognitive functioning and emotional regulation (Attia & Walsh, 2009). Therefore, weight restoration is an essential primary treatment goal. However, because patients with acute AN have considerable difficulty gaining weight outside of a highly structured treatment, many of those who seek treatment for the illness are ultimately guided to an inpatient program (Guarda, 2008).

Admission to an inpatient unit is recommended for adult patients who have lost a substantial amount of weight, particularly if the weight loss has been rapid, and for those whose weight is extremely low for their height (e.g., less than 75% ideal body weight) (Attia & Walsh, 2009). Inpatient treatment may also be appropriate for youth with AN who do not gain the expected amount of weight for their height and age (Attia & Walsh, 2009). Although some treatment providers may be reluctant to recommend inpatient treatment, data suggest that outcome is better if inpatient treatment is pursued *before* the onset of medical instability secondary to low weight (Yager, 2007).

The limited availability of specialized inpatient units that treat eating disorders, together with the significant expense of hospital-based treatments and challenges of third-party reimbursement, often make it difficult for patients to find appropriate hospital programs or to stay in hospital programs for as long as may be recommended to achieve weight restoration. The changes in U.S. health care economics of the last 20 years have dramatically shortened hospital stays, and the limited weight gain achieved by patients with AN on inpatient units raises the question of whether shorter stays and lower discharge weights may contribute to higher relapse rates (Wiseman et al., 2001).

As hospital programs have become less available, structured behavioral day treatment programs that have been developed have demonstrated efficacy in helping patients to normalize weight, albeit it at a more modest pace. One uncontrolled comparison of specialized inpatient versus day treatment behavioral programs observed an average weight gain in patients of approximately 4 pounds per week and 2 pounds per week, respectively (Guarda & Heinberg, 2004). Overall, outcomes from specialized day treatment programs are strongly associated with treatment intensity. More successful programs require patients to participate in structured treatment at least 5 days per week, 8 hours per day (Olmsted, Kaplan, & Rockert, 2003). While intensive, structured programming helps in the short-term management of AN, the long-term benefit of such interventions remains unknown (Attia & Walsh, 2009).

Outpatient treatment for acute AN may be considered for adolescents whose families are committed to intensive, structured family-based therapy aimed at weight restoration (Lock et al., 2001). Otherwise, outpatient intervention is typically indicated for the prevention of relapse following weight restoration in a structured setting or for patients with symptoms of AN that are at borderline diagnostic threshold (e.g., individuals at approximately 85% ideal body weight with associated features of AN). Weekly psychotherapy is an opportunity for patients to normalize their attitudes about weight, body shape, and eating behavior. Outpatient appointments also provide an opportunity for clinicians to monitor the weight status of patients with AN. If patients are unable to achieve or sustain a healthy weight range, clinicians should recommend an increase in session frequency to twice per week, adjunctive nutritional counseling sessions, or a return to a structured behavioral program.

Bulimia Nervosa

Many patients with uncomplicated BN do not require inpatient hospitalization. Depending on the frequency of binge–purge behaviors and severity of associated bulimic symptoms (e.g., extreme dietary restriction outside of binges, cognitive distortions regarding shape and weight), clinicians should consider biweekly psychotherapy appointments. In a standard course of CBT for BN, for example, it is recommended to start with 2 scheduled sessions per week for the first 4 weeks of treatment to help patients implement self-monitoring techniques, adopt a regular eating pattern, and break the binge–purge cycle (Fairburn, Marcus, et al., 1993). In initial biweekly IPT sessions, the clinician completes a very detailed analysis of the interpersonal context in which the eating disorder has been developed and maintained with the patient (Agras et al., 2000). After the early phase of treatment, as an individual's symptoms are remitting, psychotherapy sessions may occur on a weekly, then bimonthly basis.

If a patient with BN does not respond to an adequate trial of outpatient psychotherapy, a higher level of care should be considered. Additional indications for more structured treatment include severely impairing symptoms that have not responded to adequate trials of psychotropic medication, serious concurrent medical problems (e.g., persistent electrolyte abnormalities) or psychiatric conditions requiring an inpatient treatment independent of the eating disorder, suicidality, and severe co-occurring alcohol or drug abuse or dependence (Yager, 2007).

Though inpatient treatment has long been recognized as *the* viable alternative to outpatient care for treatment-resistant BN, recently there has been an emphasis on day treatment as an alternative along the continuum of care. Day treatment programs offer individuals with BN a cost-effective alternative to receive care in a more structured setting, while maintaining contact with their natural environment (Zipfel et al., 2002). To date, one randomized controlled trial of inpatient versus day treatment for patients with severe, chronic BN has been conducted (Zeeck et al., 2009a). Inpatient and day treatment were observed to be equally effective in reducing specific BN symptoms and general psychopathology at discharge and 3-month follow-up (Zeeck et al., 2009a). By 12-month follow-up, day treatment demonstrated an advantage in sustained improvement in binge frequency and bulimic cognitions, but no differences were noted in purging behavior or general psychopathology (Zeeck et al., 2009b). While further research in this area is needed, this study offers preliminary evidence that day treatment may provide patients with both the skills needed for alleviation of symptoms and the opportunity immediately to apply and possibly generalize these skills in their home environment.

Binge-Eating Disorder

Individuals with BED who seek treatment typically express several treatment goals, including the cessation of binge eating, the development of healthy eating patterns, and (frequently) weight loss (Devlin, Allison, Goldfein, & Spanos, 2007). While there is growing evidence that those with a BED diagnosis show greater amelioration of binge eating and associated psychopathology with specialty eating disorder treatment rather than nonspecific weight loss interventions (Wonderlich et al., 2009), there are no data regarding the relative utility of more intensive versus less intensive treatment for this group.

CONCLUSION

Although the knowledge base regarding prevalence and treatment for eating disorders is continually evolving, sufficient research exists to guide treatment at many points of care for individuals with AN, BN, and BED. Of course, many questions remain, and clinicians in practice must often rely on professional experience and practice when data fail to inform treatment decisions. One of the challenges for the field is harnessing this clinical experience in a way that furthers an empirically informed approach to care. The complementary challenge is dissemination of research findings so that clinicians in practice remain up to date and fully informed on treatment recommendations derived from the empirical research. Relatedly, expanding training opportunities in evidence-based treatments will greatly enhance our capacity to assist individuals with eating disorders most effectively in their journey to recovery.

REFERENCES

Agras, W. S., Walsh, T., Fairburn, C. G., Wilson, G. T., & Kraemer, H. C. (2000). A multicenter comparison of cognitive-behavioral therapy and interpersonal psychotherapy for bulimia nervosa. *Archives of General Psychiatry, 57*(5), 459–466.

American Psychiatric Association. (1994). *Diagnostic and statistical manual of mental disorders* (4th ed.). Washington, DC: Author.

American Psychiatric Association. (2013). *Diagnostic and statistical manual of mental disorders* (5th ed.). Arlington, VA: Author.

Andersson, G. (2009). Using the Internet to provide cognitive behaviour therapy. *Behaviour Research and Therapy, 47*(3), 175–180.

Attia, E. (2010). Anorexia nervosa: Current status and future directions. *Annual Review of Medicine, 61*, 425–435.

Attia, E., & Roberto, C. A. (2009). Should amenorrhea be a diagnostic criterion for anorexia nervosa? *International Journal of Eating Disorders, 42*(7), 581–589.

Attia, E., & Walsh, B. T. (2009). Behavioral management for anorexia nervosa. *New England Journal of Medicine, 360*(5), 500–506.

Bacaltchuk, J., & Hay, P. (2003). Antidepressants versus placebo for people with bulimia nervosa. *Cochrane Database of Systematic Reviews*(4), CD003391.

Ball, J., & Mitchell, P. (2004). A randomized controlled study of cognitive behavior therapy and behavioral family therapy for anorexia nervosa patients. *Eating Disorders, 12*(4), 303–314.

Beck, A. T. (1976). *Cognitive therapy and the emotional disorders.* New York: International Universities Press.

Becker, A.E. (2007). Culture and eating disorders classification. *International Journal of Eating Disorders, 40*(Suppl.), S111–S116.

Becker, A. E., Thomas, J. J., & Pike, K. M. (2009). Should non-fat phobic anorexia nervosa be included in DSM-V? *International Journal of Eating Disorders, 42,* 620–635.

Binford, R. B., & Le Grange, D. (2005). Adolescents with bulimia nervosa and eating disorder not otherwise specified–purging only. *International Journal of Eating Disorders, 38,* 157–161.

Bissada, H., Tasca, G. A., Barber, A. M., & Bradwejn, J. (2008). Olanzapine in the treatment of low body weight and obsessive thinking in women with anorexia nervosa: A randomized, double-blind, placebo-controlled trial. *American Journal of Psychiatry, 165*(10), 1281–1288.

Broft, A., Berner, L. A., & Walsh, B. T. (2010). Pharmacotherapy for bulimia nervosa. In C. M. Grilo & J. E. Mitchell (Eds.), *The treatment of eating disorders: A clinical handbook* (pp. 388–401). New York: Guilford Press.

Brownell, K. D. (2010). The humbling experience of treating obesity: Should we persist or desist? *Behaviour Research Therapy, 48*(8), 717–719.

Bulik, C. M., Berkman, N. D., Brownley, K. A., Sedway, J. A., & Lohr, K. N. (2007). Anorexia nervosa treatment: A systematic review of randomized controlled trials. *International Journal of Eating Disorders, 40*(4), 310–320.

Bulik, C. M., Klump, K. L., Thornton, L., Kaplan, A. S., Devlin, B., Fichter, M. M., et al. (2004). Alcohol use disorder comorbidity in eating disorders: A multi-center study. *Journal of Clinical Psychiatry, 65,* 1000–1006.

Carter, J. C., McFarlane, T. L., Bewell, C., Olmsted, M. P., Woodside, D. B., Kaplan, A. S., et al. (2009). Maintenance treatment for anorexia nervosa: A comparison of cognitive behavior therapy and treatment as usual. *International Journal of Eating Disorders, 42*(3), 202–207.

Cassin, S. E., & von Ranson, K. M. (2005). Personality and eating disorders: A decade in review. *Clinical Psychology Review, 25,* 895–916.

Castonguay, L. G., & Beutler, L. E. (2005). *Principles of therapeutic change that work.* New York: Oxford University Press.

Channon, S., DeSilva, W. P., Hemsley, D., & Perkins, R. (1989). A controlled trial of cognitive-behavioral and behavioral treatment of anorexia nervosa. *Behavioral Research and Therapy, 27,* 529-535.

Chen, E., Touyz, S. W., Beumont, P. J., Fairburn, C. G., Griffiths, R., Butow, P., et al. (2003). Comparison of group and individual cognitive-behavioral therapy for patients with bulimia nervosa. *International Journal of Eating Disorders, 33*(3), 241–254; discussion 255–256.

Commission on Adolescent Eating Disorders. (2005). Prevention of eating disorders. In D. L. Evans, E. B. Foa, R. E. Gur, H. Hendin, C. P. O'Brien, M. E. P. Seligman, et al. (Eds.), *Treating and preventing adolescent mental health disorders: What we know and what we don't know* (pp. 304–323). New York: Oxford University Press.

Cooper, P. J., & Fairburn, C. G. (1984). Cognitive behaviour therapy for anorexia nervosa: Some preliminary findings. *Journal of Psychosomatic Research, 28*(6), 493–499.

Craighead, L. W., & Agras, W. S. (1991). Mechanisms of action in cognitive-behavioral and pharmacological interventions for obesity and bulimia nervosa. *Journal of Consulting and Clinical Psychology, 59*(1), 115-125.

Craske, M. G., & Barlow, D. H. (2001). Panic disorder and agoraphobia. In D. H. Barlow (Ed.), *Clinical handbook of psychological disorders* (3rd ed., pp. 1–59). New York: Guilford Press.

Crow, S. J., & Brandenburg, B. (2010). Diagnosis, assessment, and treatment planning in bulimia nervosa. In C. M. Grilo & J. E. Mitchell (Eds.), *The treatment of eating disorders: A clinical handbook* (pp. 28–43). New York: Guilford Press.

Crow, S. J., Peterson, C. B., Swanson, S. A., Raymond, N. C., Specker, S., Eckert, E. D., et al. (2009). Increased mortality in bulimia nervosa and other eating disorders. *American Journal of Psychiatry, 166*(12), 1342–1346.

Cummins, L. H., Simmons, A. M., & Zane, N. W. (2005). Eating disorders in Asian populations: A critique of current approaches to the study of culture, ethnicity, and eating disorders. *American Journal of Orthopsychiatry, 75*(4), 553–574.

Devlin, M. J., Allison, K. C., Goldfein, J. A., & Spanos, A. (2007). Management of eating disorders not otherwise specified. In J. Yager & P. S. Powers (Eds.), *Clinical manual of eating disorders* (pp. 195–224). Washington, DC: American Psychiatric Association.

Devlin, M. J., Goldfein, J. A., Petkova, E., Jiang, H., Raizman, P. S., Wolk, S., et al. (2005). Cognitive behavioral therapy and fluoxetine as adjuncts to group behavioral therapy for binge eating disorder. *Obesity Research, 13*(6), 1077–1088.

Devlin, M. J., Goldfein, J. A., Petkova, E., Liu, L., & Walsh, B. T. (2007). Cognitive behavioral therapy and fluoxetine for binge eating disorder: Two-year follow-up. *Obesity (Silver Spring), 15*(7), 1702–1709.

de Zwaan, M. (2001). Binge eating disorder and obesity. *International Journal of Obesity and Related Metabolic Disorders, 25*(Suppl. 1), S51–S55.

Dingemans, A.E., Bruna, M. J., & van Furth, E. F. (2002). Binge eating disorder: A review. *International Journal of Obesity, 26,* 299–307.

Duncan, A. E., Neuman, R. J., Kramer, J., Kuperman, S., Hesselbroock, V., Reich, T., et al. (2005). Are there subgroups of bulimia nervosa based on comorbid psychiatric disorders? *International Journal of Eating Disorders, 37,* 19–25.

Eddy, K. T., Hennessey, M., & Thompson-Brenner, H. (2007). Eating pathology in East African women: The role of media exposure and globalization. *Journal of Nervous and Mental Disease, 195*(3), 196–202.

Eisler, I., Dare, C., Hodes, M., Russell, G., Dodge, E., & Le Grange, D. (2000). Family therapy for adolescent anorexia nervosa: The results of a controlled comparison of two family interventions. *Journal of Child Psychology and Psychiatry, 41*(6), 727–736.

Eisler, I., Dare, C., Russell, G. F., Szmukler, G., Le Grange, D., & Dodge, E. (1997). Family and individual therapy in anorexia nervosa. A 5-year follow-up. *Archives of General Psychiatry, 54*(11), 1025–1030.

Eisler, I., Simic, M., Russell, G. F., & Dare, C. (2007). A randomised controlled treatment trial of two forms of family therapy in adolescent anorexia nervosa: A five-year follow-up. *Journal of Child Psychology and Psychiatry, 48*(6), 552–560.

Eldredge, K. L., & Agras, W. S. (1996). Weight and shape overconcern and emotional eating in binge eating disorder. *International Journal of Eating Disorders, 19*(1), 73–82.

Eldredge, K. L., Agras, W. S., Arnow, B., Telch, C. F., Bell, S., Castonguay, L., et al. (1997). The effects of extending cognitive-behavioral therapy for binge eating disorder among initial treatment nonresponders. *International Journal of Eating Disorders, 21*(4), 347–352.

Fairburn, C. G. (1995). *Overcoming binge eating.* New York: Guilford Press.

Fairburn, C. G. (2008). *Cognitive behavior therapy and eating disorders.* New York: Guilford Press.

Fairburn, C. G., Cooper, Z., Doll, H. A., O'Connor, M. E., Bohn, K., Hawker, D. M., et al. (2009). Transdiagnostic cognitive-behavioral therapy for patients with eating disorders: A two-site trial with 60-week follow-up. *American Journal of Psychiatry, 166*(3), 311–319.

Fairburn, C. G., Cooper, Z., Doll, H. A., & Welch, S. L. (1999). Risk factors for anorexia nervosa: Three integrated case-control comparisons. *Archives of General Psychiatry, 56*(5), 468–476.

Fairburn, C. G., Doll, H. A., Welch, S., Hay, P. J., Davies, B. A., & O'Connor M. E. (1998). Risk factors for binge eating disorder: A community-based, case-control study. *Archives of General Psychiatry, 55*(5), 425–432.

Fairburn, C. G., Jones, R., Peveler, R. C., Carr, S. J., Solomon, R. A., O'Connor, M. E., et al. (1991). Three psychological treatments for bulimia nervosa: A comparative trial. *Archives of General Psychiatry, 48*(5), 463–469.

Fairburn, C. G., Jones, R., Peveler, R. C., Hope, R. A., & O'Connor, M. (1993). Psychotherapy and bulimia nervosa: Longer-term effects of interpersonal psychotherapy, behavior therapy, and cognitive behavior therapy. *Archives of General Psychiatry, 50*(6), 419–428.

Fairburn, C. G., Marcus, M. D., & Wilson, G. T. (1993). Cognitive-behavioral therapy for binge eating and bulimia nervosa: A comprehensive treatment manual. In C. G. Fairburn & G. T. Wilson (Eds.), *Binge eating: Nature, assessment, and treatment* (pp. 361–404). New York: Guilford Press.

Fernandez-Aranda, F., Nunez, A., Martinez, C., Krug, I., Cappozzo, M., Carrard, I., et al. (2009). Internet-based cognitive-behavioral therapy for bulimia nervosa: A controlled study. *Cyber Psychology, Behavior, and Social Networking, 12*(1), 37–41.

Foa, E. B., & Franklin, M. E. (2001). Obsessive–compulsive disorder. In D. H. Barlow (Ed.), *Clinical handbook of psychological disorders* (3rd ed., pp. 209–263). New York: Guilford Press.

Fichter, M. M., & Quadflieg, N. (2004). Twelve year course and outcome of anorexia nervosa. *Psychological Medicine, 34*, 1395–1406.

Fischer, S., Smith, G. T., & Cyders, M. A. (2008). Another look at impulsivity: A meta-analytic review comparing specific dispositions to rash action in their relationship to bulimic symptoms. *Clinical Psychology Review, 28*, 1413–1425.

Forcano, L., Fernandez-Aranda, F., Alvarez-Moya, E., Bulik, C., Granero, R., Gratacos, M., et al (2009). Suicide attempts in bulimia nervosa: Personality and psychopathological correlates, *European Psychiatry, 24*(2), 91–97.

Franko, D. L., Becker, A. E., Thomas, J. J., & Herzog, D. B. (2007). Cross-ethnic differences in eating disorder symptoms and related distress. *International Journal of Eating Disorders, 40*, 156–164.

Garner, D. G., Vitousek, K. M., & Pike, K. M. (1997). Cognitive-behavioral therapy for anorexia nervosa. In D. M. Garner & P.E. Garfinkel (Eds.), *Handbook of treatment for eating disorders* (pp. 94–144). New York: Guilford Press.

Goldschmidt, A. B., Hilbert, A., Manwaring, J. L., Wilfley, D. E., Pike, K. M., Fairburn, C. G., et al. (2010). The significance of overvaluation of shape and weight in binge eating disorder. *Behaviour Research and Therapy, 48*(3), 187–193.

Grilo, C. M. (2002). Binge eating disorder (2002). In C. G. Fairburn & K. D. Brownell (Eds.), Eating disorders and obesity (pp. 178–182). New York: Guilford Press.

Grilo, C. M. (2006). *Eating and weight disorders.* Hove, UK: Psychology Press.

Grilo, C. M., Hrabosky, J. I., White, M. A., Allison, K. C., Stunkard, A. J., & Masheb, R. M. (2008). Overvaluation of shape and weight in binge eating disorder and overweight controls: Refinement of a diagnostic construct. *Journal of Abnormal Psychology, 117*(2), 414–419.

Grilo, C. M., & Masheb, R. M. (2005). A randomized controlled comparison of guided self-help cognitive behavioral therapy and behavioral weight loss for binge eating disorder. *Behavioural Research and Therapy, 43*(11), 1509–1525.

Grilo, C. M., Masheb, R. M., & White, M. A. (2010). Significance of overvaluation of shape/weight in binge-eating disorder: Comparative study with overweight and bulimia nervosa. *Obesity (Silver Spring), 18*(3), 499–504.

Grilo, C. M., Masheb, R. M., & Wilson, G. T. (2005). Efficacy of cognitive behavioral therapy and fluoxetine for the treatment of binge eating disorder: A randomized double-blind placebo-controlled comparison. *Biological Psychiatry, 57*(3), 301–309.

Guarda, A. S. (2008). Treatment of anorexia nervosa: Insights and obstacles. *Physiology and Behavior, 94*(1), 113–120.

Guarda, A. S., & Heinberg, L. J. (2004). Inpatient and partial hospital approaches to the treatment of eating disorders. In J. K. Thompson (Ed.), *Handbook of eating disorders and obesity* (pp. 297–322). Hoboken, NJ: Wiley.

Halmi, K. A., Agras, W. S., Crow, S., Mitchell, J., Wilson, G. T., Bryson, S. W., et al. (2005). Predictors of treatment acceptance and completion in anorexia nervosa: Implications for future study designs. *Archives of General Psychiatry, 62*(7), 776–781.

Hartmann, A., Zeeck, A., & Barrett, M. S. (2010). Interpersonal problems in eating disorders. *International Journal of Eating Disorders, 43,* 619–627.

Hay, P. J., & Claudino, A. M. (2012). Clinical psychopharmacology of eating disorders: a research update. *International Journal of Neuropsychopharmacology, 15*(2), 209–222.

Herzog, D. B., & Eddy, K. T. (2007). Comorbidity in eating disorders. In S. Wonderlich, J. Mitchell, M. de Zwaan, & H. Steiger (Eds.), *Eating disorders review—Part 1* (pp. 35–50). New York: Radcliffe.

Hjern, A., Lindberg, L., & Lindblad, F. (2006). Outcome and prognostic factors for adolescent female in-patients with anorexia nervosa: 9–14 year follow-up. *British Journal of Psychiatry, 189,* 428-432.

Hoek, H. W. (2006). Incidence, prevalence and mortality of anorexia nervosa and other eating disorders. *Current Opinion in Psychiatry, 19*(4), 389–394.

Hoek, H. W., & van Hoeken, D. (2003). Review of the prevalence and incidence of eating disorders. *International Journal of Eating Disorders, 34*(4), 383–396.

Holm-Denoma, J. M., Witte, T. K., Gordon, K. H., Herzog, D.B., Franko, D. L., Fichter, M., et al. (2008). Deaths by suicide among individuals with anorexia nervosa as arbiters between competing explanations of the anorexia–suicide link. *Journal of Affective Disorders, 107,* 231-236.

Hrabosky, J. I., Masheb, R. M., White, M. A., & Grilo, C. M. (2007). Overvaluation of shape and weight in binge eating disorder. *Journal of Consulting and Clinical Psychology, 75*(1), 175–180.

Hudson, J. I., Hiripi, E., Pope, H. G., Jr., & Kessler, R. C. (2007). The prevalence and correlates of eating disorders in the National Comorbidity Survey Replication. *Biological Psychiatry, 61*(3), 348–358.

Jacobi, C., Hayward, C., de Zwaan, M., Kraemer, H.C., & Agras, W.S. (2004). Coming to terms with risk factors for eating disroders: Application for risk terminology and suggestions for a general taxonomy. *Psychological Bulletin, 130*(1), 19–65.

Javaras, K. N., Pope, H. G., Lalonde, J. K., Roberts, J. L., Nillni, Y. I., Laird, N. M., et al. (2008). Co-occurrence of binge eating disorder with psychiatric and medical disorders. *Journal of Clinical Psychiatry, 69*(2), 266–273.

Johnson, J. G., Cohen, P., Kasen, S., & Brook, J. S. (2006). Personality disorder traits evident by early adulthood and risk for eating and weight problems during middle adulthood. *International Journal of Eating Disorders, 39,* 184–192.

Johnson, J. G., Spitzer, R. L., & Williams, J. B. (2001). Health problems, impairment and illnesses associated with bulimia nervosa and binge eating disorder among primary care and obstetric gynaecology patients. *Psychologica Medicine, 31*(8), 1455–1466.

Jonas, S., Bebbington, P., McManus, S., Meltzer, H., Jenkins, R., Kuipers, E., et al. (2011). Sexual abuse and psychiatric disorder in England: Results from the 2007 Adult Psychiatric Morbidity Survey. *Psychological Medicine, 41*(4), 709–719.

Kalarchian, M. A., Marcus, M. D., Levine, M. D., Courcoulas, A. P., Pilkonis, P. A., Ringham, R. M., et al. (2007). Psychiatric disorders among bariatric surgery candidates: Relationship to obesity and functional health status. *American Journal of Psychiatry, 164*(2), 328-334; quiz 374.

Karwautz, A., Rabe-Hesketh, S., Hu, X., Ahao, J., Sham, P., Collier, D. A., et al. (2001). Individual specific risk factors for anorexia nervosa: A pilot study using discordant sister-pair design. *Psychogical Medicine, 31*(2), 317–329.

Katzman, M. A., & Lee, S. (1997). Beyond body image: The integration of feminist and transcultural theories in the understanding of self starvation. *International Journal of Eating Disorders, 22*(4), 385–394.

Kaye, W. H., Bulik, C. M., Thornton, L., Barbarich, N. C., & Masters, K. (2004). Comorbidity of anxiety disorders with anorexia nervosa and bulimia nervosa. *American Journal of Psychiatry, 161*, 2215–2221.

Kaye, W. H., Nagata, T., Weltzin, T. E., Hsu, L. K., Sokol, M. S., McConaha, C., et al. (2001). Double-blind placebo-controlled administration of fluoxetine in restricting- and restricting-purging-type anorexia nervosa. *Biological Psychiatry, 49*(7), 644–652.

Keel, P. K., & Brown, T. A. (2010). Update on course and outcome in eating disorders. *International Journal of Eating Disorders, 43*(3), 195–204.

Keel, P. K., & Klump, K. L. (2003). Are eating disorders culture-bound syndromes?: Implications for conceptualizing their etiology. *Psychological Bulletin, 129*(5), 747–769.

Keys, A., Brozek, J., Henschel, A., Mickelsen, O., & Taylor, H. L. (1950). *The biology of human starvation*. Minneapolis: University of Minnesota Press.

Klerman, G. L., Weissman, M. M., Rounsaville, B. J., & Chevron, E. S. (1984). *Interpersonal psychotherapy of depression*. New York: Basic Books.

Krysanski, V. L., & Ferraro, F. R. (2008). Review of controlled psychotherapy treatment trials for binge eating disorder. *Psychological Reports, 102*, 339–368.

Le Grange, D., Crosby, R. D., Rathouz, P. J., & Leventhal, B. L. (2007). A randomized controlled comparison of family-based treatment and supportive psychotherapy for adolescent bulimia nervosa. *Archives of General Psychiatry, 64*(9), 1049–1056.

Le Grange, D., Luow, J., Breen, A., & Katzman, M. A. (2004). The meaning of "self-starvation" in impoverished Black adolescents in South Africa. *Cultural Medicine, and Psychiatry, 28*, 439–461.

Lee, S. (1994). The diagnostic interview schedule and anorexia nervosa in Hong Kong. *Archives of General Psychiatry 51*, 251–252.

Lee, S., Ho, T. P., & Hsu, L. K. G. (1993). Fat phobic and non-fat phobic anorexia nervosa: A comparative study of 70 Chinese patients in Hong Kong. *Psychological Medicine, 23*, 999–1017.

Linehan, M. M. (1993). *Skills training manual for treating borderline personality disorder*. New York: Guilford Press.

Lock, J., Agras, W. S., Bryson, S., & Kraemer, H. C. (2005). A comparison of short- and long-term family therapy for adolescent anorexia nervosa. *Journal of the American Academy of Child and Adolescent Psychiatry, 44*(7), 632–639.

Lock, J., Le Grange, D., Agras, W. S., & Dare, C. (2001). *Treatment manual for anorexia nervosa: A family-based approach*. New York: Guilford Press.

Loeb, K. L., Wilson, G. T., Gilbert, J. S., & Labouvie, E. (2000). Guided and unguided self-help for binge eating. *Behaviour Research and Therapy, 38*(3), 259–272.

Marques, L., Alegria, M., Becker, A. E., Chen, C., Fang, A., Chosak, A., et al. (2011). Comparative prevalence, correlates of impairment, and service utilization for eating disorders across US ethnic groups: Implications for reducing ethnic disparities in health care access for eating disorders. *International Journal of Eating Disorders, 44*(5), 412–420.

Masheb, R. M., & Grilo, C. M. (2000). Binge eating disorder: A need for additional diagnostic criteria. *Comprehensive Psychiatry, 41*(3), 159–162.

Masheb, R. M., & Grilo, C. M. (2006). Eating patterns and breakfast consumption in obese patients with binge eating disorder. *Behavioural Research and Therapy, 44*(11), 1545–1553.

Mazzeo, S. E., Slof-Op't, Landt, M.C.T., van Furth, E. F., & Bulik, C. M. (2006). Genetics of eating disorders. In S. Wonderlich, J. E. Mitchell, M. deZwaan, & H. Steiger (Eds.), *Annual review of eating disorders* (pp. 17–34). Oxford, UK: Radcliffe.

McIntosh, V. V., Jordan, J., Carter, F. A., Luty, S. E., McKenzie, J. M., Bulik, C. M., et al. (2005). Three psychotherapies for anorexia nervosa: A randomized, controlled trial. *American Journal of Psychiatry, 162*(4), 741–747.

Meehan, K. G., Loeb, K. L., Roberto, C. A., & Attia, E. (2006). Mood change during weight restoration in patients with anorexia nervosa. *International Journal of Eating Disorders, 39*(7), 587–589.

Mehler, J. E., Birmingham, C. L., Crow, S. J., & Jahraus, J. P. (2010). Medical complications of eating disorders. In C. M. Grilo & J. E. Mitchell (Eds.), *The treatment of eating disorders: A clinical handbook* (pp. 66–80). New York: Guilford Press.

Miller, W. R., & Rollnick, S. (2002). *Motivational interviewing: Preparing people for change* (2nd ed.). New York: Guilford Press.

Mitchell, J. E., Crosby, R. D., Wonderlich, S. A., Crow, S., Lancaster, K., Simonich, H., et al. (2008). A randomized trial comparing the efficacy of cognitive-behavioral therapy for bulimia nervosa delivered via telemedicine versus face-to-face. *Behavioural Research and Therapy, 46*(5), 581–592.

Nathan, P. E., & Gorman, J. M. (Eds.). (2002). *A guide to treatments that work* (2nd ed.). New York: Oxford University Press.

National Institute for Clinical Excellence. (2004). Eating disorders—Core interventions in the treatment and management of anorexia nervosa, bulimia nervosa and related eating disorders. *NICE Clinical Guideline No. 9.* Available online at *www.nice.org.uk/nicemedia/pdf/cg009niceguidance.pdf.*

Nobakht, M., & Dezhkam, M. (2000). An epidemiological study of eating disorders in Iran. *International Journal of Eating Disorders, 28*(3), 265–271.

Ogden, J., & Mundray, K. (1998). The effect of the media on body satisfaction: The role of gender and size. *European Eating Disorders Review, 4,* 171–182.

Olmsted, M. P., Kaplan, A. S., & Rockert, W. (2003). Relative efficacy of a 4-day versus a 5-day day hospital program. *International Journal of Eating Disorders, 34*(4), 441–449.

Papadopoulos, F. C., Ekbom, A., Brandt, L., & Ekselius, L. (2009). Excess mortality, causes of death and prognostic factors in anorexia nervosa. *British Journal of Psychiatry, 194*(1), 10–17.

Paulson-Karlsson, G., Engstrom, I., & Nevonen, L. (2009). A pilot study of a family-based treatment for adolescent anorexia nervosa: 18- and 36-month follow-ups. *Eating Disorders, 17*(1), 72–88.

Peterson, C. B., Mitchell, J. E., Engbloom, S., Nugent, S., Pederson Mussell, M., Crow, S. J., et al. (2001). Self-help versus therapist-led group cognitive-behavioral treatment of binge eating disorder at follow-up. *International Journal of Eating Disorders, 30*(4), 363–374.

Pike, K. M., Carter, J. C., & Olmsted, M. P. (2010). Cognitive-behavioral therapy for anorexia nervosa. In C. M. Grilo & J. E. Mitchell (Eds.), *The treatment of eating disorders: A clinical handbook* (pp. 83–107). New York: Guilford Press.

Pike, K. M., Hilbert, A., Wilfley, D. E., Fairburn, C. G., Dohm, F. A., Walsh, B. T., et al. (2008). Toward an understanding of risk factors for anorexia nervosa: A case control study. *Psychological Medicine, 38*(10), 1443–1453.

Pike, K. M., & Mizushima, H. (2005). The clinical presentation of Japanese women with anorexia nervosa and bulimia nervosa: A study of the Eating Disorders Inventory–2. *International Journal of Eating Disorders, 37*(1), 26–31.

Pike, K. M., Walsh, B. T., Vitousek, K., Wilson, G. T., & Bauer, J. (2003). Cognitive behavior therapy in the posthospitalization treatment of anorexia nervosa. *American Journal of Psychiatry, 160*(11), 2046–2049.

Pike, K. M., Wilfley, D., Hilbert, A., Fairburn, C. G., Dohm, F. A., Striegel-Moore, R. H. (2006). Antecedent life events of binge eating disorder. *Psychiatric Research, 142,* 19–29.

Pope, H. G., & Hudson, J. I. (1992). Is childhood sexual abuse a risk factor for bulimia nervosa? *American Journal of Psychiatry, 149*(4), 455–463.

Raboch, J., & Faltus, F. (1991). Sexuality of women with anorexia nervosa. *Acta Psychiatrica Scandinavica, 84,* 9–11.

Reas, D. L., & Grilo, C. M. (2008). Review and meta-analysis of pharmacotherapy for binge-eating disorder. *Obesity (Silver Spring), 16*(9), 2024–2038.

Riva, G., Bacchetta, M., Baruffi, M., & Molinari, E. (2002). Virtual-reality-based multidimensional therapy for the treatment of body image disturbances in binge eating disorders: A preliminary controlled study. *IEEE Transactions on Information Technoly Biomedicine, 6*(3), 224–234.

Ro, O., Martinsen, E. W., Hoffart, A., & Rosenvinge, J. (2005). Two-year prospective study of personality disorders in adults with longstanding eating disorders. *International Journal of Eating Disorders, 37,* 112–118.

Roberto, C. A., Grilo, C. M., Masheb, R. M., & White, M. A. (2010). Binge eating, purging, or both: Eating disorder psychopathology findings from an internet community survey. *International Journal of Eating Disorders, 43*(8), 724–731.

Roberts, M. E., Tchanturia, K., Stahl, D., Southgate, L., & Treasure, J. (2007). A systematic review and meta-analysis of set-shifting ability in eating disorders. *Psychological Medicine, 37*(8), 1075–1084.

Rosen, D. S. (2010). Identification and management of eating disorders in children and adolescents. *Pediatrics, 126*(6), 1240–1253.

Russell, G. F., Szmukler, G. I., Dare, C., & Eisler, I. (1987). An evaluation of family therapy in anorexia nervosa and bulimia nervosa. *Archives of General Psychiatry, 44*(12), 1047–1056.

Safer, D. L., Telch, C. F., & Agras, W. S. (2001a). Dialectical behavior therapy adapted for bulimia: A case report. *International Journal of Eating Disorders, 30*(1), 101–106.

Safer, D. L., Telch, C. F., & Agras, W. S. (2001b). Dialectical behavior therapy for bulimia nervosa. *American Journal of Psychiatry, 158*(4), 632–634.

Santonastaso, P., Ferrara, S., & Favaro, A. (1999). Differences between binge eating disorder and non-purging bulimia nervosa. *International Journal of Eating Disorders, 25,* 215–218.

Schmidt, U., Lee, S., Beecham, J., Perkins, S., Treasure, J., Yi, I., et al. (2007). A randomized controlled trial of family therapy and cognitive behavior therapy guided self-care for adolescents with bulimia nervosa and related disorders. *American Journal of Psychiatry, 164*(4), 591–598.

Serfaty, M. A., Turkington, D., Heap, M., Ledsham, L., & Jolley, E. (1999). Cognitive therapy versus dietary counseling in the outpatient treatment of anorexia nervosa: Effects of the treatment phase. *European Eating Disorders Review, 7,* 334–350.

Shapiro, J. R., Berkman, N. D., Brownley, K. A., Sedway, J. A., Lohr, K. N., & Bulik, C. M. (2007). Bulimia nervosa treatment: A systematic review of randomized controlled trials. *International Journal of Eating Disorders, 40*(4), 321–336.

Smolak, L., & Murnen, K. (2001). Gender and eating problems. In R. Striegel-Moore & L. Smolak (Eds.), *Eating disorders: Innovative directions in research and practice* (pp. 91–110). Washington, DC: American Psychological Association Press.

Smyth, J. M., Wonderlich, S. A., Heron, K. E., Sliwinski, M. J., Crosby, R. D., Mitchell, J. E., et al. (2007). Daily and momentary mood and stress are associated with binge eating and vomiting in bulimia nervosa patients in the natural environment. *Journal of Consulting Clinical Psychology, 75*(4), 629–638.

Soh, N. L., Touyz, S. W., & Surgenor, L. J. (2006). Eating and body image disturbances across cultures: A review. *European Eating Disorders Review, 14,* 54–65.

Steinglass, J. E., Sysko, R., Glasofer, D., Albano, A. M., Simpson, H. B., & Walsh, B. T. (2011). Rationale for the application of exposure and response prevention to the treatment of anorexia nervosa. *International Journal of Eating Disorders, 44*(2), 134–141.

Steinglass, J., Sysko, R., Schebendach, J., Broft, A., Strober, M., & Walsh, B. T. (2007). The application of exposure therapy and D-cycloserine to the treatment of anorexia nervosa: A preliminary trial. *Journal of Psychiatric Practice, 13*(4), 238–245.

Steinglass, J. E., Walsh, B. T., & Stern, Y. (2006). Set shifting deficit in anorexia nervosa. *Journal of International Neuropsychological Society, 12*(3), 431–435.

Steinhausen, H. C. (2002). The outcome of anorexia nervosa in the 20th century. *American Journal of Psychiatry, 159*(8), 1284–1293.

Steinhausen, H. C., & Weber, S. (2009). The outcome of bulimia nervosa: Findings from one-quarter century of research. *American Journal of Psychiatry, 166*(12), 1331–1341.

Stice, E. (2001). Risk factors for eating pathology: Recent advances and future directions. In R. Striegel-Moore & L. Smolak (Eds.), *Eating disorders: Innovative directions in research and practice* (pp. 51–74). Washington, DC: American Psychological Association Press.

Stice, E., & Agras, W. S. (1998). Predicting onset and cessation of bulimic behaviors during adolescence: A longitudinal grouping analyses. *Behavior Therapy, 29,* 257–276.

Striegel-Moore, R. H., Fairburn, C. G., Wilfley, D. E., Pike, K. M., Dohm, F. A., & Kraemer, H. (2005). Toward an understanding of risk factors for binge eating disorder in black and white women: A community-based case-control study. *Psychological Medicine, 35*(6), 907–917.

Striegel-Moore, R. H., & Franko, D. L. (2003). Epidemiology of binge eating disorder. *International Journal of Eating Disorders, 34*(Suppl.), S19–S29.

Striegel-Moore, R. H., Silberstein, L. R., & Rodin, J. (1986). Toward an understanding of risk factors for bulimia. *American Psychologist, 41*(3), 246–263.

Strober, M., Freeman, R., DeAntonio, M., Lampert, C., & Diamond, J. (1997). Does adjunctive fluoxetine influence the post-hospital course of restrictor-type anorexia nervosa?: A 24-month prospective, longitudinal followup and comparison with historical controls. *Psychopharmacological Bulletin, 33*(3), 425–431.

Strober, M., Freeman, R., Lampert, C., Diamond, J., Teplinsky, C., & DeAntonio M. (2006). Are there gender differences in core symptoms, temperament, and short-term prospective outcome in anorexia nervosa? *International Journal of Eating Disorders, 39,* 570–575.

Sysko, R., Sha, N., Wang, Y., Duan, N., & Walsh, B.T. (2010). Early response to antidepressant treatment in bulimia nervosa. *Psychological Medicine, 40*(6), 999–1005.

Sysko, R., & Walsh, B. T. (2006). Early response to desipramine among women with bulimia nervosa. *International Journal of Eating Disorders, 39*(1), 72–75.

Sysko, R., & Walsh, B. T. (2008). A critical evaluation of the efficacy of self-help interventions for the treatment of bulimia nervosa and binge-eating disorder. *International Journal of Eating Disorders, 41*(2), 97–112.

Tanofsky-Kraff, M., & Wilfley, D. E. (2010). Interpersonal psychotherapy for BN and BED. In C. M. Grilo & J. E. Mitchell (Eds.), *The treatment of eating disorders: A clinical handbook* (pp. 271–289). New York: Guilford Press.

Tchanturia, K., Davies, H., Lopez, C., Schmidt, U., Treasure, J., & Wykes, T. (2008). Neuropsychological task performance before and after cognitive remediation in anorexia nervosa: A pilot case-series. *Psychological Medicine, 38*(9), 1371–1373.

Tchanturia, K., & Hambrook, D. (2010). Cognitive remediation therapy for anorexia nervosa. In C. M. Grilo & J. E. Mitchell (Eds.), *The treatment of eating disorders: A clinical handbook* (pp. 130-149). New York: Guilford Press.

Telch, C. F., Agras, W. S., & Linehan, M. M. (2001). Dialectical behavior therapy for binge eating disorder. *Journal of Consulting and Clinical Psychology, 69*(6), 1061–1065.

Tobin, D. L., Griffing, A., Griffing, S. (1997). An examination of subtypes of bulimia nervosa. *International Journal of Eating Disorders, 22,* 179-186.

Tozzi, F., Thronton, L. M., Mitchell, J., Fichter, M. M., Klump, K. L., Lilenfeld, L. R., et al (2006). Features associated with laxative abuse in individuals with eating disorders. *Psychosomatic Medicine, 68,* 470–477.

Varchol, L., & Cooper, H. (2009). Psychotherapy approaches for adolescents with eating disorders. *Current Opinion in Pediatrics, 21*(4), 457–464.

Vitousek, K., Watson, S., & Wilson, G. T. (1998). Enhancing motivation for change in treatment-resistant eating disorders. *Clinical Psychology Review, 18*(4), 391–420.

Vocks, S., Tuschen-Caffier, B., Pietrowsky, R., Rustenbach, S. J., Kersting, A., & Herpertz, S. (2010). Meta-analysis of the effectiveness of psychological and pharmacological treatments for binge eating disorder. *International Journal of Eating Disorders, 43*(3), 205–217.

von Ranson, K. M. (2008). Personality and eating disorders. In S. Wonderlich, J. Mitchell, M. de Zwaan, & H. Steiger (Eds.), *Eating disorders review—Part 2* (pp. 84–96). New York: Radcliffe.

Walsh, B. T., Kaplan, A. S., Attia, E., Olmsted, M., Parides, M., Carter, J. C., et al. (2006). Fluoxetine after weight restoration in anorexia nervosa: A randomized controlled trial. *Journal of the American Medical Association, 295*(22), 2605–2612.

Wilfley, D. E., Crow, S. J., Hudson, J. I., Mitchell, J. E., Berkowitz, R. I., Blakesley, V., et al. (2008). Efficacy of sibutramine for the treatment of binge eating disorder: A randomized multi-center placebo-controlled double-blind study. *American Journal of Psychiatry, 165*(1), 51-58.

Wilfley, D. E., MacKenzie, K. R., Welch, R. R., Ayres, V. E., & Weissman, M. M. (2000). *Interpersonal psychotherapy for group*. New York: Basic Books.

Wilfley, D. E., Welch, R. R., Stein, R. I., Spurrell, E. B., Cohen, L. R., Saelens, B. E., et al. (2002). A randomized comparison of group cognitive-behavioral therapy and group interpersonal psychotherapy for the treatment of overweight individuals with binge-eating disorder. *Archives of General Psychiatry, 59*(8), 713–721.

Wilson, G. T., Fairburn, C. C., Agras, W. S., Walsh, B. T., & Kraemer, H. (2002). Cognitive-behavioral therapy for bulimia nervosa: Time course and mechanisms of change. *Journal of Consulting and Clinical Psychology, 70*(2), 267–274.

Wilson, G. T., Grilo, C. M., & Vitousek, K. M. (2007). Psychological treatment of eating disorders. *American Psychologist, 62*(3), 199–216.

Wilson, G. T., Wilfley, D. E., Agras, W. S., & Bryson, S. W. (2010). Psychological treatments of binge eating disorder. *Archives of General Psychiatry, 67*(1), 94–101.

Wiseman, C. V., Sunday, S. R., Klapper, F., Harris, W. A., & Halmi, K. A. (2001). Changing patterns of hospitalization in eating disorder patients. *International Journal of Eating Disorders, 30*(1), 69–74.

Wonderlich, S. A., Gordon, K. H., Mitchell, J. E., Crosby, R. D., & Engel, S. G. (2009). The validity and clinical utility of binge eating disorder. *International Journal of Eating Disorders, 42*(8), 687–705.

Yager, J. (2007). Assessment and determination of initial treatment approaches for patients with eating disorders. In J. Yager & P. S. Powers (Eds.), *Clinical manual of eating disorders* (pp. 31–68). Washington, DC: American Psychiatric Publishing.

Yanovski, S. Z. (1993). Binge eating disorder: Current knowledge and future directions. *Obesity Research, 1*(4), 306–324.

Young, J. E., Weinberger, A. D., & Beck, A. T. (2001). Cognitive therapy for depression. In D. H. Barlow (Ed.), *Clinical handbook of psychological disorders* (3rd ed., pp. 264–308). New York: Guilford Press.

Zastrow, A., Kaiser, S., Stippich, C., Walther, S., Herzog, W., Tchanturia, K., et al. (2009). Neural correlates of impaired cognitive-behavioral flexibility in anorexia nervosa. *American Journal of Psychiatry, 166*(5), 608–616.

Zeeck, A., Weber, S., Sandholz, A., Wetzler-Burmeister, E., Wirsching, M., & Hartmann, A. (2009a). Inpatient versus day clinic treatment for bulimia nervosa: A randomized trial. *Psychotherapy and Psychosomatics, 78*(3), 152–160.

Zeeck, A., Weber, S., Sandholz, A., Wetzler-Burmeister, E., Wirsching, M., Scheidt, C. E., et al.

(2009b). Inpatient versus day treatment for bulimia nervosa: Results of a one-year follow-up. *Psychotherapy and Psychosomatics, 78*(5), 317–319.

Zemishlany, Z., & Weizman, A. (2008). The impact of mental illness on sexual dysfunction. *Advances in Psychosomatic Medicine, 29,* 89–106.

Zipfel, S., Reas, D. L., Thornton, C., Olmsted, M. P., Williamson, D. A., Gerlinghoff, M., et al. (2002). Day hospitalization programs for eating disorders: A systematic review of the literature. *International Journal of Eating Disorders, 31*(2), 105–117.

CHAPTER 8

Substance Use Disorders

Robert O. Pihl
Sherry H. Stewart

In this chapter, we review the basic and applied literature on substance use disorders. In the first section, we survey what is known about the psychopathology of substance use disorders—their nature and causes. In the second section we summarize the current state of knowledge about effective interventions (both psychological and biological) for this set of disorders. Although we make this distinction between the basic findings generally covered in the first section and the clinical/applied findings generally being covered in the second section, we believe the results of basic psychopathology research can and should help practitioners better address their clients' needs.

TYPICAL SYMPTOMS

The phrase "nosology necessarily precedes etiology" is often uttered but seldom followed. Patently, if one cannot define and measure a problem, then one cannot understand it. If one cannot understand it, then the interventions applied will be at best chaotically effective, if at all. Furthermore, the reasons a treatment (be it a physical or psychological one) is efficacious or not will be incompletely understood. Substance use disorders seem to have a definitional advantage over many other pathologies, because they imply the excessive use of a substance, which is an external and measurable behavior. Unfortunately, however, the task of defining these problems is not so simple.

DSM-IV included definitions of two forms of substance use disorders: dependence and abuse. This distinction has been dropped in DSM-5, and the two definitions have been merged into a single disorder with graded severity. Eleven symptoms are listed for this integrated definition of substance-related and addictive disorders. A person must have at least two of the following to qualify for the diagnosis: failure to complete major role obligations because of persistent substance use; repeated use of a substance in situations that are dangerous (e.g., driving when impaired); persistent use of a substance in spite of serious social or interpersonal consequences; development of tolerance; onset of withdrawal; substance is frequently used in larger amounts or for a longer period of time than intended; repeated desire or unsuccessful efforts to reduce or control use of the substance; spending large amounts of time doing things that are necessary to obtain the substance or recover from its effects; giving up important activities because of substance use; continued use of the substance in spite of the recognition that serious problems are caused by its use; and craving or strong urges to use the substance. If two or three of these criteria are present, the severity of the condition is rated as being "mild." If six or more criteria are present, the condition is rated as being "severe."

Perusal of this list of symptoms makes it immediately apparent that the amount of the drug consumed is not an issue unless it leads to "clinically significant impairment or distress." Even the old standbys of physiological tolerance and withdrawal (which, again, are measurable) can be ignored, and the focus can instead shift to psychological dependence. Hence, the heterogeneity and relative severity of substance use disorders are not well served by these concepts. It is clear that we are dealing with a plethora of differential disorders, all of which involve considerable clinical judgment and multiple pathways to the diagnostic endpoint. Thus, to assume the applicability of a single intervention would be akin to "a man standing in a bucket and trying to lift himself up by the handle."

Furthermore, the abusable substances on the list are legion. The DSM lists several classes of drugs: alcohol; sympathomimetics, such as amphetamines; caffeine; cannabis; cocaine; hallucinogens; inhalants; nicotine; opioids; phencyclidine; and sedatives/anxiolytics. These divisions are problematic because they are neither mutually exclusive (e.g., phencyclidine contains elements of both a sympathomimetic and a hallucinogen) nor collectively exhaustive. Moreover, prescribed medications, over-the-counter medications, and basically any substance used for the purpose of intoxication can be considered candidates for substance dependence and/or abuse. Furthermore, dependence can develop even if an individual is not using the drug for intoxicating purposes (e.g., using benzodiazepines to treat insomnia or narcotics for pain management). Also, clinicians must be cognizant that in addition to the preceding list, an individual can display mental disorders after exposure (which may be accidental) to a wide range of what are mostly toxic substances. Studies of individuals treated in hospital emergency wards reveal high percentages of drug-induced injury, illness, and unusual behavior. Particularly noteworthy is that the exclusion criterion "symptoms not due to the physiological effects of a substance" is fundamental to most other DSM definitions.

The definition of substance use disorders can be sweeping. Granted, the phrase "clinically significant impairment or distress" does get repeated, but in various circumstances it can simply reflect a projective test of the examiner or a convenient target to obscure other issues. Controversial issues that were debated during the revision of the chapter on substance use disorders included: the need to meld DSM-5 definitions with the World Health Organization's *International Classification of Diseases* (ICD-11), the consideration of categorical and/or dimensional definitions, the inclusion of neurobiological correlates in the definition, and the relevance of differential cultural aspects. Of particular concern to the area of substance use disorders is the issue of whether the focus should be on substances per se or shift to the concept of addictions. The latter, which was adopted in DSM-5, means that problems such as Internet addiction (which is a serious issue in Asian countries, in particular; Black, 2008) and pathological gambling should be included. In the case of pathological gambling, which is included in DSM-5, both the definition and behaviors (including neurocorrelates) are identical to some substance abuse disorders, leading some to refer to pathological gambling as an "addiction without the drug" (e.g., Potenza, 2001). Other pertinent diagnostic concerns include how to deal with high rates of comorbidity, the threshold for diagnosis, the applicability of criteria to different age groups, and putative subtypes of the disorder (Saunders, Schuckit, Sirovatka, & Regier, 2007). Consistent with both the breadth of the current definition of substance use disorders and its likely definition in the future, this class of disorders can only be described as extraordinarily robust.

PREVALENCE

The prevalence of substance use disorders—which are a compilation of dependence and abuse—has been assessed by numerous epidemiological studies. Given the wide range of these definitions, numerous problems should be and, in fact, have been determined. In effect, these disorders can be viewed as the most common of all mental disorders. However, this depends on the epidemiological survey to which one attends. For example, specific to alcohol, the Epidemiologic Catchment Area Survey of the 1980s (Regier et al., 1990) determined a lifetime diagnostic prevalence rate for alcohol dependence and abuse of 17.7 versus 12.3% for anxiety disorders and 7.8% for affective disorders. The National Comorbidity Survey (NCS) of the early 1990s, on the other hand, found lifetime rates of 23.5, 24.9, and 19.3%, respectively (Kessler et al., 1994), making anxiety disorders somewhat more prevalent than alcohol use disorders. The more recent National Comorbidity Survey Replication (NCS-R), using a sample of 10,000 respondents and data updated as of 2007, yielded lifetime prevalence estimates of, respectively, 13.2, 31.2, and 21.4% (Harvard School of Medicine, 2005). Finally, data from the National Epidemiologic Survey on Alcohol and Related Conditions (NESARC; collected between 2001 and 2002) showed, across 43,093 individuals, a lifetime prevalence of 10.3% for alcohol use disorder alone (Hasin, Stinson, Ogburn, & Grant, 2007). Rates were higher for males (13.8%)

than for females (7.1%), and the peak age was around late adolescence/early 20s. Some subsets of the population showed higher prevalence rates than others. Native Americans, for example, had a relatively high rate of 18.4%.

Surveys of college students have shown that 21–31% of them have an alcohol use disorder, 14% have nicotine dependence, and 5% have a problem with other drugs (Knight et al., 2002). Binge drinking is particularly prevalent and problematic in this population, and helps account for the high prevalence of alcohol use disorder in this group. As for cigarettes, the prevalence of smoking adults in the United States has decreased dramatically since the 1950s, when smokers constituted over one-half of all men and one-fourth of all women. In contrast, only 23.9% of men and 18% of women smoked in 2007. The addictive power of nicotine et al. (there are over 4,000 chemical compounds in cigarettes) is exemplified by the fact that in the National Health Interview Survey in 2006, 44.2% of smokers (19.9 million) had tried unsuccessfully to quit (Pleis & Lethbridge-Cejku, 2007). Marijuana (cannabis), the most commonly consumed illegal drug, is used by approximately 14% of people in the United States over the age of 12. Although this percentage has been relatively stable over the past decade, there has been an 18% increase in marijuana use disorders (Stinson, Ruan, Pickering, & Grant, 2006). In terms of other illicit drugs, the most recent Substance Abuse and Mental Health Services Administration (SAMHSA) data in 2007 show that percentages for use in the past 12 months: psychotherapeutics (6.6%), cocaine (2.3%), hallucinogens (1.5%), inhalants (0.8%), and heroin (0.1%; Hughes, Sathe, & Spagnola, 2009). It is essential to remember that use and abuse are not necessarily the same thing—even water can be an intoxicant when consumed in excessive quantities, supporting the adage that "too much of anything can lead to the suppression of something." Furthermore, the popularity of a specific drug is often relative to time and place.

COURSE

Although dogmas such as "one drink, one drunk" often proliferate when considering the course of substance misuse, this simplicity tends to flourish in direct proportion to our ignorance. Complexity is the rule. Which drug, used how and how much, with whom, under what conditions, and most significantly, by whom, all impact the course of the disorder. Hence, diagnostic issues are not trivial. The class of drug abused must be considered. With cocaine and the opiates, for example, many months after an individual has ceased use, strong cravings can be stimulated by situations previously associated with taking the drug. Thus, statistics are as high as 80% for cocaine-treated addicts relapsing within a year. The route of administration of the drug needs also to be considered. Smoking or injecting cocaine is far more nefarious than snorting, thus impacting severity and course. Also, with whom the drug is used can impact course. The individual who misuses alcohol socially or succumbs to illegal drug use only among peers is likely to have a less severe course than the private, "first thing in the morning" consumer. Another example of variation in course within a drug class is illustrated by a large national trajectory study of 18- to 26-year-olds for drinking, smoking, and marijuana use (Sher, Jackson, & Steinley, 2011). Consistent with other reports, four differential trajectories were determined: chronic high use, late-onset use, developmentally limited use, and low use. Predictably, the chronic high use group displayed the strongest risk characteristics (delinquency and sensation seeking), as well as co-usage of other drugs. Thus, understanding course necessitates the understanding of individual etiology. However, and finally, the NESARC survey (Hasin et al., 2007) reported that only 8% of individuals who qualify for a diagnosis of abuse, and 38% of those who meet criteria for dependence, ever receive treatment. This alarming statistic is a major cause for concern and likely reflects numerous factors. The primary reason, however, is most likely a lack of understanding of differential etiological pathways.

ASSOCIATED CLINICAL FEATURES

The high prevalence of substance abuse disorders resonates in a cacophony of negative ramifications that pose both direct and indirect effects. Numerous studies have made the relationship among alcohol intoxication, driving, and accidents well known. Less well known is the fact that alcohol is present in the perpetrator and, to a lesser degree, in the victim in approximately 40–50% of all murders, assaults, and rapes, and in roughly 67% of domestic violence cases (Murdoch, Pihl, & Ross, 1990). An extreme of this lack of control is found in studies that indicate having a drug or alcohol problem is a major factor in violence against women at the time of pregnancy (Chu, Goodwin, & D'Angelo, 2010). This fact seemingly contradicts to the fact that marriage per se reduces drug problems. Albeit, this protective effect of marriage is much less likely for those who have a family history of drug abuse, externalizing characteristics, and heavy use prior to marriage (Leonard & Homish, 2008). More generally, continued drug abuse can both obviate coping with daily problems in living as well as exacerbate them, hence increasing abuse in an ever increasing spiral of destruction, with the endpoint of destructiveness being suicide. Individuals with substance use disorders are at a six- to ten-fold increased risk for suicidal behavior, particularly when the substance use disorder is comorbid with personality disorders and depression (Preuss, Koller, Barnow, Eikmeier, & Soyka, 2006). Additionally, a drug such as alcohol is frequently used at the time of the suicidal act, adding a degree of disinhibition to finalize an ongoing perturbation.

Alcohol problems not only impact social functioning but they also have severe health consequences. For instance, around 1% of babies suffer from fetal alcohol spectrum disorders. In 2005, Room, Babor, and Rehm noted that 4% of the global burden of disease emanates from alcohol, and over 60 specific medical conditions are alcohol related. Table 8.1 presents the proportions of worldwide disease and accidents attributable to alcohol. Interestingly, ancient societies were also well aware of

TABLE 8.1. Major Disease and Injury Conditions Related to Alcohol and Proportions Attributable to Alcohol Worldwide

	Men	Women	Both
Malignant neoplasms			
Mouth and oropharynx cancers	22%	9%	19%
Esophageal cancer	37%	15%	29%
Liver cancer	30%	13%	25%
Breast cancer	n/a	7%	7%
Neuropsychiatric disorders			
Unipolar depressive disorders	3%	1%	2%
Epilepsy	23%	12%	18%
Alcohol use disorders: alcohol dependence and harmful use	100%	100%	100%
Diabetes mellitus	–1%	–1%	–1%
Cardiovascular disorders			
Ischemic heart disease	4%	–1%	2%
Hemorrhagic stroke	18%	1%	10%
Ischemic stroke	3%	–6%	–1%
Gastrointestinal diseases			
Cirrhosis of the liver	39%	18%	32%
Unintentional injury			
Motor vehicle accidents	25%	8%	20%
Drownings	12%	6%	10%
Falls	9%	3%	7%
Poisonings	23%	9%	18%
Intentional injury			
Self-inflicted injuries	15%	5%	11%
Homicide	26%	16%	24%

the burden of excessive consumption. In fact, the ancient Egyptians were the first to order abstinence.

The consequences of smoking are also well known to all, including addicted smokers. Smoking is currently the most preventable cause of disease and death in North America. In spite of the graphic, "in your face" warning labels that are required on cigarette packs in Canada, during cold Canadian winters throngs of intelligent individuals can be seen puffing away outdoors in huddled circles like musk ox during an Arctic blizzard. Of course, smokers is not only hurt their own health and longevity but they also compromising the health and longevity of others in the form of secondhand smoke. Studies have shown that the infant offspring of smokers have five times more of tobacco toxins in their urine than do controls. As well, children of smokers are more likely to suffer negative health effects such as asthma, to be impulsive, and to smoke as adolescents (Joseph et al., 2007).

Increased social problems and deteriorating health for the user and others is just the beginning of a potential list of possible direct negative ramifications of abusing various drugs. There is not an aspect of who we are that cannot be affected. For example, it is not uncommon for speakers listing the effects of heavy drinking to present a picture of a limp alcohol bottle to illustrate sexual dysfunction as an associated feature. The same is true for smoking, most illegal drugs, and many commonly prescribed medications, most notably the selective serotonin reuptake inhibitors. Even drugs thought to enhance sexual experience (e.g., some stimulants, ecstasy), over time, can result in a deterioration of sexual functioning. Furthermore, heavy episodic use of drugs by young adults, interacting with self-regulation difficulties and sensation seeking, has been shown to increase the prevalence of risky sexual behavior (Quinn & Fromme, 2010). Sleep is another area often impacted by heavy drug use. The most profound effect is typically among stimulant abusers, whose disrupted sleep patterns rival those of the bipolar patient in an acute manic phase. Alcohol, which is often taken to promote sleep and is beneficial for falling asleep, actually disturbs the many chemical processes that control sleep and can result in sleep deprivation. Furthermore, heavy drinking can narrow air passages, thus promoting and exacerbating sleep apnea. Even general use of alcohol, cigarettes, and marijuana by teens has respective odds ratios for insufficient sleep of 1.64, 1.45, and 1.52, respectively (McKnight-Eily et al., 2011). Sleep deprivation diminishes most waking activities, with school and work performance being obvious activities that suffer. Concerning the latter, increasingly employers are eliminating illegal drug users from the workforce through mandatory drug testing. Employers are also becoming cognizant of statistics showing that heavy users of even legal drugs have increased absenteeism, health problems, and accidents on the job.

Illegal drugs present severe direct and indirect consequences. In regard to direct ramifications, both the type and the degree vary between drugs. For example, drugs such as opiates, when compared to alcohol, result in fewer negative health consequences if one does not consider indirect effects. Indirect effects, on the other hand, are another matter. First, criminalization of some drugs results in de facto expulsion from normal society. Second, these drugs pose an increased risk of overdose and death, due primarily to the lack of quality control and the manner of consumption typically associated with them. And, finally, individuals addicted to these drugs often resort to criminal behavior to maintain their addiction. In the United States, approximately 1 of every 18 men is in prison and 70% of prisoners are non-white. Moreover, 55% of federal prisoners are serving drug sentences (Bureau of Justice, 2008). Thus, it appears that, there is currentlya preference for viewing addiction as criminal behavior rather than as mental illness.

In accordance with the adage "Pharmacology is the art of selective poisoning," most drugs, when used heavily, have negative neurological sequelae. Prime examples of such risky drugs are alcohol, methamphetamines, and ecstasy. In fact, the effects of these and other drugs add to the confusion in determining the possible brain bases for addictive behaviors, since cause and consequence of use obviously confuse the interpretation of any research finding with addicts.

In summary, in this section, we have reviewed a large number of associated clinical features that frequently are seen in individuals with substance use disorders, including physical health ramifications, social and interpersonal problems, sleep difficulties, sexual problems, suicidality, and impairments in work and school functioning. In clinical practice, it is crucial that these associated features be assessed at baseline, in addition to assessment of substance use disorder symptoms, for treatment planning with an individual client. We also recommend that these associated features be monitored throughout the course of treatment to ensure that patients are responding as their substance use disorder symptoms improve. Some of these associated features may require treatment in their own right, if they are not merely secondary consequences of the substance misuse.

COMORBIDITY

Substance abuse disorders seldom occur in isolation. Rather, it is often the case that more than one drug is abused (homotypic comorbidity) and/or the substance abuse co-occurs with another diagnosable mental disorder (heterotypic comorbidity). The previously mentioned NESARC, while controlling for sociodemographic conditions, determined representative co-occurring lifetime and 12-month odds ratios for the following various alcohol use disorders (abuse and dependence) and other mental health disorders: drug use disorder, 10.4/9.0 (lifetime vs. 12-month odds ratio); drug dependence, 15.9/15.0; mood disorder, 2.4/2.2; anxiety disorder, 2.3/1.9; bipolar I disorder, 3.5/2.7; and antisocial personality disorder 6.5/2.9. In fact, all 19 disorders subsumed under the categories of drug use disorder, mood disorder, anxiety disorder, and personality disorder resulted in significant lifetime odds ratios (Hasin et al., 2007). However, 12-months data may be more accurate in regard to actual temporal co-occurrence, as the disorders are likely to be less contemporaneous over a lifetime. In terms of homotypic co-occurrence, Falk, Hsiao-Ye, and Hiller-Sturmhöfel (2008), who also analyzed NESARC data, found that over the past year, 29% of individuals with alcohol use disorders had abused other drugs. The percentages for drug use disorders were as follows: 9.9%, cannabis; 2.4%, opioids; 2.5%, cocaine; 1.3%, hallucinogens; and 1.2%, amphetamines.

"Polydrug use," in which substances are used concomitantly, is also quite common. For example, 58% of heavy drinkers smoke (Hughes et al., 2009), and the correlation between cocaine and alcohol dependence is .84 (Helzer & Pryzbeck, 1988). These relationships are hardly random. While cocaine addicts often say that they drink to "come down," the combination of cocaine and alcohol actually produces cocaethylene, which is more excitatory than either cocaine or alcohol taken alone. So much for self-report! Certain situations, such as rave attendance, virtually guarantee polydrug use (Barrett, Gross, Garand, & Pihl, 2005). Furthermore, recent trends, such as using energy drinks and stimulants (mostly alcohol) to enhance the high, are quickly growing in popularity (Price, Hilchey, Darredeau, Fulton, & Barrett, 2010).

Traditionally, it has been assumed that the comorbidity of disorders emanates when one disorder leads to a second or third disorder, and so on, and/or when there is a common underlying risk factor for the disorders. In the case of substance abuse there are four possibilities (Mueser, Drake, & Wallach, 1998): Substance abuse leads to other disorders; other disorders lead to substance abuse; substance abuse and other disorders bidirectionally increase risk; or substance abuse and other disorders have common underlying risk factors. In clinical practice, where substance abuse problems are typically both underdiagnosed and not treated, there seems to be a preference for the model in which other disorders increase vulnerability to substance abuse. Even when this model is true, it is possible that the substance abuse can function to maintain the "primary" disorder and, therefore, lack of diagnoses and treatment for drug abuse can undermine the therapeutic endeavor. For example, a person starts abusing a drug because of depression, but the ramifications of the drug use inevitably result in dysphoria, which promotes the continuation of depression, creating a vicious cycle in which one disorder maintains the other over time. Perhaps the most significant error in current practice is the pervasive blindness to common underlying vulnerabilities that, very often, should be the focus of treatment. A study by Conrod, Pihl, Stewart, and Dongier (2000) demonstrates this point. Drug-dependent women from the general population ($n = 298$) completed a large battery of psychological tests and symptom rating scales. A factor analysis yielded four distinct factors: anxiety sensitivity, hopelessness, sensation seeking, and impulsivity. A cluster analysis, which is presented in Figure 8.1, illustrates how the drug-dependent women performed in each of these factors. Significantly, there was a strong relationship between the cluster into which each woman fell, the type of drug on which they were dependent, and their co-occuring mental disorder. For example, the odds ratios for women in the anxiety sensitive cluster (vs. the other clusters) were 3.0 for anxiolytic dependence, 2.1 for simple phobia, 1.9 for generalized anxiety disorder, and 5.8 for somatization disorder. The odds ratios for women in the hopelessness dimension were 2.9 for opioid dependence, 1.9 for recurrent depression, 2.7 for major depressive episode, 2.1 for panic disorder/agoraphobia, and 2.6 for social phobia. Women in the sensation-seeking cluster were 4.3 times more likely to be alcohol dependent. Impulsive women, on the other hand, were 2.7 times more likely to be alcohol dependent. In addition, the impulsive women were 1.8 times more likely to be cocaine dependent and 2.8 times more likely to be diagnosed with antisocial personality disorder. While these findings suggest some shared underlying factor that is common to the development of these differential disorders, their sequence of appearance is unknown. A report

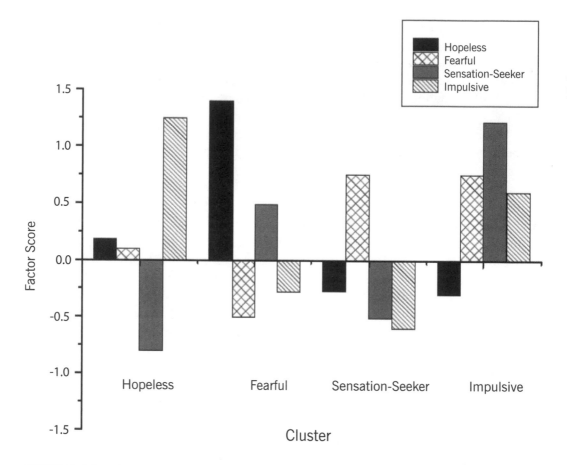

FIGURE 8.1. Motivational profiles of five subtypes of female substance abusers: Factor scores on four dimensions of personality. Adapted from Conrod, Pihl, and Stewart (2000). Copyright 2000 by the American Psychological Association. Adapted by permission.

(Ferguson, Boden, & Harwood, 2009) from a 25-year longitudinal birth cohort study in New Zealand—after controlling for confounding factors—determined that in both men and women alcohol problems preceded depression. In contrast, a review of the literature suggests that depression more often precedes alcohol problems among women (Sabourin & Stewart, 2009).

In addition to co-occurring disorders, there are behavioral profiles that, although not necessarily reaching the threshold for diagnoses, support the earlier conclusion of differential pathways. Profiles with extremes of externalizing and internalizing behaviors have been linked to substance abuse. For example, sons of alcoholics who are known to be at four to nine times increased risk for developing the disorder often display externalizing patterns. When compared to controls, they as a group have been found to display autonomic hyperreactivity to stress and novelty, reduced academic achievement, relative deficits on cognitive tests, and general impaired behavioral regulation (Pihl, 2010). Yet prediction based on these behaviors alone remains precarious. How these profiles and other risk factors, such as parents' antisociality or poor parenting, or mothers' depression, or peer relationships, impact risk is the topic of etiology.

ETIOLOGY

From the previous discussion, it should be eminently clear that substance abuse represents differential disorders with a potentially large number of distinct etiological pathways. The fact that this is also true for a single drug needs to be highlighted and must be actively considered even for treatments directed at a specific drug. Additionally, one needs to underscore the likely interaction between various pathways to abuse. The knowledge of these pathways is essential for clinicians, since their interventions should be based on what they think is wrong. The fact that most substance-abusing individuals are never treated, and that clinicians tend to focus their treatment on a co-occurring disorder of which they are more knowledgeable, are due directly to a lack of understanding about substance abuse/dependence. Alcohol is a prime example of this and is therefore featured in the following sections. However, irrespective of the drug, etiological information does exist on genetic, biochemical, behavioral and social levels.

Genes

The explosive growth in molecular genetics has heightened enthusiasm for discovery of the specific genes implicated in the heritability findings of traditional family, twin, and adoption studies for practically all mental disorders, as well as seemingly social behaviors such as divorce. In the area of substance abuse, genetics work has covered all existing drugs and the area currently defies generalization due to the large number of genes that have been related to it. Furthermore, enthusiasm for various target genes frequently seems to shift, thus increasing the trepidation to produce conclusions. Perhaps the situation in drug abuse is akin to that in schizophrenia, where recent work has found mutant genes in 15–20% of subjects studied. However, the exact genes implicated have varied from one individual (family) to the next. Nonetheless, most of the variants were related to genes involved in brain development (Walsh et al., 2008). Perhaps the most comprehensive work regarding substance abuse has been derived from the massive Collaborative Study on the Genetics of Alcoholism. Predictably, and consistent with previous knowledge, this study found that genes affecting alcohol metabolism are implicated in alcoholism, as are genes that affect receptors, such as gamma-aminobutyric acid (GABA), acetylcholine, and dopamine (Edenberg & Foround, 2006). Yet the large number of genes implicated in 51 determined chromosomal regions, many of which are involved in other addictions and disorders, is perplexing. This suggests, at best, some form of polygenic contribution (Johnson et al., 2006). These genes are known to function in cellular signaling (both between and within cells), brain development, cell adhesion, and varying cell functions. Exactly how these genes contribute to vulnerability, in whom, and for what remain complex, unanswered questions.

Both twin and adoption studies have shown and continue to show generally high heritability for substance abuse disorders. Some sample estimates of heritability include the following: alcohol, 51–73% (Tyndale 2003); smoking, 0–60% (Kendler, 2001); cannabis, 30–80% (Agrawal & Lynskey, 2006); and stimulants, opiates, sedatives, and psychedelics; 30–50% (Tsuang et al., 1998). Thus, genes play an undeniable role in enhancing one's risk for substance abuse, but it would be erroneous to conclude that there are specific genes for addictions just as for any behavior. Of course, the crucial issue is the question of which propensities and limitations are affected by genes via neurological functioning and interactions with environmental events. It is the latter that in many situations trigger gene expression, finally signaling the death toll to the nature–nurture debate.

The Brain and Addiction

Various drugs have differential effects on brain functioning. Furthermore, pharmacokinetics, such as dose and route of administration, greatly affect responsivity. For example, injecting or smoking stimulants (e.g., cocaine) result in a significantly more robust response than snorting them. Furthermore, the baseline functioning of these brain systems related to genetic vulnerability, among other possibilities, is thought greatly to determine the level of response. Models organized according to theoretical system groupings provide some explanatory power. The cue for reward/psychomotor/activation system primarily involving the mesocorticolimbic dopamine system, the anxiety/threat/inhibition system (which is mostly GABA mediated and involves an extended limbic network from the amygdala through the orbitofrontal cortex), and the cognitive control system (which primarily involves the prefrontal cortex but also includes pathways to and from the cerebellum through the limbic system)—as well as their interactions that represent relevant models. Of course, these putative systems are highly complex, involving numerous neurotransmitters and neuromodulators that individually and collectively also impact addiction. The cue for the reward system is activated by stimulants, the threat system is inhibited by anxiolytics, and the cognitive system can be both dampened and facilitated by various drugs. Imaging studies have revealed that when subjects are challenged with alcohol, amphetamine, or cocaine, the cue for reward system is activated via dopamine release (Leyton, 2007). This activation is associated with feelings of euphoria, energy, and general positive affect. Hence, it is easy to see why these drugs are abused (at least initially) and why stimuli associated with this situation, both directly and advantageously, are easily conditioned to elicit drug craving. Similar hedonic responses to cigarette smoking have been reported and are also related to the release of dopamine, although the brain area involved is not precisely the same as for other stimulants (Barrett, Boileau, Okker, Pihl, & Dagher, 2004). Notably, individuals who are more at risk for developing problems with stimulants due to family history or the presence of particular biological markers display a dopamine response with greater amplitude than that of controls (Boileau et al., 2003; Leyton, 2007), and with repeated drug exposure both conditioned (Boileau et al., 2007) and sensitized dopamine responses are developed (Boileau et al., 2006). These findings support the proposition of individual differential sensitivities to drug effects and, hence, differential likelihoods to develop addictions. Furthermore, these stimulant responders are distinct from controls and threat-sensitive individuals in that they exhibit less amygdala activation in response to fearful stimuli (Glahn, Lovallo, & Fox, 2007) and show general orbital–frontal activation instead (Heitzig, Nigg, Yau, Zubita, & Zucker, 2008).

A surfeit of imaging studies with threat-sensitive individuals demonstrate extreme ongoing activation of emotional circuitry to fear/threat-provoking stimuli (Feldman-Barrett, & Wager, 2006). Unfortunately, though, there is a relative absence of drug challenge studies designed to assess the neurological aspects of this response. A commonly used approach has been stress response dampening studies, in which anxiolytics (including alcohol) demonstrate reductions in autonomic (Stewart & Pihl, 1994) and subjective–emotional responsivity to threat stimuli, particularly among threat sensitive individuals. Descriptively, these individuals report their drug experience as "relaxing," as "a relief," and as the obviation of a negative state, and they report heightened levels of anxiolytic drugs (including alcohol) use to cope with their negative affective states (e.g., Stewart, Karp, Pihl, & Peterson, 1997). These two models appear to reflect, in the first case, positive reinforcement, and in the second, negative reinforcement. Both models are, however, modified by the third model (i.e., the cognitive model).

A less well recognized yet particularly important point in developing motivation for change in any kind of therapy is the recognition that drug use–misuse has benefits for the individual. Clearly, two of the previous models are based on reinforcing aspects of drug use. Drugs can lubricate social functioning, provide identification for the adolescent, self-medicate dysphoric/anxious states, promote strong positive feelings, and improve cognitive functioning. With respect to the latter, college students with prescriptions for stimulant drugs, supposedly for the treatment of attention-deficit/hyperactivity disorder (ADHD), are highly likely to sell these drugs to others (Darredeau, Barrett, Jardin & Pihl, 2007). Incidentally, these drugs have pharmacological profiles similar to cocaine and therefore produce indistinguishable effects (Volkow & Swanson, 2003). In the immediate sense, these stimulant drugs are often used as study aids among the university population. This raises the intriguing question of whether this form of performance enhancement can be considered cheating.

An ongoing interactive circularity affects brain functioning and gene expression. We are increasingly learning that what we think about and how we cope with various environmental events determines the activity of genes and brain function-ing. There are more examples of how cognitive-behavioral interventions and pla-cebo drugs alter brain function, often producing brain images that illustrate those factors thought to be causative of the disorder. Importantly, this means that risk, irrespective of genetic–brain susceptibility, can be altered–controlled by a strong cognitive-inhibitory propensity. For example, individuals who display a particular high-risk response when challenged with alcohol can have that biological response muted by a prior learning experience (Brunelle & Pihl, 2007).

Cognitive Factors

As noted in the previous section on the brain and addiction, some substances of abuse have positively reinforcing consequences, such as feelings of euphoria, while others have negatively reinforcing consequences, such as anxiolytic or analgesic effects, or reductions in social inhibitions (Greeley & Oei, 1999; Pomerlau, Fager-strom, Marks, Tate, & Pomerleau, 2003). Social learning theory posits that these positive and negative reinforcement effects of substance use are learned through direct and indirect experiences (Maisto, Carey, & Bradizza, 1999). Expectancies about the outcomes of engaging in substance use are then formed. Expectancies can be thought of as "if–then" statements regarding the expected outcome of a behavior such as substance use (e.g., "If I were to drink alcohol, then I would feel very calm and relaxed"). Basic research has repeatedly shown that expectancies can influ-ence postdrug consumption behavior over and above actual drug effects (Testa et al., 2006), and that outcome expectancies exert powerful influences on subsequent substance use behavior (e.g., Fromme, Stroot, & Kaplan, 1993; Valdivia & Stewart, 2005). Outcome expectancies have been shown to develop before children have even had any direct experiences with substances (Miller, Smith, & Goldman, 1990). Expectancies can develop through observation of parents' or peers' substance use, or through advertising and media influences (Dunn & Yniguez, 1999). Prospective research suggests that children may begin drinking at least partly because of these indirectly acquired alcohol outcome expectancies (Christiansen, Smith, Roehling, & Goldman, 1989).

   Another important cognitive variable in the social learning model of substance use disorders (Maisto et al., 1999) is self-efficacy expectancies. In this context, "self-efficacy" is the belief that one can cope successfully without using substances, or that one has the ability to refuse the drug if it is offered. For example, a woman who does not believe she has the skills to relax on her own, without the use of substances, following a conflict with her partner is said to be particularly prone to developing a substance use disorder (O'Connor & Stewart, 2010). Recent prospec-tive research has shown that lack of drinking refusal self-efficacy in teens is pre-dictive of problem drinking 1 year later. Specifically, teens with lower self-efficacy about their ability to refuse drinks offered by others were found to be at increased risk for problem drinking (Connor, George, Gullo, Kelly, & Young, 2011). According to social learning theory, self-efficacy expectancies and outcome expectancies may interact: When positive outcome expectancies are combined with low levels of self-efficacy, substance use is particularly likely to occur (Marlatt & Gordon, 1985). Thus, both outcome expectancies and self-efficacy expectancies should be targeted in substance use disorder treatment (Marlatt & Gordon, 1985).

Stress

The roles of stress in contributing to the onset and maintenance of substance abuse and dependence have received considerable research attention over the years. First, it appears that early stress can increase vulnerability to the development of substance misuse. Animal models have shown that early stress can lead to enduring changes in neurotransmitter systems (e.g., dopamine) within limbic brain structures that contribute to a propensity to self-administer large amounts of drugs such as cocaine, amphetamine, and alcohol. For example, one study with mice indicated that early stress led to higher operant responding for alcohol in adulthood, and that this effect of early stress was mediated by alterations in dopamine and glutamate neurotransmission (Campbell, Szumlinksi, & Kippin, 2009).

Stress can also trigger relapse to substance abuse in recovered substance abusers (Marlatt & Gordon, 1985; Wang, You, Rice, & Wise, 2007). Interestingly, stress activates dopamine release (Lataster et al., 2011) in a manner similar to the dopamine release observed in response to drug administration (Leyton, 2007). This stress-induced dopamine release can act as a conditioned cue, triggering drug craving (Sinha, 2007), drug seeking, and ultimately drug relapse (Volkow, 2011). Thus, psychological treatments should focus on helping the client develop alternative skills for coping with stress and teaching techniques to deal with stress-induced urges and cravings to use, in order to prevent relapse. In terms of implications for pharmacotherapies, these results suggest that drugs targeting the stress response and those minimizing craving through impacts on the dopamine system are likely to be helpful in the treatment of substance use disorders (Sinha, 2007), as we outline later in the section on treatment.

Social–Familial Factors

The cultural variation in drug use and response is profound, even among groups with the same genetic heritage. For example, as opposed to the typical finding of increased aggressiveness when intoxicated, there are cultures in which people in fact show significantly less aggression when under the influence (MacAndrew & Edgerton, 1969). In areas of the world where cocaine and heroin are grown (and the former processed), abuse is miniscule in comparison to North American and European societies. Rather than relying on the notion of genetic differences, Reinarman (2005) has argued that the nature of our mass consumption, individualistic, hedonistic, and competitive culture provides more powerful explanations. Whereas genetic–biological studies typically begin with families with histories of abuse, within society are subcultures that are more at risk, and that are relatively immune to the disorder, despite equivalent biological vulnerability. Populations at higher risk for abuse than the general population include adolescents, the ghettoized poor, the disenfranchised, males, and the less educated. Religiosity, on the other hand, has consistently been shown to reduce risk significantly. One's family and peers represent small societies with concomitant beliefs and attitudes. This is important given that parental and peer modeling are powerful inducements in initiating and maintaining drug use. Numerous studies have indicated that this is clearly the case in regard to alcohol, cigarettes, and even illicit drugs. Yet another familial aspect of drug taking also deserves consideration: the propensity to treat all problems— undiagnosed and unspecified—with drugs. "Dr. Mom" supplies the palliatives in the form of medicines of dubious value. Physicians write prescriptions for what can be best determined as "problems in living." Thus, both facto teach avoidance without coping. Chemical agents offer an immediate remedy for the slightest twinge in one's psyche. Overall, family plays a crucial role in substance abuse. For this reason, therapy with adolescent drug abusers often requires family involvement in order to deal with not only the issues and angst of the adolescent but also family attitudes and practices. We return to the role of social and familial factors when we consider interventions later in the chapter.

Interactions

It would be inadequate to assume that any of the earlier sections on etiology is singularly explanatory. Cause is a multifactorial, multilevel, interactional process. For example, gene expression is altered by environmental events, and vice versa. Antisocial behavior—a common precursor to substance abuse—can result from just such a scenario. Caspi et al. (2002), for instance, showed that a polymorphism of a gene related to antisocial behavior had an effect if the individual was maltreated as a child. In this case, the specific genotype putatively altered one's sensitivity to environmental events ultimately resulting in the phenotypic expression of antisocial behavior. More recently, Ornish et al. (2008) demonstrated, in what they refer to as a "pilot study," that strict and comprehensive lifestyle changes over 3 months (primarily involving diet, exercise, and stress management) resulted in an up-regulation of 48 and down-regulation of 453 selected gene transcripts.

Gene–environment effects are not simply additive. The heritability of smoking increased from zero for men born before 1910 to 60% for those born after 1940, as smoking became less of a normative behavior (Kendler, 2001). Then there are the learned associations that develop by virtue of taking many drugs. For instance, Volkow et al. (2006) showed in a positron emission tomographic (PET) study that when cocaine addicts watch a video of cocaine being used, they release significantly more dopamine than when watching a video about nature. Prosaically put, "You can take the drug from the addict but the craving lives on."

TREATMENT

Just as there are myriad etiological factors and multiple pathways to the development of substance use disorders, there are also numerous approaches to treating
substance abuse and dependence. For some with severe physiological dependence
on a substance, treatment may begin with an inpatient stay for "detoxification"
involving medical management of withdrawal symptoms (Morgan, 1981). For those
treated on an outpatient basis, various other medications are available to target the
different brain systems involved in addiction, as described earlier in this chapter.
And given the importance of social factors in addiction etiology, as well as the powerful roles of cognition and learning, a variety of cognitive-behavioral therapy techniques have been advanced to assist those with substance use disorders. Family and
couple therapies have been developed and evaluated in the treatment of this set of
disorders given the etiological and maintaining roles of family factors, as discussed
earlier. We look at each of these approaches in turn and at the evidence for their
efficacy across a variety of forms of substance use disorder (e.g., abuse vs. dependence; alcohol vs. nicotine vs. illicit drug dependence). We conclude by considering
some general principles of change in the treatment of individuals with substance
use disorders.

Although we do have effective treatments that help many people with substance use disorders, available treatments could be much more effective. Unfortunately, as noted earlier, many people with substance use disorders fail to seek treatment (Hasin et al., 2007). And when they do seek treatment, the positive gains of
treatment are not always lasting—rates of relapse are alarmingly high in the area of
substance use disorders (Marlatt, Larimer, Baer, & Quigley, 1993). We discuss some
recent efforts to remedy this situation, for example, the development of relapse prevention approaches designed to help those with substance use disorders maintain
their treatment gains in the longer term. And we consider recent efforts to match
treatments (whether they be biomedical or psychosocial) better to the underlying
pathways to substance abuse and dependence, in an effort to improve treatment
outcome. Since one barrier to treatment engagement can be individuals' failure to
recognize they have a problem and need to change, we begin with an approach
designed to get people with substance use disorders to commit to the work required
to overcome an addiction, namely, motivational interviewing.

Motivational Interviewing

The first step in recovery from a substance use disorder is for the affected individual to recognize that he or she does have a problem with the substance and needs
assistance to overcome the problem. People with substance use disorders, however,
arrive at treatment at different "stages of change" or states of readiness to tackle
their substance misuse (Miller & Rollnick, 2002; Prochaska, DiClemente, & Norcross, 1997). Many people with substance use disorders arrive at treatment in the

precontemplation stage (e.g., attending treatment session due to partner's threat of leaving) or contemplation (e.g., just beginning to consider that they have a problem with substances) stage rather than the preparation or action stages that are required for successful treatment (Prochaska & DiClemente, 1992). A therapist cannot help a person who is not yet ready to change his or her substance use behavior (Miller, 1985). In fact, research has shown that if a client's readiness to change his or her substance use behavior is low, the treatment outcome is less than optimal (Gonzalez, Schmitz, & DeLaune, 2006).

Poor engagement with treatment among substance abusers, as evidenced by signs such as failure to complete homework, medication noncompliance, or missed therapy sessions, has traditionally been viewed by therapists as evidence of "resistance" (Westra & Dozois, 2006). However, others have suggested that these behaviors may be signs of ambivalence about change (Engle & Arkowitz, 2006). On the one hand, those with substance use disorders are attracted to substances for their many reinforcing properties (e.g., stimulants' activating effects in the brain reward system; anxiolytic drugs' dampening of the threat system, as discussed earlier in this chapter). On the other hand, they are aware of the severe negative consequences of continued substance use, such as financial and relationship troubles, health issues, and problems with employers. Some argue that this ambivalence must be resolved prior to the client being able to commit to a more active treatment, such as the biological or psychological treatments we discuss next in this chapter.

A specific psychological technique called "motivational interviewing" (Miller & Rollnick, 1991, 2002) has been developed to help those with substance abuse/dependence improve their motivation to change and move toward a stage in which they are ready to put in the effort required to change their problematic use of alcohol/drugs. Motivational interviewing is directed at exploring and resolving ambivalence about change in order to increase clients' engagement with the treatment process, enhance compliance, and ultimately improve response rates. In motivational interviewing, the therapist encourages clients to explore their own feelings and thoughts about the possibility of changing their substance use. The therapist does not advocate for change, but instead helps clients to become more effective advocates for their own change (Westra & Dozois, 2006). One way to accomplish this is to increase client self-change statements. For example, the therapist uses techniques to steer the client toward talking less about continuing substance misuse and more about change.

Motivational interviewing can be used as a stand-alone intervention or as a "prelude" (i.e., brief preparatory intervention) prior to other treatments such as cognitive-behavioral therapy (CBT) or biological treatments (see below). When used as a stand-alone intervention, the idea is that many clients actually have the tools to make changes in their substance use behavior, and all they need to be able to make the necessary changes is to resolve their ambivalence about making changes. When used as a prelude to other treatments, motivational interviewing focuses only on resolving the client's ambivalence about change. Other treatments such as CBT (to be discussed next) then provide the client with the skills to make those changes (Arkowitz & Westra, 2004; Bux & Irwin, 2006). The treatment outcome literature suggests that when brief courses of motivational interviewing are used as preludes to other substance use disorder treatments, very promising outcomes can be achieved (see review by Burke et al., 2003). Such treatment preludes also improve treatment attendance (see review by Walitzer, Dermen, & Connors, 1999). And motivational interviewing appears more effective when used as a prelude to CBT than when used as a stand-alone treatment (see review by Burke, Arkowitz, & Menchola, 2003). In short, motivational interviewing is a valuable technique in the treatment of substance use disorders, particularly when used as a prelude to other, more active, skills-based interventions (see review by O'Connor & Stewart, 2010). One such set of skills-based interventions is CBT, which we discuss next.

Cognitive-Behavioral Therapy

CBT is a time-limited psychotherapy that is based in social learning theory (Bandura, 1977). As noted earlier, social learning theory emphasizes the roles of outcome expectancies and self-efficacy expectancies in contributing to substance abuse. Given the importance of outcome expectancies, one CBT technique to treat substance use disorders is "expectancy challenge" (Darkes & Goldman, 1993)—helping the client gather evidence against, and critically evaluate the veracity and utility of, these expected positive consequences of engaging in alcohol or drug use. Self-efficacy expectancies are enhanced through techniques such as training in drink/drug refusal skills, which can specifically increase individuals' belief in their ability to refuse the substance if it is offered (Connor et al., 2011). More generally, in CBT, self-efficacy is enhanced through coping skills training (discussed next), because greater knowledge and experience with adaptive coping skills can increase clients' belief in their ability to cope without use of the substance.

Coping skills training, a core component of CBT for substance use disorders, is designed to remediate any skills deficits and to enhance clients' sense of self-efficacy. Clients are taught specific cognitive and behavioral techniques they can employ when faced with triggers to use the substance in their daily lives. These triggers can be intrapersonal (e.g., positive or negative mood states, stress) or interpersonal (e.g., a conflict with a spouse). To counter interpersonal triggers, clients may be taught assertiveness and drink/drug refusal skills, for example. To counter intrapersonal triggers, clients are taught skills, for example, in urge management, stress management, and increasing pleasant activities (Monti, Kadden, Rohsenow, Cooney, & Abrams, 2002).

Another commonly component in CBT for substance use disorder is cue exposure (Monti et al., 2002). According to social learning theory, certain cues such as specific internal states (e.g., stress) or places become conditioned with substance use. Exposure to these cues can trigger a craving or urge to use the substance (Abrams & Niaura, 1987). Thus, cue exposure treatment involves repeatedly exposing clients to cues that typically trigger their substance use, and teaching them to cope with these urges without the use of substances. The repeated exposure should reduce the strength of the urges elicited in response to future cues. More recent developments in CBT for substance use disorders include components involving mindful awareness and acceptance. For example, clients are taught skills in "urge surfing"—noticing and accepting urges to use substances, without fighting or giving in to them, and learning to let them pass (Witkiewitz, Marlatt, & Walker, 2005).

The treatment goal in CBT is typically selected by the client in collaboration with the therapist, be it abstinence or controlled use (Sobell & Sobell, 1993). Both of these treatment goals appear to be equally effective, at least in the area of alcohol use disorder treatment (Marlatt et al., 1993). However, neither can be considered a cure given high relapse rates (Barlow, Durand, & Stewart, 2009).

Many successfully treated people with substance use disorder eventually relapse. For example, as many as 70–80% of treated alcoholics relapse over the long term (Marlatt et al., 1993). Thus, CBT for substance use disorders typically includes techniques focused on "relapse prevention." "Lapse incidents"—times when the individual striving for abstinence uses the drug, or when the person striving for controlled use engages in heavy substance use—are dealt with as occurrences from which the person can recover. Instead of viewing these lapse episodes as inevitably leading to more substance use, people undergoing CBT for a substance use disorder are encouraged to see the lapse as an episode brought on by stress or by a situation that can be changed. They are taught to view lapses as learning experiences rather than as the beginning of an inevitable road to relapse (Marlatt & Gordon, 1985; Witkiewitz et al., 2005).

CBT is among the most effective and commonly employed treatments for alcohol use disorders (e.g., Finney & Monahan, 1996; O'Connor & Stewart, 2010; Oei, Lim, & Young, 1991; Stewart & Conrod, 2005; Swindle, Peterson, Paradise, & Moos, 1995). There is also mounting evidence for the efficacy of CBT in the treatment of nicotine dependence (Hall, Munoz, & Reus, 1994) and illicit substance use disorders such as methamphetamine (Rawson, Gonzales, & Brethen, 2002) or cocaine (Carroll et al., 2004) use. Numerous randomized controlled trials have demonstrated CBT efficacy to be comparable to alternative therapies such as motivational enhancement treatment or 12-step programs, to be discussed later (e.g., Project MATCH Research Group, 1997, 1998). In addition to the empirical support for CBT, there is also high client satisfaction with CBT for substance use disorders (Donovan, Kadden, DiClemente, & Carroll, 2002).

Social Context Interventions

As noted in the previous section on motivational interviewing, there has been a great deal of recent focus within treatment for substance use disorders on the importance of clients' motivation to change. One such innovation involves motivating substance abusers by considering their broader social context. This trend involves recognition of how the client's broader social community, including friends' and family members' behaviors and communication styles, contributes to the maintenance of his or her substance use disorders. This trend also recognizes how the client's social context can be used to advantage in motivating and promoting change in his or her substance use behavior (Stewart & Conrod, 2005). For example, in family therapy with adolescent substance abusers, family attitudes and practices relative to substance use are a treatment target (Kaminer & Slesnick, 2006). As another example, communication difficulties that contribute to problematic beliefs that maintain substance abuse are a therapy target in the behavioral couple therapy approach for alcoholism (Fals-Stewart, O'Farrell, Birchler, Cordova, & Kelley, 2005). Family members may also be taught helpful ways to assist the client with treatment compliance (e.g., taking his or her medications to treat their substance use disorder; Fals-Stewart et al., 2005)). Similarly, in the community reinforcement approach (Meyers, Villanueva, & Smith, 2005), a spouse, friend, or relative who is not a substance abuser is recruited to participate in relationship therapy to help the substance-abusing client improve his or her relationship skills. In addition, new recreational and social activities are used to help the client replace substance use with socially reinforcing activities (Meyers et al., 2005).

Social context is also a very important component of the most popular model for the treatment of substance abuse, namely, the 12-step approach first developed by Alcoholics Anonymous (AA). Specifically, the social support provided through group meetings may be one important key to the efficacy of this approach (Barlow et al., 2009). People who regularly participate in AA group meetings and follow the guidelines (e.g., acknowledging their addiction to alcohol; the requirement of complete abstinence; spiritual component) are more likely to have a positive outcome (Emrick, Tonigan, Montgomery, & Little, 1993). In fact, people who fully participate in AA have outcomes similar to those who receive CBT treatment (Ouimette, Finney, & Moos, 1997). Unfortunately though, a large number of people who begin AA eventually drop out: One-half drop out after 4 months, and three-fourths after 12 months (Alcoholics Anonymous, 1990). The reliance of the 12-step approach on spirituality and its adoption of a disease model of addiction can be stumbling blocks for many with substance use disorders. Thus, while AA and other 12-step treatments such as Narcotics Anonymous can be very helpful for those who engage fully with the approach, other treatments are needed for the large numbers of people with a substance use disorder who do not respond to this approach (Barlow et al., 2009).

Treatment Matching in Psychotherapy

Given the marked heterogeneity in substance-abusing clients and the unique pathways to substance abuse and dependence highlighted at the outset of this chapter, recent efforts have been made to match treatments to the particular needs of individual clients—a notion known as "treatment matching." For example, the

National Institute on Alcohol Abuse and Alcoholism initiated a study called Project MATCH (Matching Alcoholism Treatment to Client Heterogeneity). The goal of this project was to determine whether specific client characteristics would predict response to three specific alcoholism treatments: CBT, a motivational enhancement therapy, or a 12-step approach. The main finding of the study was that overall the three treatments performed similarly and well in treating alcoholic clients (Project MATCH Research Group, 1997). And initial analyses were disappointing in that they suggested few specific matching effects (see review by Conrod, Stewart, et al., 2000). Nonetheless, more recent analyses of Project MATCH data are promising. For example, Witkiewitz, Hartzler, and Donovan (2010) showed that in outpatient settings, individuals with low levels of motivation to change their substance use at baseline benefited more from motivational enhancement techniques than from CBT.

A more recent set of treatment matching studies was performed in Canada and the United Kingdom (Conrod, Stewart, et al., 2000). This new approach focused on matching on substance-abusing clients' personality traits and reasons for substance use. The personality profiles targeted in this approach were the four discussed earlier in this chapter as motivating substance use, but for different reasons: anxiety sensitivity, hopelessness, impulsivity, and sensation seeking. Motivational enhancement and CBT techniques were used to create specific brief treatments for each type of substance abuser. For example, sensation seekers were taught skills to help them meet their needs for excitement in less risky ways than substance abuse. In contrast, anxiety-sensitive substance abusers were taught cognitive and behavioral skills that manage anxiety better than substance abuse. In the first study to test this approach, adult women substance abusers recruited from the community were randomly assigned to receive one of the following three interventions: (1) a motivation-matched intervention involving personality-specific motivational and coping skills training (e.g., an anxiety-sensitive person, receiving an intervention specifically designed for anxiety-sensitive substance abusers); (2) a motivation-mismatched intervention targeting a theoretically different personality profile (e.g., an anxiety-sensitive substance abuser receiving an intervention designed for a sensation seeker); or (3) a motivational control intervention in which clients watched a film about substance abuse, then had a supportive discussion with a therapist. At 6-month follow-up, only the matched intervention was superior to the motivational control intervention in terms of reducing the frequency and severity of problematic substance use (Conrod, Stewart, et al., 2000). More recently, this approach has been shown to be effective in reducing alcohol use and misuse in young people when delivered in a group context in schools (Conrod, Stewart, Comeau, & Maclean, 2006). Moreover, this approach shows promise in treating symptoms of several mental health disorders that are so commonly comorbid with substance use disorders (Castellanos & Conrod, 2006). These results indicate promise for treatment-matching approaches that match clients to treatments at the level of personality risk factors for substance misuse (Barlow et al., 2009).

Biological Treatments

In addition to the myriad psychosocial treatments for substance use disorder discussed thus far, numerous biological approaches are also available. For example, some of the available medications block the pleasurable effects of the drug, while others create an aversive reaction when the drug is ingested. We look next at a few commonly used medications in the treatment of various forms of substance use disorder.

Aversive Treatment

One method for treating people with substance use disorders is for the clinician to administer a drug that makes ingestion of the abused substance very unpleasant. This leads to aversive learning and avoidance of the abused substance by the client. The best known example of this type of medication is disulfiram, which is used in the treatment of those with alcohol dependence (Gallant, 1999). Disulfiram prevents the breakdown of a by-product of alcohol—acetaldehyde—if the alcoholic patient should consume alcohol. The resulting buildup of acetaldehyde causes the patient to experience nausea, vomiting, and elevated respiration and heart rate. The usual regimen is to have patients take the medication in the morning, before they are confronted with strong urges to drink (Nathan, 1993). Compliance issues are a major concern with this form of treatment (see Barlow et al., 2009). For these reasons, some of the psychosocial approaches discussed earlier, such as motivational interviewing or behavioral couple therapy, can help clients increase their internal or external motivations to remain compliant with their medication regimen.

Antagonist Treatments

Earlier in this chapter, we discussed how many substances of abuse produce pleasurable effects (e.g., euphoria) through their effects on the brain, such as the dopamine reward system. One form of medication for the treatment of some types of substance use disorder exerts its therapeutic actions by blocking these pleasurable effects; this class of drugs called "antagonists" blocks or cancels out the effects of the substance of abuse (Barlow et al., 2009). A well-known example is the opiate antagonist naltrexone. For example, naltrexone has been investigated in the treatment of alcohol dependence. It prevents alcohol's positive reinforcing effects by blocking the release of dopamine in the nucleus accumbens (O'Malley, 1996; Stewart, Collins, Blackburn, Ellery, & Klein, 2005). It also reduces cravings (Crockford & el-Guebaly, 1998). Laboratory-based research shows that naltrexone blocks alcohol-induced pleasurable stimulation in human participants (Peterson, Conrod, Vassileva, Gianoulakis, & Pihl, 2006). Treatment research suggests that naltrexone can enhance an overall treatment approach to alcoholism that includes psychotherapy (O'Malley et al., 1992). Similarly, when used in the treatment of opiate dependence, naltrexone has only limited success unless it is used in conjunction with a structured treatment program (Goldstein, 1994). In summary, antagonist drugs such as naltrexone help some individuals with substance dependence, assisting them to reduce cravings, and they are best used as an adjunct to effective psychotherapeutic techniques (Barlow et al., 2009).

Agonist Substitution

Another method for treating substance use disorders with medication is to offer the patient a drug that has a similar chemical makeup to the drug of abuse but is safer in terms of its overall negative consequences. This is known as "agonist substitution." Two well-known examples are nicotine replacement therapy in the treatment of cigarette dependence and methadone maintenance therapy in the treatment of opiate dependence. Agonist substitution can be considered a form of "harm reduction" treatment (Roberts & Marlatt, 1999), because it involves trading a more harmful behavior for a much less harmful alternative.

With nicotine replacement therapy for the treatment of cigarette smoking, the addictive drug in the tobacco smoke (nicotine) is provided to the client in the form of gum or a nicotine patch. This can be considered a harm reduction treatment because, although nicotine itself can have harmful effects (e.g., increased blood pressure), the nicotine gum and patch lack the carcinogens contained in cigarette smoke. Moreover, the dose is decreased over time to reduce nicotine withdrawal. Both forms of nicotine replacement therapy have been shown to be successful in helping people quit smoking (Hatsukami et al., 2000; Tiffany, Cox, & Elash, 2000). However, nicotine replacement therapy should be used in combination with a comprehensive psychosocial treatment program, because a substantial proportion of smokers relapse to smoking after they discontinue use of the nicotine gum or patch (Cepeda-Benito, 1993). Recent research suggests that nicotine replacement therapy combined with physical exercise may be beneficial in helping people not only quit smoking but also prevent weight gain following smoking cessation (Prappavessis et al., 2007).

Methadone is an opioid receptor agonist with a relatively long half-life (Eap, Buclin, & Baumann, 2002). Methadone administration is helpful in the treatment of opiate dependence, because high doses alleviate cravings and withdrawal symptoms related to opiate use. Moreover, when people take methadone, cross-tolerance to other opiates develops, so that patients cannot experience euphoria if they administer the opiate of abuse while taking methadone, since methadone already occupies the receptors (Epstein, Renner, Ciraulo, Knapp, & Jaffe, 2005; McKim, 2006). Methadone thus provides negative reinforcement for remaining abstinent (by alleviating aversive opioid withdrawal symptoms) and prevents positive reinforcement (by preventing euphoria if the client uses other opiates while taking the medication; Fulton, 2011). Methadone maintenance therapy is the most widely known and best researched treatment for opiate dependence (Krambeer, von McKnelly, Gabrielli, & Penick, 2001). When methadone is combined with psychotherapy, not only do many clients reduce their use of opiates such as heroin but other harmful effects are also reduced. For example, methadone maintenance treatment is associated with decreased criminality (as patients are not engaging in as much crime to procure drugs) and decreased risk for HIV/AIDS and hepatitis (through reduced exposure to unsafe injection practices; Millson et al., 2007; Murray, 1998). On the negative side, many patients in methadone maintenance treatment continue to abuse other drugs (Fulton, Barrett, Stewart, & MacIssac, 2012). And even if patients do benefit, some remain addicted to methadone for the rest of their lives (O'Brien, 1996). But most professionals agree that this is a positive harm reduction outcome, since methadone, for example, has far fewer negative consequences than heroin (Fulton, 2011).

Other Medications

Pharmacotherapeutic management of withdrawal symptoms may take place during detoxification. For example, a severely alcohol-dependent patient might be administered a benzodiazepine medication during the withdrawal phase to prevent dangerous seizures or to help minimize discomfort (Brown, Anton, Malcolm, & Ballenger, 1988; McCreery & Walker, 1993).

Another medication for the treatment of alcohol dependence that does not readily fall into any of the categories discussed earlier is acamprosate. This medication exerts its therapeutic effects via its impact on the GABA and glutamate neurotransmitter systems (Gordis, 2000). A recent meta-analysis of placebo-controlled trials of the efficacy of acamprosate in the treatment of alcohol dependence showed acamprosate to be superior to placebo in both abstinence rates and cumulative days abstinent (Dranitsaris, Selby, & Negrete, 2009).

Treatment Matching in Pharmacotherapy

While a number of pharmacotherapies are effective in the treatment of substance use disorders, meta-analyses reveal only modest effect sizes for these various approaches (Mann & Hermann, 2010). For example, in the treatment of alcohol dependence, both naltrexone and acamprosate are effective relative to placebo, but both have relatively modest effects overall (Dranitsaris et al., 2009). Some have argued that this may be because these drugs are tested in heterogeneous samples, in which the assumption that "one [treatment] size fits all" is simply untenable (Mann & Hermann, 2010). Researchers in Europe are currently testing the possibility that naltrexone may work best for a subtype of alcoholic that shows greater reactivity to pictures of alcohol cues and carries a specific variant of the mu-opioid receptor gene. In contrast, they propose that magnetic resonance spectroscopy of brain glutamate levels may detect potential acamprosate responders. These exciting hypotheses are currently being tested in a study called Project PREDICT (Mann et al., 2009).

GENERAL PRINCIPLES OF CHANGE
IN TREATMENT OF SUBSTANCE USE DISORDERS

To conclude this chapter, we now consider seven principles of change that emerge from our review of the literature. These are intended to serve as a guide to helping clinicians of different orientations focus on important issues in the treatment of clients with substance use disorder.

First, it is essential to motivate the client to desire to undertake the challenges necessary to overcome his or her substance use disorder (Miller & Rollnick, 2002). For example, a client who attends an assessment session because his wife has been nagging him to go but sees no need himself to change his drug taking habits will need to develop a stronger motivation for change if he is to overcome his substance use problem. Motivational enhancement interventions can be helpful for those undergoing pharmacotherapy for a substance use disorder in terms of motivating clients to stick to the prescribed medication regimen (Miller & Rollnick, 2002).

Second is the importance of challenging expectancies (decreasing positive outcome expectancies and increasing self-efficacy expectancies; Marlatt & Gordon, 1985). For example, a teenage problem drinker needs to develop strong drink refusal self-efficacy expectancies to equip her for dealing with peer pressure to use alcohol. Third, the successful treatment of substance use disorders involves helping clients develop more adaptive coping skills for dealing with their own individual triggers to use substances (Monti et al., 2002). For some, this may involve stress management training, while for others the focus may be on increasing alternative pleasant activities. Fourth, urges should be a target of intervention (Sinha, 2007), either through the use of cue exposure (Monti et al., 2002) or through newer acceptance-based techniques, like training in "urge surfing" (Witkiewitz et al., 2005).

Fifth, there should be recognition of and planning for the high rates of relapse that are so characteristic of the substance use disorders. Specifically, relapse prevention (Marlatt & Gordon, 1985) should be a component of treatment planning to ensure that the inevitable lapse does not progress into a full-scale relapse. Sixth, it is crucial to consider the client's broader social context within the treatment (Stewart & Conrod, 2005). Social support can be directly incorporated into the treatment by involving family members or supportive peers in the therapy (e.g., as in family therapy, behavioral couple treatment, 12-step facilitation) or via recommending that clients in individual treatment garner social support in the recovery process. Social support can be helpful even in pharmacotherapy for substance use disorders, as discussed in relation to having the spouse involved in positively assisting with medication compliance in the behavioral couple therapy approach (Fals-Stewart et al., 2005).

The seventh and final principle of change in the treatment of substance use disorders involves the importance of matching the intervention to the underlying pathway to addiction involved. For example, an anxiety-prone individual who is misusing substances to manage her anxiety has very different treatment needs than a sensation seeker who is misusing substances for the excitement and high he so enjoys. We believe that this principle applies as much to pharmacotherapy selection as to the selection of techniques in psychosocial treatments such as CBT. Just as appropriate matching of client subtypes to treatments (e.g., Conrod, Stewart, et al., 2000; Witkiewitz et al., 2010), has been shown to improve efficacy of psychosocial interventions, efficacious pharmacotherapies for those with substance use disorders are likely to be advanced substantially by a more "personalized medicine" approach in which the specific pathway to addiction is considered in medication selection for a given patient (Mann & Hermann, 2010).

REFERENCES

Abrams, D. B., & Niaura, R. S. (1987). Social learning theory of alcohol use and abuse. In H. Blane & K. Leonard (Eds.), *Psychological theories of drinking and alcoholism* (pp. 131–180). New York: Guilford Press.

Agrawal, A., & Lynskey, M. (2006). The genetic epidemiology of cannabis use, abuse, and dependence: A review. *Addiction, 101,* 801–812.

Alcoholics Anonymous. (1990). *Comments on A.A.'s triennial surveys.* New York: Alcoholics Anonymous World Services.

American Psychiatric Association. (2013). *Diagnostic and statistical manual of mental disorders* (5th ed.). Arlington, VA: Author.

Arkowitz, H., & Westra, H. A. (2004). Motivational interviewing as an adjunct to cognitive behavioral therapy for depression and anxiety. *Journal of Cognitive Psychotherapy, 18,* 337–350.

Bandura, A. (1977). *Social learning theory.* Engelwood Cliffs, NJ: Prentice-Hall.

Barlow, D. H., Durand, V. M., & Stewart, S. H. (2009). *Abnormal psychology: An integrative approach* (2nd ed.). Toronto: Nelson.

Barrett, S., Boileau, I., Okker, J., Pihl, R. O., & Dagher, A. (2004). The hedonic response to cigarette smoking is proportional to dopamine release in the human striatum as measured by positron emission tomography and [^{11}C] raclopride. *Synapse, 54,* 65–71.

Barrett, S., Gross, S., Garand, I., & Pihl, R. O. (2005). Patterns of simultaneous polysubstance use in Canadian rave attendees. *Substance Use and Misuse, 40,* 1525–1538.

Black, J. (2008). Issues for DSM-V: Internet addiction. *American Journal of Psychiatry, 165,* 306–307.

Boileau, I., Assaad, J.-M., Pihl, R. O., Benkelfat, C., Leyton, M., Diksic, M., et al. (2003). Alcohol promotes dopamine release in the human nucleus accumbens. *Synapse, 49,* 226–231.

Boileau, I., Dagher, A., Leyton, M., Gunn, R. N., Baker, G. B., Diksic, M., et al. (2006). Modeling sensitization to stimulants in humans: A [^{11}C]raclopride/PET study in healthy volunteers. *Archives of General Psychiatry, 63,* 1386–1395.

Boileau, I., Dagher, A., Leyton, M., Gunn, R. N., Baker, G. B., Diksic, M., et al. (2007). Conditioned dopamine release in humans: A PET [^{11}C]raclopride/PET study with amphetamine. *Journal of Neuroscience, 27,* 3998–4003.

Brown, M. E., Anton, R. F., Malcolm, R., & Ballenger, J. C. (1988). Alcohol detoxification and withdrawal seizures: Clinical support for a kindling hypothesis. *Biological Psychiatry, 23,* 507–514.

Brunelle, C., & Pihl, R.O. (2007). Effects of conditioned reward and non reward cues on the heart rate response to alcohol intoxication in male social drinkers. *Alcoholism: Clinical and Experimental Research, 31,* 383–389.

Bureau of Justice. (2008). *Prison statistics.* Washington, DC: U.S. Department of Justice.

Burke, B. L., Arkowitz, H., & Melanchola, M. (2003). The efficacy of motivational interviewing:

A meta-analysis of controlled clinical traits. *Journal of Consulting and Clinical Psychology, 71,* 843–861.

Bux, D. A., & Irwin, T. W. (2006). Combining motivational interviewing and cognitive behavioral skills training for the treatment of crystal methamphetamine abuse/dependence. *Journal of Gay and Lesbian Psychotherapy, 10,* 143–152.

Campbell, J. C., Szumlinski, K. K., & Kippin, T. E. (2009). Contribution of early environmental stress to alcoholism vulnerability. *Alcohol, 43,* 547–554.

Carroll, K. M., Fenton, L. R., Ball, S. A., Nich, C., Frankforter, T. L., Shi, J., et al. (2004). Efficacy of disulfiram and cognitive behavior therapy in cocaine dependent outpatients. *Archives of General Psychiatry, 62,* 264–272.

Caspi, A., McClay, J., Moffitt, T., Mill, J., Martin, J., Craig, I., et al. (2002). Role of genotype in the cycle of violence in maltreated children. *Science, 297,* 851–854.

Castellanos, N., & Conrod, P. J. (2006). Brief interventions targeting personality risk factors for adolescent substance misuse reduce depression, panic, and risk-taking behaviors. *Journal of Mental Health, 15,* 645–658.

Cepada-Benito, A. (1993). Meta-analytic review of the efficacy of nicotine chewing gum in smoking treatment programs. *Journal of Consulting and Clinical Psychology, 61,* 822–830.

Christiansen, B. A., Smith, G. T., Roehling, P. V., & Goldman, M. S. (1989). Using alcohol expectancies to predict adolescent drinking behavior after one year. *Journal of Consulting and Clinical Psychology, 57,* 93–99.

Chu, S. Y., Goodwin, M. M., & D'Angelo, D. V. (2010). Physical violence against U. S. women around the time of pregnancy, 2004–2007. *American Journal of Preventive Medicine, 28,* 317–322.

Connor, J. P., George, S. M., Gullo, M. J., Kelly, A. B., & Young, R. M. (2011). A prospective study of alcohol expectancies and self-efficacy as predictors of young adolescent alcohol misuse. *Alcohol and Alcoholism, 46,* 161–169.

Conrod, P., Pihl, R. O., Stewart, S., & Dongier, M. (2000). Validation of a system of classifying female substance abusers on the basis of personality and motivational risk factors for substance abuse. *Psychology of Addictive Behaviors, 14,* 243–256.

Conrod, P. J., Stewart, S. H., Comeau, M. N., & Maclean, M. (2006). Efficacy of cognitive behavioral interventions targeting personality risk factors for youth alcohol misuse. *Journal of Clinical Child and Adolescent Psychology, 35,* 550–563.

Conrod, P. J., Stewart, S. H., Pihl, R. O., Côté, S., Fontaine, V., & Dongier, M. (2000). Efficacy of brief coping skills interventions that match different personality profiles of female substance abusers. *Psychology of Addictive Behaviors, 14,* 231–242.

Crockford, D. N., & el-Guebaly, N. (1998). Psychiatric comorbidity in pathological gambling: A critical review. *Canadian Journal of Psychiatry, 43,* 43–50.

Darkes, J., & Goldman, M. S. (1993). Expectancy challenge and drinking reduction: Experimental evidence for a meditational process. *Journal of Consulting and Clinical Psychology, 61,* 344–353.

Darredeau, C., Barrett, S., Jardin, B., & Pihl, R.O. (2007). Patterns and predictors of medication compliance, diversion, and misuse in adult prescribed methylphenidate users. *Human Psychopharmacology: Clinical and Experimental, 22,* 529–536.

Donovan, D. M., Kadden, R. M., DiClemente, C. C., & Carroll, K. M. (2002). Client satisfaction with three therapies in the treatment of alcohol dependence: Results from Project MATCH. *American Journal on Addiction, 11,* 291–307.

Dranitsaris, G., Selby, P., & Negrete, J. C. (2009). Meta-analyses of placebo-controlled trials of acamprosate for the treatment of alcohol dependence: Impact of the combined pharmacotherapies and behavior interventions study. *Journal of Addiction Medicine, 3,* 74–82.

Dunn, M. E., & Yniguez, R. M. (1999). Experimental demonstration of the influence of alcohol advertising on the activation of alcohol expectancies in memory among fourth- and fifth-grade children. *Experimental and Clinical Psychopharmacology, 7,* 473–483.

Eap, C. B., Buclin, T., & Baumann, P. (2002). Interindividual variability of clinical pharmacokinetics of methadone: Implications for the treatment of opioid dependence, *Clinical Pharmacokinetics, 41*, 1153–1193.

Edenberg, H., & Foround, T. (2006). The genetics of alcoholism: Identifying specific genes through family studies. *Biology, 11*, 386–396.

Emrick, C. D., Tonigan, J. S., Montgomery, H., & Little, L. (1993). Alcoholics Anonymous: What is currently known? In B. S. McCrady & W. R. Miller (Eds.), *Research on Alcoholics Anonymous: Opportunities and alternatives* (pp. 41–76). New Brunswick, NJ: Rutgers Center of Alcohol Studies.

Engle, D. E., & Arkowitz, H. (2006). *Ambivalence in psychotherapy: Facilitating readiness to change.* New York: Guilford Press.

Epstein, S., Renner, J. A., Ciraulo, D. A., Knapp, C. M., & Jaffe, J. H. (2005). Opioids. In H. R. Kranzler & D. A. Ciraulo (Eds.), *Clinical manual of addiction psychopharmacology* (pp. 55–110). Arlington, VA: American Psychiatric Publishing, Inc.

Falk, D., Hsiao-Ye, Y., & Hiller-Sturmhöfel, S. (2008). An epidemiological analysis of co-occurring alcohol and drug use and disorders: Findings from the National Epidemiologic Survey of Alcohol and Related Conditions (NESARC). *Alcoholism Research and Health, 31*, 100–110.

Fals-Stewart, W., O'Farrell, T. J., Birchler, G. R., Cordova, J., & Kelley, M. L. (2005). Behavioral couples therapy for alcoholism and drug abuse: Where we've been, where we are, and where we're going. *Journal of Cognitive Psychotherapy, 19*, 229–246.

Feldman-Barrett, L., & Wager, T. (2006). The structure of emotion. *Current Directions in Psychological Science, 15*, 79–83.

Ferguson, D., Boden, J., & Harwood, J. (2009). Tests of causal links between alcohol abuse or dependence and major depression. *Archives of General Psychiatry, 66*, 260–266.

Finney, J. W., & Monahan, S. C. (1996). The cost-effectiveness of treatment for alcoholism: A second approximation. *Journal of Studies on Alcohol, 57*, 229–243.

Fromme, K., Stroot, E., & Kaplan, D. (1993). Comprehensive effects of alcohol: Development and psychometric assessment of a new expectancy questionnaire. *Psychological Assessment, 5*, 19–26.

Fulton, H. G. (2011). *Substance use and psychiatric characteristics of prescription opioid users in a low-threshold methadone maintenance treatment program in Nova Scotia.* Unpublished doctoral dissertation, Dalhousie University, Halifax, Canada.

Fulton, H. G., Barrett, S. P., Stewart, S. H., & MacIsaac, C. (2012). Prescription opioid misuse: Characteristics of earliest and most recent memory of hydromorphone use. *Journal of Addiction Medicine, 6*, 137–144.

Gallant, D. (1999). Alcohol. In M. Gallanter & H. D. Kleber (Eds.), *Textbook of substance abuse treatment* (2nd ed., pp. 151–164). Washington, DC: American Psychiatric Press.

Glahn, D., Lovallo, W., & Fox, P. (2007). Reduced amygdala activation in young adults at high risk of alcoholism: Studies from the Oklahoma Family Health Patterns Project. *Biological Psychiatry, 61*, 1306–1309.

Goldstein, A. (1994). *Addiction: From biology to drug policy.* New York: Freeman.

Gonzalez, V. M., Schmitz, J. M., & DeLaune, K. A. (2006). The role of homework in cognitive-behavioral therapy for cocaine dependence. *Journal of Consulting and Clinical Psychology, 74*, 633–637.

Gordis, E. (2000). Research refines alcohol treatment options. *Alcohol Research and Health, 24*, 53–61.

Greeley, J., & Oei, T. (1999). Alcohol and tension reduction. In K. E. Leonard & H. T. Blane, (Eds), *Psychological theories of drinking and alcoholism* (2nd ed., pp. 14–53). New York: Guilford Press.

Hall, S. M., Munoz, R. F., & Reus, V. I. (1994). Cognitive-behavioral intervention increases abstinence rates for depressive-history smokers. *Journal of Consulting and Clinical Psychology, 62*, 141–146.

Harvard School of Medicine. (2005). National Comorbidity Survey (NCS) and National Comorbidity Survey Replication (NCS-R). Retrieved June 9, 2009, from *www.hcp.med.harvard.edu/ncs/index.php*.

Hasin, D., Stinson, F., Ogburn, E., & Grant, B. (2007). Prevalence, correlates, disability, and comorbidity of DSM-IV alcohol abuse and dependence in the United States. *Archives of General Psychiatry, 64*, 830–842.

Hatsukami, D. K., Grillo, M., Boyle, R., Allen, S., Jensen, J., Bliss, R., et al. (2000). Treatment of spit tobacco users with transdermal nicotine system and mint snuff. *Journal of Consulting and Clinical Psychology, 68*, 241–249.

Heitzig, M., Nigg, J., Yau, W., Zubita, J., & Zucker, R. (2008). Affective circuitry and risk for alcoholism in late adolescence: Differences in fronto striatal responses between vulnerable and resilient children of alcoholic parents. *Alcoholism: Clinical and Experimental Research, 32*, 414–426.

Helzer, J., & Prysbeck, T. (1988). The occurrence of alcoholism with other psychiatric disorders in the general population and its impact on treatment. *Journal of Studies on Alcohol, 49*, 219–224.

Hughes, A., Sathe, N., & Spagnola, K. (2009). *State estimates of substance use from the 2006–2007 National Surveys on Drug Use and Health* (NSDUH Series H-35, HHS Publication No. SMA 09–4362). Rockville, MD: Office of Applied Studies, Substance Abuse and Mental Health Services Administration.

Johnson, C., Drgon, T., Liu, Q.-R., Walther, D., Edenberg, H., Rice, J., et al. (2006). Pooled association genome scanning for alcohol dependence using 104,268 SNPs: Validation and use to identify alcoholism vulnerability loci in unrelated individuals from the collaborative study on the genetics of alcoholism. *American Journal of Medical Genetics B: Neuropsychiatric Genetics, 141*, 844–853.

Joseph, D. V., Jackson, J. A., Westaway, J., Taub, N. A., Petersen, S. A., & Wailoo, M. P. (2007). Effect of parental smoking on cotinine levels in newborns. *Archives of Disease in Childhood: Fetal and Neonatal Edition, 92*, F484–F488.

Kaminer, Y., & Slesnick, N. (2006). Evidence-based cognitive-behavioral and family therapies for adolescent alcohol and other substance use disorders. In M. Galanter (Ed.), *Alcohol problems in adolescents and young adults: Epidemiology, neurobiology, prevention, and treatment* (pp. 383–405). New York: Springer.

Kendler, K. (2001). Twin studies of psychiatric illness. *Archives of General Psychiatry, 58*, 1005–1014.

Kessler, R.C., McGonagle, A., Zhao, S., Nelson, C.B., Hughes, M., Eshleman, S., et al. (1994). Lifetime and 12–month prevalence of DSM-III-R psychiatric disorders in the United States: Results from the National Comorbidity Survey. *Archives of General Psychiatry, 51*, 8–19.

Knight, J., Wechsler, H., Kuo, M., Seibring, M., Weitzman, E., & Schuckit, M. (2002). Alcohol abuse and dependence among U.S. college students. *Journal of Studies on Alcohol, 63*, 263–270.

Krambeer, L. L., von McKnelly, W., Jr., Gabrielli, W. R., Jr., & Penick, E. C. (2001). Methadone therapy for opioid dependence. *American Family Physician, 15*, 2404–2410.

Lataster, J., Collip, D., Ceccarini, J., Haas, D., Booij, L., van Os, J., et al. (2011). Psychosocial stress is associated with in vivo dopamine release in human ventromedial prefrontal cortex: A positron emission tomography study using [^{18}F]fallypride. *NeuroImage, 58*, 1081–1089.

Leonard, K. E., & Homish, G. G. (2008). Predictors of heavy drinking and drinking problems over the first 4 years of marriage. *Psychology of Addictive Behaviors, 22*, 25–35.

Leyton, M. (2007). Conditioned and sensitized responses to stimulant drugs in humans. *Progress in Neuropsychopharmacology and Biological Psychiatry, 31*, 1601–1613.

MacAndrew, C., & Edgerton, R. (1969). *Drunken comportment: A social explanation.* Chicago: Aldine.

Maisto, S., Carey, K., Bradizza, C. (1999). Social learning theory. In K. Leonard & H. Blane (Eds.),

Psychological theories of drinking and alcoholism (2nd ed., pp. 106–163). New York: Guilford Press.

Mann, K., & Hermann, D. (2010). Individualized treatment in alcohol dependent patients. *European Archives of Psychiatry and Clinical Neuroscience, 260*(Suppl. 2), S116–S120.

Mann, K., Kiefer, F., Smolka, M., Gann, H., Wellek, S., Heinz, A., & the PREDICT Study Research Team. (2009). Searching for responders to acamprosate and naltrexone in alcoholism treatment: Rationale and design of the Predict Study. *Alcoholism: Clinical and Experimental Research, 33,* 674–683.

Marlatt, G. A., & Gordon, J. R. (Eds.). (1985). *Relapse prevention.* New York: Guilford Press.

Marlatt, G. A., Larimer, M. E., Baer, J. S., & Quigley, L. A. (1993). Harm reduction for alcohol problems: Moving beyond the controlled drinking controversy. *Behavior Therapy, 24,* 461–504.

McCreery, J. M., & Walker, R. D. (1993). Alcohol problems. In D. L. Dunner (Ed.), *Current psychiatric therapy* (pp. 92–98). Philadelphia: Saunders.

McKim, W. A. (2006). *Drugs and behavior: An introduction to behavioral pharmacology* (6th ed.). Upper Saddle River, NJ: Pearson/Prentice-Hall.

McKnight-Eily, L. R., Eaton, D. K., Lowry, R., Croft, J. B., Presley-Cantrell, L., & Perry, G. S. (2011). Relationships between hours of sleep and health risk behaviors in US adolescent students. *Preventive Medicine, 53,* 271–273.

Meyers, R., Villanueva, M., & Smith, J. E. (2005). The community reinforcement approach: History and empirical justification. *Journal of Cognitive Psychotherapy, 19*(3), 247–260.

Miller, P. M., Smith, G. T., & Goldman, M. S. (1990). Emergence of alcohol expectancies in childhood: A possible critical period. *Journal of Studies on Alcohol, 51,* 343–349.

Miller, W. R. (1985). Motivation for treatment: A review with special emphasis on alcoholism. *Psychological Bulletin, 119,* 322–348.

Miller, W. R., & Rollnick, S. (1991). *Motivational interviewing: Preparing people for change.* New York: Guilford Press.

Miller, W. R., & Rollnick, S. (2002). *Motivational interviewing: Preparing people for change* (2nd ed.). New York: Guilford Press.

Millson, P., Challacombe, L., Villeneuve, P. J., Strike, C. J., Fischer, B., Myers, T., et al. (2007). Reduction in the injection-related HIV risk after 6 months in a low-threshold methadone treatment program. *AIDS Education and Prevention, 19,* 124–136.

Monti, P. M., Kadden, R. M., Rohsenow, D. J., Cooney, N. L., & Abrams, D. B. (2002). *Treating alcohol dependence: A coping skills training guide* (2nd ed.). New York: Guilford Press.

Morgan, H. W. (1981). *Drugs in America: A social history, 1800–1980.* Syracuse, NY: Syracuse University Press.

Mueser, K. T., Drake, R. E., & Wallach, M. A. (1998). Dual diagnosis: A review of etiological theories. *Addictive Behaviors, 23*(6), 717–734.

Murdoch, D., Pihl, R. O., & Ross, D. (1990). Alcohol and crimes of violence: Present issues. *International Journal of Addictions, 25,* 1059–1075.

Murray, J. B. (1998). Effectiveness of methadone maintenance for heroin addiction. *Psychological Reports, 83,* 295–302.

Nathan, P. E. (1993). Alcoholism: Psychopathology, etiology, and treatment. In P. B. Sutker & H. E. Adams (Eds.), *Comprehensive handbook of psychopathology* (pp. 451–476). New York: Plenum.

O'Brien, C. P. (1996). Recent developments in the pharmacotherapy of substance abuse. *Journal of Consulting and Clinical Psychology, 64,* 677–686.

O'Connor, R. M., & Stewart, S. H. (2010). Substance use disorders. In D. McKay, J. S. Abramowitz, & S. Taylor (Eds.), *Cognitive-behavioral therapy for refractory cases: Turning failure into success* (pp. 211–229). Washington, DC: American Psychological Association.

Oei, T. P. S., Lim, B., & Young, R. M. (1991). Cognitive processes and cognitive behavior therapy in the treatment of problem drinking. *Journal of Addictive Disorders, 10,* 63–80.

O'Malley, S. S. (1996). Opioid antagonists in the treatment of alcohol dependence: Clinical efficacy and prevention of relapse. *Alcohol and Alcoholism, 31*(Suppl. 1), 77–81.

O'Malley, S. S., Jaffe, A. J., Chang, G., Schottenfeld, R. S., Meyer, R. E., & Rounsaville, B. (1992). Naltrexone and coping skills therapy for alcohol dependence: A controlled study. *Archives of General Psychiatry, 49,* 881–887.

Ornish, D., Magbama, M., Weidner, G., Weinberg, V., Kemp, C., Green, C., et al. (2008). Changes in prostate gene expression in men undergoing an intensive nutrition and lifestyle intervention. *Proceedings of the National Academy of Sciences, 105,* 8369–8374.

Ouimette, P. C., Finney, J. W., & Moos, R. H. (1997). Twelve-step and cognitive-behavioral treatment for substance abuse: A comparison of treatment effectiveness. *Journal of Consulting and Clinical Psychology, 65,* 230–240.

Peterson, J. B., Conrod, P. J., Vassileva, J., Gianoulakis, C., & Pihl, R. O. (2006). Differential effects of naltrexone on cardiac, subjective, and behavioral reactions to acute ethanol intoxication. *Journal of Psychiatry and Neuroscience, 31,* 386–393.

Pihl, R. O. (2010). Mental disorders are brain disorders: You think? *Canadian Psychologist, 51*(1), 40–49.

Pleis, J. R., & Lethbridge-Cejku, M. (2007). Summary health statistics for U.S. adults: National Health Interview Survey, 2006. *Vital and health statistics: Series 10. Data from the National Health Survey, 235,* 1–153.

Pomerleau, O. F., Fagerstrom, K. O., Marks, J. L., Tate, J. C., & Pomerleau, C. S. (2003). Development and validation of a self-rating scale for positive and negative reinforcement smoking: The Michigan Nicotine Reinforcement Questionnaire. *Nicotine and Tobacco Research, 5,* 711–718.

Potenza, M. N. (2001). The neurobiology of pathological gambling. *Seminars in Clinical Neuropsychiatry, 6,* 217–226.

Prappavessis, H., Cameron, L., Baldi, J. C., Robinson, S., Borrie, K., Harper, T., et al. (2007). The effects of exercise and nicotine replacement therapy on smoking rates in women. *Addictive Behaviors, 32,* 1416–1432.

Preuss, U. W., Koller, G., Barnow, S., Eikmeier, M., & Soyka, M. (2006). Suicidal behavior in alcohol dependent subjects: The role of personality disorders. *Alcoholism: Clinical and Experimental Research, 30,* 866–877.

Price, S. R., Hilchey, C. A., Darredeau, C., Fulton, H. G., & Barrett, S. P. (2010). Energy drink co-administration is associated with increased reported alcohol ingestion. *Drug and Alcohol Review, 29,* 331–333.

Prochaska, J. O., & DiClemente, C. C. (1992). The transtheoretical approach. In J. C. Norcross, & M. R. Goldfried (Eds.), *Handbook of psychotherapy integration* (pp. 300–334). New York: Basic Books.

Prochaska, J. O., DiClemente, C. C., & Norcross, J. C. (1997). In search of how people change: Applications to addictive behaviors. In G. A. Marlatt, & G. R. VandenBos (Eds.), *Addictive behaviors: Readings on etiology, prevention, and treatment* (pp. 671–696). Washington, DC: American Psychological Association.

Project MATCH Research Group. (1997). Matching alcoholism treatments to client heterogeneity: Project MATCH post-treatment drinking outcomes. *Journal of Studies on Alcohol, 58,* 7–29.

Project MATCH Research Group. (1998). Matching alcoholism treatments to client heterogeneity: Treatment main effects and matching effects on drinking during treatment. *Journal of Studies on Alcohol, 59,* 631–639.

Quinn, P. D., & Fromme, K. (2010). Self-regulation as a protective factor against risky drinking and sexual behavior. *Psychology of Addictive Behaviors, 24,* 376–385.

Rawson, R. A., Gonzales, R., & Brethen, P. (2002). Treatment of methamphetamine use disorders: An update. *Journal of Substance Abuse Treatment, 23,* 145–150.

Regier, D., Farmer, M., Rae, D., Locke, B., Keith, S., Judd, L., et al. (1990). Co-morbidity of mental disorders with alcohol and other drug abuse: Results from the Epidemiologic Catchment Area Study. *Journal of the American Medical Association, 264,* 2511–2518.

Reinarman, C. (2005). Between genes and addiction: A critique of genetic determinism. *Drugs and Alcohol Today, 5,* 32–33.

Roberts, L. J., & Marlatt, G. A. (1999). Harm reduction. In P. J. Ott & R. E. Tarter (Eds.), *Sourcebook on substance abuse: Etiology, epidemiology, assessment, and treatment* (pp. 389–398). Needham Heights, MA: Allyn & Bacon.

Room, R., Babor, T., & Rehm, J. (2005). Alcohol and public health. *Lancet, 365,* 519–530.

Sabourin, B. C., & Stewart, S. H. (2009). Patterns of depression–substance use disorder comorbidity in women seeking addictions treatment. In J. Gallivan & S. Cooper (Eds.), *Pathways, bridges, and havens: Psychosocial determinants of women's health* (pp. 160–177). Sydney, NS, Canada: Cape Breton University Press.

Saunders, J., Schuckit, M., Sirovatka, P., & Regier, D. (Eds.). (2007). *Diagnostic issues in substance use disorders: Refining the research agenda for DSM-V.* Arlington, VA: American Psychiatric Association.

Sher, K. J., Jackson, K. M., & Steinley, D. A. (2011). Alcohol use trajectories and the ubiquitous cat's cradle: Cause for concern? *Journal of Abnormal Psychology, 120,* 322–335.

Sinha, R. (2007). Imaging stress- and cue-induced drug and alcohol craving: Association with relapse and clinical implications. *Drug and Alcohol Review, 26,* 25–31.

Sobell, M. B., & Sobell, L. C. (1993). *Problem drinkers: Guided self-change.* New York: Guilford Press.

Stewart, S. H., Collins, P., Blackburn, J. R., Ellery, M., & Klein, R. N. (2005). Heart rate increase to alcohol administration and video lottery terminal (VLT) play. *Psychology of Addictive Behaviors, 19,* 94–98.

Stewart, S. H., & Conrod, P. J. (2005). State of the art in cognitive-behavioral interventions for substance use disorders: Introduction to the special issue. *Journal of Cognitive Psychotherapy, 19,* 195–198.

Stewart, S., Karp, J., Pihl, R., & Peterson, R. (1997). Anxiety sensitivity and self-reported reasons for drug use. *Journal of Substance Abuse, 9,* 223–240.

Stewart, S., & Pihl, R.O. (1994). Effects of alcohol administration on psychophysiological and subjective–emotional responses to aversive stimulation in anxiety sensitive women. *Psychology of Addictive Behaviors 8,* 29–42.

Stinson, F., Ruan, W., Pickering, R., & Grant, B. (2006). Cannabis use disorders in the USA: Prevalence, correlates, and co-morbidity. *Psychological Medicine, 36,* 1447–1460.

Swindle, R. W., Peterson, K. A., Paradise, M. J., & Moos, R. H. (1995). Measuring substance abuse program treatment orientations: The Drug and Alcohol Program Treatment Inventory. *Journal of Substance Abuse, 7,* 61–78.

Testa, M., Fillmore, M. T., Norris, J., Abbey, A., Curtin, J. J., Leonard, K. E., et al. (2006). Understanding alcohol expectancy effects: Revisiting the placebo condition. *Alcoholism: Clinical and Experimental Research, 30,* 339–348.

Tiffany, S. T., Cox, L. S., & Elash, C. A. (2000). Effects of transdermal nicotine patches on abstinence-induced and cue-elicited craving in cigarette smokers. *Journal of Consulting and Clinical Psychology, 68,* 233–240.

Tsuang, M., Lyons, M., Meyer, J., Doyle, T., Eisen, S., Goldberg, J., et al. (1998). Co-occurrence of abuse of different drugs in men: The role of drug-specific and shared vulnerabilities. *Archives of General Psychiatry, 55,* 967–972.

Tyndale, R. F. (2003). Genetics of alcohol and tobacco use in humans. *Annals of Medicine, 35,* 94–121.

Valdivia, I., & Stewart, S. H. (2005). A further examination of the psychometric properties of the Comprehensive Effects of Alcohol Questionnaire. *Cognitive Behaviour Therapy, 34,* 22–33.

Volkow, N. D. (2011, October). *The brain and dual diagnosis* [Keynote lecture at the II International

Congress of Dual Disorders: Addictive Behaviors and Other Mental Disorders], Barcelona, Spain.

Volkow, N. D., & Swanson, J. M. (2003). Variables that affect the clinical use and abuse of Ritalin in the treatment of ADHD. *American Journal of Psychiatry, 160,* 1909–1918.

Volkow, N. D., Wang, G.-J., Telang, F., Fowler, J. S., Logan, J., Childress, A.-R., et al. (2006). Cocaine cues and dopamine in dorsal striatum: Mechanism of craving in cocaine addiction. *Journal of Neuroscience, 26,* 6583–6588.

Walitzer, K. S., Dermen, K. H., & Connors, G. J. (1999). Strategies for preparing clients for treatment. *Behavior Modification, 23,* 129–151.

Walsh, T., McClellan, J. M., McCarthy, S. E., Addington, A. M., Pierce, S. B., Cooper, G. M., et al. (2008). Rare structural variants disrupt multiple genes in neurodevelopmental pathways in schizophrenia. *Science, 25*(5875), 539–543.

Wang, B., You, Z.-B., Rice, K. C., & Wise, R. A. (2007). Stress-induced relapse to cocaine seeking: Roles for the CRF2 receptor and CRF-binding protein in the vental tegmental area of the rat. *Psychopharmacology, 193,* 283–294.

Westra, H. A., & Dozois, D. J. A. (2006). Preparing clients for cognitive behavioral therapy: A randomized pilot study of motivational interviewing for anxiety. *Cognitive Therapy and Research, 30,* 481–498.

Witkiewitz, K., Hartzler, B., & Donovan, D. (2010). Matching motivation enhancement treatment to client motivation: Re-examining the motivation matching hypothesis. *Addiction, 105,* 1403–1413.

Witkiewitz, K., Marlatt, G. A., & Walker, D. (2005). Mindfulness-based relapse prevention for alcohol and substance use disorders. *Journal of Cognitive Psychotherapy, 19,* 211–228.

CHAPTER 9

Personality Disorders

Jeffrey J. Magnavita
Abigail D. Powers
Jacques P. Barber
Thomas F. Oltmanns

S uccessful interactions with other people are governed by a variety of psychological mechanisms and adaptive patterns that, taken together, constitute our
personalities. "Personality" refers to enduring patterns of thinking, feeling, perception, and behavior that define the person and distinguish him or her from other
people. Included in these patterns are preferred ways of expressing or not expressing emotion, as well as patterns of thinking about ourselves and other people. In
healthy individuals, there is a balance between self and other functions, and difficulties may ensue when these are not in balance. When repetitive maladaptive patterns bring the person into repeated conflict with others, when they prevent the person from forming attachments or maintaining close relationships with others, and
when they interfere with establishing and pursuing reasonable personal goals, an
individual's personality may be considered disordered. Personality disorders (PDs)
represent a wide spectrum of maladaptive styles of perceiving, relating to, and feeling and thinking about the world. Because of these problems, PDs are among the
most ubiquitous and disruptive forms of psychopathology.

Our goal in this chapter is to provide a review of general knowledge on PDs
and to highlight important considerations in the treatment of individuals with PDs.
First, we discuss common features of PDs and outline how such features may operate differently across the disorders. We then address classification issues related to
PDs, including how PDs relate to normal personality traits, and what factors may

275

affect conceptualization and diagnosis of these disorders. We also review epidemiological and general etiology factors related to PDs. Finally, we conclude with a perspective on what basic and applied research is still needed to enhance our understanding of and ability to treat individuals with PD. We consider treatment implications throughout the chapter. Because it is impossible exhaustively to cover the diverse treatment implications for all PDs in a single chapter, we focus particularly on general principles of therapeutic change that cut across all theoretical orientations and can be applied differentially in the treatment of any individual with personality pathology.

TYPICAL SYMPTOMS AND ASSOCIATED FEATURES

The dividing line between trait disturbances, or subsyndromal presentations, that might not meet diagnostic threshold and personality pathology is difficult to identify. We all have our quirks and idiosyncrasies, and there are many different ways to manage relationships with other people. For example, it is often helpful to be skeptical of the things other people do and say. When does a tendency to be suspicious of other people's motives cross the line into being a characteristic of paranoid PD and, beyond that, when does the problem actually meet criteria for delusional disorder? Self-confidence is another admirable quality, but it can lead to problems if it escalates into full-blown grandiosity. The capacities necessary to maintain a realistic and stable sense of self include multiple domain areas, such as perception, cognition, affective regulation, and defensive style. In many ways, the distinctions among healthy traits, eccentricity, and personality pathology are contextual and depend on the person's ability to adapt to the demands of different situations. Part of that ability to adapt relies on a stable self-identity, one that can remain relatively intact regardless of the changing demands of the environment. Variety and flexibility in interpersonal behavior are also undoubtedly helpful. One's capacity to handle stress and regulate his or her emotions in the face of difficult experiences is important. These are all areas in which people with personality dysfunction may show impairment; they often make their own social problems worse (often unwittingly) by persistently responding in ways that do not suit the social challenges that they face.

Most forms of mental disorder, such as anxiety disorders and mood disorders, are "ego-dystonic"; that is, people with these disorders are distressed by their symptoms and uncomfortable with their situations. PDs, however, are usually "ego-syntonic." Often individuals with PDs have developed a familiarity with their patterns of dysfunction, which are not associated with distress or anxiety. Instead, they feel like familiar modes of behaving and relating, as if they are accepted as part of the self. Some clinicians would argue that these individuals do not have *insight* into the nature of their own problems, that they have a difficult time understanding the perspective of others and are not capable of "mentalization" (or the ability to understand the mental state of self or others) (Fonagy, 2004) in more severe presentations. In many cases, those with PDs create distress in those with whom they have close relationships, such as family, peers, and coworkers. In other words, externalization is a common defense; when trouble occurs, the person with a PD usually blames it on others and often is not distressed him- or herself.

The specific symptoms that define PDs represent maladaptive variations in several of the important domains of personality. These include motives, perceptual processes, affective–cognitive schemas regarding the self and others, attachment patterns, temperament, and defensive organization. We have organized our description of typical symptoms around these issues, which run through the broad mixture of specific symptoms that define different types of personality pathology.

Social Motivation

The concept of a "motive" refers to a person's desires and goals (Emmons, 1997). Motives (either conscious or unconscious) describe the way people would like things to be, and they help to explain *why* people behave in a particular fashion. For example, a man might have neglected to return a telephone call because he wanted to be alone (rather than because he forgot that someone had called). Two useful constructs in understanding human personality are "affiliation"—the desire for close relationships with other people—and "power"—the desire for impact, prestige, or dominance (Winter, John, Stewart, Klohnen, & Duncan, 1998). Individual differences with regard to these motives have an important influence on a person's general health and adjustment.

Many of the symptoms of personality pathology can be described in terms of maladaptive variations with regard to needs for affiliation and power. One particularly important issue is the absence of motivation for affiliation. The need for intimacy and closeness is based on our evolutionarily adapted need to maintain attachment to our caregivers. Humans are relational at their core (Bowlby, 1969). However, while most people enjoy spending time with other people and want to develop intimate relationships with friends and family members, some people do not. Some patients with PD prefer isolation or are so anxious that they are not able to act on their longings. Severely diminished or absent motivation for social relationships is another pervasive theme that serves to define certain kinds of PD.

Exaggerated motivation for power (and achievement) also contributes to the picture that describes some PDs. For example, some people are preoccupied with a need for admiration and the praise of others, called "narcissism." They think of themselves as privileged people and insist on special treatment. In other cases, excessive devotion to work and professional accomplishment can lead some individuals to ignore friends and family members, as well as the pursuit of leisure activities. This lack of balance can have a serious disruptive effect on the person's social adjustment.

Cognitive Perspectives Regarding Self and Others

Our social world also depends on mental processes that determine knowledge of ourselves and other people (Wilson, 2009). Distortions of these mechanisms are associated with PDs. One central issue involves our image of ourselves. When we are able to maintain a realistic and stable image of ourselves, we can plan, negotiate, and evaluate our relationships with other people. Knowing (and having confidence in) our own values and opinions is a necessary prerequisite for making independent decisions without the assistance or reassurance of others. Self-image is also intimately connected to mood states. If we vacillate between unrealistically positive and negative views of ourselves, our moods will swing dramatically. We may also need constant reassurance from others and be too dependent on their opinions as a means of maintaining our own self-esteem. We have to be able to evaluate our own importance. Of course, it is useful to think of ourselves in positive terms (and many maintain a positive "halo"), but extreme grandiosity can be disruptive. Perhaps even more damaging is a pattern in which people see themselves as socially inept or inferior to other people.

Another issue involves our image of others. When we misperceive the intentions, motives, or abilities of other people, our relationships can be severely disturbed. Paranoid beliefs are one example. Some people believe, without good reason, that others are exploiting, deceiving, or otherwise trying to harm them. Unreasonable fears of being abandoned, criticized, or rejected are also examples of distorted perception of others' intentions. Working effectively in a group of people also requires realistic appraisal of the talents and abilities of others. In order to cooperate with other people, we must be able to appreciate their competence. Those with PDs often run into problems, because they misperceive other people in varied ways (as being threatening or uncaring, or incompetent). These perceptual distortions are often derived from internal schema that might include beliefs encoded from earlier developmental experiences, such as "The world is unsafe" or "I am bad"; these beliefs and self–other representations are then used as pattern recognition tools for current relationships (Beck, Freeman, & Davies, 2004; Summers & Barber, 2009; Westen & Cohen, 1993).

Many elements of social interaction also depend on being able to appraise the nature of our relationships with other people, then to make accurate judgments about appropriate and inappropriate behaviors. The many aspects involved include the ability to interpret facial emotion, to hear the nuance of tone and prosody of speech, and generally to pick up on the emotional tenor being communicated. For example, a successful relationship with a sexual partner involves knowing when intimacy is expected and when it should be avoided. This capacity to manage the elements of self–other relationships and regulate the need for intimacy and autonomy is a critical function of an adaptive personality system (Magnavita, 2004). Those with PDs often have persistent problems in regulating social distance (either becoming too intimate or maintaining too much distance from others). Finally, another important element of interpersonal perception is the ability to "empathize" with others—to anticipate and decipher their emotional reactions and use that knowledge to guide our own behavior (Gallese, Keysers, & Rizzolatti, 2004). Deficits in the ability to understand the emotions of other people represent another of the core features of many PDs.

Temperament and Personality Traits

If motivation helps to explain *why* people behave in certain ways, temperament and personality traits describe *how* they behave. "Temperament" refers to a person's most basic, neurobiologically endowed, characteristic styles of relating to the world, especially those styles that are evident during the first year of life (e.g., Caspi & Roberts, 1999). Definitions of temperament typically include dimensions such as activity level and emotional reactivity. These factors vary considerably in level or degree from one infant to the next and have important implications for later development, such as social and academic adjustment when the child eventually enters school. For example, children who demonstrate a "lack of control" when they are very young are much more likely than their peers to experience problems with hyperactivity, distractibility, and conduct disorder when they are adolescents (Cohen, Crawford, Johnson, & Kasen, 2005). Young children who are extremely shy are more likely to be anxious and socially inhibited in subsequent years (Eisenberg et al., 1998).

Experts disagree about the basic dimensions of temperament and personality. Some theories are relatively simple, using only three or four dimensions. Others are more complicated and consider as many as 30 or 40 traits. One theory that has come to be widely accepted is known as the five-factor model (FFM) of personality (e.g., Trull & Widiger, 2008). The basic traits (also known as "domains") included in this model are Neuroticism, Extraversion, Openness to Experience, Agreeableness, and Conscientiousness. We return to consider these domains and specific "facets" of personality when we discuss dimensional perspectives on classification later in this chapter. Taken as a whole, the FFM provides a relatively comprehensive description of any person's behavior.

Defensive Organization

Another important aspect of personality pathology is the constellation of "defense mechanisms" that each patient uses. These mechanisms refer to mental strategies that the person employs, typically without awareness, often to cope with reality and to maintain a positive view of the self, and to prevent the experience of anxiety or distress. While these styles of perceiving and thinking about challenging events and interpersonal crises have typically been given more emphasis by clinicians working within a psychodynamic tradition, they do describe important styles that provide a valuable perspective for all therapists and investigators (Paulhus, Fridhandler, & Hayes, 1997).

Defenses are viewed as being unique to the person, even among those who fit the overall criteria for the various PDs described later in the chapter. They presumably represent the basic molecules of adaptive patterns. As many clinicians have observed in the context of therapy, each individual has a unique constellation of defenses, and those constellations can change when the individual faces considerable stress (Magnavita, 1997). For example, an individual with an obsessive–compulsive personality might use isolation of affect, intellectualization, rationalization, and repression of emotions. Under high stress, where the system is challenged, this person may revert to previous patterns of behavior that include explosive affect, withdrawal, and obsessive and ruminative thinking. The construct of defense has considerable empirical support (Cramer, 2008; Soldz & Vaillant, 1998; Perry et al., 1998). For example, in a review of social psychology research related to defense mechanisms, Baumeister, Dale, and Sommer (1998) found ample research evidence to suggest that individuals use a number of defenses in daily life, including reaction formation, projection, isolation, and denial. Although there are many ways of describing and organizing different forms of defense, one popular model arranges them into four categories, beginning with the most primitive: (1) psychotic, (2) immature, (3) neurotic, and (4) mature (Vaillant, 1995, 2000). The consideration of defenses can allow researchers and clinicians to attain a more nuanced profile that goes beyond the relatively simple consideration of lists of symptoms that define each specific type of personality pathology.

Disturbance in Interpersonal Functioning

The concept of social dysfunction plays an important role in the definition of PDs, as well as in their assessment (Bender, Morey, & Skodol, 2011). Subjective distress and social impairment provide a large part of the justification for defining these problems as mental disorders. If the maladaptive personality characteristics described in the diagnostic manual interfere with a person's ability to get along with other people and perform social roles, they become more than just a collection of eccentric traits or peculiar habits. They can then be viewed as a form of harmful dysfunction (Kendell, 2002; Wakefield, 1999).

Several lines of evidence indicate that personality pathology is associated with impaired social and occupational functioning. In clinical samples, PDs are typically associated with impaired social functioning and increased interpersonal conflict (e.g., Skodol et al., 2002; Zanarini, Frankenburg, Hennen, Reich, & Silk, 2006). Some researchers also report higher levels of social impairment and interpersonal conflict among people with PDs in community samples (e.g., Bagge et al., 2004; Jackson & Burgess, 2004; Oltmanns, Melley, & Turkheimer, 2002; Ro & Clark, 2009). PDs also play an important role in many cases of marital discord (Whisman, Tolejko, & Chatav, 2007). One troubling aspect of marital conflict associated with PDs is partner aggression, particularly among individuals with borderline and antisocial PD (Holtzworth-Munroe & Stuart, 1994; Mauricio, Tein, & Lopez, 2007). It has been theorized that this tendency toward violence with partners may be a result of the presence of impulsivity or angry hostility in these disorders (Holtzworth-Munroe, 2000).

In addition to interpersonal and social difficulties, personality traits and personality pathology are also related to problems in several other dimensions of functioning. Among such problems are health and general medical issues for both younger and older adults. Patients with PDs consume more mental and physical health care resources than do people without PDs (Jackson & Burgess, 2002; Pilkonis, Blehar, & Prien, 1997). One study that assessed PDs in primary practice settings found that patients with high scores on PD questionnaires reported increased numbers of outpatient, emergency, and inpatient visits in the previous 6 months (Hueston, Werth, & Mainous, 1999). PDs are also associated with a greater likelihood of having a number of serious medical conditions, including cardiovascular disease, stroke, arthritis, and obesity (El-Gabalawy, Katz, & Sareen, 2010; Frankenburg & Zanarini, 2006; Lee et al., 2010; Pietrzak, Wagner, & Petry, 2007). These data are consistent with previous suggestions that personality variables play an important role in relation to various long-term aspects of physical health (Friedman, Hawley, & Tucker, 1994; Shen, McCreary, & Myers, 2004).

Another serious consequence related to having a PD is suicide, one of the world's leading causes of death (De Leo et al., 2001). Research suggests that roughly 30–40% of completed suicides are committed by individuals with PDs (Duberstein & Conwell, 1997). Although evidence varies, some studies suggest that specific personality traits, including negative affectivity, hostility, and impulsivity, are important predictors of suicidal behavior (Brittlebank et al., 1989; Nock et al., 2009; Yen et al., 2009). Comorbidity between PDs and other mental disorders, such as major depression or substance use disorders, also increases one's risk for suicidal acts (Yen et al., 2003). For example, using data from the National Epidemiological Survey on Alcohol and Related Conditions (NESARC), a longitudinal survey of psychopathology in U.S. adults, Bolton, Pagura, Enns, Grant, and Sareen (2010) found that the presence of PDs increased risk of suicide attempts among individuals with major depressive disorder, even when past suicidal behavior was controlled. Borderline PD has a particularly strong relationship with suicidal behavior and acts, and as we discuss later in this chapter, treatment protocols often focus on this explicitly in relation to borderline pathology (Critchfield, Levy, Clarkin, & Kernberg, 2008; Linehan, 1987; Oldham, 2006). These suicidal gestures are often viewed as attempts to gain attention from others (rather than as genuine suicide attempts) (Kernberg, 2001), but the gestures are dangerous nontheless and certainly cannot be ignored.

Sexual dysfunction and sleep problems, two other symptoms that commonly cause distress for individuals with various forms of psychopathology, have received little attention from researchers who study PDs. Evidence of the relationship between sexual dysfunction and PDs is almost nonexistent (see Zemishlany & Weizman, 2008, for a review). As we discussed previously, however, individuals with PDs frequently have dysfunctional interpersonal relationships, and that dysfunction is most evident in close, intimate relationships. Furthermore, certain PDs have symptoms specifically tied to intimacy problems, ranging from fear of abandonment and extreme clinginess to complete disinterest in sexual relationships. Therefore, the extent of sexual dysfunction may vary by disorder. There is a similar lack of research on sleep disturbance in PDs. Because sleep problems are strongly related to major depression (sleep disturbance is one of the diagnostic criteria for depression; American Psychiatric Association, 2013) and depression is often comorbid with PDs, it makes sense that sleep could also be a problem area for individuals with PDs. More research is needed in these areas before definitive conclusions can be drawn.

Clinical Implications

Heterogeneity of symptoms across different forms of personality pathology can have important consequences for the conceptualization and treatment of PDs. For example, absence of motivation for social relationships is a well-known theme for patients with schizoid or paranoid PD. Individuals with avoidant PD are different. They have a strong internal desire for connections with other people but are frequently unable to overcome their rejection sensitivity and seek out social relationships. It may seem that they are less motivated to engage with other people, but the reasons for their isolation are different from those that affect an individual with schizoid PD. Because avoidant patients desire interpersonal connections, treatment focused on reducing anxiety and increasing social contact is more beneficial for them than for patients with schizoid features.

It may be easier to consider separate symptoms or features in terms of a broader constellation of pathology when planning treatment. For example, motivation for power is related to one's self-image, image of others, and the way that individual then relates in interpersonal or intimate interactions. An individual with obsessive–compulsive PD may be conceptualized in terms of an excessive need for power; this may be motivated by a desire for the control and order that comes from professional accomplishments and cannot as easily be found in emotional or interpersonal experiences. This focus on professional success then comes at the cost of development in other areas, such as family relationships. Furthermore, the need for power might negatively impact work relationships and undermine productivity or job stability. By understanding motivating factors and interpersonal consequences, and how they relate to specific personality dysfunction, a practicing clinician may be better able to determine an appropriate treatment plan.

Because all PDs can be associated with specific sets of distorted beliefs called "schemas" (Beck et al., 2004), addressing these misperceptions is likely to be an important aspect of the therapist's role throughout the course of treatment. Reality testing is a commonly used technique with PD patients across all orientations and treatment approaches. Practicing clinicians must decide how confrontational to become when challenging misperceptions (Summers & Barber, 2009). This style may depend partly on theoretical orientation, but individual differences in the patient with PD and the unique personality dysfunction are also important to consider when determining a treatment approach. We discuss this in more detail later in the chapter.

How to address defenses in the context of therapy should also be considered in terms of unique patient characteristics. The first step is to identify a patient's defenses, then decide how to address those defenses in the context of therapy. It can be difficult to decide when to confront defenses and when to work around them. Clinicians often take a more supportive approach when patients have significant difficulty with emotional stability and handling internal and external stress. Regardless of theoretical approach, it is essential for clinicians to remain aware of how defenses are used and to be cognizant of how they become manifest under stress or when more actively addressed.

In relation to all the symptoms and features of PDs, it is also important to keep emotional regulation and capacity for emotional experience in mind. Certain PDs, such as borderline PD, are specifically characterized by difficulty with emotion regulation. Emotional awareness and stability are important factors across the spectrum of personality pathology, and it is beneficial to help patients learn to regulate their own emotions in healthy ways. Although the specific approach may vary across orientation, a general therapeutic goal should be to help patients with PD to identify what triggers an extreme emotional reaction in a specific situation. By tracking down those triggers, patients gain awareness and are more able to choose how to approach the situation in new ways.

The comorbidity between PDs and physical health outcomes should also be kept in mind when conceptualizing a PD case and planning treatment. Physical and mental health problems often complicate the treatment of one another, and a thorough initial assessment of physical health conditions should be taken before treatment begins. PD patients often do not adhere to medical recommendations. Helping a patient understand the importance of taking medication regularly, follow physician orders regarding a chronic medical condition, or engage in healthy lifestyle choices may be a necessary part of treatment that a practicing clinician might not otherwise use. Similarly, addressing sleep difficulties and providing basic education in sleep hygiene techniques may also prove beneficial to some patients with personality dysfunction (see Dautovich, McNamara, Williams, Cross, & McCrae, 2010, for a review of nonpharmacological treatment options for sleeplessness).

The strong interpersonal dysfunction associated with personality pathology makes it especially important to assess the nature of family relationships and social support of patients with PD. Action must be taken if the individual is in a violent relationship, either as perpetrator or victim. Therapists will also likely need to help patients with PD understand how healthy relationships work and find ways to enhance positive support in their lives. Finally, it is essential to assess specifically for suicidal ideation, both before treatment begins and during its course, because personality pathology is associated with increased risk for suicidal acts.

CLASSIFICATION

DSM-5 includes two different approaches to the classification of personality disorders. The main body of the manual describes the traditional categorical approach (American Psychiatric Association, 2013). Each of 10 specific types of personality disorder is defined by a set of characteristic symptoms. People who meet the general criteria for a personality disorder and who also exhibit enough symptoms to pass the diagnostic threshold for a specific type of disorder would qualify for a diagnosis. Those who do not meet this somewhat arbitrary threshold do not have a disorder, according to this perspective. We will refer to this approach as the *categorical definition of personality disorders*.

The workgroup charged with revising the classification of personality disorders proposed a dramatic change for DSM-5 (Krueger, Eaton, Clark, et al., 2011; Skodol et al., 2011). Their proposal emphasized the description of maladaptive personality traits using a set of 25 dimensional scales. We will refer to this approach as the *dimensional definition of personality disorders*, and it will be described later in this chapter. The new dimensional definition was ultimately rejected, but it is included in Section III of the manual, along with other conditions that require further consideration. For now, the categorical model remains the official DSM-5 approach to defining personality disorders.

DSM-5 PD Categories

The DSM-5 categorical system for personality disorders includes 10 types that are organized into three clusters on the basis of broadly defined characteristics. In order to qualify for a PD diagnosis using the categorical definition of PDs, a person must fit the general definition of PD (which applies to all 10 subtypes) and must also meet the specific criteria for a particular type of PD. The specific criteria comprise a list of characteristic features and behaviors that define the disorder. The general definition of PD emphasizes the duration of the pattern and the social impairment associated with the traits in question. The problems must be part of "an enduring pattern of inner experience and behavior that deviates markedly from the expectations of the individual's culture" (American Psychiatric Association, 2013, p. 646). The pattern must be evident in two or more of the following domains: cognition (e.g., ways of thinking about the self and other people), emotional responses, interpersonal functioning, or impulse control. This pattern of maladaptive experience and behavior must also be

- Inflexible and pervasive across a broad range of personal and social situations.
- The source of clinically significant distress or impairment in social, occupational, or other important areas of functioning.
- Stable and of long duration, with an onset that can be traced back at least to adolescence or early adulthood.

The authors of DSM-5 provide descriptions of 10 specific forms of PD organized in three clusters. In the following pages we give brief descriptions of these PD subtypes. The first three types are paranoid, schizoid, and schizotypal PDs. The behavior of people who fit these subtypes is typically odd, eccentric, or asocial. All three types (Cluster A) share similarity with the symptoms of schizophrenia. One implicit assumption is that these types of PD may represent behavioral traits or interpersonal styles on the same spectrum as schizophrenia, and they are sometimes referred to as "schizophrenia spectrum disorders."

Paranoid PD

Paranoid PD is characterized by the pervasive tendency to be inappropriately suspicious of other people's motives and behaviors. People who fit the description for this disorder are constantly on guard and hypervigilant. They expect other people to try to harm them, and they take extraordinary precautions to avoid being exploited or injured. People who are paranoid are inflexible in the way that they view the motives of other people, making it difficult for them to develop relationships or choose situations in which they can trust other people.

Paranoid PD should be distinguished from psychotic disorders such as schizophrenia and delusional disorder. The pervasive suspicions of people with paranoid PD do not always reach delusional proportions. In other words, their fears are generally reality based but represent an exaggeration, as opposed to a delusion based on extreme distortion.

Schizoid PD

Schizoid PD is defined in terms of a pervasive pattern of indifference to other people, coupled with a diminished range of emotional experience and expression. These people tend to be loners; they prefer social isolation to interactions with friends or family. Other people see them as being cold and aloof. By their own report, they do not experience strong subjective emotions such as sadness, anger, or happiness. They may appear "old" or "eccentric."

Schizotypal PD

Schizotypal PD centers on peculiar patterns of behavior rather than the emotional restriction and social withdrawal associated with schizoid PD. Many of these idiosyncratic behaviors take the form of perceptual and cognitive disturbance. People with this disorder may report bizarre or autistic fantasies and unusual perceptual experiences. Their speech may be slightly difficult to follow, because they use words in an odd or eccentric way or express themselves in a vague or disjointed manner. Their affective expressions may be constricted in range, as in schizoid PD, or they may be silly and inappropriate.

In spite of their odd or unusual behaviors, people with schizotypal PD are not necessarily psychotic or out of touch with reality. Their bizarre fantasies are generally not delusional, and their unusual perceptual experiences are not sufficiently real or compelling to be considered hallucinations.

The next group includes antisocial, borderline, histrionic, and narcissistic PDs (Cluster B). According to DSM-IV, these disorders are characterized by dramatic, emotional, or erratic behavior, and all are associated with marked difficulty in sustaining interpersonal relationships.

Antisocial PD

Antisocial PD is defined in terms of a persistent pattern of irresponsible and antisocial behavior that begins during childhood or adolescence and continues into the adult years. The DSM-IV definition is based on features that indicate a pervasive pattern of disregard for, and violation of, the rights of others. Once the person has become an adult, these difficulties include persistent failure to perform responsibilities associated with occupational and family roles. Conflict with others when one perceives he or she has been slighted is also common. These individuals can show irritability and aggression toward their spouses and children, as well as people outside the home. They can be impulsive, reckless, and irresponsible, showing little regard for the consequences of their actions.

Borderline PD

Borderline PD is a diffuse category whose essential feature is a pervasive pattern of instability in mood and interpersonal relationships. Individuals with borderline PD are often intolerant of being alone. They can form intense, unstable relationships with others and are often seen as manipulative. Their "manipulative" behavior is usually an adaptive strategy to maintain an attachment they perceive as vital to their survival. Their mood may shift rapidly and inexplicably from depression to anger to anxiety over a pattern of several hours. Intense anger is common and may be accompanied by temper tantrums, physical assault, or suicidal threats and parasuicidal behavior.

Many clinicians consider identity disturbance to be the diagnostic hallmark of borderline PD (Westen & Cohen, 1993). People with this disturbance presumably have great difficulty maintaining an integrated image of self that simultaneously incorporates positive and negative features. Therefore, they alternate between thinking of themselves in unrealistically positive terms and unrealistically negative terms at different moments in time. When they are focused on their own negative features, they have a deflated view of themselves and may become seriously depressed. They frequently express uncertainty about issues such as personal values, sexual preferences, and career alternatives. Chronic feelings of emptiness and boredom may also be present.

Histrionic PD

Histrionic PD is characterized by a pervasive pattern of excessive emotionality and attention-seeking behavior. Individuals with histrionic PD thrive on being the center of attention. They are often seen as self-centered, vain, and demanding, and they constantly seek approval from others. When interacting with other people, their behavior is often inappropriately sexually seductive or provocative. Their emotions tend to be shallow and may vacillate erratically. They reactions in situations may frequently be seen as exaggerated beyond what others would expect.

Many features of histrionic PD overlaps with other types of PD, especially borderline PD. Those with either disorder can be show heightened emotionality and display behavior that appears manipulative. Unlike people with borderline PD, however, people with histrionic PD have an essentially intact sense of their own identity and a better capacity for stable relationships.

Narcissistic PD

Narcissistic PD is conceptualized primarily by a pervasive pattern of grandiosity, need for admiration, and a limited capacity to respond with empathy to others. Narcissistic individuals often have a greatly exaggerated sense of their own importance. They tend to be preoccupied with their own achievements and abilities. Because they lack a well-developed sense of others and are overly concerned with themselves, they often ignore the feelings of others and are seen as being arrogant or haughty.

There is a considerable amount of overlap between narcissistic PD and borderline PD. Both types of people feel that other people should recognize their needs and do special favors for them. They may also react with anger if they are criticized. One distinction between these personality characterizations reflects the inflated sense of self-importance found in narcissistic PD and the deflated or devalued sense of self found in borderline PD (Ronningstam & Gunderson, 1991).

The last group includes avoidant, dependent, and obsessive–compulsive PDs (Cluster C). The common element in all three disorders is presumably anxiety or fearfulness. This description fits most easily with the avoidant and dependent types. In contrast, obsessive–compulsive PD is more accurately described in terms of preoccupation with rules and lack of emotional warmth than in terms of anxiety.

Avoidant PD

Avoidant PD is characterized by a pervasive pattern of social discomfort, fear of negative evaluation, and timidity. People with this disorder tend to be socially isolated when outside their own family circle because they are afraid of criticism. Unlike people with schizoid PD, they want to be liked by others but are extremely shy— easily hurt by even minimal signs of disapproval from other people. This rejection sensitivity makes them avoid social and occupational activities that require significant contact with other people.

Avoidant PD is often indistinguishable from generalized social phobia. In fact, some experts have argued that they are probably two different ways of defining the same condition (Frances, First, & Pincus, 1995; Reich, 2000). Others have argued that people with avoidant PD have more trouble than people with social phobia in relating to other people (Millon & Martinez, 1995). People with avoidant PD are presumably more socially withdrawn and have very few close relationships, because they are so shy. People with social phobia may have a lot of friends, but they are afraid of performing in front of them. This distinction is relatively clear when social phobia is defined narrowly in terms of a particular kind of situation, such as public speaking. It is much more difficult to make if the social phobia becomes more generalized.

Dependent PD

Dependent PD centers on a pervasive pattern of submissive and clinging behavior. People with this disorder are afraid of separating from other people on whom they are dependent for advice and reassurance. Often unable to make everyday decisions on their own, they feel anxious and helpless when they are alone. Like people with avoidant PD, they are easily hurt by criticism, extremely sensitive to disapproval, and lacking in self-confidence. One difference between avoidant and dependent PD involves the point in a relationship at which people experience the most difficulty. People who are avoidant have trouble initiating a relationship (because they are fearful). People who are dependent have trouble being alone or separating from other people with whom they already have a close relationship.

Obsessive–Compulsive PD

Obsessive–compulsive PD is defined by a pervasive pattern of orderliness, perfectionism, and mental and interpersonal control, at the expense of flexibility, openness, and efficiency. The central features of this disorder may involve a marked need for control and lack of tolerance for uncertainty (Gibbs, South, & Oltmanns, 2003). Individuals with this disorder set ambitious standards for their own performance that frequently are so high as to be unattainable. Many would be described as "workaholics." In other words, they are so devoted to work that they ignore friends, family members, and leisure activities. They are so preoccupied with details and rules that they lose sight of the main point of an activity or project. Intellectual endeavors are favored over feelings and emotional experience. These individuals are excessively conscientious, moralistic, and judgmental, and tend to be intolerant of emotional behavior in other people.

Problems with the Categorical Definition of PDs

The categorical approach treats PDs as discrete categories, and it assumes that there are sharp boundaries between normal and abnormal personalities. In fact, many people with serious personality problems do not fit the official subtypes. According to the DSM-5 categorical definitions, a person must exhibit at least a certain number of symptoms in order to meet the diagnostic criteria for each disorder. For example, borderline PD is defined in terms of nine features, and the person must exhibit at least five of them to be given a diagnosis, so there are 250 possible and unique ways to receive a diagnosis of borderline PD. Obsessive–compulsive PD lists eight features, and the person must exhibit at least four of them. Antisocial PD lists seven features (to be present as an adult), and the person must exhibit at least three of them (in addition to showing evidence of conduct disorder before age 15). These thresholds were established in a more or less arbitrary way; they have not been validated empirically. What should a clinician make of the patient who exhibits three symptoms of borderline PD, therefore falling short of an official diagnosis? Does that person not have a mental disorder? What about patients who exhibit selected features of several different kinds of PD, without having enough features of any specific PD to qualify for a diagnosis? The diagnosis of PD not otherwise specified has typically been used to describe these patients.

A related issue with the categorical description of PDs is the considerable overlap among categories. At least 50% of patients who meet the diagnostic criteria for one PD also meet the criteria for another disorder (e.g., Coid, Yang, Tyrer, Roberts, & Ullrich, 2006). To some extent, this overlap is due to the fact that similar symptoms are used to define more than one disorder. For example, impulsive and reckless behaviors are part of the definition of both antisocial and borderline PDs. Also, as previously mentioned, social withdrawal is used to define schizoid, schizotypal, and avoidant PD. However, this may also be due to the arbitrary definition of those disorders and the lack of organizational principles underlying their descriptions. A comprehensive and well-established theory of personality and psychopathology would be beneficial to organize this field (Magnavita, 2002).

There is also extensive overlap between PDs and other mental disorders. Approximately 75% of people who qualify for a PD diagnosis also meet criteria for a syndrome such as major depression, substance dependence, or anxiety disorder (e.g., Dolan-Sewell, Krueger, & Shea, 2001). This overlap may also be viewed from the other direction: Many people who are treated for a disorder such as depression or alcoholism also meet the criteria for a PD (e.g., Barber et al., 1996). Borderline PD appears to be the most common PD among patients treated at mental health facilities (both inpatient and outpatient settings). Averaged across studies, the evidence suggests that this disorder is found among slightly more than 30% of all patients treated for psychological disorders (Lyons, 1995; Zimmerman, Rothschild, & Chelminski, 2005).

In large part because of the issue of comorbidity, many experts favor the development of an alternative classification system for PDs, one that would be based on a dimensional view of personality pathology grounded in extensive research on the basic elements of personality (Clark, 2007; Widiger & Trull, 2007). Such a dimensional system would also have a stronger theoretical basis than the arbitrary nosology for personality disorders that is represented in the categorical system in DSM-5 (Krueger, Eaton, Derringer, et al., 2011). A dimensional system might provide a more complete description of each person, and it would be more useful with patients who fall on the boundaries between different types of PD. It might also be easier to use than the traditional categorical approach.

The Dimensional Alternative in DSM-5

Many leading PD experts believe that the classification of PDs will be dramatically improved if it is based on empirically validated personality traits (Markon, Krueger, & Watson, 2005). One important suggestion has been to use the FFM as the basic structure for a comprehensive description of personality problems (Widiger & Trull, 2007). This approach would require the clinician to consider information regarding 30 personality facets (six for each of the five domains of Neuroticism, Extraversion, Openness, Agreeableness, and Conscientiousness). This system would be economical compared to making a judgment regarding the presence of 80 PD features in DSM-IV (approximately eight features for each of the 10 PD categories).

Many PDs are defined in terms of maladaptive variations on the kinds of traits described in the FFM (Widiger & Simonsen, 2005). Problems may arise in association with extreme variations in either direction (high or low). Dramatically elevated levels of anger—hostility, impulsiveness, and excitement seeking—are particularly important, as are extremely low levels of trust, compliance, and tender-mindedness. Although some forms of PD are associated with high levels of anxiousness and vulnerability, people with antisocial PD frequently exhibit unusually low levels of anxiety and concern about danger.

The workgroup that was charged with revising the classification of personality disorders for DSM-5 proposed a model that represents a substantial change from the previous system (Skodol et al., 2011). Their proposal, which we call the dimensional PD model, was ultimately rejected in favor of retaining the traditional categorical model. Nevertheless, the dimensional PD model is listed in Section III of DSM-5, and many experts believe that it will eventually replace the categorical PD model, after it has been studied more extensively.

According to the PD workgroup's proposal, the diagnosis of personality disorders is based on a two-part process. First, the clinician is asked to make a judgment regarding impairment in personality functioning as defined by problems with the person's view of self and others (identity and self-direction) as well as difficulties with maintaining interpersonal relationships (empathy and intimacy). Problems identified in these areas serve as general markers for the presence of a personality *disorder*; it is the key decision point in deciding whether to assign a diagnosis. This judgment replaces the categorical model's general criteria for PDs, which are often ignored and have been criticized for being vague and unreliable. In fact, many experts have argued that the most important consideration regarding assessment of personality pathology is overall level of severity rather than specific types of PDs (Tyrer et al., 2011). The dimensional system for rating level of personality functioning is relatively straightforward, and it might be efficient and effective in that role.

The second step in the proposed dimensional process specifies the nature or form of the disorder using ratings of pathological personality traits. What *kind* of personality problem does the person exhibit? The organization of these traits generally follows the FFM, but the broad domains are labeled in a way that emphasizes the maladaptive nature of characteristics associated with PDs (Krueger, Eaton, Clark, et al., 2011). For example, the domain known as agreeableness in the FFM is called antagonism in the new model. Altogether, the proposed system includes consideration of 25 core traits. The primary domains in the DSM-5 dimensional approach to defining PDs are the following (with specific facets or traits for each domain presented in parentheses):

- Negative affect (emotional lability, anxiousness, separation insecurity, submissiveness, hostility, perseveration)
- Detachment (withdrawal, intimacy avoidance, anhedonia, depressivity, restricted affectivity, suspiciousness)
- Antagonism (agreeableness, manipulativeness, deceitfulness, grandiosity, attention seeking, callousness)
- Disinhibition (irresponsibility, impulsivity, distractibility, risk taking, rigid perfectionism)
- Psychoticism (unusual beliefs and experiences, eccentricity, cognitive and perceptual dysregulation)

The clinician's task involves selecting and rating the traits in this list that best describe the nature of the personality problems that are related to the person's impaired personal and social functioning.

The dimensional model places primary emphasis on ratings of the maladaptive traits, but it also retains 6 of the 10 specific types of PD from the categorical model: antisocial, avoidant, borderline, narcissistic, obsessive–compulsive, and schizotypal PD. Traits replace diagnostic criteria for each PD in the categorical system. By including some of the types, the dimensional system retains some continuity with the categorical system, which mental health professionals already know. The types may provide a useful shorthand in communicating with other professionals and in conceptualizing certain kinds of problems because they bring to mind familiar or prototypical combinations of several maladaptive traits.

Other forms of PD will be identified in the dimensional system using a new

diagnosis called Personality Disorder Trait Specified (or PDTS). In order to qualify for this diagnosis, the person must exhibit significant impairment in self or
interpersonal functioning, as well as one or more pathological personality traits.
This system replaces four of the categorical types with simplified trait ratings.
Paranoid PD, for example, would be described by a high rating on suspiciousness, histrionic PD would be described by a high rating on attention seeking,
and dependent PD would be described by a high rating on submissiveness. This
system makes it easier to describe problems exhibited by people with a variety of
maladaptive traits because it avoids the need to assign more than one type of PD
diagnosis. Furthermore, people who exhibit a few symptoms that would be below
the diagnostic threshold in the categorical system are easily described with one
set of ratings.

Notice that the trait descriptors actually help explain the overlap or comorbidity
that has been observed for many of the PD types. One example involves borderline
and antisocial PD. Many people qualify for a diagnosis of both disorders using the
categorical system. The borderline and antisocial types share several maladaptive
traits involving antagonism (e.g., hostility) and disinhibition (impulsivity). They are
most clearly distinguished by the fact that people with borderline PD are also high
on traits involving negative affectivity (e.g., emotional lability, anxiousness, and
depressivity). Again, the relative simplicity of the trait-based approach offers an
advantage over the categorical approach.

One attractive feature is that the alternative dimensional models for PDs recognize explicitly the continuous nature of these phenomena. Rather than assume
that a person either does or does not have a PD, dimensional models place their
emphasis on measuring the extent or degree to which the person exhibits a certain personality characteristic, such as impulsivity or negative emotionality. This
advantage is intuitively appealing, but it might also be somewhat misleading when
we consider the way such a system must be used in clinical practice. Therapists
will ultimately need to make certain important decisions that are fundamentally
categorical in nature, such as whether a person needs treatment, and whether that
treatment should be reimbursed financially. The DSM-5 Committee, as it worked on
developing the dimensionally based system, opted for the new focus on the level of
personality functioning as a mechanism for making decisions about the presence of
disorder. It remains to be seen whether this aspect of the proposal will ultimately
pass subsequent tests that focus on its reliability and validity.

Clinical Implications

The previous section on classification demonstrates even further the heterogeneity
across various forms of personality pathology, as well as the variability that can
occur within a given PD. The frequent presence of comorbid mental disorders, such
as depression and substance use disorders, adds to this complexity. This diversity

makes it essential that personality pathology is assessed and considered as part of the larger case formulation. In general, if a patient presents with several mental disorders, then this should be a sign to the clinician that the potential for personality dysfunction is contributing to these clinical symptoms.

The constellation of clinical syndromes and relational disturbances with which a patient comes into therapy can have serious implications for treatment, and practicing clinicians should know that personality dysfunction can hinder treatment progress (Crits-Cristoph & Barber, 2007; Magnavita, 2004). For example, the treatment approach a clinician selects for a depressed patient with comorbid avoidant PD is likely to be different than the approach with a patient who has a narcissistic PD or does not have comorbid personality pathology at all. In a study exploring the differential effects of cognitive and interpersonal psychotherapy on the treatment of depression, Barber and Muenz (1996) found that positive response to treatment was dependent on the type of personality pathology diagnosed. Depressed individuals with avoidant pathology were more likely to respond to cognitive therapy, whereas depressed individuals with obsessive personality pathology were more likely to respond to interpersonal therapy. Even within a given PD, treatment may need to be tailored to fit the unique interpersonal problems of each patient (Crits-Christoph & Barber, 2007). There is limited research on treatment matching for individuals with PDs, but this study demonstrated the role personality pathology can play in determining treatment response. Regardless of treatment approach or orientation, clinicians working with patients with comorbid mental disorders may want to do some focused work on pathological personality patterns, in addition to the evidence-based treatment used for disorders such as depression. Length of treatment must also be considered. Treatment generally takes longer when comorbid personality pathology is present (Critchfield & Benjamin, 2006; Tyrer, Gunderson, Lyons, & Tohen, 1997).

There are many limitations to the classification system for personality disorders, and a PD "diagnosis" is unlikely to provide all the information that a clinician needs. There may be times when a patient's symptoms fall short of a diagnosis of PD, but a subthreshold presentation still has important implications for treatment. If a client engages in impulsive, dangerous behavior and has difficulty managing emotional reactions, these features must be kept in mind, even if the person's personality patterns and symptoms do not reach the diagnostic threshold for borderline PD. It is also possible that personality dysfunction may be difficult to detect in the beginning stages of treatment. Individuals with avoidant, dependent, or obsessive–compulsive PDs, which are characterized by constricted emotions, often seek treatment because of depression or anxiety. Because they do not generally engage in the attention-getting behaviors (e.g., angry outbursts), their personality dysfunction can be overlooked. A thorough history of how patients are functioning in all aspects of their lives can be valuable in ensuring that these kinds of issues do not go unnoticed (Crits-Christoph & Barber, 2007; Magnavita, 1997). Ongoing assessment and refinement of case conceptualization is necessary throughout the course of treatment, since a patient's level of functioning and overall relational ability may change. An individual who appears to function rather well may, as treatment unfolds, present as being more fragile or unstable than the original presentation suggested. Conversely, some patients who initially present as disturbed may quickly restabilize with treatment.

The severity of personality dysfunction must also be kept in mind when determining the best treatment approach. The more severe the personality dysfunction, the more likely the practicing clinician will have to use a multimodal treatment approach (Millon, Grossman, Meagher, Millon, & Everly, 1999). This might include individual treatment in combination with psychopharmacological treatment, family support, couple therapy, or the use of community resources such as brief hospitalizations. Determining whether outpatient care is sufficient for a client with severe personality dysfunction is critical. Does the practicing clinician have the resources to provide treatment safely to this patient? Or is more intensive inpatient care needed? One evidenced-based approach to the treatment of patients with borderline PD (Linehan, 1993), which we discuss in more detail later in the chapter, requires that therapists work in a team to provide care. This approach is used to ensure the safety of the patients, who are often parasuicidal, and both that therapists are getting the support they need when working with such a difficult population (Linehan et al., 2006).

Practicing clinicians may also find it helpful to consider personality pathology in terms of presenting personality trait characteristics (in addition to specific symptoms for categorical types). Dramatically elevated levels of anger–hostility and excitement seeking or extremely low levels of trust, compliance, and tendermindedness would contribute differently to the therapeutic relationship and treatment progress. Although some forms of PD are associated with high levels of anxiousness and vulnerability, people with antisocial PD frequently exhibit unusually low levels of anxiety and concern about danger. This low level of anxiety is not necessarily captured by symptoms for antisocial PD and could be missed by a clinician unfamiliar with antisocial pathology (Harris & Rice, 2006). With this in mind, the use of a structured measure to identify maladaptive variants of personality traits could be an extremely useful tool for clinicians when conceptualizing a patient with PD and planning treatment (Krueger, Derringer, Markon, Watson, & Skodol, 2012; Widiger, Lynam, Miller, & Oltmanns, 2012).

EPIDEMIOLOGY

PDs are considered to be among the most common forms of psychopathology when considered as a general category (i.e., any of the 10 DSM-5 PDs). Several epidemiological studies in the United States and in Europe have used semistructured diagnostic interviews to assess PDs in samples of people living in the community.

Prevalence in Community Samples

In studies that have examined community-based samples of adults, the overall lifetime prevalence for having at least one PD (any type) varies between 10–14% (Lenzenweger, Lane, Loranger, & Kessler, 2007; Trull, Jahng, Tomko, Wood, & Sher, 2010). While this figure tends to be relatively consistent from one study to the next, prevalence rates for specific types of PD vary quite a bit. The highest prevalence rates, usually found to be associated with obsessive–compulsive, antisocial, and avoidant PDs, may affect 3 or 4% of adults.

The most precise information available regarding the prevalence of PDs in community samples concerns the antisocial type specifically (Moran, 1999). In two large-scale epidemiological studies of mental disorders, structured interviews were conducted with several thousand participants. The overall lifetime prevalence rate for antisocial PD (men and women combined) was 3% in both studies (Kessler et al., 1994; Robins & Regier, 1991). More recent research supports this estimated prevalence rate (Coid et al., 2006).

Gender Differences

The overall prevalence of PDs is approximately equal in men and women (Lenzenweger et al., 2007; Torgersen, Kringlen, & Cramer, 2001; Weissman, 1993). There are, however, consistent gender differences with regard to at least one specific disorder: Antisocial PD is unquestionably much more common among men than among women, with prevalence rates of approximately 5% reported for men and 1% for women (Coid et al., 2006; Kessler et al., 1994; Robins & Regier, 1991). Thus, antisocial PD is actually an alarmingly common problem among adult males in the United States.

Epidemiological evidence regarding gender differences for the other types of PD is much more ambiguous. In the DSM-5 (American Psychiatric Association, 2013), borderline and dependent PD are described as being diagnosed more frequently in women than in men, but the evidence is not strong (Oldham, Skodol, & Bender, 2009). There has also been some speculation that paranoid and obsessive–compulsive PD may be somewhat more common among men than women (Coid et al., 2006), although there is not enough empirical evidence to draw any clear conclusions.

It is not clear whether differential prevalence rates exist (with the exception of antisocial PD); there is some evidence to suggest that PD symptoms may differentially affect men and women across many domains of functioning. For example, some borderline symptoms, such as affective instability, unstable relationships, and stress-related paranoia, may be more relevant to borderline pathology in women, whereas impulsivity may be more relevant to borderline pathology in men (Boggs et al., 2005). Other mental disorders also may be represented differently in male and female patients with borderline PD. In a national epidemiological sample, Grant et al. (2008) found that borderline males showed higher rates of comorbid substance use disorders, while females showed higher rates of comorbid depression and anxiety, in particular posttraumatic stress disorder. Differences in patterns of comorbid disorders may result from differences in how borderline men and women manifest impulsivity, with men showing more substance abuse, while women may engage in more disordered eating (Trull, Sher, Minks-Brown, Durbin, & Burr, 2000; Zlotnick, Rothschild, & Zimmerman, 2002).

Age Differences

Longitudinal studies of community samples are also important with regard age, but they have been limited to those extending from adolescence into young adulthood. For example, Cohen and her colleagues (2005) reported that the amount of personality pathology exhibited by participants in the Children in the Community Study (CIC) decreased steadily from adolescence into young adulthood (Cohen, 2008). That pattern is, of course, very interesting, but it leaves open the possibility that different patterns might emerge as participants progress through middle-age and into later life (Moffitt, 2007).

Evidence regarding the prevalence of specific PDs in later life comes exclusively from *cross-sectional* comparisons of younger and older people, using DSM thresholds to decide whether or not each person qualifies for a specific PD diagnosis. Unfortunately, relatively little evidence has been collected in longitudinal studies. Rather, these developmental inferences are drawn on the basis of cross-sectional comparisons between younger and older participants. The evidence is not overwhelming, but several studies indicate that paranoid, schizoid, and obsessive–compulsive PDs are more prevalent in older people than in younger people (Abrams & Horowitz, 1999). In contrast, borderline and antisocial PDs are less prevalent in older people than in younger people (e.g., Samuels et al., 2011). This pattern is interesting, but considerable caution must be exercised in drawing conclusions about patterns of change on the basis of this evidence. Cross-sectional studies necessarily compare people from different age groups who are living in different contexts. Differences in the extent of social isolation or dependence might reflect variation in life circumstances for younger and older adults rather than true developmental changes in the prevalence of specific personality problems (Oltmanns & Balsis, 2011).

The tentative evidence that has been reported suggests the possibility that the prevalence of certain features of personality pathology may change over the lifespan. For example, one 10-year follow-up evaluation of almost 300 patients with borderline PD, recruited during inpatient treatment between the ages of 18 and 35, found that marked improvement in some types of symptoms was frequently accompanied by persistent problems in other areas (Zanarini et al., 2007). Major improvements were most often seen in self-mutilation and suicidal behaviors. Problems managing anger and dysphoria, and interpersonal difficulties related to fears of abandonment and dependency were the most stable symptoms of BPD.

The DSM-5 general definition specifies that a PD must begin by adolescence, and the assumption is that these characteristics are stable over time. Based on evidence provided by several follow-up studies with young adults, we now know that this assumption regarding stability is exaggerated (Samuel et al., 2011). Many patients with PD do improve over time, but longitudinal studies have not been conducted in later life. No one has studied a community sample of middle-aged or older adults for a sufficiently long period of time to determine whether new cases appear (Oltmanns & Balsis, 2011). Therefore, if the issue is considered in terms of relatively large-scale epidemiological evidence, we do not know whether there is such a thing as late-onset PD.

Although some argue against the diagnosis of PDs in children, others believe that choosing to ignore their existence does a disservice by allowing these children to suffer needlessly (Freeman & Reinecke, 2007). A number of clinical researchers, however, believe that in certain cases children should be diagnosed with a PD only after a through assessment has been completed. It is probably best when considering the diagnosis of a PD in children or adolescence to use a systemic framework that examines the child's or adolescent's personality within the context of family, community, and cultural systems, and to view the personality as an adaptation to these relational and cultural forces (Magnavita, 2005b, 2007). A more extensive review of this topic is beyond the scope of this chapter, and readers who are interested should refer to the Freeman and Reinecke volume cited earlier. When conducting treatment planning with children and adolescents it is critical to include the family system (Magnavita & MacFarlane, 2004).

Examples of late-onset PD have been reported in the literature. For example, Bernstein, Reich, Zanarini, and Siever (2002) described the case of a 45-year-old woman who first sought treatment when in her late 30s. She received medication for the treatment of depression but was later hospitalized when she experienced suicidal ideation and engaged in wrist cutting. Several hospitalizations followed, and she eventually received a diagnosis of borderline PD. After a brief description of the case, three experts discussed the diagnosis. Perhaps the most interesting aspect of this discussion is the fact that none of the experts considered seriously the possibility that her disorder emerged in middle age. Rather, they speculated that her problems went unnoticed earlier in her life because she had not been in treatment. The prevailing assumption in this discussion is that if more careful observations had been made several years earlier, features of the disorder would have been identified. The possibility that goes largely unmentioned is that her problems emerged when she was an adult. Of course, another important possibility that should always be kept in mind is that the personality symptoms were a result of her depressive episode. It can be unclear whether a clinician is detecting a PD or manifestations of another mental disorder that exacerbates some trait (Klein, Kotov, & Bufferd,

2010). In a recent study of treatment for depression, Barber, Barrett, Gallop, Rynn, and Rickels (2012) diagnosed presence of PD by asking depressed patients to think about whether they reported PD symptoms when they were not depressed. This resulted in a smaller number of actual PD diagnoses.

Why is the field so committed to the apparently unquestioned assumption that PDs must begin early in a person's life? Part of the explanation may be due to the long-standing assumption that personality remains stable over the lifespan. Of course, this is a controversial topic, and current evidence suggests that personality structure is not completely stable (Roberts, Walton, & Viechtbauer, 2006). And PDs may be much less stable than previously assumed. Follow-up studies suggest that some symptoms may remit over time (Gunderson et al., 2000, 2011; Zanarini et al., 2005), although negative outcomes are still related to borderline pathology even at subthreshold levels (Blum et al., 2008). We do not know whether some PD symptoms may emerge later in life, with or without a foundation in related personality traits. It may be that for some, personality dysfunction may emerge under certain conditions and in certain contexts. For example, for some individuals, going to prison results in the emergence of what is considered an antisocial PD, which may be the result of adaptation to the extreme demands of prison. There are also anecdotal reports about individuals who go from being unknown to being famous and developing narcissistic PD. When considering these and other examples, it is often useful to think of this phenomenon as the expression of a complex system (Magnavita, 2005b) called "personality systematics" (Magnavia, 2011).

Another related issue involves the fact that the onset of a PD is difficult to identify. It is certainly true that the onset of more florid symptoms, such as hallucinations or washing rituals or prominent drinking problems, might be easier to pinpoint in time. But many forms of psychopathology have symptoms that emerge gradually. And many disorders are preceded by an extended prodromal period that is difficult to identify.

In the absence of a substantial literature regarding age of onset and PDs, we turn to the literature on personality traits. These studies show some evidence of change, which most often is gradual (Roberts et al., 2006). If we think of PDs as correlates of these personality traits, we have to consider the possibility or the likelihood that the presentation of PDs may change similarly. Furthermore, when we think in terms of latent traits or propensities to behave in a certain way that becomes manifest (and perhaps troublesome) within a particular social context (which can change across the life course), it seems reasonable to argue that sudden onset is unusual or unexpected. That is different than saying, however, that late onset is impossible.

Ethnicity

There is very limited epidemiological research on ethnic or racial differences among individuals with PDs. One large-scale study (Lenzenweger et al., 2007) reported no significant racial differences among the PDs. In other epidemiological studies, race/ethnicity is often simply controlled in analyses. With the few empirical studies that have found differences, findings are mixed. As part of the Collaborative Longitudinal Personality Disorders Study (CLPS), Chavira et al. (2003) examined the relationship between ethnicity and four PDs (i.e., avoidant, schizotypal, borderline, and obsessive–compulsive). The results showed higher rates of schizotypal PD among African Americans and higher rates of borderline PD among Hispanics compared to European Americans. Other research supports the association between schizotypal PD and African American women (Pulay et al., 2009). Alternatively, a more recent meta-analysis of studies of the association between PDs and race/ethnicity demonstrated that blacks were significantly less likely to be diagnosed with a PD than whites, although whether there is actually less prevalence of personality pathology among these individuals, or whether PDs are less likely to be diagnosed cannot be determined from available evidence (McGilloway, Hall, Lee, & Bhui, 2010). No differences between Asian or Hispanic groups and white groups were found. Clearly, without more research, we cannot draw any specific conclusions about the role of ethnicity in understanding PDs. As with any form of psychopathology, however, it is critical to keep cultural factors in mind when conceptualizing a case, planning treatment, and implementing an intervention.

Clinical Implications

Personality pathology is common across both clinical and community populations. It is therefore critical to assess for PDs during the initial assessment process, while keeping in mind potential gender, age, and ethnicity differences. PD symptoms may manifest differently in men and women, and they may also have different comorbid pathology (Grant et al., 2008); differences in comorbid pathology can affect how treatment may proceed or what interventions one chooses as a clinician. With regard to age, the clinical presentation of certain disorders may also change over the lifespan and could further impact treatment decisions or focus. Changes in the presentation of personality dysfunction may be subtle and difficult to detect, making it especially important for practicing clinicians to be aware of how psychopathology is likely to look in the age groups they treat. More generally, practicing clinicians should always consider the sociocultural context of the patient, including ethnicity, education level, and socioeconomic status, and how those factors may affect a patient's ability to participate fully in treatment. African Americans, for example, often show mistrust for the American health care system and may present with paranoia about the care they will receive (Whaley, 2001). There is also a particularly strong stigma against mental health treatment among many African Americans. If they do seek treatment, these patients may be ashamed of their condition or hide treatment information from family or friends (Alvidrez, 1999; Sirey et al., 2001). It may be necessary as a clinician to address these kinds of concerns during therapy. Understanding such concerns can help in the development of a strong therapeutic relationship and promote motivation to continue treatment.

COURSE AND OUTCOME

Lifespan perspectives on psychopathology have played a crucial role in shaping the classification of many forms of psychopathology. Established views of major mental disorders, such as schizophrenia and bipolar disorder, are based on careful descriptions that include close attention to the course of the disorders over extended periods of time. Kraepelin's early recognition of the distinction between dementia praecox and manic–depressive psychosis hinged largely on the different patterns these disorders follow over time rather than on the presence of specific symptoms during periods of acute disturbance. Therefore, it is important to consider the available evidence regarding the course of PDs from childhood to adulthood and later life.

Childhood Antecedents

Temporal stability is one of the most important assumptions about PDs. As we discussed briefly in the previous section, a few longitudinal studies have made substantial contributions to our understanding of continuity of personality pathology, and they have focused largely on the period of the lifespan ranging from childhood through adolescence and young adulthood (Paris, 2003; Skodol, 2008). For example, the CIC study followed a large, community-based sample of children (average age at baseline = 14) over three decades, assessing personality pathology at five separate periods, until participants were on average 38 years old (Cohen, 2008). Several papers from this innovative study have demonstrated that various types of PD are associated with the subsequent development of social impairment, as well as the onset of other forms of psychopathology (Cohen et al., 2005).

Stability (from Adolescence to Young Adulthood)

Another important study concerned with the stability of PDs over time is the CLPS, which included careful assessments in a sample of approximately 700 psychiatric patients between the ages of 18 and 45 in treatment at five different clinics (Skodol, Gunderson, et al., 2005). Patients were followed over a period of 10 years. Reports from this group of investigators have demonstrated that the symptoms of PDs are not as stable as previously believed and may be a function of the method of assessment. On the other hand, functional impairment associated with personality pathology was found to be extensive and relatively more stable in comparison to PD symptoms (e.g., Blum et al., 2008; Skodol, Pagano, et al., 2005).

The CIC study also continued to collect information regarding the prevalence and stability of PDs among adolescents (Bernstein, Ahluvalia, Pogge, & Handels-man, 1997). This investigation is particularly important, because it did not depend solely on subjects who had been referred for psychological treatment and it was concerned with the full range of PDs. The rate of PDs was relatively high in this sample: Of the adolescents, 17% received a diagnosis of at least one PD. Categorically defined diagnoses were not particularly stable; fewer than half of the adolescents who originally qualified for a PD diagnosis met the same criteria 2 years later. Nevertheless, many of the study participants continued to exhibit similar problems over the next 8 years. Viewed from a dimensional perspective, the maladaptive traits that represent the core features of the disorders remained relatively stable between adolescence and young adulthood (Crawford, Cohen, & Brook, 2001).

Burnout (in Clinical Samples)

Several studies have examined the stability of PDs among people who have received professional treatment for their problems, especially those who have been hospitalized for schizotypal or borderline PD. Many patients treated for these problems are still significantly impaired several years later, but the disorders are not uniformly stable (Grilo et al., 2005; Paris, 2003). Recovery rates are relatively high among patients with a diagnosis of borderline PD. If patients initially treated during their early 20s are followed up when they are in their 40s and 50s, only about 1 person in 4 would still qualify for a diagnosis of borderline PD. The long-term prognosis is less optimistic for schizotypal and schizoid PDs. People with these diagnoses are likely to remain socially isolated and occupationally impaired. It may be the case that this Cluster A disorder has the greatest neurobiological vulnerability and is less likely to benefit from available treatment.

ETIOLOGY

Evidence regarding causal factors involved in the development and maintenance of PDs points to a complicated set of interactions involving genetic factors and environmental events (Kendler et al., 2008). Most studies of these issues have focused on specific types of PDs rather than the entire spectrum of personality pathology.

Genetic Factors

The most extensive research on genetic factors in PDs has been on schizotypal PD, because of its associations with schizophrenia and psychotic spectrum disorders; schizotypal PD symptoms have similarities with prodromal schizophrenic symptoms (e.g., see Parnas, Licht, & Bovet, 2005). Twin studies have examined genetic contributions to schizotypal PD from a dimensional perspective in which schizotypal personality traits are measured with questionnaires. Evidence points to a significant genetic contribution (Linney et al., 2003). Family studies point to the same conclusion; the first-degree relatives of schizophrenic patients are considerably more likely than people in the general population to exhibit features of schizotypal PD (Kendler et al., 1993).

There has also been some genetic research on borderline PD, which also is one of the most widely studied PDs. Genetic factors seem to play a less salient role in the etiology of borderline PD when it is viewed in terms of the syndrome defined in DSM (Torgersen, 1994). This does not mean, however, that genes are irrelevant to the development of this set of problems, because the fundamental personality traits that serve to define the disorder, such as neuroticism and impulsivity, are clearly influenced by genetic factors (Livesley, 2008; Skodol et al., 2002).

Several investigators have also used twin and adoption studies to examine the contributions of genetic and environmental factors to the development of antisocial PD, and of criminal behavior more generally. The adoption strategy is based on the study of adoptees: people who were separated from their biological parents at an early age and raised by adoptive families. Several adoption studies have found that the development of antisocial behavior is determined by an interaction between genetic factors and adverse environmental circumstances (Rhee & Waldman, 2002). In other words, both types of influence are important. The highest rates of conduct disorder and antisocial behavior are found in the offspring of antisocial biological parents, raised in an adverse adoptive environment (Cadoret Yates, Ed, Woodworth, & Stewart, 1995; Yates, Cadoret, & Troughton, 1999).

Environmental Adversity

Many researchers are interested in the role of environmental adversity in the development of PDs. With antisocial PD, adoption studies indicate that genetic factors interact with environmental events to produce patterns of antisocial and criminal behavior (Rhee & Waldman, 2002). There is also evidence that environmental factors contribute to the onset of other types of personality pathology (MacMillan et al., 2001).

What kinds of events might be involved in this process? Obvious candidates include childhood abuse and neglect. Longitudinal data on adolescents reported by Johnson, Cohen, Brown, Smailes, and Bernstein (1999) and Johnson et al. (2001) explored the relation between childhood maltreatment and personality pathology, including only documented cases of physical abuse, sexual abuse, and emotional neglect. Children who experienced childhood abuse or neglect were four times more likely than those who had not been mistreated to develop symptoms of PDs as young adults. Physical abuse was most closely associated with subsequent antisocial PD; sexual abuse, with borderline PD; and childhood neglect, with antisocial, borderline, narcissistic, and avoidant PD. Other research with male Veterans Administration (VA) patients also found a link between childhood maltreatment and risk for PDs (Ruggiero, Bernstein, & Handelsman, 1999). These studies were not able to show whether childhood abuse is associated with specific characteristics of PD. However, an increasing body of research indicates an association between early trauma exposure and increased risk for adult psychotic symptoms (Morrison, Frame, & Larkin, 2003; Read et al., 2005). For example, Berenbaum, Valera, and Kerns (2003) found that child abuse was associated with certain schizotypal symptoms, including ideas of reference, magical thinking, unusual perceptual experiences, and paranoid ideation.

Other research has suggested a link between the experience of childhood abuse and borderline symptoms (Fonagy & Bateman, 2008). This model is supported by studies of the families of patients with borderline PD and by comparisons with the literature on social development in monkeys that examined the effects of separating infants from their mothers. Studies of patients with borderline PD do point toward the influence of widespread problematic relationships with their parents. Adolescent girls with borderline PD report pervasive lack of supervision; frequent witnessing of domestic violence; and being subjected to inappropriate behavior by their parents and other adults, including verbal, physical, and sexual abuse (Helgeland & Torgersen, 2004; Pally, 2002). The extent and severity of abuse vary widely across individuals. Many patients describe multiple forms of abuse by more than one person. These data (both retrospective and longitudinal) support the argument that maladaptive patterns of parenting and family relationships increase the probability that a person will develop certain types of PD.

Clinical Implications

While there is relatively little research on etiological factors related to PDs, the treatment considerations that emerge may be particularly critical to understand regardless of the treatment method being used. We discuss a few here.

Because of the link between childhood trauma and PDs, thorough evaluation of lifetime trauma exposure, with a particular focus on childhood maltreatment, is encouraged when treating patients with PDs. Especially if the patient has experienced trauma, there may be comorbid symptoms of posttraumatic stress disorder that need attention during the course of treatment. Because the trauma may also be minimized or romanticized by the patient in treatment, it may be necessary to help him or her face the severity of the trauma experienced. Family history of psychiatric conditions should also be assessed, especially considering genetic factors for antisocial and schizotypal PDs.

For practicing clinicians who work with children, it is also critical to be aware of the developmental precursors to personality dysfunction. As Cohen et al. (2005) found in the CIC study, behavioral and conduct disorder, when not transient, often lead to the development of PD in adolescence and adulthood. Children with chronic developmental problems need to have increased attention, with preventive treatment aimed toward helping them avoid chronic personality dysfunction.

Understanding the nature of developmental relationships in patients with PD may also be particularly informative, because those relationships likely contributed to current dysfunctional images of self and others (Magnavita, 2000). This can be valuable regardless of theoretical orientation and does not have to take away from a general emphasis on "the present," which is characteristic of some of the current PD treatments, such as dialectical behavior therapy (DBT). Descriptions of current relationships with family and friends also provide clinicians with an idea of what social support is present for the patient and what environmental factors may impede treatment progress. There is no clear etiological pathway to developing PD, but it is beneficial to keep in mind the general contribution of family and traumatic experiences.

TREATMENT

Treatment of PDs is invariably difficult. It has been particularly challenging for investigators to provide clear, evidence-based principles grounded in solid empirical evidence, because PDs are heterogeneous. Treatment procedures for people with PDs are especially difficult to design and evaluate for three principal reasons. First, as previously mentioned, people with these disorders frequently do not have insight into the nature of their problems. Thus, they are unlikely to seek treatment, and if they do, they frequently terminate treatment prematurely. Second, pure forms of PD are relatively rare. Most people with PDs who are in treatment also exhibit comorbid forms of other mental disorders, such as depression or drug addiction. Third, people with PDs have difficulty establishing and maintaining meaningful, stable interpersonal relationships of the sort required for psychotherapy.

The field of PD treatment is advancing, and a number of evidence-based approaches have been developed for personality disorders (Magnavita, 2010). Three therapeutic approaches have been specifically developed for the treatment of borderline PD: DBT (Linehan, 1987; Robins, Rosenthal, & Cuper, 2010); mentalization-based therapy (MBT; Bateman & Fonagy, 2006; Fonagy & Target, 2006); and transference-focused psychotherapy (TFP; Clarkin, Yeomans, & Kernberg, 2006). Schema-focused therapy (Young, 1994) has also proven to be effective for borderline PD. Short-term dynamic psychotherapy (Davanloo, 1980; Mc Cullough Valliant, 1997; Magnavita, 1997; Messer & Abbass, 2010) has been shown to be effective, especially for certain anxious and dramatic forms of PD. Psychodynamic group therapy delivered in a partial hospital setting, which is an underutilized cost-effective treatment (Piper, 2008), is also effective in the treatment of PDs (Piper, Rosie, & Joyce, 1996). Each of these approaches may offer useful strategies and techniques for working with a spectrum of individuals with PDs.

Some of these approaches seem more effective when used with patients with specific types of PDs. For example, DBT (Linehan, 1993) was developed for individuals with borderline PD and seems most effective for those with parasuicidal behavior (Linehan, Heard, & Armstrong, 1993). In some randomized control trials, DBT has specifically shown greater efficacy than treatment as usual in reducing hospitalizations, suicidal acts, impulsive behavior, and overall treatment retention (Linehan et al., 2006; Verheul et al., 2003), although there is evidence that other PD treatments show similar results (McMain et al., 2009; see Crits-Christoph & Barber, 2007; Magnavita, 2010, for a review of the literature). Treatment also may involve the use of antipsychotic or antidepressant medication, most often for patients with schizotypal or borderline PD. A few controlled studies indicate that pharmacological treatment can be beneficial (Ingenhoven, Lafay, Rinne, Passchier, & Duivenvoorden, 2010). More research is needed to determine the differential benefits of these treatment methods and what factors clinicians should consider when planning treatment.

Beyond specific treatment options, many general therapeutic principles of change are essential to effective intervention regardless of the therapist's theoretical orientation (Castonguay & Beutler, 2006). Two groups of researchers have reviewed the research literature and identified a number of common principles that may be particularly important to keep in mind in the treatment of individuals with PDs. Some of the principles include a strong therapeutic relationship; honest communication about the limits of therapy and difficulty of change; emphasis on goal-oriented, structured therapy sessions; and a general focus on increasing adaptive ways of thinking and behaving, and decreasing maladaptive thinking–behavior patterns (Critchfield & Benjamin, 2006; Linehan, Davison, Lynch, & Sanderson, 2005).

Clinical Implications

Develop a Collaborative Relationship

Probably the most vexing part of working with persons with personality dysfunction is that they typically experience widespread difficulties in social and interpersonal relationships. The standard way that clinicians develop a collaborative relationship is not likely to be effective. Nevertheless, the importance of a strong therapeutic alliance is clear. The therapeutic relationship can be used as a model for how healthy relationships might work.

The clinician will likely need to tend to the therapeutic alliance regularly, with particular attention to therapeutic ruptures, an inevitable part of the treatment process that affects the therapeutic relationship over time (Muran & Safran, 2002). Some research suggests that an explicit focus on the nature of the therapeutic relationship in therapy can have a positive effect on outcome (Clarkin et al., 2001), although there is still limited evidence on what client-specific factors must be kept in mind when using such an approach. The focus of the therapeutic relationship may differ by type of PD (Critchfield & Benjamin, 2006) or nature of the presenting problems (e.g., Summers & Barber, 2009). For example, a strong, positive alliance may greatly benefit individuals with PDs, who often alienate others and have difficulty with developing close relationships, such as a person with paranoid PD. Alternatively, individuals with borderline PD may easily develop a strong attachment to their therapist but have difficulty managing the relationship. In these cases, attention might best be focused on establishing relational boundaries, demonstrating appropriate distance in the relationship, and modeling the integration of positive and negative aspects of an interpersonal relationship.

Critchfield and Benjamin (2006) describe a number of principles that can help the development and maintenance of a positive therapeutic relationship with patients with PD, including expression of empathy, positive regard, and patience in sessions, as well as adoption of a flexible stance toward treatment (while maintaining appropriate boundaries). Therapeutic flexibility may be particularly important when working patients with PD because PDs involve such a heterogeneous group of conditions and are related to so many kinds of relationship difficulties.

No single style or therapeutic approach fits every patient with a PD, but these principles reach across all theoretical orientations. It is imperative for clinicians to assess the needs and capacities of each individual and modify the treatment as needed. It may be helpful for therapists to take a more experimental attitude when working with patients with PD and be able to shift flexibly between treatment approaches, and even integrate them at times based on a patient's response to treatment. It is also important to limit unacceptable behavior in therapy and model appropriate expression of thoughts or emotions (Seibel & Dowd, 2001). Practicing clinicians may find that patients with borderline pathology push the limits of therapy more than people with any other PD, so this point is particularly relevant in the treatment of these individuals. Finally, explicitly addressing patients' expectations for success, discussing the limits of therapy, and conveying understanding about the difficulty of change helps to ensure that patients do not hold unrealistic expectations that the therapist can never meet. In brief, there is a need in some cases to provide ongoing education about therapy (e.g., Linehan, 1993).

Emphasis on Working toward Explicit Mutually Agreed-Upon Goals

Psychotherapists should consider an active stance in helping patients organize their complaints and distress into clear and understandable goals, which become benchmarks toward which to work. Many individuals with personality dysfunction are unaware of the nature and the impact of their dysfunctional patterns and therefore do not generally seek treatment for these problems. They may enter treatment with relational disturbances or clinical syndromes such as depression, or they may be in treatment because the courts or family members referred them. The therapist must accept patients as they are and formulate goals consistent with their wishes. As treatment unfolds, the psychotherapist can begin to shift by expanding or narrowing the focus of treatment when the patient appears to be ready for such change. Regardless of therapeutic orientation, detailed analyses of the precipitating factors and consequences of problematic behaviors are an important first step in gaining a thorough picture of the patient's difficulty and what will need to be addressed in the context of therapy (Linehan, 1993). Related to this, education about the patterns discovered and how treatment can help is necessary. For example, a patient with dependent PD should understand how the dependent patterns interfere with goal attainment and ultimate satisfaction, and how facing unpleasant affective states allows growth to proceed.

While determining treatment goals may seem to be relatively straightforward, the implementation of PD treatment is often thrown off course. Remember that individuals with PDs are characteristically rigid and inflexible in their patterns of thinking and behaving, and they often feel comfortable with these patterns. It is common, and often needed, for therapists to spend a great deal of therapy time discussing a patient's desire for change, reviewing treatment goals and the reason those goals were determined, and assessing level of distress or dysfunction with current behavior. This process can look very different, depending on the PD patient. Therapists may have a particularly difficult time with therapy impasses or unfocused treatment when working with patients with borderline PD (Linehan et al., 1993; Kernberg, Yeomans, Clarkin, & Levy, 2008; Fonagy & Bateman, 2008). Structure and consistency are essential in the treatment of patients with borderline PD, however, because their lives are almost always filled with chaos outside of therapy. Avoidant patients, on the other hand, may remain distant during sessions or even avoid therapy as a way to avoid facing their fears; if a clear pattern emerges, this behavior could then be addressed in an empathetic way by the therapist.

To ensure progress toward treatment goals, it is critical that clinicians take an active therapeutic stance (Critchfield & Benjamin, 2006; Linehan, 1993). Because of their tendency perceptually to misperceive or distort the intentions of others, patients with PD generally do not do well with an overly detached, passive therapeutic stance (e.g., Kernberg, 1996). A balance must be sought between controlling the process and letting it stagnate, which will result in premature termination. Furthermore, active monitoring of a patient's response to treatment is essential. If the patient is not responding, the psychotherapist and patient should collaborate about changing treatment goals.

Focus on Increasing Adaptive Thinking/Behaving and Decreasing Maladaptive Thinking/Behavior

One of the criteria for a diagnosis of PD is the presence of maladaptive patterns of thinking or behaving in cognition, emotional responses, interpersonal functioning, and/or impulse control. Whether or not these tie explicitly to treatment goals, part of the therapist's role is to facilitate more adaptive ways of thinking about the self and others, manage emotional reactions, and tolerate distress. At the same time, it is essential to avoid reinforcing negative behaviors. Some of this can be done in the context of the therapeutic relationship, but it is also important for the therapist to relate newly learned behaviors to the patient's everyday life (Linehan, 1993). While most treatments for psychopathology share the focus of altering affect, cognition, and behavior in one way or another, affect may be a particularly critical focus in PD treatment (Critchfield & Benjamin, 2006; Summers & Barber, 2009).

CONCLUSION

PDs are among the most common and debilitating of conditions presented in clinical practice and medical offices. The classification of PDs, although problematic in many ways, continues to be an essential conceptual framework for organizing a spectrum of various types and structures of dysfunctional personality. Their negative impact is far-reaching, affecting many aspects of individuals' lives, with a particularly detrimental impact on interpersonal relationships. Pathological personality traits often begin in childhood or adolescence, and those early traits are associated with an increased risk for the subsequent development of PD and other mental disorders (Cohen, Chen, Crawford, Brook, & Gordon, 2007). PDs are commonly comorbid with other psychopathology, such as major depression or substance use disorders. They can also have a negative impact on the course of such disorders and make treatment adherence difficult (Fournier et al., 2008), although there is also evidence that PDs can be helpful in treatment (Barber & Muenz, 1996; Milrod, Leon, Barder, Markowitz, & Graf, 2007). In some cases, PDs also represent the beginning stages of the onset of a more serious form of psychopathology. Paranoid and schizotypal PDs, for example, sometimes precede the onset of schizophrenic disorders.

While the devastating impact of PDs on general functioning and well-being is clear, there are a number of limitations in the current basic research. First, much of the work described earlier focuses on a single PD (i.e., borderline PD) or a group of PDs, and does not provide data on the full range of personality pathology. Combining what we know about general personality traits and PDs, and exploring interactions among personality traits (e.g., high Neuroticism, low Conscientiousness, and low Agreeableness) may be one way to advance our basic knowledge of PDs. The way PDs are measured also varies across studies, making it difficult to make specific conclusions about etiological or sociocultural factors in relation to PDs, or to determine the particular impact of a given PD feature. Furthermore, many of the longitudinal studies up to now have been restricted to small clinical samples with only younger adults. There is a great need to expand PD research into middle adulthood and later life (Oltmanns & Balsis, 2011). The presentation of personality pathology may change as individuals' age. There is growing evidence of risk for negative physical health outcomes associated with PDs, and these outcomes occur much more frequently in older adults (Frankenburg & Zanarini, 2006).

This is an unusual time for PD researchers and clinicians, as clearly demonstrated by the fact that DSM-5 includes two alternative systems for classifying PDs. The categorical system for PDs remains the primary system and is located in the main body of the diagnostic manual. The dimensional system for PDs is included in Section III of DSM-5 ("Emerging Measures and Models"). Dimensional classification systems have the advantage of being better able to account for similarities and differences in people with various combinations of personality traits and do not require the assumption of arbitrary boundaries between normal and abnormal personality. Although this is different from the categorical method currently used by clinicians, it may be equally or even more useful when trying to conceptualize patients and determine treatment.

PDs are heterogeous, challenging conditions to diagnose and treat. There is still a great deal we need to learn about the etiology, course, and consequences of PDs. There is also a long way to go in validating empirically supported treatments for patients with PD. However, the importance of understanding and treating personality pathology in clinical practice cannot be overemphasized. PDs are extremely costly to our health care system, and evidence shows that when PDs are treated, there are significant reductions in health care utilization for up to 3 years following completion of treatment (Davies & Campling, 2003). The variability among individuals with PDs makes it much too difficult to expect that one theoretical model or therapeutic technique can satisfy that diversity. By using general principles of change and common themes that run across orientations as our guide, we can better understand what makes treatment effective for each unique individual. As we think about next steps for the field, it will be imperative to move beyond the barriers of a single theoretical orientation and investigate the therapeutic elements associated with treatment efficacy and how effectiveness varies with different patients.

REFERENCES

Abrams, R., & Horowitz, S. (1999). Personality disorders after age 50: A meta-analytic review of the literature.In A. Rosowsky, R. Abrams, & R. Zweig (Eds.), *Personality disorders in older adults: Emerging issues in diagnosis and treatment* (pp. 55–68). Mahwah, NJ: Erlbaum.

Alvidrez, J. (1999). Ethnic variations in mental health attitudes and service use among low-income African American, Latina, and European American young women. *Community Mental Health Journal, 35,* 515–530.

American Psychiatric Association. (2013). *Diagnostic and statistical manual of mental disorders* (5th ed.). Arlington, VA: Author.

Bagge, C., Nickell, A., Stepp, S., Durrett, C., Jackson, K., & Trull, T. (2004). Borderline personality disorder features predict negative outcomes 2 years later. *Journal of Abnormal Psychology, 113,* 279–288.

Barber, J., & Muenz, L. (1996). The role of avoidance and obsessiveness in matching patients to cognitive and interpersonal psychotherapy: Empirical findings from the Treatment for Depression Collaborative Research Program. *Journal of Consulting and Clinical Psychology, 64,* 951–958.

Barber, J. P., Barrett, M. S., Gallop, R., Rynn, M., & Rickels, K. (2012). Short term dynamic therapy vs. pharmacotherapy for major depressive disorder. *Journal of Clinical Psychiatry, 73*(1), 66–73.

Barber, J. P., Frank, A., Weiss, R. D., Blaine, J., Siqueland, L., Moras, K., et al. (1996). Prevalence of personality disorder diagnoses among cocaine/crack dependents in the NIDA study. *Journal of Personality Disorders, 10,* 297–311.

Bateman, A., & Fonagy, P. (2006). *Mentalization-based treatment for borderline personality disorder: A practical guide.* New York: Oxford University Press.

Baumeister, R., Dale, K., & Sommer, K. (1998). Freudian defense mechanisms and empirical findings in modern social psychology: Reaction formation, projection, displacement, undoing, isolation, sublimnation, and denial. *Journal of Personality, 66,* 1081–2023.

Beck, A. T., Freeman, A., & Davies, D. D. (2004). *Cognitive therapy of personality disorders* (2nd ed.). New York: Guilford Press.

Bender, D. S., Morey, L. C., & Skodol, A. E. (2011). Toward a model for assessing level of personality functioning in DSM-5: Part I. A review of theory and methods. *Journal of Personality Assessment, 93,* 332–346.

Berenbaum, H., Valera, E., & Kerns, J. (2003). Psychological trauma and schizotypal personality disorder. *Journal of Abnormal Psychology, 117,* 502–519.

Bernstein, D., Ahluvalia, T., Pogge, D., & Handelsman, L. (1997). Validity of the Childhood Trauma Questionnaire in an adolescent psychiatric population. *Journal of the American Academy of Child and Adolescent Psychiatry, 36,* 340–348.

Bernstein, M. E., Reich, D., Zanarini, M. C., & Siever, L. J. (2002). "Late-onset" borderline personality disorder: A life unraveling. *Harvard Review of Psychiatry, 10,* 292–301.

Blum, N., St. John, D., Pfohl, B., Stuart, S., McCormick, B., Allen, J., et al. (2008). Systems training for emotional predictability and problem solving (STEPPS) for outpatients with borderline personality disorder: A randomized controlled trial and 1=year follow-up. *American Journal of Psychiatry, 165,* 468–478.

Boggs, C., Morey, L., Skodol, A., Shea, M., Sanislow, C., Grilo, C., et al. (2005). Differential impairment as an indicator of sex bias in the DSM-IV criteria for four personality disorders. *Psychological Assessment, 17,* 492–496.

Bolton, J., Pagura, J., Enns, M., Grant, B., & Sareen, J. (2010). A population-based longitudinal study of risk factors for suicide attempts in major depressive disorder. *Journal of Psychiatry Research, 44*(13), 817–826.

Bowlby, J. (1969). *Attachment and loss.* New York: Penguin.

Brittlebank, A., Cole, A., Hassanyeh, F., Kenny, M., Simpson, D., & Scott, J. (1989). Hostility, hopelessness, and deliberate self-harm: A prospective follow-up study. *Acta Psychiatrica Scandinavica, 81,* 280–283.

Cadoret, R., Yates, W., Ed, T., Woodworth, G., & Stewart, M. (1995). Genetic environmental interactions in the genesis of aggressivity and conduct disorders. *Archives of General Psychiatry, 52,* 916–924.

Caspi, A., & Roberts, B. (1999). Personality change and continuity across the life course. In L. A. Pervin & O. P. John (Eds.), *Handbook of personality theory and research* (pp. 300–326). New York: Guilford Press.

Castonguay, L., & Beutler, L. (2006). *Principles of therapeutic change that work.* New York: Oxford University Press.

Chavira, D., Grilo, C., Shea, M. T., Yen, S., Gunderson, J., & Morey, L., et al. (2003). Ethnicity and four personality disorders. *Comprehensive Psychiatry, 44,* 483–491.

Clark, L. A. (2007). Assessment and diagnosis of personality disorder: Perennial issues and an emerging reconceptualization. *Annual Review of Psychology, 58,* 227–257.

Clarkin, J. F., Foelsch, P. A., Levy, K. N., Hill, J. W., Delaney, J. C., & Kernberg, O. F. (2001). The development of psychodynamic treatment for patients with borderline personality disorder: A preliminary study of behavior change. *Journal of Personality Disorders, 15,* 487–495.

Clarkin, J. F., Yeomans, F., & Kernberg, O. F. (2006). *Psychotherapy for borderline personality: Focusing on object relations.* New York: Wiley.

Cohen, P. (2008). Child development and personality disorder. *Psychiatric Clinics of North America, 31*(3), 477–493.

Cohen, P., Chen, H., Crawford, T. N., Brook, J. S., & Gordon, K. (2007). Personality disorders in early adolescence and the development of later substance use disorders in the general population. *Drug and Alcohol Dependence, 88,* S71–S84.

Cohen, P., Crawford, T. N., Johnson, J. G., & Kasen, S. (2005). The Children in the Community Study of developmental course of personality disorder. *Journal of Personality, 19,* 466–486.

Coid, J., Yang, M., Tyrer, P., Roberts, A., & Ullrich, S. (2006). Prevalence and correlates of personality disorder among adults aged 16 to 74 in Great Britain. *British Journal of Psychiatry, 188,* 423–431.

Cramer, P. (2008). Seven pillars of defense mechanism theory. *Social and Personality Psychology Compass, 2,* 1963–1981.

Crawford, T., Cohen, P., & Brook, J. (2001). Dramatic–erratic personality disorder symptoms: Continuity from early adolescence into adulthood. *Journal of Personality Disorders, 15,* 319–335.

Critchfield, K. L., & Benjamin, L. S. (2006). Principles for psychosocial treatment of personality disorder: an integration of participant, relationship, and treatment domains. In L. Castonguay & L. Beutler (Eds.), *Principles of therapeutic change that work* (pp. 253–271). New York: Oxford University Press.

Critchfield, K. L., Levy, K. N., Clarkin, J. F., & Kernberg, O. F. (2008). The relational context of aggression in borderline personality disorder: Using attachment style to predict forms of hostility, *Journal of Clinical Psychology, 64*(7), 67–82.

Crits-Christoph, P., & Barber, J.P. (2007). Psychological treatments for personality disorders. In P.E. Nathan & J.M. Gorman (Eds.), *A guide to treatments that works* (3rd ed., pp. 641–658). New York: Oxford University Press.

Dautovich, N., McNamara, J., Williams, J., Cross, N., & McCrae, C. (2010). Tackling sleeplessness: Psychological treatment options for insomnia. *Nature and Science of Sleep, 10*(2), 23–37.

Davanloo, H. (Ed.). (1980). *Short-term dynamic psychotherapy.* New York: Aronson.

Davies, S., & Campling, P. (2003). Therapeutic community treatment of personality disorder: Service use and mortality over 3 years' follow-up. *British Journal of Psychiatry, 182,* s24–s27.

De Leo, D., Padoani, W., Scocco, P., Lie, D., Bille-Brahe, U., Arensman, E., et al. (2001). Attempted and completed suicide in older subjects: Results from the WHO/EURO Multicentre Study of Suicidal Behaviour. *International Journal of Geriatric Psychiatry, 16,* 300–310.

Dolan-Sewell, R., Krueger, R., & Shea, M. T. (2001). Co-occurrence with syndrome disorders. In J. L. Livesley (Ed.), *Handbook of personality disorders: Theory, research, and treatment* (pp. 84–106). New York: Guilford Press.

Duberstein, P., & Conwell, Y. (1997). Personality disorders and completed suicide: A methodological and conceptual review. *Clinical Psychology: Science and Practice, 4,* 359–376.

Eisenberg, D., Davis, R., Ettner, S., Appel, S., Wilkey, S., Van Rompay, M., et al. (1998). Trends in alternative medicine use in the United States, 1990–1997. *Journal of the American Medical Association, 280,* 1569–1575.

El-Gabalawy, R., Katz., L., & Sareen, J. (2010). Comorbidity and associated severity of borderline personality disorder and physical health conditions in a nationally representative sample. *Psychosomatic Medicine, 72,* 641–647.

Emmons, R. (1997). Motives and goals. In R. Hogan, J. Johnson, & R. Stephan (Eds.), *Handbook of personality psychology* (pp. 485–512). San Diego, CA: Academic Press.

Fonagy, P. (2004). *Psychotherapy for borderline personality disorder: Menatlization-based treatment.* New York: Oxford University Press.

Fonagy, P., & Bateman, A. (2008). The development of borderline personality disorder—a mentalizing model. *Journal of Personality Disorders, 22,* 4–21.

Fonagy, P., & Target, M. (2006). The mentalization-based approach to self pathology. *Journal of Personality Disorders, 20,* 544 – 576.

Fournier, J. C., DeRubeis, R. J., Shelton, R. C., Gallop, R., Amsterdam, J. D., & Hollon, S. D. (2008). Antidepressant medications v. cognitive therapy in people with depression with or without personality disorder. *British Journal of Psychiatry, 192,* 124–129.

Frances, A., First, M., & Pincus, H. (1995). *DSM-IV guidebook.* Washington, DC: American Psychiatric Press.

Frankenburg, F., & Zanarini, M. (2006). Obesity and obesity-related illnesses in borderline patients. *Journal of Personality Disorders, 20,* 71–80.

Freeman, A., & Reinecke, M. A. (Eds.). (2007). *Personality disorders in children and adolescents.* Hoboken, NJ: Wiley.

Friedman, H., Hawley, P., & Tucker, J. (1994). Personality, health, and longevity. *Current Directions in Psychological Science, 3*(2), 37–41.

Gallese, V., Keysers, C., & Rizzolatti, G. (2004). A unifying view of the basis of social cognition. *Trends in Cognitive Science, 7,* 287–292.

Gibbs, N., South, S., & Oltmanns, T. (2003). Attentional coping style in obsessive–compulsive personality disorder: A test of the intolerance of uncertainty hypothesis. *Personality and Individual Differences, 34,* 41–57.

Grant, B., Chou, S., Goldstein, R., Huang, B., Stinson, F., Saha, T., et al. (2008). Prevalence, correlates, disability, and comorbidity of DSM-IV borderline personality disorder: Results from the Wave 2 National Epidemiological Survey on Alcohol and Related Conditions. *Journal of Clinical Psychiatry, 69,* 533–545.

Grilo, C., Sanislow, C., Shea, M., Skodol, A., Stout, R., Gunderson, J., et al. (2005). Two-year prospective naturalistic study of remission from major depressive disorder as a function of personality disorder comorbidity. *Journal of Consulting and Clinical Psychology, 73,* 78–85.

Gunderson, J. G. (2010). Revising the borderline diagnosis for DSM-V: An alternative proposal. *Journal of Personality Disorders, 24,* 694–708.

Gunderson, J. G., Shea, M. T., Skodol, A. E., McGlashan, L. T. H., & Keller, M. B. (2000). The collaborative longitudinal personality disorders study: Development, aims, design, and sample characteristics. *Journal of Personality Disorders, 14,* 300–315.

Gunderson, J. G., Stout, R. L., McGlashan, T. H., Shea, M. T., Morey, L. C., Grio, C. M., et al. (2011). Ten-year course of borderline personality disorder: Psychopathology and function from the Collaborative Longitudinal Personality Disorders Study. *Archives of General Psychiatry, 68*(8) 827–837.

Harris, G. T., & Rice, M. E. (2006). Treatment of psychopathy: A review of empirical findings. In C. J. Patrick (Ed.), *Handbook of psychopathy* (pp. 555–572). New York: Guilford Press.

Helgeland, M., & Torgersen, S. (2004). Developmental antecedents of borderline personality disorder. *Comprehensive Psychiatry, 45,* 138–147.

Holtzworth-Munroe, A. (2000). A typology of men who are violent toward their female partners: Making sense of the heterogeneity in husband violence. *Current Directions in Psychological Science, 9*(4), 140–143.

Holtzworth-Munroe, A., & Stuart, G. L. (1994). Typologies of male batterers: Three subtypes and the differences among them. *Psychological Bulletin, 116*(3), 476–497.

Hueston, W., Werth, J., & Mainous, A. (1999). Personality disorder traits: Prevalence and effects on health status in primary care patients. *International Journal of Psychiatry in Medicine, 29,* 63–74.

Ingenhoven, T., Lafay, P., Rinne, T., Passchier, J., & Duivenvoorden, H. 2010. Effectiveness of pharmacotherapy for severe personality disorders: meta-analyses of randomized controlled trials. *Journal of Clinical Psychiatry. 71,* 14–25.

Jackson, H. J., & Burgess, P. M. (2000). Personality disorders in the community: A report from the Australian National Survey of Mental Health and Wellbeing. *Social Psychiatry and Psychiatric Epidemiology, 35,* 531–538.

Jackson, H. J., & Burgess, P. M. (2002). Personality disorder in the community: Results from the Australian National Survey of Mental Health and Wellbeing Part II. Relationships between personality disorder, Axis I mental disorders and physical conditions with disability and health consultations. *Social Psychiatry and Psychiatric Epidemiology, 37*(6), 251–260.

Johnson, J., Cohen, P., Smailes, E., Skodol, A., Brown, J., & Oldham, J. (2001). Childhood verbal abuse and risk for personality disorders in adolescence and early adulthood. *Comprehensive Psychiatry, 42,* 16–23.

Johnson, J., Cohen, P., Brown, J., Smailes, E., & Bernstein, D. (1999). Childhood maltreatment increases risk for personality disorders during early adulthood. *Archives of General Psychiatry, 56,* 600–606.

Kendell, R. E. (2002). The distinction between personality disorder and mental illness. *British Journal of Psychiatry, 180,* 110–115.

Kendler, K., Aggen, S., Czajkowski, N., Roysamb, E., Tambs, K., et al. (2008). The structure of genetic and environmental risk factors for DSM-IV personality disorders: A multivariate twin study. *Archives of General Psychiatry, 65,* 1438–1446.

Kendler, K., McGuire, M., Gruenberg, A., O'Hare, A., Spellman, M., & Walsh, D. (1993). The Roscommon Family Study, III: Schizophrenia-related personality disorders in relatives. *Archives of General Psychiatry, 50*(10), 781–788.

Kernberg, O. (1996). A psychoanalytic theory of personality disorders. In J. F. Clerkin & M. F. Lenzenweger (Eds.), *Major theories of personality disorder* (pp. 106–137). New York: Guilford Press.

Kernberg, O. (2001). The suicidal risk in severe personality disorders: Differential diagnosis and treatment. *Journal of Personality Disorders, 15,* 195–208.

Kernberg, O., Yeomans, F., Clarkin, J., & Levy, K. (2008). Transference focused psychotherapy: Overview and update. *International Journal of Psychoanalysis, 89,* 601–620.

Kessler, R., McGonagle, K., Zhao, S., Nelson, C., Hughes, M., Eshleman, S., et al. (1994). Lifetime and 12–month prevalence of DSM-III-R psychiatric disorders in the United States. *Archives of General Psychiatry, 51,* 8–19.

Klein, D. N., Kotov, R., & Bufferd, S. J. (2011). Personality and depression: Explanatory models and review of the evidence. *Annual Review of Clinical Psychology, 7,* 269–295.

Krueger, R. F., Derringer, J., Markon, K. E., Watson, D., & Skodol, A. E. (2012). Initial construction of a maladaptive personality trait model and inventory for DSM-5. *Psychological Medicine, 42*(9), 1879–1890.

Krueger, R., Eaton, N., Clark, L., Watson, D., Markon, K., Derringer, J., Skodol, A., & Livesley, J. (2011). Deriving an empirical structure of personality pathology for DSM-5. *Journal of Personality Disorders, 25,* 170–191.

Krueger, R. F., Eaton, N. R., Derringer, J., Markon, K. E., Watson, D., & Skodol, A. E. (2011). Personality in DSM-5: Helping delineate personality disorder content and framing the metastructure. *Journal of Personality Assessment, 93,* 325–331.

Lee, H. B., Bienvenu, J., Cho, S., Ramsey, C., Bandeen-Roche, K., Eaton, W., et al. (2010). Personality disorders and traits as predictors of incident cardiovascular disease: Findings from the 23-year follow-up of the Baltimore ECA Study. *Psychosomatics, 51,* 289–296.

Lenzenweger, M. F., Lane, M. C., Loranger, A. W., & Kessler, R. C. (2007). DSM-IV personality disorders in the National Comorbidity Survey Replication. *Biological Psychiatry, 62,* 553–564.

Linehan, M. (1987). Dialectical behavior therapy for borderline personality disorder: Theory and method. *Bulletin of the Menninger Clinic, 51,* 261–276.

Linehan, M. M. (1993). *Cognitive behavioral treatment of borderline personality disorder.* New York: Guilford Press.

Linehan, M. M., Comtois, K. A., Murray, A. M., Brown, M. Z., Gallop, R. J., Heard, H. L., et al. (2006). Two-year randomized controlled trial and follow-up of dialectic behavior therapy vs. therapy by experts for suicidal behaviors and borderline personality disorder. *Archives of General Psychiatry, 63,* 757–766.

Linehan, M. M., Davison, G., Lynch, T., & Sanderson, C. (2005). Technique factors in treating personality disorders. In L. Castonguay & L. Beulter (Eds.), *Principles of therapeutic change that work* (pp. 239–252). New York: Oxford University Press.

Linehan, M. M., Heard, H. L., & Armstrong, H. E. (1993). Naturalistic follow-up of a behavioral treatment for chronically parasuicidal borderline patients. *Archives of General Psychiatry, 50,* 971–974.

Linney, Y. M., Murray, R. M., Peters, E. R., MacDonald, A. M., Rijsdijk, F., & Sham, P. C. (2003). A quantitative genetic analysis of schizotypal personality traits. *Psychological Medicine, 33,* 803–816.

Livesley, J. (2008). Toward a genetically-informed model of borderline personality disorder. *Journal of Personality Disorders, 22,* 42–71.

Lyons, M. J. (1995). Epidemiology of personality disorders. In M. T. Tsuang, M. Tohen, & G. E. P. Zahner (Eds.), *Textbook in psychiatric epidemiology* (pp. 407–436). New York: Wiley.

MacMillan, H., Fleming, J. E., Streiner, D. L., Lin, E., Boyle, M. H., Jamieson, E., et al. (2001). Childhood abuse and lifetime psychopathology in a community sample. *American Journal of Psychiatry, 158,* 1878–1883.

Magnavita, J. J. (1997). *Restructuring personality disorders: A short-term dynamic approach.* New York: Guilford Press.

Magnavita, J. J. (2000). *Relational therapy for personality disorders.* New York: Wiley.

Magnavita, J. J. (2002). *Theories of personality: Contemporary approaches to the science of personality.* Hoboken, NJ: Wiley.

Magnavita, J. J. (2004). *Handbook of personality disorders: Theory and practice.* Hoboken, NJ: Wiley.

Magnavita, J. J. (2005a). *Personality-guided relational therapy: A unified approach.* Washington, DC: American Psychological Association.

Magnavita, J. J. (2005b). Systems theory foundation of personality, psychopathology, and psychotherapy. In S. Strack (Ed.), *Handbook of personology and psychopathology* (pp. 140–163). Hoboken, NJ: Wiley.

Magnavita, J. J. (2007). A systemic family perspective on child and adolescent personality disorders. In A. Freeman & M. A. Reinecke (Eds.), *Personality disorders in childhood and adolescence* (pp. 131–181). Hoboken, NJ: Wiley.

Magnavita, J. J. (Ed.). (2010). *Evidence-based treatment of personality dysfunction.* Hoboken, NJ: Wiley.

Magnavita, J. J. (2011). Reflections on personality systematics and a unified clinical science. In L. L'Abate (Ed.), *Paradigms in theory construction* (pp. 207–216). New York: Springer.

Magnavita, J. J., & MacFarlane, M. (2004). Family treatment of personality disorders: Historical overview and current perspectives. In, M. M. MacFarlane (Ed.), *Family treatment of personality disorders: Advances in clinical practice* (pp. 3–39). New York: Haworth Press.

Markon, K., Krueger, R., & Watson, D. (2005). Delineating the structure of normal and abnormal personality disorder: An integrative hierarchical approach. *Journal of Personality and Social Psychology, 88,* 139–157.

Mauricio, A. M., Tein, J.-Y., & Lopez, F. G. (2007). Borderline and antisocial personality scores as mediators between attachment and intimate partner violence. *Violence and Victims, 22*(2), 139–157.

McCullough Valliant, L. (1997). *Changing character: Short-term anxiety regulating psychotherapy for regulating defenses, affects and attachment.* New York: Basic Books.

McGilloway, A., Hall, R., Lee, T., & Bhui, K. (2010). A systematic review of personality disorder, race and ethnicity: Prevalence, aetiology and treatment. *BMC Psychiatry, 10,* 33.

McMain, S. F., Links, P. S., Gnam, W. H., Guimond, T., Cardish, R. J., Korman, L., et al. (2009). A randomized trial of dialectical behavior therapy versus general psychiatric management for borderline personality disorder. *American Journal of Psychiatry, 166,* 1365–1374.

Messer, S. B., & Abbass, A. A. (2010). Evidence-based psychodynamic therapy with personality disorders. In J. J. Magnavita (Ed.), *Evidence-based treatment of personality dysfunction: Principles, methods, and processes* (pp. 79–111). Washington, DC: American Psychological Association.

Millon, T., Grossman, S., Meagher, S., Millon, C., & Everly, G. (1999). Theoretical personalities. In W. J. Livesley (Ed.), *Handbook of personality disorders: Theory, research, and treatment* (pp. 39–59). New York: Guilford Press.

Millon, T., & Martinez, A. (1995). Avoidant personality disorder. In W. J. Livesley (Ed.), *The DSM-IV personality disorders* (pp. 218–233). New York: Guilford Press.

Milrod, B., Leon, A., Barder, J., Markowitz, J., & Graf, E. (2007). Do comorbid personality disorders moderate panic-focused psychotherapy?: An exploratory examination of the American Psychiatric Association practice guidelines. *Journal of Clinical Psychiatry, 68,* 885–891.

Moffitt, T. E. (2007). A review of research on the taxonomy of life-course persistent versus adolescence-limited antisocial behavior. In D. J. Flannery, A. T. Vazsonyi, & I. D. Waldman (Eds.), *The Cambridge handbook of violent behavior and aggression* (pp. 49–74). New York: Cambridge University Press.

Moran, P. (1999). *Antisocial personality disorder: An epidemiological perspective.* London: Gaskell.

Morrison, A., Frame, L., & Larkin, W. (2003). Relationship between trauma and psychosis: A review and integration. *British Journal of Clinical Psychology, 42,* 331–353.

Muran, J. C., & Safran, J. D. (2002). A relational approach to psychotherapy: Resolving ruptures in the therapeutic alliance. In F. W. Kaslow (Ed.), *Comprehensive handbook of psychotherapy* (pp. 253–281). New York: Wiley.

Nock, M., Hwang, I., Sampson, N.., Kessler, R., Angermeyer, M., Beautrais, A., et al. (2009). Cross-national analysis of the associations among mental disorders and suicidal behavior: Findings from the WHO World Mental Health Surveys. *PLoS Medicine, 6*(8), e1000123.

Oldham, J. (2006). Borderline personality disorder and suicidality. *American Journal of Psychiatry, 163,* 20–26.

Oldham, J. M., Skodol, A. E., Bender, D. S. (2009). Future directions: Toward DSM-V. In J. M. Oldham, A. E. Skodol, & D. S. Bender (Eds.), *Essentials of personality disorders* (pp. 381–392). Arlington, VA: American Psychiatric Publishing.

Oltmanns, T. F., & Balsis, S. (2011). Personality pathology in later life: Questions about the measurement, course, and impact of disorders. *Annual Review of Clinical Psychology, 7,* 321–349.

Oltmanns, T. F., Melley, A., & Turkheimer, E. (2002). Impaired social function and symptoms of personality disorders assessed by peer and self-report in a nonclinical sample. *Journal of Personality Disorders, 16,* 437–452.

Pally, R. (2002). The neurobiology of borderline personality disorder: The synergy of "nature and nurture." *Journal of Psychiatric Practice, 8*(3), 133–142.

Paris, J. (2003). Personality disorders over time: Precursors, course and outcome. *Journal of Personality Disorders, 17,* 479–488.

Parnas, J., Licht, D., & Bovet, P. (2005). Cluster A personality disorders: A review. In M. Maj, H. S. Akiskal, J. E. Mezzich, & A. Okasha (Eds.), *Personality disorders, Volume 8* (pp. 1–124). Chichester, UK: Wiley.

Paulhus, D. L., Fridhandler, B., & Hayes, S. (1997). Psychological defense: Contemporary theory and research. In R. Hogan, J. A. Johnson, & S. R. Briggs (Eds.), *Handbook of personality psychology* (pp. 543–579). San Diego, CA: Academic Press.

Perry, J., Hoglend, P., Shear, K., Vaillant, G. E., Horowitz, M., Kardos, M. E., et al. (1998). Field trial of a diagnostic axis for defense mechanisms for DSM-IV. *Journal of Personality Disorders, 12*, 56–68.

Pietrzak, R., Wagner, J., & Petry, N. (2007). DSM-IV personality disorders and coronary heart disease in older adults: Results from the national epidemiological survey on alcohol and related conditions. *Journal of Gerontology B: Social Sciences, 62*, 295–299.

Pilkonis, P., Blehar, M., & Prien, R. (1997). Introduction to the special feature: Research directions for the personality disorders. *Journal of Personality Disorders, 11*, 201–204.

Piper, W. E. (2008). Underutilization of short-term group therapy: Enigmatic or understandable? *Psychotherapy Research, 18*, 127–138.

Piper, W. E., Rosie, J. S., & Joyce, A. S. (1996). *Time-limited day treatment for personality disorders: Integration of research and practice in a group program.* Washington, DC: American Psychological Association.

Pulay, A., Stinson, F., Dawson, D., Goldstein, R., Chou, P., et al. (2009). Prevalence, correlates, disability, and comorbidity of DSM-IV schizotypal personality disorder: Results from the Wave 2 National Epidemiologic Survey on Alcohol and Related Conditions. *Journal of Clinical Psychiatry, 11*(2), 53–67.

Read, J., van Os, J., Morrison, A. P., & Ross, A. (2005). Childhood trauma, psychosis, and schizophrenia: A literature review with theoretical and clinical implications. *Acta Psychiatrica Scandinavica, 112*, 330–350.

Reich, J. (2000). The relationship of social phobia to avoidant personality disorder: A proposal to reclassify avoidant personality disorder based on empirical findings. *European Psychiatry, 15*, 151–159.

Rhee, S., & Waldman, I. (2002). Genetic and environmental influences on antisocial behavior: A meta-analysis of twin and adoption studies. *Psychological Bulletin, 128*, 490–529.

Ro, E., & Clark, L.A. (2009). Psychosocial functioning in the context of diagnosis: Assessment and theoretical issues. *Psychological Assessment, 21*, 313–324.

Roberts, B., Walton, K., & Viechtbauer, W. (2006). Patterns of mean-level change in personality traits across the life course: A meta-analysis of longitudinal studies. *Psychological Bulletin, 132*, 1–25.

Robins, L., & Regier, D. (1991). *Psychiatric disorders in America: The Epidemiological Catchment Area Study.* New York: Free Press.

Robins, C. J., Rosenthal, M. Z., & Cuper, P. F. (2010). Dialectic behavior therapy. In J. J. Magnavita (Ed.), *Evidence-based treatment of personality dysfunction: Principles, methods, and processes* (pp. 49–78). Washington, DC: American Psychological Association.

Ronningstam, E., & Gunderson, J. (1991). Differentiating borderline personality disorder from narcissistic personality disorder. *Journal of Personality Disorders, 5*, 225–232.

Ruggiero, J., Bernstein, D., & Handelsman, L. (1999). Traumatic stress in childhood and later personality disorders: A retrospective study of male patients with substance abuse. *Psychiatric Annals, 29*, 713–721.

Samuel, D., Hopwood, C., Ansell, E., Morey, L., Sanislow, C., Markowitz, J. C., et al. (2011). Comparing the temporal stability of self-report and interview assessed personality disorder. *Journal of Abnormal Psychology, 120*, 670–680.

Seibel, C. A., & Dowd, E. T. (2001). Personality characteristics associated with psychological reactance. *Journal of Clinical Psychology, 57*(7), 963–969.

Shen, B., McCreary, C., & Myers, H. (2004). Independent and mediated contributions of personality, coping, social support, and depressive symptoms to physical functioning outcome among patients in cardiac rehabilitation. *Journal of Behavioral Medicine, 27*, 39–62.

Sirey, J., Bruce, M., Alexopoulos, G., Perlick, D. A., Friedman, S., & Meyers, B. (2001). Stigma as a barrier to recovery: Perceived stigma and patient-rated severity of illness as predictors of antidepressant drug adherence. *Psychiatric Services, 52,* 1615–1620.

Skodol, A. E. (2008). Longitudinal course and outcome of personality disorders. *Psychiatric Clinics of North America, 31,* 495–503.

Skodol, A. E., Bender, D. S., Morey, L. C., Clark, L. A., Oldham, J. M., Alarcon, R. D., et al. (2011). Personality disorder types proposed for DSM-5. *Journal of Personality Disorders, 25,* 136–169.

Skodol, A. E., Gunderson, J. G., McGlashan, T. H., Dyck, I. R., Stout, R. L., Bender, D. S., et al. (2002). Functional impairment in patients with schizotypal, borderline, avoidant, or obsessive-compulsive personality disorders. *American Journal of Psychiatry, 159,* 276–283.

Skodol, A. E., Gunderson, J. G., Shea, M. T., McGlashan, T. H., Morey, L. C., Sanislow, C. A., et al. (2005). The Collaborative Longitudinal Personality Disorders Study (CLPS): Overview and implications. *Journal of Personality Disorders, 19*(5), 487–504.

Skodol, A. E., Pagano, M. E., Bender, D. S., Shea, M., Gunderson, J. G., Yen, S., et al. (2005). Stability of functional impairment in patients with schizotypal, borderline, avoidant, or obsessive–compulsive personality disorder over two years. *Psychological Medicine, 35,* 443–451.

Soldz, S., & Vaillant, G. E. (1998). A 50–year longitudinal study of defense use among inner city men: A validation of the DSM-IV defense axis. *Journal of Nervous and Mental Disease, 186,* 104–111.

Summers, R. J., & Barber, J. P. (2009). *Dynamic psychotherapy: A guide to evidence based practice.* New York: Guilford Press.

Torgersen, S. (1994). Genetics in borderline conditions. *Acta Psychiatica Scandinavica, 89*(379, Suppl.), 19–25.

Torgersen, S., Kringlen, E., & Cramer, V. (2001). The prevalence of personality disorders in a community sample. *Archives of General Psychiatry, 58,* 590–596.

Trull, T., Sher, K., Minks-Brown, C., Durbin, J., & Burr, R. (2000). Borderline personality disorder and substance use disorders: A review and integration. *Clinical Psychology Review, 20,* 235–253.

Trull, T. J., Jahng, S., Tomko, R. L., Wood, P. K., & Sher, K. J. (2010). Revised NESARC personality disorder diagnoses: Gender, prevalence, and comorbidity with substance dependence disorders. *Journal of Personality Disorders, 24,* 412–426.

Trull, T. J., & Widiger, T. A. (2008). Geology 102: More thoughts on a shift to a dimensional model of personality disorders. *Social and Personality Psychology Compass, 2*(2), 949–967.

Tyrer, P., Gunderson, J., Lyons, M., & Tohen, M. (1997). Extent of comorbidity between mental state and personality disorders. *Journal of Personality Disorders, 11,* 242–259.

Vaillant, G. E. (1995). *The wisdom of the ego.* Cambridge, MA: Harvard University Press.

Vaillant, G. E. (2000). Defense mechanisms. In A. E. Kazdin (Ed.), *Encyclopedia of psychology* (Vol. 2, pp. 454–457). Washington, DC: American Psychological Association.

Verheul, R., van den Bosch, L. M., Koeter, M. W., Deridder, M. A., Stijnen, T., & Brink, W. (2003). Dialectic behaviour therapy for women with borderline personality disorder: 12-month, randomized clinical trial in The Netherlands. *British Journal of Psychiatry, 182,* 135–148.

Wakefield, J. C. (1999). Evolutionary versus prototype analyses of the concept of disorder. *Journal of Abnormal Psychology, 108,* 374–399.

Weissman, M. (1993). The epidemiology of personality disorders: A 1990 update. *Journal of Personality Disorders, S1,* 44–62.

Whaley, A. L. (2001). Cultural mistrust and the clinical diagnosis of paranoid schizophrenia in African American patients. *Journal of Psychopathology and Behavioral Assessment, 23,* 93–100.

Whisman, M. A., Tolejko, N., & Chatav, Y. (2007). Social consequences of personality disorders: Probability and timing of marriage and probability of marital disruption. *Journal of Personality Disorders, 21,* 690–695.

Widiger, T. A., Lynam, D. R., Miller, J. D., & Oltmanns, T. F. (2012). Measures to assess maladaptive variants of the five-factor model. *Journal of Personality Assessment, 94*(5), 450–455.

Widiger, T. A., & Simonsen, E. (2005). Alternative dimensional models of personality disorder: Finding a common ground. *Journal of Personality Disorders, 19*, 110–130.

Widiger, T. A., & Trull, T. J. (2007). Plate tectonics in the classification of personality disorder: Shifting to a dimensional model. *American Psychologist, 62*, 71–83.

Wilson, T. (2009). Know thyself. *Perspectives on Psychological Science, 4*, 384–389.

Winter, D. G., John, O. P., Stewart, A. J., Klohnen, E. C., & Duncan, L. E. (1998). Traits and motives: Toward an integration of two traditions in personality research. *Psychological Review, 105*, 230–250.

Yates, W., Cadoret, R., & Troughton, E. (1999). The Iowa Adoption Studies: Methods and results. In M. LaBuda (Ed.), *On the way to individuality: Current methodological issues in behavioral genetics* (pp. 95–125). Hauppauge, NY: Nova Science.

Yen, S., Shea, T., Sanislow, C., Skodol, A., Grilo, C., et al. (2009). Personality traits as protective predictors of suicide attempts. *Acta Psychiatrica Scandinavica, 120*, 222–229.

Yen, S., Shea, M. T., Pagano, M., Sanislow, C. A., Grilo, C. M., McGlashan, T. H., et al. (2003). Axis I and II disorders as predictors of prospective suicide attempts: Findings from the Collaborative Longitudinal Personality Disorders Study. *Journal of Abnormal Psychology, 113*(3), 375–381.

Young, J. E. (1994). *Cognitive therapy for personality disorders: A schema-focused approach* [Practitioner's Resource Series]. Sarasota, FL: Professional Resource Press/Professional Resource Exchange.

Zanarini, M., Frankenburg, F., Hennen, J., Reich, B., & Silk, K. (2005). The McLean study of adult development (MSAD): Overview and implications of the first six years of prospective follow-up. *Journal of Personality Disorders, 19*, 505–523.

Zanarini, M., Frankenburg, F., Reich, D., Silk, K., Hudson, J., & McSweeney, L. (2007). The subsyndromal phenomenology of borderline personality disorder: A 10-year follow-up study. *American Journal of Psychiatry, 164*, 929–935.

Zanarini, M. C., Frankenburg, F. R., Hennen, J., Reich, D. B., & Silk, K. R. (2006). Prediction of the 10-year course of borderline personality disorder. *American Journal of Psychiatry, 163*, 827–832.

Zemishlany, Z., & Weizman, A. (2008). The impact of mental illness on sexual dysfunction. *Advances in Psychosomatic Medicine, 29*, 89–106.

Zimmerman, M., Rothschild, L., & Chelminski, I. (2005). The prevalence of DSM-IV personality disorders in psychiatric outpatients. *American Journal of Psychiatry, 162*, 1911–1918.

Zlotnick, C., Rothschild, L., & Zimmerman, M. (2002). The role of gender in the clinical presentation of patients with borderline personality disorder. *Journal of Personality Disorders, 16*(3), 277–282.

CHAPTER 10

Bipolar Disorder

Sheri L. Johnson
Allison J. Applebaum
Michael W. Otto

Bipolar disorder is a severely disabling and recurrent condition. While its genetic etiology has been recognized, it has also been shown to be responsive to psychosocial treatment (Johnson & Leahy, 2004; Otto & Miklowitz, 2004). For example, research has documented the benefits of psychotherapy for bipolar depression even after antidepressant medications and mood stabilizers did not provide relief (cf. Miklowitz et al., 2007). In this chapter, we review current knowledge about the phenomenology and etiology, as well as the pharmacological and social interventions that have received empirical support in the treatment of bipolar disorder.

PHENOMENOLOGY

Bipolar disorder is complex on many fronts: Symptoms vary from the extreme highs of mania to the lows of depression, and comorbid conditions are the norm rather than the exception. The severity of symptoms can contribute to high rates of occupational and social problems, and of particular concern, rates of completed suicide far exceed those in the general population. Here we provide a brief summary of the definitions and symptomatology of the different forms of the disorder, as well as the associated clinical features, epidemiology, and most common comorbid conditions.

Typical Symptoms and Course

Bipolar disorders are defined on the basis of manic symptoms of varying severity and duration. DSM-5 criteria define a "manic episode" as a period of 1 week (unless interrupted by hospitalization) of excessively expansive, euphoric, or irritable mood and increases in activity and energy accompanied by three or more of the following symptoms: unusually high self-esteem, racing thoughts, distractibility, little need for sleep, pressured speech, increases in goal-directed activity, and reckless behavior (American Psychiatric Association, 2013). "Hypomanic episodes" are defined by a less intense period of mood elevation: Although symptom criteria are parallel, hypomanic episodes do not reach the duration or marked impairment of a full manic episode.

Three major forms of bipolar disorder (BD) are recognized in the DSM. Most of the treatment literature focuses on bipolar I disorder (BD), defined by at least one episode of mania. Bipolar II disorder (BD II) is defined by at least one hypomanic, but not full manic, episode and one or more depressive episodes. Cyclothymic disorder is defined by chronic fluctuations between high and low moods that are not severe enough to qualify as hypomanic or depressive episodes, yet persist for 2 years (1 year in children and adolescents).

There is a need for treatment outcome researchers to focus on the broader spectrum of bipolar disorders. The notion that BD II has a less chronic course is not borne out by recent research. Limited research is available on treatment options for this subtype (Shen et al., 2008).

Across the BD spectrum, treatment is complicated, in that the disorder most commonly includes both (hypo) manic and depressive symptoms. In a 13-year prospective study, subsyndromal symptoms of depression were present during half of the weeks of follow-up (Judd et al., 2002). Although many patients experience chronic depressive symptoms, there is considerable heterogeneity in the severity of depressive symptoms. Community epidemiological studies document that 25–35% of people with BD do not evidence major depressive episodes during their lifetime (see Cuellar, Johnson, & Winters, 2005, for review). Because depressive symptoms often motivate people to seek treatment, clinic samples tend to comprise people who experience both manic and depressive symptoms.

Although treatment is undoubtedly helpful, rates of relapse even within treated samples diagnosed with BD are high—as many as one-half of patients with BD relapse within the first year after an episode (Keller et al., 1986), and three-fourths of patients relapse within 4 to 5 years (Gitlin, Swendsen, Heller, & Hammen, 1995; Tohen, Waternaux, & Tsuang, 1990). Between episodes, most patients experience subsyndromal symptoms (Judd et al., 2002).

Associated Clinical Features

One of the most intriguing aspects of BD is the extreme variability in outcomes. BD is overrepresented among highly accomplished, creative groups (Jamison, 1993).

Nonetheless, functional outcomes are poor for many people with the disorder. BDs are the ninth leading medical cause of global disability (World Health Organization, 2001). Even when asymptomatic, persons with BDs often report low quality of life across psychological, physical, and social domains (Brissos, Dias, & Kapczinski, 2008).

In studies of occupational functioning, one major study of BD I and BD II found that only 42% of patients were working either full- or part-time (Suppes et al., 2001), and another found that 74% of patients with BD had moderate impairment or poor outcomes a full year after hospital discharge (Harrow, Goldberg, Grossman, & Meltzer, 1990). Although many patients continue to recover in the year after hospitalization, problems with social and occupational functioning appear to endure in about half of people even after symptoms remit (Keck et al., 1998).

Social functioning also appears to be highly variable. On average, though, people with BD report lower levels of support than those without psychological disorders, and perceptions of social support appear to decline over the course of the illness (Romans & McPherson, 1992). A burgeoning literature focuses on the effects of BD on significant others, documenting high rates of caregiver burden and even elevated rates of major depressive disorder among close family members of those struggling with the illness (Perlick et al., 2007). The disorder is also associated with high rates of family conflict (Simoneau, Miklowitz, & Saleem, 1998), as well as marital dissatisfaction, separation, and divorce (Coryell et al., 1993).

Suicide is all too common in BD. In one sample of people hospitalized for BD, completed suicide was found to occur at 15 times the rates observed in the general population (Harris & Barraclough, 1997). In a 20-year study of 7,000 psychiatric outpatients (Brown, Beck, Steer, & Grisham, 2000), persons with BD were found to have the highest risk for completed suicide of psychiatric groups in the sample. Among 406 patients hospitalized for BD, 11% committed suicide over a 40-year period (Angst, Gerber-Werder, & Gamma, 2005). It is important for clinicians to be aware that BD II and cyclothymia are related to high rates of suicidality (Moreno & Andrade, 2005).

Epidemiology

BD I and BD II are estimated to affect between 1 and 3% of the population (Kessler, Chiu, Demler, & Walters, 2005). Findings from an epidemiological study in the Netherlands suggest that as many as 4.2% of people experience cyclothymia (Regeer et al., 2004). Rates of disorder are fairly consistent across cultures, although there has been some indication that countries with high levels of fish oil consumption (possibly related to the role of omega-3 fatty acids as a mood stabilizer) may be characterized by lower rates of BD diagnoses (Noaghiul & Hibbeln, 2003).

The average age of onset for BD is during adolescence, and earlier age of onset has been found to predict a worse course of illness and greater risk of suicidality (Perlis et al., 2004). Women and men are equally likely to receive a diagnosis of the disorder (Kessler et al., 1994), although women report more episodes of depression than do men (Leibenluft, 1996).

Comorbidity

Manic symptoms are highly likely to be comorbid with other medical and psychiatric syndromes. Both types of comorbidity have important implications for outcomes.

In regard to medical comorbidity, BD has been related to high rates of medical illness (Krishnan, Mast, Ficker, Lawhorne, & Lichtenberg, 2005). Standardized mortality rates for cardiovascular disease are highly elevated in people with BD compared to the general population (Laursen, Munk-Olsen, Nordentoft, & Mortensen, 2007), a pattern that is observed for both BD I and BD II (Fiedorowicz et al., 2009). People with BD have been found to have 40% higher general medical costs than those observed among age- and gender-matched medical outpatients (Simon & Unützer, 1999).

In regard to psychiatric comorbidity, a number of disorders commonly co-occur with BD. Indeed, within a community epidemiological sample, hypomanic symptoms were more related to childhood externalizing disorders, anxiety disorders, and substance abuse than to depressive symptoms (Kessler et al., 2005). In community studies, it has been estimated that 61% of participants with BD meet lifetime diagnostic criteria for alcohol or substance abuse or dependence (Regier et al., 1990) and more than half meet lifetime diagnostic criteria for anxiety disorders (Simon et al., 2004). Eating disorders also commonly co-occur with BD (McElroy et al., 2001), as does childhood attention deficit disorder (Nierenberg et al., 2005).

Many studies overestimate the occurrence of comorbid personality disorders by assessing personality symptoms during mood episodes. In one study of people who had achieved remission from episodes of BD I, 28.8% met diagnostic criteria for a personality disorder. The most common were histrionic and obsessive–compulsive personality disorders (George, Miklowitz, Richards, Simoneau, & Taylor, 2003).

Clinical Implications

A number of clinical implications can be derived from research on the phenomenology of BD. In addition to assessing the symptoms associated with this disorder, clinicians should systematically evaluate occupational, social, and medical functioning. Not only could this allow therapists to provide care aimed at improving broad domains of clients' life quality, but it might also reduce risk for relapse or recurrence of symptoms. As mentioned earlier, risk for relapse, even when remission has been achieved, is very high. It is therefore important for clinicians to educate clients about such risk, to teach them about self-monitoring of symptoms (including subsyndromal symptoms), and to arrange for follow-up assessment and treatment sessions after the completion of a treatment episode. As we describe later in the chapter, specific interventions have been developed to address the important issue of relapse prevention. Irrespective of his or her theoretical orientation and professional background, it is also crucial for the clinician working with BD to evaluate (and be ready to address) clients' risk for suicide. He or she should be especially concerned about risk for suicidality for clients with early onset of BD, which, needless to say, points to the importance of assessing when clients began to suffer from manic and/or depressive symptoms. Furthermore, it is important to assess comorbid conditions and to consider these in treatment planning. Less response to treatment has been found for those experiencing comorbid anxiety (Feske et al., 2000), attention-deficit/hyperactivity disorder (Masi et al., 2004), substance use disorders (Tohen et al., 1990), or personality disorders (Dunayevich et al., 2000). Despite these replicable findings, few researchers have grappled with ways to enhance treatment for these more complex forms of disorder. In one study, Weiss et al. (2007) provided a group intervention for persons with BD and comorbid substance use disorders. Despite significant improvement in substance use indices, the group's mania symptoms did not improve. This early work serves as an important reminder of the difficulty of effectively treating BD when serious comorbid conditions are present.

ETIOLOGY

Genetic Factors

There is strong evidence for the heritability of BD. In the best of a series of twin studies, participants were recruited from the community, and diagnoses were verified using structured interviews. In such studies, heritability estimates as high as 85% were obtained (McGuffin et al., 2003). Although few adoption studies are available, such studies also suggest that BD is highly heritable (Wender et al., 1986).

Intriguingly, the heritability for manic and depressive symptoms within BD appears to be separable. One twin study found that 71% of the genetic liability to mania was distinct from that of depression (McGuffin et al., 2003). Hence, people with a lifetime history of mania may vary considerably in their genetic propensity toward depression.

Upon learning about the highly genetic nature of the disorder, many people with BD wonder whether their children might develop the disorder. A meta-analysis of 17 studies suggested that children of parents with BD have a fourfold increase in risk for developing a mood disorder compared to children of parents without a psychiatric diagnosis (LaPalme, Hodgins, & LaRoche, 1997). For concerned parents, it is worth noting that most offspring will not develop BD, and that many researchers are focused on early prevention programs.

Although there has been considerable effort to identify specific polymorphisms associated with disorder, findings have been highly mixed, and nonreplications have been all too common. Segurado and colleagues (2003) took considerable care to consider both published and unpublished data to avoid the positive biases often inherent in whether a result is published. They gathered 18 original datasets, each with more than 20 probands affected by BD, to examine genetic regions associated with BD. Their meta-analysis, weighted for sample size, provided the strongest support for four out of 120 regions implicated in BD: 14q 9p-q, 10q, 18p-q, and 8q. Even these four regions were not replicated in more than 10 of the 18 studies. Hence, early studies provide support for a few key regions, but most researchers assume that any given polymorphism explains a very small proportion of the risk for disorder.

Psychosocial Risk Factors

A range of psychological and social variables have been found to predict the course of disorder, such as negative life events (Ellicott, Hammen, Gitlin, Brown, & Jamison, 1990) and expressed emotion (Miklowitz, Goldstein, Neuchterlein, Snyder, & Mintz, 1988). In describing psychosocial predictors, it is important to note that these factors often differentially influence bipolar depression versus mania. We first discuss medication nonadherence, which frequently appears to explain manic and depressive relapse. We then review key psychosocial predictors of bipolar depression and, finally, manic symptoms.

Medication Adherence

Rates of medication nonadherence in BD are high. About half of people with BD discontinue mood stabilizer medications within 2 months of an episode (Scott & Pope, 2002). Over long periods, 80% of patients have at least some periods of nonadherence (Weiss et al., 1998). Patients who discontinue medications, particularly if they do so rapidly, are at a greatly increased risk of relapse and suicide (Tondo & Baldessarini, 2000).

Some of the reasons for nonadherence are likely to be similar to those for other disorders, such as forgetfulness, not understanding the need for medications, or diminished motivation over time. Beyond this, issues specific to BD include the significant side effects of medications (e.g., weight gain, fatigue, cognitive dysfunction), missing high moods, concerns about stigma related to medication, and lack of information about the disorder (Johnson & Fulford, 2008).

Psychosocial Predictors of Bipolar Depression

The symptomatology and neurobiology of unipolar and bipolar depression have many strong parallels (Cuellar et al., 2005). Accordingly, many of the variables that have been shown robustly to predict unipolar depression, such as neuroticism, also appear to predict bipolar depression (Lozano & Johnson, 2001). Prospective studies indicate that negative life events predict increases in bipolar depression over time (see Johnson, 2005a, for review). Similarly, low perceived social support predicts increases in bipolar depression over time (L. Johnson, Lundström, Åberg-Wistedt, & Mathé, 2003). "Expressed emotion" (EE), defined by family criticism, hostility, or overinvolvement toward the patient with BD, has been found to be detrimental for the course of symptoms of BD (Butzlaff & Hooley, 1998), and particularly predictive of depressive symptoms within BD (Yan, Hammen, Cohen, Daley, & Henry, 2004). Overly negative cognitive styles have been found to be present in people with BD in a broad range of studies, and to correlate with the severity of previous and current depressive symptoms (Cuellar et al., 2005). Furthermore, negative cognitive styles and low self-esteem predict increases in bipolar depression over time (Johnson & Fingerhut, 2004). In summary, psychosocial models of unipolar depression appear to be applicable to understanding bipolar depression.

Psychosocial Predictors of Manic Symptoms

Many of the variables that predict bipolar depression do not predict the course of manic symptoms. For example, in prospective studies, no direct effects have been obtained for negative life events (see Johnson, 2005a, for review) or social support (Johnson, Winett, Meyer, Greenhouse, & Miller, 1999) as predictors of mania. Although negative cognitive styles are often documented in BD, they are most likely to be found during depressed rather than well periods (Johnson & Kizer, 2002), they more consistently predict depression than mania (Johnson & Fingerhut, 2004; but see Alloy, Reilly-Harrington, Fresco, Whitehouse, & Zechmeister, 1999), and they can be explained by the presence of depressive history rather than manic history (Alloy et al., 1999). Hence, not all forms of psychosocial disruption appear to help understand mania. Available models highlight two types of predictors of mania: goal dysregulation and sleep deprivation/schedule disruption.

GOAL DYSREGULATION

The goal dysregulation model suggests that mania may result from excessive goal engagement secondary to increased sensitivity of the dopaminergic reward pathways (Johnson, 2005b). People with a history of mania describe themselves as more sensitive to rewards on the Carver and White (1994) self-report Behavioral Activation Scales (BAS; see Johnson, Edge, Holmes, & Carver, 2012, for review); that is, they endorse feeling more energized and excited by opportunities to pursue goals, and more excited by having success in achieving goals. Importantly, BAS levels appear to be stably high, even when symptoms of mania are not present (Meyer, Johnson, & Winters, 2001). Risk for the disorder also appears to be correlated with heightened psychophysiological reactivity to positive stimuli in some studies (Harmon-Jones et al., 2008). Although many studies have focused on positive reactivity to achieving goals, people with BD also appear to experience high levels of frustration when goals are thwarted (Wright, Lam, & Brown, 2008), which helps link reward sensitivity conceptually to the irritable symptoms of mania. Beyond cross-sectional studies, BAS scores predicted increases in manic symptoms over 6 months in a BP I sample (Meyer et al., 2001). Excess reward sensitivity and goal focus may heighten reactivity to success, such that manic symptoms would be more likely to occur after life events involving goal attainment. Goal attainment life events predict increases in manic, but not depressive, symptoms (cf. Johnson et al., 2008). Such effects were apparent even after researchers controlled for baseline levels of manic symptoms and excluded life events that could have been caused by patients' symptoms. In summary, studies with a range of measures suggest that reward sensitivity is elevated in BD, and that this reward sensitivity can help predict the course of BD.

A growing literature has focused on the cognitive aspects of being highly reward-oriented. Several of these cognitive studies suggest that people with BD emphasize goals and endorse more extreme life ambitions than do people without BD, even during remission (Johnson, Eisner, & Carver, 2009; Lam, Wright, & Smith, 2004). Beyond these trait-like features of cognition, it also appears that people who are prone to mania may react with greater shifts in cognition in the face of positive moods. Confidence appears particularly high after positive mood inductions (Mansell & Lam, 2006). People diagnosed with the disorder also appear to overinterpret the meaning of hypomanic symptoms, taking them as signs to move forward and conquer goals (Jones & Day, 2008). Heightened confidence appears to predict relapse into manic episodes; that is, Lam, Wright, and Sham (2005b) found that persons with BD who endorsed overly positive views of self were more likely to relapse over a 6-month period. It has been suggested that these high levels of confidence then promote engagement in more ambitious and demanding goals (Johnson, 2005b). This overly busy, overly active engagement in pursuing new goals has been found to predict an increased risk of manic symptoms within the next 2 months (Lozano & Johnson, 2001). Hence, we next discuss clinical approaches toward goal regulation, as well as those that focus on cognitive features of mania.

SCHEDULE DISRUPTION

Researchers have focused on sleep deprivation, as well as more general schedule disruption, as a trigger of manic symptoms. Drawing on the clinical observation that manic episodes are often preceded by life events that involved sleep disruption, such as transmeridian flights or childbearing, Wehr, Sack, and Rosenthal (1987) suggested that sleep disruption might be one mechanism through which life events influence symptom generation. Congruently, experimental studies of sleep deprivation suggest that a single night of sleep deprivation can trigger manic symptoms for more than 10% of people with BD (Barbini et al., 1998).

Beyond sleep deprivation, Ehlers, Frank, and Kupfer (1988) suggested that a range of social timekeepers ("social *zeitgebers*") might interfere with daily rhythms (e.g., a job with shifting work hours). One measure, the social rhythm metric (SRM), has been most widely used to test the constancy of the daily schedule (Monk, Frank, Potts, & Capfer, 1990). In one study, SRM scores were found to be lower among persons with BD (Ashman et al., 1999). In another study, the SRM total score was not found to be lower, but the number of regular activities was lower among persons with BD compared to healthy controls (Jones, Tai, Evershed, Knowles, & Bentall, 2006). Children of parents with BD have also been found to demonstrate disrupted sleep patterns, although they do not appear to manifest deficits in social *zeitgebers* (Jones et al., 2006). Hence a series of studies has found that some aspect of social rhythm is impaired in BD, although the precise nature of the disruption remains a bit unclear.

To test the life event component of the social *zeitgebers* model, Malkoff-Schwartz and colleagues (1998, 2000) conducted two studies using careful interviews to assess life events in the 8 weeks before bipolar episodes. Patients reported more life events involving social rhythm disruption (events that affect sleep or wake times, or daily routines) before the onset of mania than before depression. Taken together with the previous findings, it appears that sleep deprivation and schedule disruption may trigger increases in manic symptoms.

In summary, the variables hypothesized to influence the onset of mania include goal dysregulation and sleep/schedule disruption. As discussed below, some of these risk factors are amenable to modification through psychosocial intervention.

TREATMENT

Pharmacological Treatments

Mood stabilizers are recommended to stabilize acute episodes and to prevent recurrence. Lithium (brand names Eskalith, Lithobid) has been used as a mood stabilizer for 30 years. Anticonvulsants, such as divalproex (brand name Depakote) and lamotrigine (brand name Lamictal), as well as atypical antipsychotic medications such as olanzapine (Zyprexa) and risperidone (Risperdal) also provide mood stabilization. For acute episodes, U.K. and U.S. treatment guidelines suggest use of lithium, valproate, or antipsychotic medication (American Psychiatric Association, 2002; Goodwin, 2003). For longer-term maintenance treatment, U.S. guidelines recommend lithium or valproate, but U.K. guidelines recommend lithium, valproate, or olanzapine as first-line approaches.

In practice, mood-stabilizing medications are often combined with antidepressants or anxiolytic agents. Despite the popularity of antidepressant and benzodiazepine medications, there is little evidence of the efficacy of benzodiazepines for bipolar episodes (Simon et al., 2004), and researchers have found that when added to a mood stabilizer regimen, antidepressants are no more effective than placebo (Nemeroff et al., 2001). In addition, antidepressants can trigger manic episodes in patients with BD when taken without a mood stabilizer (Ghaemi, Lenox, & Baldessarini, 2001). Hence, antidepressant and benzodiazepine medications are not recommended as first-line approaches to BD. Lamotrigine appears helpful for relapse prevention (Brown et al., 2006) but not for acute treatment of bipolar depression (Calabrese et al., 2008). An ongoing focus of research, then, is the identification of pharmacological strategies to address bipolar depression.

Despite advances in pharmacotherapy, recurrences of mood episodes and chronic subsyndromal symptoms, particularly depressive symptoms, appear to be normative aspects of BD despite medication use (e.g., Gitlin et al., 1995). Given these data, researchers have focused on psychological treatments that might be used as adjuncts to mood stabilizers.

Psychosocial Treatment

At the outset of considering psychosocial treatments for BD, it is important to note that despite being based on different theoretical orientations, there is a surprising degree of similarity among current empirically supported treatments. Most treatments include psychoeducation about BD and the importance of medication adherence, and rehearsal of methods for the early detection of symptoms. To these basic elements, treatments may add training in problem solving, stress management, cognitive interventions, activity and sleep management, amelioration of negative interpersonal/family interactions, and goal regulation.

For each of these current BD treatments, we provide an overview of the intervention, and the evidence concerning depression and mania outcomes. Where evidence is available, we also note findings regarding mechanisms of change. We conclude our review of treatment outcome studies by identifying principles of change that can guide the clinician to tailor interventions based on the specific treatment goal and risk factors for a particular patient. Beyond the psychological interventions noted here, researchers have tested innovative system-level interventions in tandem with psychoeducation (see Simon et al., 2005).

Psychoeducation and Relapse Prevention Programs

Several psychoeducation programs have been developed. Beyond basic education about BD, many of these programs incorporate a range of strategies designed to prevent relapse. For example, Perry, Tarrier, Morriss, McCarthy, and Limb (1999) tested a 12-session version of individual cognitive-behavioral therapy (CBT) designed to foster early symptom detection and treatment seeking for 69 outpatients who had experienced bipolar relapse during the past 12 months. Patients were asked to review a list of prodromal symptoms to identify the most common ones during their episodes. They were also encouraged to keep a diary of prodromal symptoms, so as to become more skilled at distinguishing symptoms from everyday mood variations, and to note potential triggers. Simple strategies to respond to emergent symptoms, such as calling the doctor, were written on a small, laminated card to be carried in the wallet. This intervention was compared to treatment as usual. Assessments were conducted during the active study phase and through an 18-month follow-up. Results indicated a significant improvement in the length of time until manic, but not depressive, relapse among patients who received CBT.

In a larger study, Colom and colleagues (2009) examined the impact of group psychotherapy for 120 BD I and BD II outpatients in remission. Patients were randomized to receive structured, group-based psychoeducation or nondirective group therapy as adjuncts to standard medication treatment. Psychoeducation included six sessions focused on BD and its course, two sessions focused on symptom detection, six sessions focused on education about different medication classes, and five sessions focused on avoiding triggers (e.g., substance abuse, sleep disruption) and coping with early symptoms. The group treatment significantly reduced the number of episodes and hospitalizations per patient, and increased the time to depressive, as well as manic–hypomanic–mixed, recurrences. The psychoeducation intervention continued to be associated with diminished rates of recurrence and hospitalization in a 5-year follow-up of 99 patients.

Several studies have examined variables that might help to explain these positive treatment effects. For example, researchers have shown that psychoeducation improves knowledge about the disorder (Bauer, McBride, Chase, Sachs, & Shea, 1998). Indeed, Peet and Harvey (1991) showed that even viewing a 12-minute videotape and receiving written materials improved knowledge of BD. Beyond improving knowledge of disorder, psychoeducation also seems to enhance medication adherence. Cochran (1984) found that a 6-week cognitive-behavioral intervention for patients with BD improved adherence and decreased adherence-related hospitalizations compared to a control group. Psychoeducation has also been found to improve medication adherence as measured by lithium blood serum levels (Colom et al., 2005).

Cognitive-Behavioral Therapy

A range of CBT manuals have been developed (cf. Lam, Jones, Hayward, & Bright, 1999; Otto et al., 2009). The relative emphases in these manuals differ, but all of the CBT manuals include psychoeducation about BD. They also focus on identifying maladaptive negative thoughts about the self and teaching skills to challenge these overly negative thoughts. Many also include interventions to improve treatment engagement, and to target the overly positive thoughts that might be present during mania. The manual by Lam et al. (1999) provides a more extensive set of strategies to support self-calming during early stages of mania and diminish excessive goal engagement, and the Otto et al. (2009) manual provides treatment modules (e.g., anger management, anxiety management, assertiveness training) that can be added as needed to complement the core treatment elements. To aid the application of these and related strategies, self-help books (e.g., Jones, Hayward, & Lam, 2002) are available.

In terms of evidence for CBT, Lam and colleagues (2003) conducted a randomized controlled trial of brief individual CBT (12–18 sessions within the first 6 months, and two booster sessions in the second 6 months of care) relative to standard pharmacological care. Patients who received CBT had significantly fewer bipolar episodes, higher social functioning, and less depression during the first year of follow-up than did patients in the control group. In a 2-year follow-up study, significant advantages were seen for CBT efficacy in reducing depressive, but not manic, symptoms (Lam et al., 2005).

Scott, Garland, and Moorhead (2001) tested a broad CBT intervention that supplemented traditional cognitive interventions with strategies to help regulate activities and sleep. Patients were randomly assigned to CBT or to a waiting-list condition, and assessments were conducted at 6- and 18-month follow-up. Significant improvements in global functioning, depressive symptoms, and depressive relapse rates were reported among patients who received CBT, while overall reductions in manic symptoms were not significant.

Findings of one study suggest that improvements in depressive symptoms are not explained by the psychoeducation component of CBT. In one small study, patients were randomly assigned to receive six sessions of psychoeducation alone or six sessions of psychoeducation followed by 14 sessions of CBT. Patients who received the CBT demonstrated greater decreases in depressive symptoms than did those who received psychoeducation alone (Zaretsky, Lancee, Miller, Harris, & Parikh, 2008).

Given the early, promising results for CBT in the treatment of bipolar depression, it is important to consider whether such findings transfer well to community settings. One large-scale study focused on the effectiveness of CBT within a community context. Scott et al. (2006) examined the impact of 22 sessions of CBT versus treatment as usual in 253 patients. The overall results were disappointing; the groups did not differ in symptom severity levels or time to episode recurrence over an 18-month follow-up. Although findings described below (Miklowitz, Otto, Frank, Reilly-Harrington, Wisniewski, et al., 2007) suggest that CBT might be effective in reducing bipolar depressive symptoms when offered in community mental health centers, other, smaller studies also fail to document significant effects of CBT (Patelis-Siotis et al., 2001).

In summary, findings for CBT have not been uniform. Several studies, though, suggest that CBT can be helpful, particularly in the management of bipolar depressive symptoms. Questions remain about generalizability to community settings. Evidence has not been supportive of the efficacy of all forms of CBT for the treatment of manic symptoms, although in one major trial, Lam and colleagues' (1999) cognitive manual did appear helpful in reducing manic symptoms.

Family and Marital Therapy

Drawing on the links between EE and the course of the disorder, researchers have considered whether family or marital approaches can help reduce bipolar symptoms. The best-studied approach, family-focused therapy (FFT), provides psychoeducation for patients and their family members, and draws on family interventions that have effectively improved family communication and delayed relapse in schizophrenia (e.g., Hogarty et al., 1991). The family components include communication enhancement training, in which patients rehearse expressing positive and negative feelings, listening, and requesting changes in others' behaviors, and problem-solving skills training, in which patients learn to identify, define, and solve specific family problems (Miklowitz & Goldstein, 1997).

Miklowitz, George, Richards, Simoneau, and Suddath (2003) randomly assigned 101 patients with BD to receive FFT or less intensive clinical management (CM) as adjuncts to standard pharmacotherapy. Patients and their family members completed 21 sessions and were evaluated every 3–6 months for 2 years. Compared to CM, FFT was associated with lower levels of symptoms and longer time before relapse. Significant interactions between time and treatment were observed for depression but not for mania scores.

Similar support for FFT was found by Rea et al. (2003). In a randomized clinical trial of FFT versus individual treatment, 53 patients with a recent manic episode who were receiving mood stabilizers were assessed every 3 months during treatment and at 1-year follow-up. Patients who received FFT experienced fewer relapses and hospitalizations than did those who received individual treatment. It is not clear whether improvements were specific to depression, though, because analyses collapsed across mania and depression.

Some research has been conducted on the mechanisms of change for family therapy. Honig, Hofman, Hilwiq, Noorthoorn, and Ponds (1995) found that a family therapy program significantly reduced EE from spouses married to patients with BD. More specifically, Simoneau, Miklowitz, Richards, Saleem, and George (1999) examined the impact of FFT compared to CM with two sessions of family education on communication between family members of those with BD. Although FFT did not change negative family interactions, it was associated with more positive nonverbal family communication compared to CM. Improvements in positive nonverbal communication were correlated with improvements in mood. Davenport, Ebert, Adland, and Goodwin (1977) found that family therapy also reduced the risk of marital dissolution for patients with BD. Findings are consistent with the idea that one mechanism involved in family treatment is improvement in family communication and functioning.

Because FFT also includes psychoeducation, one might expect that another mechanism would be enhanced medication adherence. Findings do suggest that persons who receive FFT demonstrate better medication adherence than do those who receive CM (Miklowitz et al., 2003).

It is important to note that some forms of family therapy other than FFT have not been shown to produce changes in manic or depressive symptoms (Miller, Solomon, Ryan, & Keitner, 2004; van Gent & Zwart, 1991). For example, Clarkin et al. (1990) tested the efficacy of 15 sessions of marital therapy among 19 patients and did not observe significant symptom differences compared to medication management alone. FFT is distinguished from these other approaches by its longer duration, as well as more structured exercises concerning family communication, more education about BD, and more specific strategies for responding to symptoms. FFT does appear to promote better control over depressive symptoms, as well as improvements in medication adherence. Findings to date do not provide strong support for FFT as a mania prevention intervention.

Interventions to Improve Sleep, Interpersonal Functioning, and Schedules

Two types of approaches have evolved regarding sleep and schedule disruption. One set of findings, largely from case studies, have focused specifically on improving sleep. A second set of studies, which includes large-scale randomized controlled trials, focuses on interpersonal and social rhythm therapy (IPSRT), designed more broadly to improve social rhythms and reduce life stress. We begin by describing the more specific sleep intervention work and then consider the research on IPSRT.

Wehr et al. (1998) theorized that a light–dark cycle that mirrors the natural rhythm of the sun might help protect sleep and thereby reduce symptoms in BD. Accordingly, they asked a person with BD to rest in bed in a dark room for 14 hours per night. Over a 19-month period, the dark period was gradually reduced to 10 hours. Symptoms were tracked daily for several years before the intervention and throughout the 19 months of the intervention. The intervention successfully improved sleep, activity, and mood symptoms. In other case studies (Totterdell & Kellett, 2008; Wirz-Justice, 2006) and uncontrolled studies (Barbini et al., 2005), researchers have achieved good results by encouraging people with BD to extend time spent in bed or to develop better sleep habits.

Beyond these interventions focused on sleep, substantial research has focused on changing social rhythms more broadly. Shen et al. (2008) randomly assigned 71 participants with high scores on a measure of risk for mania to either a schedule regulation program or a control group. The experimental group did demonstrate improvement in social rhythm scores, but these changes did not result in diminished manic or depressive symptoms over time. Findings from the study are somewhat difficult to interpret, though, because the relatively mild symptom status of participants at baseline may have provided less room for symptom improvement during the study.

Considerable research has been conducted on IPSRT, which focuses on three potential triggers of bipolar symptoms: medication noncompliance, social rhythm disruption, and interpersonal difficulties (Frank, 2005). Similar to traditional interpersonal therapy (Klerman, Weissman, Rounsaville, & Chevron, 1984), IPSRT focuses on four types of interpersonal problems: grief (extended to cover grief over the "lost healthy self" with the diagnosis of BD), interpersonal conflicts, role transitions (i.e., changes in one's employment situation), and interpersonal deficits (i.e., social isolation). Hence, IPSRT is designed to address many of the triggers involved in the course of bipolar symptoms, including medication adherence, schedule disruption, negative life events, and low social support.

Frank et al. (1997) examined the efficacy of individual IPSRT as an adjunct to medication treatment. Patients were randomly assigned to receive either IPSRT or

CM (symptom and medication monitoring). Perhaps because of the small sample size ($N = 38$), differences in mean symptoms were not observed between groups, even though manic and depressive symptoms remitted more quickly for those in the IPSRT condition than for those in the CM condition.

In a larger study, Frank et al. (2005) examined the effects of acute and maintenance versions of IPSRT as adjuncts to medication management. They randomly assigned 175 acutely ill participants to receive either IPSRT or clinical management. IPSRT was administered as acute therapy (weekly sessions for several months) or maintenance therapy (monthly for 2 years), leading to four combinations of acute/maintenance treatment: CM/CM, CM/IPSRT, IPSRT/IPSRT, and IPSRT/CM. Findings from the study were mixed, in that acute IPSRT treatment led to longer periods before recurrence, but maintenance IPSRT did not yield improvements in symptoms compared to CM.

As with FFT, some research has examined the mechanisms through which IPSRT produces change. In the previously described studies of IPSRT (Frank et al., 1997, 2005) patients who received IPSRT achieved greater stability of daily routines than did those who received CM. Although two studies have suggested that greater stability of daily routines does not result in symptom improvements (Frank et al., 1997; Shen et al., 2008), the findings of the 2005 Frank et al. study indicate that improvement in social rhythms during the acute phase is predictive of less likelihood of relapse. Hence, more severe baseline symptoms, longer follow-up, and larger sample sizes might be needed to detect the effects of social rhythm improvements.

In summary, IPSRT appears helpful as an acute treatment but not as a maintenance treatment. Despite some null findings, improvement in social rhythms predicted outcomes in acute IPSRT within the largest study to date.

An Intervention to Address Goal Regulation

Building on the finding that there is a link between goal dysregulation and mania, Johnson and Fulford (2009) examined the feasibility of a mania prevention treatment program designed to improve goal regulation skills for those with BD. In an open trial with 10 participants, the program led to reductions in manic symptoms and overly ambitious goal setting from baseline to termination. No controlled data are available, though. Although promising, this treatment awaits further testing.

Comparison of Different Forms of Therapy

Given the findings for CBT, IPSRT, and FFT, a key question is whether these three treatments differ in their efficacy. In the large-scale Systematic Treatment Enhancement Program (STEP) for BD protocol, 293 patients with bipolar I or bipolar II disorder drawn from 15 study sites were randomized to receive either intensive psychosocial treatment (up to 30 sessions of CBT, IPSRT, or FFT over 9 months) or a three-session psychoeducational intervention (collaborative care; CC) as adjuncts to pharmacotherapy. All patients were experiencing bipolar depression, so the focus of the analysis was on the reduction of depressive symptoms. All three intensive psychosocial treatments were more effective than CC in enhancing the odds and timing of recovery from bipolar depression (Miklowitz, Otto, Frank, Reilly-Harrington, Wisniewski, et al., 2007). The three intensive interventions did not differ in their efficacy. Findings, then, suggest an advantage of intensive psychotherapy compared to very brief psychoeducation.

Principles of Change

Given the range of available treatment options and the relatively comparable level of evidence for many of these treatments, clinicians may want to tailor their choice of treatment to the patient by considering principles of change; that is, the best treatment options likely depend on whether the goal is reducing manic or depressive relapse, and the particular social and psychological risk factors for a given patient.

In Table 10.1, we consider principles of change and specific interventions that might address each domain. Psychoeducation has the strongest long-term support and might be considered a first line of psychological intervention early in the course of disorder, or for those patients who have not yet received solid information about their disorder and treatment options. Several options have been found to reduce depressive symptoms, so for depression treatment, the clinician might choose treatments based on whether a patient demonstrates interpersonal difficulties, social rhythm disturbances, family conflict, or negative cognitive styles. Early detection and intervention strategies have been applied successfully to preventing the occurrence and severity of manic relapse.

CONCLUSION

BD is one of the most debilitating of mental illnesses. People diagnosed with this disorder are at high risk for recurrent episodes and incur substantial losses to their social and occupational worlds. Their risk for suicide is higher than rates observed across most psychiatric disorders. Clearly, there is a need for treatment development and innovation.

Medication treatments have provided the first line of treatment in the fight against symptoms, and every major treatment guideline recommends medication as the best way not only to reduce acute symptoms but also to protect against recurrence over time. Even with such medications, though, rates of relapse remain disappointingly high.

Although genetic heritability is clearly the major force involved in whether

TABLE 10.1. Principles of Change in Psychological Treatment Approaches for Bipolar Disorder

Principles of change	Examples of specific guidelines
Improve awareness of symptoms.	Teach patient to routinely review symptoms, so as to be alert to the signs and symptoms of an incipient mood episode.
Increase motivation for medication adherence.	Teach patient about course of disorder and role of mood stabilizers as a relapse prevention treatment (i.e., to be taken even in the absence of symptoms).
Increase treatment engagement.	Educate patient, care providers, and support network about efficacy of specific psychosocial treatment. Establish strong rapport, provide forum for discussing the meaning and hardships associated with illness. Provide education and support to improve motivation for treatment. Teach strategies to enhance regular medication regimens, including techniques to prevent forgetfulness and to manage side effect of medications.
Reduce risk factors for episodes.	Teach patient about the dangers of substance abuse for symptom management; consider behavioral strategies to help reduce substance abuse. Teach skills to manage stress and/or anxiety comorbidity.
Improve family functioning.	Teach communication skills to patient and his or her family (e.g., constructive expression of both positive and negative feelings, listening, assertiveness training).
Develop plans to foster appropriate support from close others and treatment providers if mood episodes emerge.	Consider use of treatment contracts that specify actions of providers and others (e.g., preferred hospital should severe mood episodes be encountered).
Promote regular sleep–wake cycles and activity cycles.	Teach patient sleep hygiene skills, help them extend resting period in bed, and enhance stability of daily routines.
Diminish excessive engagement in overly ambitious goal pursuit and practice self-calming skills after goal-attainment life events.	Help patient learn to avoid periods of overly confident risk-taking and frenetic goal engagement. Help patient learn to avoid acting on surges of confidence present after small successes.
Address interpersonal stress and social isolation.	Help patient identify core interpersonal goals for change, identify goals for change, and use behavioral strategies to promote change.
Address maladaptive thoughts.	Identify and challenge overly negative self-relevant thoughts with use of cognitive strategies similar to those employed for unipolar depression.

a person develops the disorder, genetic models are less helpful in predicting the course of disorder. Medication nonadherence can trigger increases in depressive and manic symptoms. Psychological variables have been found to predict the course of disorder. Negative life events, negative cognitive styles, and family criticism are related to a more severe pattern of depressive symptoms over time. Schedule and sleep disruption, as well as various facets of goal dysregulation, appear to predict increases in mania over time. Each of these variables can be considered a potential treatment target.

A growing body of evidence supports the efficacy of specific psychosocial treatments for BD. Psychoeducation, training in medication adherence, and early symptom monitoring appear to have significant relapse prevention effects. CBT has been found to reduce depression significantly, and there is evidence for the prevention of mania during the first year after treatment, but not the second, with one of the available CBT manuals. Family treatment has been shown to enhance a range of outcomes but to influence depression most directly. Several different treatments have been designed to enhance sleep, with good outcomes in case reports. IPSRT integrates interventions to address both schedule disruption and interpersonal stressors. IPSRT has been found to provide symptom relief when offered as an acute treatment, but not as a maintenance treatment. A recently developed intervention strives to enhance goal regulation, but no controlled data are available. The large-scale STEP study suggests that CT, FFT, and IPSRT performed comparably in reducing depressive symptoms.

Beyond the encouraging findings relative to symptoms, several studies suggest that psychotherapies can bolster social and occupational functioning; that is, brief psychoeducation (Bauer et al., 1998; van Gent et al., 1991), FFT (Miklowitz et al., 2003), and CBT (Lam et al., 2003; Miklowitz, Otto, Frank, Reilly-Harrington, Kogan, et al., 2007) have been found to improve social functioning. Marital therapy has been found to reduce rates of marital dissolution. IPSRT also improved occupational functioning as an acute treatment but did not achieve these effects as a maintenance treatment (Frank et al., 2008). More work is needed, though, given the extreme occupational and social distress associated with this disorder.

In summary, the findings from the host of treatment outcome studies are encouraging, in that a range of mechanisms have been targeted, with beneficial effects on a broad range of outcomes. Notwithstanding the significance of these gains, there is fundamental need for more precise studies of the mechanisms involved in symptom generation and for treatments that more directly target these mechanisms. For example, it remains unclear whether sleep or schedule disruption are better predictors of outcome, and knowing this would certainly shape treatment targets. Very few longitudinal studies have examined cognitive predictors of manic symptoms (see Lam et al., 2005, for an exception). Such analyses of which variables are most predictive could help refine treatment targets.

Overall, treatment outcome research on BD has achieved a great deal. The early findings suggest that a host of treatments can be helpful. Psychoeducation can enhance medication adherence and diminish symptoms. More specific interventions are designed to address other mechanisms involved in the course of the disorder. These basic findings on treatment outcome in BD, then, set the stage for more careful integration of specific mechanisms with intervention studies, and extension of research to a broader range of outcomes and populations.

REFERENCES

Alloy, L. B., Reilly-Harrington, N., Fresco, D. M., Whitehouse, W. G., & Zechmeister, J. S. (1999). Cognitive styles and life events in subsyndromal unipolar and bipolar disorders: Stability and prospective prediction of depressive and hypomanic mood swings. *Journal of Cognitive Psychotherapy, 13,* 21–40.

American Psychiatric Association. (2002). *Practice guideline for the treatment of patients with bipolar disorder* (2nd ed.). Washington, DC: Author.

American Psychiatric Association. (2013). *Diagnostic and statistical manual of mental disorders* (5th ed.). Arlington, VA: Author.

Angst, J., Angst, F., Gerber-Werder, R., & Gamma, A. (2005). Suicide in 406 mood-disordered patients with and without long-term medication: A 40 to 44 year follow-up. *Archives of Suicide Research, 9,* 279–300.

Ashman, S. B., Monk, T. H., Kupfer, D. J., Clark, C. H., Myers, F. S., Frank, E., et al. (1999). Relationship between social rhythms and mood in patients with rapid cycling bipolar disorder. *Psychiatry Research, 86,* 1–8.

Barbini, B., Benedetti, F., Colombo, C., Dotoli, D., Bernasconi, A., Cigala-Fulgosi, M., et al. (2005). Dark therapy for mania: A pilot study. *Bipolar Disorders, 7,* 98–101.

Barbini, B., Colombo, C., Benedetti, F., Campori, E., Bellodi, L., & Smeraldi, E. (1998). The unipolar–bipolar dichotomy and the response to sleep deprivation. *Psychiatry Research 79,* 43–50.

Bauer, M. S., McBride, L., Chase, C., Sachs, G., & Shea, N. (1998). Manual-based group psychotherapy for bipolar disorder: A feasibility study. *Journal of Clinical Psychiatry, 59,* 449–455.

Brissos, S., Dias, V., & Kapczinski, F. (2008). Cognitive performance and quality of life in bipolar disorder. *Canadian Journal of Psychiatry, 52,* 517–524.

Brown, E. B., McElroy, S. L., Keck, P. E., Deldar, A., Adams, D. H., Tohen, M., et al. (2006). A 7 week, randomized, double-blind trial of olanzapine/fluoxetine combination versus lamotrigine in the treatment of bipolar I depression. *Journal of Clinical Psychiatry, 67,* 1025–1033.

Brown, G. K., Beck, A. T., Steer, R. A., & Grisham, J. R. (2000). Risk factors for suicide in psychiatric outpatients: A 20–year prospective study. *Journal of Consulting and Clinical Psychology, 68,* 371–377.

Butzlaff, R. L., & Hooley, J. M. (1998). Expressed emotion and psychiatric relapse: A meta-analysis. *Archives of General Psychiatry 55,* 547–552.

Calabrese, J. R., Huffman, R. F., White, R. L., Edwards, S., Thompson, T. R., Ascher, J. A., et al. (2008). Lamotrigine in the acute treatment of bipolar depression: Results of five double-blind, placebo-controlled clinical trials. *Bipolar Disorders, 10,* 323–333.

Carver, C. S., & White, T. L. (1994). Behavioral inhibition, behavioral activation, and affective responses to impending reward and punishment: The BIS/BAS scales. *Journal of Personality and Social Psychology, 67,* 319–333.

Clarkin, J. F., Glick, I. D., Haas, G. L., Spencer, J. H., Lewis, A. B., Peyser, J. (1990). A randomized clinical trial of inpatient family intervention: V. Results for affective disorders. *Journal of Affective Disorders, 18,* 17–28.

Cochran, S. D. (1984). Preventing medical noncompliance in the outpatient treatment of bipolar affective disorders. *Journal of Consulting and Clinical Psychology, 52,* 873–878.

Colom, F., Vieta, E., Sanchez-Moreno, J., Martinez-Aran, A., Reinares, M., Goikolea, J. M., et al. (2005). Stabilizing the stabilizer: Group psychoeducation enhances the stability of serum lithium levels. *Bipolar Disorders, 7,* 32–36.

Colom, F., Vieta, E., Sanchez-Moreno, J., Palomino-Otiniano, R., Reinares, M., Goikolea, J. M., et al. (2009). Group psychoeducation for stabilised bipolar disorders: 5-year outcome of a randomised clinical trial. *British Journal of Psychiatry, 194,* 260–265.

Coryell, W., Scheftner, W., Keller, M., Endicott, J., Maser, J., & Klerman, G. L. (1993). The enduring psychosocial consequences of mania and depression. *American Journal of Psychiatry, 150,* 720–727.

Cuellar, A., Johnson, S. L., & Winters, R. (2005). Distinctions between bipolar and unipolar depression. *Clinical Psychology Review, 25,* 307–339.

Davenport, Y. B., Ebert, M. H., Adland, M. L., & Goodwin, F. K. (1977). Couples group therapy as adjunct to lithium maintenance of the manic patient. *American Journal of Orthopsychiatry, 47,* 495–502.

Dunayevich, E., Sax, K. W., Keck, P. E., McElroy, S. L., Sorter, M. T., McConville, B. J., et al. (2000). Twelve-month outcome in bipolar patients with and without personality disorders. *Journal of Clinical Psychiatry, 61,* 134–139.

Ehlers, C. L., Frank, E., & Kupfer, D. J. (1988). Social zeitgebers and biological rhythms: A unified approach to understanding the etiology of depression. *Archives of General Psychiatry, 45,* 948–952.

Ellicott, A., Hammen, C., Gitlin, M., Brown, G., & Jamison, K. (1990). Life events and the course of bipolar disorder. *American Journal of Psychiatry, 147,* 1194–1198.

Feske, U., Frank, E., Mallinger, A. G., Houck, P. R., Fagiolini, A., & Shear, M. K. (2000). Anxiety as a correlate of response to the acute treatment of bipolar I disorder. *American Journal of Psychiatry, 157,* 956–962.

Fiedorowicz, J. G., Solomon, D. A., Endicott, J., Leon, A. C., Li, C., Rice, J. P., et al. (2009). Manic/hypomanic symptom burden and cardiovascular mortality in bipolar disorder. *Psychosomatic Medicine, 71,* 598–606.

Frank, E. (2005). *Treating bipolar disorder: A clinician's guide to interpersonal and social rhythm therapy.* New York: Guilford Press.

Frank, E., Cyranowski, J. M., Rucci, P., Shear, M. K., Fagiolini, A., Thase, M., et al. (2002). Clinical significance of lifetime panic spectrum symptoms in the treatment of patients with bipolar I disorder. *Archives of General Psychiatry, 59,* 905–911.

Frank, E., Hlastala, S., Ritenour, A., Houck, P., Tu, X. M., Mark, T. H., et al. (1997). Inducing lifestyle regularity in recovering bipolar disorder patients. *Biological Psychiatry, 41,* 1165–1173.

Frank, E., Kupfer, D., Thase, M. E., Mallinger, A. G., Swartz, H. A., Fagiolini, A. M., et al. (2005). Two-year outcomes for interpersonal and social rhythm therapy in individuals with bipolar I disorder. *Archives of General Psychiatry, 62,* 996–1004.

Frank, E., Soreca, I., Swartz, H. A., Fagiolini, A. M., Mallinger, A. G., Thase, M. E., et al. (2008). The role of interpersonal and social rhythm therapy in improving occupational functioning in patients with bipolar I disorder. *American Journal of Psychiatry, 165,* 1559–1565.

George, E. L., Miklowitz, D. J., Richards, J. A., Simoneau, T. L., & Taylor, D. O. (2003). The comorbidity of bipolar disorder and axis II personality disorders: Prevalence and clinical correlates. *Bipolar Disorders, 5,* 115–122.

Ghaemi, S. N., Lenox, M. S., & Baldessarini, R. J. (2001). Effectiveness and safety of long-term antidepressant treatment in bipolar disorder. *Journal of Clinical Psychology, 62,* 565–569.

Gitlin, M. J., Swendsen, J., Heller, T. L., & Hammen, C. (1995). Relapse and impairment in bipolar disorder. *American Journal of Psychiatry, 152,* 1635–1640.

Goodwin, G. M., for the Consensus Group of the British Association for Psychopharmacology. (2003). Evidence-based guidelines for treating bipolar disorder: Recommendations from the British Association for Psychopharmacology. *Journal of Psychopharmacology, 17,* 149–173.

Harmon-Jones, E., Abramson, L. Y., Nusslock, R., Sigelman, J. D., Urosevic, S., Turonie, L. D., et al. (2008). Effect of bipolar disorder on left frontal cortical responses to goals differing in valence and task difficulty. *Biological Psychiatry, 63,* 693–698.

Harris, E. C., & Barraclough, B. (1997). Suicide as an outcome for mental disorders: A meta-analysis. *Britich Journal of Psychiatry, 170,* 205–208.

Harrow, M., Goldberg, J., Grossman, L., & Meltzer, H. (1990). Outcome in manic disorders. A naturalistic follow-up study. *Archives of General Psychiatry, 47*, 665–671.

Hogarty, G. E., Anderson, C. M., Reiss, D. J., Kornblith, S. J., Greenwald, D. P., & Ulrich, R. F. (1991). Family psychoeducation, social skills training, and maintenance chemotherapy in the aftercare of schizophrenia. *Archives of General Psychiatry 48*, 340–347.

Honig, A., Hofman, A., Hilwiq, M., Noorthoorn, E., & Ponds, R. (1995). Psychoeducation and expressed emotion in bipolar disorder: Preliminary findings. *Psychiatry Research, 28*, 299–301.

Jamison, K. (1993). *Touched with fire: Manic depressive illness and the artistic temperament.* New York: Free Press.

Johnson, L., Lundström, O., Åberg-Wistedt, A., & Mathé, A. A. (2003). Social support in bipolar disorder: Its relevance to remission and relapse. *Bipolar Disorders, 5*, 129–137.

Johnson, S. L. (2005a). Life events in bipolar disorder: Towards more specific models. *Clinical Psychology Review, 25*, 1008–1027.

Johnson, S. L. (2005b). Mania and dysregulation in goal pursuit. *Clinical Psychology Review, 25*, 241–262.

Johnson, S. L., Cuellar, A., Ruggero, C., Perlman, C., Goodnick, P., White, R., et al. (2008). Life events as predictors of mania and depression in bipolar I disorder. *Journal of Abnormal Psychology 117*, 268–277.

Johnson, S. L., Edge, M. D., Holmes, M. K., & Carver, C. S. (2012). The behavioral activation system and mania. *Annual Review of Clinical Psychology, 8*, 243–267.

Johnson, S. L., Eisner, L., & Carver, C. (2009). Elevated expectancies among persons diagnosed with bipolar disorders. *British Journal of Clinical Psychology, 48*, 217–222.

Johnson, S. L., & Fingerhut, R. (2004). Negative cognitions predict the course of bipolar depression, not mania. *Jouranl of Cognitive Psychotherapy, 18*, 149–162.

Johnson, S. L., & Fulford, D. C. (2008). Development of the treatment attitudes questionnaire in bipolar disorder. *Journal of Clinical Psychology, 64*, 466–481.

Johnson, S. L., & Fulford, D. (2009). The Goals Program: A mania prevention intervention. *Behaviour Research and Therapy, 40*, 103–113.

Johnson, S. L., & Kizer, A. (2002). Bipolar and unipolar depression: A comparison of clinical phenomenology and psychosocial predictors. In I. H. Gotlib & C. L. Hammen (Eds.), *Handbook of depression* (pp. 141–165). New York: Guilford Press.

Johnson, S. L., & Leahy, R. L. (Eds.). (2004). *Psychological treatment of bipolar disorder.* New York: Guilford Press.

Johnson, S. L., Winett, C. A., Meyer, B., Greenhouse, W. J., & Miller, I. (1999). Social support and the course of bipolar disorder. *Journal of Abnormal Psychology, 108*, 558–566.

Jones, S. H., & Day, C. (2008). Self appraisal and behavioural activation in the prediction of hypomanic personality and depressive symptoms. *Personality and Individual Differences, 45*, 643–648.

Jones, S., Hayward, P., & Lam, D. (2002). *Coping with bipolar disorder: A guide to living with manic depression.* Oxford, UK: One World.

Jones, S. H., Tai, S., Evershed, K., Knowles, R., & Bentall, R. (2006). Early detection of bipolar disorder: A pilot familial high-risk study of parents with bipolar disorder and their adolescent children. *Bipolar Disorders, 8*, 362–372.

Judd, L. L., Akiskal, H. S., Schetteler, P. J., Endicott, J., Maser, J., Solomon, D. A., et al. (2002). The long-term natural history of the weekly symptomatic status of bipolar I disorder. *Archives of General Psychiatry, 59*, 530–537.

Keck, P., McElroy, S., Strakowski, S., West, S., Sax, K., Hawkins, J., et al. (1998). Twelve-month outcome of patients with bipolar disorder following hospitalization for a manic or mixed episode. *American Journal of Psychiatry, 155*, 646–652.

Keller, M., Lavori, P., Coryell, W., Andreasen, N., Endicott, J., Clayton, P., et al. (1986). Differential outcome of pure manic, mixed/cycling, and pure depressive episodes in patients with bipolar illness. *Journal of the American Medical Association, 255*, 3138–3142.

Kessler, R. C., Chiu, W. T., Demler, O., & Walters, E. E. (2005). Prevalence, severity, and comorbidity of 12-month DSM-IV disorders in the National Comorbidity Survey Replication. *Archives of General Psychiatry, 62*, 617–627.

Kessler, R., McGonagle, K., Zhao, S., Nelson, C., Hughes, M., Eshleman, S., et al. (1994). Lifetime and 12-month prevalence of DSM-III-R psychiatric disorders in the United States: Results from the National Comorbidity Survey. *Archives of General Psychiatry, 51*, 8–19.

Klerman, G., Weissman, M., Rounsaville, B., & Chevron, E. (1984). *Interpersonal psychotherapy for depression.* New York: Basic Books.

Krishnan, M., Mast, B., Ficker, L., Lawhorne, L., & Lichtenberg, P. (2005). The effects of preexisting depression on cerebrovascular health outcomes in geriatric continuing care. *Journals of Gerontology A: Biological Sciences and Medical Sciences, 60*, 915–919.

Lam, D. H., Jones, S. H., Hayward, P., & Bright, J. A. (1999). *Cognitive therapy for bipolar disorder: A therapist's guide to concepts, methods, and practice.* Chichester, UK: Wiley.

Lam, D. H., Watkins, E. R., Hayward, P., Bright, J., Wright, K., & Kerr, N. (2003). A randomized controlled study of cognitive therapy of relapse prevention for bipolar affective disorder: Outcome of the first year. *Archives of General Psychiatry, 60*, 145–152.

Lam, D., Wright, K., & Sham, P. (2005). Sense of hyper-positive self and response to cognitive therapy in bipolar disorder. *Psychological Medicine, 35*, 69–77.

Lam, D., Wright, K., & Smith, N. (2004). Dysfunctional assumptions in bipolar disorder. *Journal of Affective Disorders, 79*, 193–199.

LaPalme, M., Hodgins, S., & LaRoche, C. (1997). Children of parents with bipolar disorder: A meta-analysis of risk for mental disorders. *Canadian Journal of Psychiatry, 42*, 623–631.

Laursen, T. M., Munk-Olsen, T., Nordentoft, M., & Mortensen, P. B. (2007). Increased mortality among patients admitted with major psychiatric disorders: A register-based study comparing mortality in unipolar depressive disorder, bipolar affective disorder, schizoaffective disorder, and schizophrenia. *Journal of Clinical Psychiatry, 68*, 899–907.

Leibenluft, E. (1996). Women with bipolar illness: Clinical and research issues. *American Journal of Psychiatry, 153*, 163–173.

Lozano, B., & Johnson, S. L. (2001). Can personality traits predict increases in manic and depressive symptoms? *Journal of Affective Disorders, 63*, 103–111.

Malkoff-Schwartz, S., Frank, E., Anderson, B. P., Hlastala, S. A., Luther, J. F., & Sherrill, J. T. (2000). Social rhythm disruption and stressful life events in the onset of bipolar and unipolar episodes. *Psychological Medicine, 30*, 1005–1016.

Malkoff-Schwartz, S., Frank, E., Anderson, B., Sherrill, J. T., Siegel, L., & Patterson, D. (1998). Stressful life events and social rhythm disruption in the onset of manic and depressive bipolar episodes: A preliminary investigation. *Archives of General Psychiatry, 55*, 702–707.

Mansell, W., & Lam, D. (2006). "I won't do what you tell me!": Elevated mood and the assessment of advice-taking in euthymic bipolar I disorder. *Behaviour Research and Therapy, 44*, 1787–1801.

Masi, G., Perugi, G., Toni, C., Millepiedi, S., Mucci, M., Bertini, N., et al. (2004). Predictors of treatment nonresponse in bipolar children and adolescents with manic or mixed episodes. *Journal of Child and Adolescent Psychopharmacology, 14*, 395–404.

McElroy, S., Altshuler, L., Suppes, T., Keck, P., Frye, M., Denikoff, K., et al. (2001). Axis I psychiatric comorbidity and its relationship to historical illness variables in 288 patients with bipolar disorder. *American Journal of Psychiatry, 158*, 420–426.

McGuffin, P., Rijsdijk, F., Andrew, M., Sham, P., Katz, R., & Cardno, A. (2003). The heritability of bipolar affective disorder and the genetic relationship to unipolar depression. *Archives of General Psychiatry, 60,* 497–502.

Meyer, B., Johnson, S. L., & Winters, R. (2001). Responsiveness to threat and incentive in bipolar disorder: Relations of the BIS/BAS scales with symptoms. *Journal of Psychopathology and Behavioral Assessment, 23,* 133–143.

Miklowitz, D. J., George, E. L., Richards, J. A., Simoneau, T. L., & Suddath, R. L. (2003). A randomized study of family-focused psychoeducation and pharmacotherapy in the outpatient management of bipolar disorder. *Archives of General Psychiatry, 60,* 904–912.

Miklowitz, D. J., & Goldstein, M. J. (1997). *Bipolar disorder: A family-focused treatment approach.* New York: Guilford Press.

Miklowitz, D. J., Goldstein, M. J., Nuechterlein, K. H., Snyder, K. S., & Mintz, J. (1988). Family factors and the course of bipolar affective disorder. *Archives of General Psychiatry, 45,* 225–231.

Miklowitz, D. J., Otto, M. W., Frank, E., Reilly-Harrington, N. A., Kogan, J. N., Sachs, G. S., et al. (2007). Intensive psychosocial intervention enhances functioning in patients with bipolar depression: Results from a 90-month randomized controlled trial. *American Journal of Psychiatry, 164,* 1340–1347.

Miklowitz, D. J., Otto, M. W., Frank, E., Reilly-Harrington, N. A., Wisniewski, S. R., Kogan, J. N., et al. (2007). Psychosocial treatments for bipolar depression: A one-year randomized trial from the Systematic Treatment Enhancement Program. *Archives of General Psychiatry, 64,* 419–427.

Miller, I., Solomon, D. A., Ryan, C. E., & Keitner, G. I. (2004). Does adjunctive family therapy enhance recovery from bipolar I mood episodes? *Journal of Affective Disorders, 82,* 431–436.

Monk, T. H., Frank, E., Potts, J. M., & Kupfer, D. J. (2002). A simple way to measure daily lifestyle regularity. *Journal of Sleep Research, 11,* 183–190.

Moreno, D. H., & Andrade, L. H. (2005). The lifetime prevalence, health service utilization, and risk for suicide of bipolar spectrum subjects, including subthreshold categories in the Sao Paulo ECA Study. *Journal of Affective Disorders, 87,* 231–241.

Nemeroff, C., Evans, D., Gyulai, L., Sachs, G., Bowden, C., Gergel, I., et al. (2001). Double-blind, placebo-controlled comparison of imipramine and paroxetine in the treatment of bipolar depression. *American Journal of Psychiatry, 158,* 906–912.

Nierenberg, A., Miyahara, S., Spencer, T., Wisniewski, S., Otto, M., Simon, N., et al. (2005). Clinical and diagnostic implications of lifetime attention deficit/hyperactivity disorder comorbidity in adults with bipolar disorder: Data from the first 1000 STEP-BD participants. *Biological Psychiatry, 57,* 1467–1473.

Noaghiul, S., & Hibbeln, J. R. (2003). Cross-national comparisons of seafood consumption and rates of bipolar disorders. *American Journal of Psychiatry, 160,* 2222–2227.

Otto, M., & Miklowitz, D. (2004). The role and impact of psychotherapy in the management of bipolar disorder. *CNS Spectrums, 9,* 27–32.

Otto, M. W., Reilly-Harrington, N. A., Kogan, J. N., Henin, A., Knauz, R. O., & Sachs, G. S. (2009). *Managing bipolar disorder: A cognitive-behavioral approach (Therapist guide).* New York: Oxford University Press.

Patelis-Siotis, I., Young, L. T., Robb, J. C., Marriott, M., Bieling, P. J., Cox, L. C., et al. (2001). Group cognitive behavioral therapy for bipolar disorder: A feasibility and effectiveness study. *Journal of Affective Disorders, 65,* 145–153.

Peet, M., & Harvey, N. S. (1991). Lithium maintainence: 1. A standard education program for patients. *British Journal of Psychiatry, 158,* 197–200.

Perlick, D. A., Rosenheck, R. A., Miklowitz, D. J., Chessick, C., Wolff, N., Kaczynski, R., et al. (2007). Prevalence and correlates of burden among caregivers of patients with bipolar disorder enrolled in the Systematic Treatment Enhancement Program for Bipolar Disorder. *Bipolar Disorders, 9,* 262–273.

Perlis, R. H., Miyahara, S., Marangell, L. B., Wisniewski, S. R., Ostacher, M., Delbello, M. P., et al. (2004). Long-term implications of early onset in bipolar disorder: Data from the first 1000 participants in the Systematic Treatment Enhancement Program for Bipolar Disorder (STEP-BD). *Biological Psychiatry, 55*, 875–881.

Perry, A., Tarrier, N., Morriss, R., McCarthy, E., & Limb, K. (1999). Randomized controlled trial of efficacy of teaching patients with bipolar disorder to identify early symptoms of relapse and obtain treatment. *British Medical Journal, 16*, 149–153.

Rea, M. M., Tompson, M., Miklowitz, D. J., Goldstein, M. J., Hwang, S., & Mintz, J. (2003). Family focused treatment vs. individual treatment for bipolar disorder: Results of a randomized clinical trial. *Journal of Consulting and Clinical. Psychology, 71*, 482–492.

Regeer, E. J., Have, M., Rosso, M. L., Hakkaart-van Roijen, L., Vollebergh, W., & Nolen, W. A. (2004). Prevalence of bipolar disorder in the general population: A reappraisal study of the Netherlands Mental Health Survey and Incidence Study. *Acta Psychiatrica Scandinavica, 110*, 374–382.

Regier, D. A., Farmer, M. E., Rae, D. S., Locke, B. Z., Keith, S. J., Judd, L. L., et al. (1990). Comorbidity of mental disorders with alcohol and other drug abuse: Results from the Epidemiologic Catchment Area (ECA) Study. *Journal of the American Medical Association, 264*, 2511–2518.

Romans, S. E., & McPherson, H. M. (1992). The social networks of bipolar affective disorder patients. *Journal of Affective Disorders, 25*, 221–228.

Scott, J., Garland, A., & Moorhead, S. (2001). A pilot study of cognitive therapy in bipolar disorders. *Psychological Medicine, 31*, 459–467.

Scott, J., Paykel, E., Morriss, R., Bentall, R., Kinderman, P., Johnson, T., et al. (2006). Cognitive-behavioural therapy for severe and recurrent bipolar disorders: Randomized controlled trial. *British Journal of Psychiatry, 188*, 313–320.

Scott, J., & Pope, M. (2002). Nonadherence with mood stabilizers: Prevalence and predictors. *Journal of Clinical Psychiatry, 63*, 384–390.

Segurado, R., Detera-Wadleigh, S. D., Levinson, D. F., Lewis, C. M., Gill, M., Nurnberger, J. I., Jr., et al. (2003). Genome scan meta-analysis of schizophrenia and bipolar disorder, part III: Bipolar disorder. *American Journal of Human Genetics, 73*, 49–62.

Shen, G., Sylvia, L., Alloy, L., Barrett, F., Kohner, M., Iacoviello, B., et al. (2008). Lifestyle regularity and cyclothymic symptomatology. *Journal of Clinical Psychology, 64*, 482–500.

Simon, G. E., Ludman, E. J., Unützer, J., Bauer, M. S., Operskalski, B., & Rutter, C. (2005). Randomized trial of a population-based care program for people with bipolar disorder. *Psychological Medicine, 35*, 13–24.

Simon, G., & Unützer, J. (1999). Health care utilization and costs among patients treated for bipolar disorder in an insured population. *Psychiatric Services, 50*, 1303–1308.

Simon, N., Otto, M., Weiss, R., Bauer, M., Miyahara, S., Wisniewski, S., et al. (2004). Pharmacotherapy for bipolar disorder and comorbid conditions: Baseline data from STEP-BD. *Journal of Clinical Psychopharmacology, 24*, 512–520.

Simoneau, T. L., Miklowitz, D. J., Richards, J. A., Saleem, R., & George, E. L. (1999). Bipolar disorder and family communication: Effects of a psychoeducational treatment program. *Journal of Abnormal Psychology, 108*, 588–597.

Simoneau, T. L., Miklowitz, D. J., & Saleem, R. (1998). Expressed emotion and interactional patterns in the families of bipolar patients. *Journal of Abnormal Psychology, 107*, 497–507.

Suppes, T., Leverich, G. S., Keck, P. E., Nolen, W. A., Denicoff, K. D., Altshuler, L. L., et al. (2001). The Stanley Foundation Bipolar Treatment Outcome Network: II. Demographics and illness characteristics of the first 261 patients. *Journal of Affective Disorders, 67*, 45–59.

Tohen, M., Waternaux, C. M., & Tsuang, M. T. (1990). Outcome in mania: A 4-year prospective follow-up of 75 patients utilizing survival analysis. *Archives of General Psychiatry, 47*, 1106–1111.

Tondo, L., & Baldessarini, R. J. (2000). Reducing suicide risk during lithium maintenance treatment. *Journal of Clinical Psychiatry, 61*, 97–104.

Totterdell, P., & Kellett, S. (2008). Restructuring mood in cyclothymia using cognitive behavioral therapy: An intensive time-sampling study. *Journal of Clinical Psycology, 64*, 501–518.

van Gent, E. M., & Zwart, R. M. (1991). Psychoeducation of partners of bipolar manic patients. *Journal of Affective Disorders, 21*, 15–18.

Wehr, R., Turner, E., Shimada, J., Lowe, C., Barker, C., & Leibenluft, E. (1998). Treatment of a rapidly cycling bipolar patient by using extended bed rest and darkness to stabilize the timing and duration of sleep. *Biological Psychiatry, 43*, 822–828.

Wehr, T. A., Sack, D. A., & Rosenthal, N. E. (1987). Sleep reduction as a final common pathway in the genesis of mania. *American Journal of Psychiatry, 144*, 210–214.

Weiss, R. D., Greenfield, S. F., Najavits, L. M., Soto, J. A., Wyner, D., Tohen, M., et al. (1998). Medication compliance among patients with bipolar disorder and substance use disorder. *Journal of Clinical Psychiatry, 59*, 172–174.

Weiss, R. D., Griffin, M. L., Kolodziej, M. E., Greenfield, S. F., Najavits, L. M., Daley, D. C., et al. (2007). A randomized trial of integrated group therapy versus group drug counseling for patients with bipolar disorder and substance dependence. *American Journal of Pyschiatry, 164*, 100–107.

Wender, P. H., Kety, S. S., Rosenthal, D., Schulsinger, F., Ortmann, J., & Lunde, I. (1986). Psychiatric disorders in the biological and adoptive families of adopted individuals with affective disorders. *Archives of General Psychiatry, 43*, 923–929.

Wirz-Justice, A. (2006). Biological rhythm disturbances in mood disorders. *International Clinical Psychopharmacology, 21*, S11–S15.

World Health Organization. (2001). *The World Health Report: Mental Health: New Understanding, New Hope.* Geneva, Switzerland: World Health Organization.

Wright, K. A., Lam, D., & Brown, R. G. (2008). Dysregulation of the behavioral activation system in remitted bipolar I disorder. *Journal of Abnormal Psychology, 117*, 838–848.

Yan, L. J., Hammen, C., Cohen, A. N., Daley, S. E., & Henry, R. M. (2004). Expressed emotion versus relationship quality variables in the prediction of recurrence in bipolar patients. *Journal of Affective Disorders, 83*, 199–206.

Zaretsky, A. E., Lancee, W., Miller, C., Harris, A., & Parikh, S. V. (2008). Is CBT more effective than psychoeducation in the treatment of bipolar disorder? *Canadian Journal of Psychiatry, 53*, 441–448.

CHAPTER 11

The Positive Symptoms
of Schizophrenia

Craig Steel
Til Wykes

T here have been various attempts to understand the presence of "insanity" throughout history. These ideas have been embedded within the social and cultural perspectives of the day. Thus, the ancient Greeks developed ideas associated with the hereditary and biological bases of mental disorders. In contrast, the European Middle Ages saw the rise of a religious perspective and the attribution of witchcraft and demonic possession to those who exhibited unusual and bizarre behaviors.

The modern psychiatric classification of schizophrenia stems from the European psychiatrist Emil Kraepelin who, in 1896, first used the term "dementia praecox." This disorder was associated with many of the symptoms that form the basis of the current diagnosis of schizophrenia. However, Kraepelin viewed the disorder as one that developed within early adulthood and had a fixed deterioration. The term "schizophrenia" was put forward by a Swiss psychiatrist Eugen Bleuler (1908), based on the Greek words *schiz* (split) and *phren* (mind), referring to a "split-mind." This classification was based on the "breaking of associative threads" and referred to problems within a wide range of psychological functions, including communication and action. Also, Bleuler suggested a wider age range within the potential onset of the disorder than did Kraepelin, and did not view the course as one of inevitable deterioration.

CLASSIFICATION

Since this early classification of schizophrenia, psychiatric diagnoses have evolved through the various versions of ICD *(International Classification of Diseases)* and

DSM *(Diagnostic and Statistical Manual of Mental Disorders).* During these developments, the diagnosis of schizophrenia has remained one of the core psychotic disorders. There are, however, a number of other psychiatric diagnoses associated with the presence of psychotic symptoms (see further discussion of these symptoms below). These include schizoaffective disorder, schizophreniform disorder, delusional disorder, substance-induced psychotic disorder, bipolar disorder, and psychotic depression. Of course, distinct diagnostic criteria for each of these disorders can be found within ICD and DSM. As a generic example, schizophrenia is associated with more negative symptoms, few affective symptoms, and longer duration than other psychotic disorders. A significant affective component to an individual presentation is likely to lead to a diagnosis of schizoaffective disorder or bipolar disorder.

A large number of clinical researchers have for some time questioned the validity and usefulness of the diagnosis of schizophrenia. The debate continues with reference to the current diagnostic criteria, as detailed in DSM-5 and ICD-11. The main difficulties involve two related questions: (1) Is schizophrenia a valid scientific category (i.e., valid distinction between schizophrenia and other psychotic disorders)? and (2) Does a diagnosis of schizophrenia prove useful in terms of prognosis and treatment response? Van Os, Linscott, Myin-Germeys, Delespaul, and Krabbendam (2009) discussed a number of studies that raised doubts over both of these points. First, overlap between the symptoms associated with the varied psychotic disorders is such that there is poor diagnostic specificity; that is, although hallucinations and delusions are more commonly associated with schizophrenia than with bipolar disorder, this distinction actually provides very limited power to predict diagnoses. There are also major doubts as to the usefulness of the diagnosis of schizophrenia in the prediction of outcome. Van Os et al. argued that future science would benefit from recognizing the common elements within what are currently a number of discrete diagnoses that represent a "cluster of psychotic disorders." They suggested that a number of symptom dimensions and different types of onset need to be considered when trying to understand the varied types of psychotic presentation. One of the major considerations here is the potential of a continuum of the varied psychotic symptoms, such as delusions and hallucinations. We consider this issue with reference to specific symptoms below.

TYPICAL SYMPTOMS

There are five core characteristics within the DSM-5 diagnostic criteria for schizophrenia: delusions, hallucinations, disorganized speech, grossly disorganized or catatonic behavior, and negative symptoms (e.g., affective flattening). In order to be diagnosed with this disorder, an individual must have experienced two or more of these symptoms for a significant proportion of time within the preceding month. The individual must also have experienced marked social or occupational dysfunction and have suffered behavioral disturbance for at least 6 months. Based on these diagnostic criteria, it is important to note that two individuals diagnosed with schizophrenia may exhibit completely distinct symptom profiles. Delusions and hallucinations are often referred to as the *positive* symptoms of schizophrenia (the focus of this chapter), because their presence is considered to be an excess of normal functioning. The third and fourth symptoms are often categorized as *disorganized* symptoms, while the fifth is referred to as *negative* symptoms (covered by Kring & Smith in Chapter 12, this volume), because they are considered a reduction in normal functioning.

This chapter outlines the varied presentations associated with the positive symptoms of schizophrenia, that is, delusions and hallucinations, along with the etiology and issues associated with intervention. Issues related to clinical associated features, epidemiology, course, and comorbidity for schizophrenia are covered in the chapter on negative symptoms. It is important for clinicians to note that these core positive symptoms may present without the individual suffering from any significant levels of distress or impact on functioning. Therefore, while these symptoms are seen as the defining features of schizophrenia, the diagnostic criteria of behavioral and social/occupational disturbance must not be forgotten. This makes the disorder distinct from emotional disorders in which distress is an inherent part of the defining characteristics.

It is important to note that hallucinations and delusions occur in a large number of individuals who have not been diagnosed with schizophrenia. Although some of these are diagnosed with other mental health problems (e.g., schizoaffective, bipolar, or borderline personality disorders), many others have no diagnosis. Much of our current understanding of these "symptoms" occurs within a framework that cuts across diagnostic boundaries.

Hallucinations

Hallucinations are frequently considered to be sensory perceptions of stimuli that are not really there. They may occur in any sensory modality; however, auditory hallucinations are the most common. Although the perceived auditory stimuli may be heard as general noises or music, they are most often heard in the form of a voice, or voices. They may be judged to originate from either inside or outside the head; may be experienced as male, female, or alien voices; and they may be either single or multiple voices. The type of communication originating from the voice may come in many forms, including "voices commenting," in which the perceived voice makes frequent comments on the actions and thoughts of the voice hearer, and "command hallucinations," in which the voice hearer is given direct instruction on how to act.

The work of Marius Romme and Sandra Escher in the late 1980s helped to highlight the relatively prevalent occurrence of voice hearing, and to challenge the psychiatric view of voices being a symptom of an illness. Their seminal work started with Romme, a social psychiatrist, and one of his voice-hearing patients appearing on a Dutch television program and inviting viewers to phone in if they had heard voices. Hundreds of viewers responded, with the majority having never received psychiatric attention. This event opened up a research program highlighting how the voice hearers who had remained outside of the psychiatric system had learned to integrate voice hearing into their daily lives (Romme & Escher, 1989). There is now considerable evidence that around 3% of people will experience voice hearing at some point during their lives (Johns et al., 2004). Voice hearers from within and outside the psychiatric system have been shown to develop relationships with their voices, and an understanding of these relationships can be an important part of a therapeutic intervention (see below).

Advances in neuroimaging technology have enabled researchers to show an association between voice hearing and activation of the left primary auditory cortex and the right middle temporal gyrus (Bentaleb, Beauregard, Liddle, & Stip, 2002). Because this region of the brain has also been associated with the production of inner speech, it may be that auditory hallucinations are the product of a misattribution of internally generated stimuli to an external source. The possibility of such a misattribution is supported by studies that highlight problems in "source monitoring" within individuals suffering from the positive symptoms of psychosis. Such studies typically involve asking participants to remember the original source of words generated by either themselves or an experimenter. Those diagnosed with schizophrenia are more likely to misattribute a self-generated word that originated from the experimenter (Brebion et al., 2000). Although these studies highlight a possible route from internal perception to hallucinatory experience, they do not account for the level of distress that may be associated with voice hearing. The idiosyncratic belief as to the origin of their voices has been shown to be critical in determining individual emotional reactions (see the section below on cognitive-behavioral models).

Implications for Treatment

Given that auditory hallucinations are an internal experience, the clinician only has the individual's self-report as a source of evidence. The clinician should be mindful that voice hearers may not wish to discuss their experiences, and that a level of trust may need to be gained. Problems with engagement may include voice hearers being concerned that they may be forced to receive inpatient psychiatric treatment or have their medication increased, if they discuss their voices. This clinician can address this issue overtly by stating whether these assumptions are correct. It may also be the case that the voice is telling the voice hearer not to discuss anything with the clinician, and may even threaten violence or death. The clinician, who may not be in a position to know this information until the patient's trust is gained, should therefore be mindful of this possibility and observe any discomfort or anxiety when inquiring about voice content.

Although an individual may be diagnosed with schizophrenia and experience auditory hallucinations, the clinician should not assume that the hallucinations are a source of significant distress. A careful assessment is needed to assess the most significant problems, and whether the hallucinations are involved. Also, the patient may experience a number of different voices attributed to different individuals. Some of these voices may be friendly and helpful, while others may be more threatening and cause distress. In either scenario, appearing to assume that the patient would be better off not hearing any voices may distance the clinician from the goals of the patient.

Delusions

Delusions, the most common symptom associated with a diagnosis of schizophrenia, are present in around 75% of patients receiving hospital care (Maher, 2001). Traditional psychiatry has defined a "delusion" as a fixed false belief that is held in the face of evidence to the contrary (Jaspers, 1913). The most recent edition of the DSM (American Psychiatric Association, 2013) uses criteria based on the same approach, with a delusion being defined as a belief that is not held within a person's culture or subculture. The underlying assumption within this perspective is that a delusion is "un-understandable" and cannot be made sense of with reference to normal thought process. However, recent research within the field of cognitive-behavioral therapy (CBT) questions this assumption (see further discussion below).

A delusional belief can often be understood within the context of hallucinatory experiences. For example, a belief that one is the son of God may be fueled by the experience of hearing a voice that tells one so. The most common of these beliefs, "delusions of persecution," characterizes the presentation of *paranoid schizophrenia*. Such delusions typically involve the belief that one is being spied on and/ or is under threat due to some kind of organized conspiracy against him or her. The sufferer may feel threatened by government agencies, God or the Devil, neighbors, or family members. "Delusions of grandeur" are associated with a belief that one is a powerful and/or famous figure (e.g., Jesus); it is quite common for such individuals also to believe that they are being persecuted, and that the persecution is a result of their (famous) identity. In another form of this symptom, "delusions of control," individuals believe their thoughts and actions are being controlled by an outside agent. A body of research highlights a possible neuropsychological basis for this specific symptom (see Frith, 1992). A commonly reported experience in schizophrenia is that certain external events are perceived to contain special messages, for example, within a news broadcast, or within the lyric of a song on the radio. These are termed *delusions of reference*.

As with auditory hallucinations, it is important to consider whether the symptoms associated with a diagnosis of schizophrenia are found within a nonclinical population, and if so, what this means regarding clinical interventions. Several surveys have highlighted the prevalence of beliefs in the paranormal and other unusual beliefs within the nonclinical population. One important study highlighted how the beliefs of a psychiatric population could not be distinguished from those of new religious movements on the basis of content alone, but only by consideration of the dimensions of controllability and distress (Peters, Day, McKenna, & Orbach, 1999). A more specific approach has highlighted the prevalence of paranoid beliefs within the general population, and how they seem to occur within a continuum, from mildly self-conscious beliefs associated with social anxiety to more extreme conspiracy theories (Freeman et al., 2005).

Reasoning processes have been extensively researched within individuals diagnosed with schizophrenia. Findings suggest that, within a laboratory situation, such individuals may "jump to conclusions" on the basis of limited evidence, and be more likely abandon their original conclusions when faced with contradictory evidence. This reasoning style is consistent with cognitive theories that suggest the positive symptoms of schizophrenia are the product of increased reliance on currently occurring information, and a relative failure to integrate this information with what has happened in the past, in order to make sense of the current situation (Hemsley, 1994).

Attribution theory has also been used in an attempt to understand paranoid delusions (Bentall, Corcoran, Howard, Blackwood, & Kinderman, 2001). Studies have shown that the normal "self-serving bias," in which nonclinical individuals attribute blame for negative events to an outside source, is exaggerated in those suffering from persecutory delusions. These theories have contributed to more generic cognitive models of psychosis and their associated interventions (see the section below on cognitive-behavioral models).

Implications for Treatment

The clinician needs to establish a level of trust to enable the client to disclose his or her beliefs. As well as being fearful of how the clinician may respond, it may be that the client may have incorporated the clinician and the psychiatric system into a paranoid belief. As with hallucinations, the clinician should not be too distracted by the level of conviction a patient exhibits for a belief that has been diagnosed as delusional. A wider assessment should be conducted in order to clarify the clinical problems of most significance.

It is important for the clinician to remember that a full assessment of an individual who presents with the symptoms of psychosis involves assessment of issues beyond the symptoms themselves. The symptoms may be having an impact on a number of factors, including social functioning, employment, sleep, drug and alcohol use, cognitive functioning, and beliefs about treatment. All such information should be gathered, whether or not it seems directly related to psychotic symptoms.

A number of psychiatric tools have been designed to assess the positive symptoms of psychosis. The most widely used within research is the Positive and

Negative Symptom Scale (PANSS; Kay et al., 1989), which incorporates a comprehensive assessment of symptoms and functioning. However, the specific assessment of hallucinations and delusions is limited to an individual item for each symptom, with the rating predominantly loaded toward frequency of hallucinations, and bizarreness and conviction of delusional belief. As discussed earlier, these criteria are not directly associated with emotional distress (Steel et al., 2007) and simplify each symptom to a unitary dimension. This latter point is particularly relevant to delusions, which have been argued to occur within a number of dimensions, each of which needs individual assessment. Harrow, Rattenbury, and Stoll (1988) refer to three dimensions within delusions: conviction, preoccupation, and the awareness of others people's reaction to one's beliefs. Most importantly it is argued that an individual's ratings on these dimensions may vary over time. More recently, the Psychotic Symptom Rating Scales (PSYRATS; Haddock, McCarron, Tarrier, & Faragher, 1999) has enabled assessment of the varied dimensions of delusional belief, including conviction, preoccupation, and distress.

ETIOLOGY

Considerable numbers of researchers have attempted to clarify the etiology of schizophrenia. Given that, treatment has predominantly been the domain of the medical profession until recently, the majority of this research has been conducted within a biological perspective. Various approaches, discussed below, have been adopted to highlight and understand the hereditary aspect of the disorder. The findings have contributed to what is widely accepted to be a genetic vulnerability. This approach has evolved into what is termed a diathesis–stress model, in which an underlying biological vulnerability is only triggered should the individual be exposed to a critical level of environmental stress. This model has the flexibility to include a wide range of stressors as potential triggers, including family stress, emotional disorders, and the experience of trauma.

Stress Sensitivity

The idea that psychosocial stress may contribute to the onset of psychotic symptoms has been discussed for several decades (see Zubin & Spring, 1977). A wide range of evidence supports this general relationship, including the higher prevalence of schizophrenia within those classified as having low socioeconomic status, those living in urban area, and those having an increased level of stressful life events in the months preceding the onset of psychosis (Bebbington et al., 1993). More specifically, there is evidence that individuals who are already diagnosed with schizophrenia and live within a high stress (or "expressed emotion") family environment are more prone to relapse (Brown, Carstairs, & Topping, 1958).

One of the major mediating systems involved in stress responses is the hypothalamic–pituitary–adrenal (HPA) axis, which regulates the release of cortisol. There is evidence that stress sensitivity (i.e., heightened levels of cortisol release) occur within individuals diagnosed with schizophrenia (Walker & Diforio, 1997). However, there are some inconsistent results in relation to this theory, likely due to the lack of clarity as to what constitutes a stressful experience. Future research will benefit from integrating a psychological approach that has refined the categorization of stressful events to include the differential impact on the HPA axis.

While there is growing evidence of some form of sensitivity to stress in individuals diagnosed with schizophrenia, it is unlikely that this will prove to be a simple linear relationship. In fact, there is evidence that exposure to certain stress events sensitizes and increases reactions to future exposure to stressful events. Also, it is possible that a number of the potential neurological markers of a diagnosis of schizophrenia (e.g., altered HPA axis, smaller hippocampus) may be the product of prolonged stressful or traumatic events during development (Read, 2001).

Prevalence of Stressful and Traumatic Events

While there is strong evidence that individuals who are prone to schizophrenia, and those already diagnosed with the disorder, are stress-sensitive, another body of research suggests that these people are likely to have suffered a higher level of stressful and traumatic life events than a nonclinical population. Although this issue has been of interest for some time, only relatively recently have large scale epidemiological studies provided relevant, high-quality data (e.g., Bebbington et al., 2004; Janssen et al., 2004; Shevlin, Dorahy, & Adamson, 2007). Findings suggest that people diagnosed with schizophrenia are more likely to have suffered a wide range of stressful life events: being bullied, being brought up in care homes, suffering a serious illness or assault, and having been sexually abused. More specifically, data from the British National Psychiatric Survey suggests that people exhibiting symptoms consistent with a diagnosis of schizophrenia were 15 times more likely than the control group to have been sexually abused.

Given these issues, it is perhaps not surprising that individuals diagnosed with schizophrenia have relatively high levels (25–40%) of comorbid posttraumatic stress disorder (PTSD; see Grubaugh et al., 2011, for a review). However, there is likely more than one potential relationship between stressful life events and schizophrenia. It may be that different forms of this relationship underlie the development of different types of psychotic presentation.

Several studies have shown that specific symptoms hallucinations and delusions are associated with increased levels of stressful life events, ranging from combat exposure to childhood sexual abuse. The relationship between specific traumatic events and specific forms of psychotic presentation remains poorly understood. One possibility is that the content of the stressful events are not relevant, and that they act as a general stressor that induces a biological reaction (HPA axis), which in turn produces a vulnerability to random anomalous experiences.

It may then be the idiosyncratic interpretation of these anomalous experiences that results in a presentation of schizophrenia (see the section below on cognitive-behavioral models).

However, a growing body of evidence suggests a more direct link between earlier life events and the content of positive symptoms. One view is that people suffer from intrusive trauma-related memories of past events in a similar manner to a presentation of PTSD, but it is the appraisal of these experiences that may lead to psychosis (Morrison, Frame, & Larkin, 2003; Steel, Fowler, & Holmes, 2005). For example, someone may experience intrusive memories of a past assault but not identify it as a memory. The person concludes that it is a premonition of a future assault sent by the Devil, which may be categorized as "thought insertion," characteristic of a delusional belief. Or someone may hear the voice of the father who abused him or her but not recognize it as a specific memory, and therefore attribute it to an external source, which may be classified as a "hallucinatory experience."

Another possible relationship specifically between hallucinations and trauma occurs not at the level of repeated memory but at the level of a match between the specific emotional experience suffered during a trauma and the emotional content of a hallucination (Hardy et al., 2005). An example would be an individual suffering intense threat during a physical attack, and the content of his or her hallucination being a threat of violence. There is also the possibility of psychotic symptoms themselves being a traumatic experience that forms the basis of intrusive memories, or "flashbacks," which continue to occur during remission of psychosis. These are likely to include moments during psychosis when the individual feared for his or her life. This type of postpsychotic PTSD (Shaw, McFarlane, Bookless, & Air, 2002) may also include intrusive memories of having been held in a psychiatric hospital against their will, or forcibly medicated, which can be experienced as very threatening.

Treatment Implications

There are clear and direct implications for treatment resulting from a history of stressful or traumatic life events. However, it is likely that the clinician will be unaware of such a history in their clients, because assessment of trauma history is rarely conducted within psychiatric services. Given this situation, clinicians should be mindful of the high prevalence of such events and (if appropriately trained) conduct such an assessment relatively early in the course of intervention. Clearly, individuals who have been abused are likely to find it particularly difficult to establish trust within a therapeutic relationship, and this should be acknowledged. There is also the possibility that clients may previously have disclosed their trauma history but not been believed, which further complicates the development of trust. More specifically, the clinician should be mindful of the setting of the clinical sessions. If this occurs within a psychiatric institution, the client may have experienced traumatic events within such an institution that contribute to heightened vigilance, triggering stressful memories and avoidance. This should be dealt with as early as possible by discussing openly whether this issue is relevant to the particular client, and how best to deal with it.

Once a thorough assessment has been conducted, the clinician needs to consider what should be the primary target for intervention. While this is best discussed collaboratively with the client, the clinician needs to decide the extent to which symptoms of PTSD are present, and how they are best treated. It may be that the client would benefit most from therapeutic work aimed specifically at PTSD or other consequences of a history of sexual abuse. Although it is beyond the scope of this chapter to discuss these treatment options at length, it is worth highlighting the debate over the use of "reliving" therapy for individuals diagnosed with schizophrenia. This type of therapy is a routine part of CBT for PTSD (Ehlers & Clark, 2000) and involves the client talking through the traumatic experience in intense detail. Many clinicians consider this form of therapy to be too emotionally intense for people with schizophrenia, and fear that it could exacerbate symptoms. There is currently no evidence to guide clinicians on this issue.

Neurotransmitters

Although "brain chemistry" has long been associated with a range of mental health problems, only relatively recently have researchers been able to associate the action of specific neurotransmitters with psychotic symptoms. In fact, the accidental discovery of the sedative effect of antihistamines within a psychotic population led to the development of the first antipsychotic drug, chlorpromazine. The dopaminergic activity that was shown to be associated with this medication led to the proposal of dopamine dysregulation underlying positive symptoms. Later studies refined the hypothesis specifically to the dopamine D_2 receptor.

Support for the dopamine hypothesis is based on the fact that all drugs shown to have antipsychotic effects have been shown to impact the dopamine system. Also, although antipsychotic drugs alleviate positive symptoms for some individuals, they also produce side effects such as muscle tremors, similar to those found in Parkinson's disease, which has been associated with low levels of dopamine. In fact, a medication widely used in the treatment of Parkinson's disease, L-dopa, acts by stimulating dopamine activity and has been associated with the onset of psychotic symptoms in some individuals. These findings suggest a continuum of dopamine activity and associated clinical symptoms. Another argument in support of the dopamine hypothesis is the fact that amphetamines are dopamine agonists, and their sustained use has been associated with both onset and exacerbation of positive symptoms (Curran, Byrappa, & McBride, 2004).

We should note, however, that no antipsychotic drugs have an impact on the dopamine system alone, and it is likely that therapeutic effects are achieved through a combined impact on a number of neurotransmitters, including serotonin. In fact, one of the newer drugs considered to be highly effective for "treatment-resistant" schizophrenia, clozapine, has a relatively low impact on the dopamine system. Another puzzling issue is the fact that although antipsychotic medication can take 4–6 weeks to have an impact on clinical symptoms, it has been shown to have an impact on dopamine activity within a matter of hours.

An interesting advance in dopamine theory directly links neurotransmitter activity with conscious experience, and provides a basis for the raw experience within a delusion of reference. Kapur (2003) states that dopamine is associated with attaching salience to a specific stimulus. Therefore, if there is excess dopamine activity, then a sense of salience will be attached to random stimuli, producing the experiences reported within delusions of reference (e.g., the numbers in the car registration seeming to contain a message specifically for the patient). However, the interaction between biological and psychological processes needs to be considered to understand why such an experience may be distressing for any individual. This perspective enables a clinician to view medication and psychological interventions as complementary rather than competitive; that is, while medication may work by "dampening" down the biological basis of unusual perceptual experiences, the psychological input focuses on how to make sense of such experiences.

Genetic Factors

While the biological abnormalities underlying a presentation of schizophrenia remain to be clarified, there is considerable evidence of a hereditary component to the disorder. Numerous studies over many decades have explored the prevalence of the disorder among the family members of an individual with a confirmed diagnosis. As with other disorders, a common research method employed when considering the role of genetics is to compare monozygotic (MZ) and dizygotic (DZ) twins. Thus, if one MZ twin has been diagnosed with schizophrenia, there is a 44% likelihood that the other will be also (Gottesman, McGuffin, & Farmer, 1987). This rate reduces to 12% for DZ twins, highlighting the potential role of genetics as a vulnerability factor in the development of schizophrenia. Offspring of one parent who has been diagnosed with schizophrenia are estimated to have a 9% likelihood of developing the disorder, almost 20 times higher than the 0.5% figure associated with the general public.

As with all research methodologies, the twin study method is open to critique. One possibility is that MZ twins share a greater similarity in environmental factors than do DZ twins. This may be due to their being treated in a more similar fashion by other people. Also, MZ twins have other biological links that are not based on genetic similarity, such as having likely shared the same placenta during birth, unlike DZ twins. Such issues are avoided through adoption studies, in which children are removed from mothers at a very early age. Although conducted some time ago, the seminal study reported by Heston (1966) is still a good example of this method. Heston followed 97 children who had been adopted, 47 of whom were from mothers diagnosed with schizophrenia, for a 36-year period. Around 17% of the group whose mothers had been diagnosed were found to exhibit symptoms, compared to none of the control group. The findings of these and other studies, when combined, show an increase in the prevalence of a diagnosis depending on how close a genetic link there is to the individual with schizophrenia (Gottesman et al., 1987).

A related discipline has been the identification of "genetic markers" through the study of characteristics associated with a diagnosis of schizophrenia. For example, there are a number of specific areas of cognitive functioning in which individuals with schizophrenia and their closely related family members have been shown to differ from the normal population. It is argued that the gene(s) responsible for poor cognitive functioning in specific tasks may also be associated with the presence of psychotic symptoms, even though these symptoms may not have been activated in the relative. Thus, if the gene associated with a specific area of cognitive functioning can be identified, then this may be considered a genetic marker. A specific example in which both diagnosed individuals and close relatives show deficits is the startle reflex (Kumari, Das, Zachariah, Ettinger, & Sharma, 2005).

Clinical Implications

The strength of evidence for a genetic component in schizophrenia suggests that a full assessment should include a family history of severe mental health problems. However, it should be remembered that even the closest of genetic links (MZ twins) suggest a concordance rate of less than 50%, and that this leaves a large percentage of variance to be determined by environmental factors. Also, despite what a patient reports as the psychiatric history of family members, the clinician cannot assume that the patient concludes that he or she suffers from a biologically based condition. Patients' beliefs regarding how and why they are suffering with current problems, and what those problems should be called, should be assessed at an early stage. While patients, of course, are entitled to have their perspective on their current problems taken seriously, the clinician should also be aware of the role of stigma in actively deterring individuals from adopting a diagnosis of schizophrenia. Therefore, during the assessment of family history, the clinician should assess not only the presence or absence of psychiatric disorder but also how that disorder would be experienced from the current patient's perspective. For example, witnessing erratic and violent behavior from a father diagnosed with schizophrenia may lead patients to assume that this is how they would behave if they also suffered from the disorder. Thus, the clinician needs to assess what the meaning of being diagnosed with schizophrenia would be for any individual.

Medication

Antipsychotic medications are known to be effective but are also associated with side effects such as drowsiness, weight gain, and extrapyramidal side effects, and these all need to be balanced when considering individual cases. In terms of groupings, antipsychotic drug comparisons have shown mixed results. Several studies have recently investigated first- and second-generation antipsychotic medications in real-life settings, with the assumption that the newer antipsychotic medications would prove to be more potent and produce fewer side effects. The trials took place in the United States (Clinical Antipsychotic Trials of Intervention Effectiveness [CATIE] schizophrenia project), in the United Kingdom (Cost Utility of the Latest Antipsychotic Drugs in Schizophrenia Study [CUtLASS]), and across Europe (European First-Episode Schizophrenia Trial [EuFEST]). No study provided unequivocal evidence, but it was clear that the second-generation antipsychotic medications were not superior and that, counter to all expectations, when asked, patients did not necessarily prefer them (Jones et al., 2006; Kahn et al., 2008; Lewis et al., 2006; Lieberman et al., 2005). The only medication that did seem to be more effective was clozapine. In the longer-term follow-up to the CATIE trial, investigations of treatment choices clearly indicated that many patients were not on one medication but on many, even though this was not recommended. Level of psychopathology is often the reason for considering treatment changes, as are indicators of metabolic functioning. But the CATIE study also highlighted an important issue—that many people (74%) discontinued their treatment over an 18-month period, with half the people discontinuing treatment before 6 months (Lewis & Liberman, 2008). It is also clear that some medications, although they may be tolerated most of the time, have high side effect burdens. For instance, in the CATIE study, olanzapine was the best-tolerated medication, but it had important side effects, such as weight gain. Other studies have also revealed that low doses of first-generation (and therefore cheaper) antipsychotic medications are no less effective than newer drugs. The convergence of these results is striking, particularly because these government-funded studies were carefully carried out, with high-quality statistical analyses. Furthermore, work by Leucht and colleagues (2009) investigated the efficacy of second- and first-generation antipsychotic medications and included 150 randomized controlled trials, with more than 21,000 participants. They showed that the group of medications known as second-generation were not homogeneous, and that only four of the nine compounds were better than first-generation drugs, and were also associated with side effects. Their suggestion is that the choice of antipsychotic medication should be based on the profile of side effects (and their acceptability to service users), the efficacy of the compound, and the cost of the drug itself to the health services.

Antipsychotic medications are not without risks to health, and some have specific, presubscription recommendations to test patients for abnormalities that might be exacerbated by some drugs. Other medications, such as clozapine, require ongoing monitoring with blood tests in order to prevent agranulocytosis. Although this monitoring is sometimes onerous at the beginning of treatment, its frequency declines over time and is usually tolerated by patients.

Clinical Implications

For all medication regimens there needs to be a therapeutic relationship between the patient and health care professional. Many patients do not adhere to the regimen prescribed, and a careful discussion of the risks and benefits, as well as an understanding by the clinician that for the patient the risk of admission may be a trade-off with the side effect burden, is crucial. Patients do not have to accept an illness model of the disorder to be adherent, and it is therefore not essential that patients show "insight." One psychological therapy that tried to improve medication adherence did show promise in the early studies but has not proved to have robust effects in more recent, bigger trials (Kemp, Hayward, Applewhaite, Everitt, & David, 1996; Gray et al., 2006).

Cognitive Functioning

For many years it has been recognized that many people diagnosed with schizophrenia have cognitive deficits, both before the onset (Cannon et al., 2002) and throughout the course of the disorder. These cognitive problems are also important variables in predicting the level of future functioning. So people with poor memory are less likely to have a job, and they have fewer friends and are more likely to live in supported accommodations and be dependent on expensive psychiatric support services. We also know that even when we provide excellent rehabilitation services cognitive problems limit the ability of people with schizophrenia to take advantage of these opportunities. In comparison to people with better memory or better attention they are less likely to be in supported work programs and less likely to have improved their social skills with a social skills program. This correlation between cognitive problems and poorer outcomes suggests that cognitive problems should be a target for intervention. Psychological theories also suggest that cognitive deficits underpin the development of the symptoms of schizophrenia (e.g., Frith, 1992; Hemsley, 1987; Goldman-Rakic, 1991; Cohen & Servan-Schreiber, 1992). Furthermore, a vulnerability stress model indicates that cognitive problems may constitute a vulnerability factor that contributes to the emergence of psychotic symptoms in the face of a stressor. While there have been mixed results from studies investigating the relationships between cognition and symptoms, there does seem to be good evidence to suggest a reasonably strong association with negative symptoms (O'Leary et al., 2000), with more inconsistent and modest associations with disorganized and especially positive symptoms (e.g., Johnson-Selfridge & Zalewski, 2001; Cuesta & Peralta, 1995).

Deficits are wide-ranging, and global intellectual functioning is generally poorer than would be expected on the basis of family and environmental factors (Aylward, Walker, & Bettes, 1984). In addition, a number of specific, additional cognitive deficits are frequently apparent, particularly in working and long-term memory, executive function, attention, processing speed, and social cognition, although cognitive profiles are rather heterogeneous. Performance in many of these cognitive domains lies more than one standard deviation below normal functioning.

Clinical Implications

Cognitive treatments for deficits in attention, memory, and planning have been developed over the last 10 years but are rarely generally available to patients. The therapy has been tested in a large number of studies, and the most recent meta-analyses show that it has had modest effects (McGurk, Twamley, Sitzer, McHugo, & Mueser, 2007; Wykes, Huddy, Cellard, McGurk, & Czobor, 2011). Cognitive rehabilitation techniques are varied and available both individually and in groups, as computerized or paper-and-pencil programs, and with a therapist present or absent. All these factors vary and the different programs developed have not really shown clear differences in their outcomes. It is likely that some programs require higher levels of functioning to be effective, and this is particularly the case for those that are free standing and require less therapist support. Therapists are provided with specific training and usually are social care workers, occupational therapists, nurses, or psychologists.

Computerized therapies have been imported from other therapeutic work (e.g., brain injury or dementia) and although they may be useful, they are not devised with this specific population of patients in mind. There are also therapies that involve educational software (e.g., NEAR program; Medalia, Revheim, & Casey, 2000). These therapies try to find educational software that purports to improve particular areas of cognitive functioning highlighted as problematic within an assessment.

Cognitive remediation therapies also differ in their targets and methods used. Some therapies specifically try to improve the skills necessary to increase cognition through practice. Other therapies include practice, as well as strategic training, on when and where to use specific information-processing skills. Others go so far as training in "metacognition," which is the ability to be aware of what one knows and when to implement this knowledge.

Most therapies involve three main techniques: errorless learning, self-monitoring, and scaffolding. The first technique, "errorless learning," is a process that provides tasks that are relatively easy to complete, allowing a very high rate of success. This can be carried out either by simplifying the tasks or by therapists providing learning supports that allow the participant to achieve 100% success using the strategies. Another strategy used in most cognitive remediation therapies is "self-monitoring," in which the participant is encouraged to follow verbal instructions that are first uttered by the therapist, repeated by the participant out loud, then repeated them covertly. This allows participants to overcome any memory problems and to consider whether they are keeping to the task instructions. "Scaffolding" describes a process whereby the individual is allowed to perform at the edge of competence, so that most tasks are performed well but do require high levels of engagement. This is essential because participants become bored if the tasks are too easy, and disengage if the tasks are too challenging.

In the version of cognitive remediation therapy used in the studies by Wykes and colleagues (2011), tasks begin at easy levels to improve participant engagement, then proceed to more difficult levels in which participants are still capable, to increase patients' chances of success. The therapist supports the use of strategies in the early stages (e.g., chunking for memory), and at later stages the participant uses them overtly, then covertly. Self-monitoring, scaffolding (supporting tasks at the edge of competence) and errorless learning are the main underpinning clinical strategies. Each session is filled with a variety of tasks so that within-session generalization can also occur for specific strategies. The therapy covers cognitive flexibility, memory, and planning tasks. Therapy is delivered to individuals at least 3 days per week, until 40 sessions are completed. Therapy is based on three general clinical principles: (1) teaching (or facilitating learning of) new, efficient information-processing strategies; (2) individualized therapy; and (3) aiding the transfer of cognitive gains into the real world through an emphasis on the use of strategies in the real-world situations.

Studies of therapies have also shown that by improving patients' cognition, it is possible to improve other functioning. For example, patients have shown improvement in social functioning and symptoms (Wykes et al., 1999, 2003, 2007). These improvements are also tangible, so that when teamed up with a rehabilitation program, there are more people working, and earning more money (McGurk, Mueser, Feldman, Wolfer, & Pascoris, 2007; Bell, Zito, Greig, & Wexler, 2008).

Cognitive-Behavioral Models

The early application of psychological models to schizophrenia was predominantly a simplistic application of learning theory that gave rise to basic behavioral interventions. However, the development of cognitive-behavioral models for affective disorders had a significant impact on psychosis research in the late 1990s. This work highlighted the extent to which the development and maintenance of a psychotic presentation could be understood with reference to psychological processes already associated with anxiety and depression. The traditional psychiatric view of schizophrenia was challenged, in that therapists were encouraged to engage directly with the content of psychotic symptoms. Two influential cognitive models of the positive symptoms of psychosis have been proposed by Garety, Kuipers, Fowler, Freeman, and Bebbington (2001) and Morrison (2001). Both models incorporate the role of negative core beliefs, hypervigilance for threat, scanning for confirmatory evidence, and safety behaviors. In essence, they concur that a psychotic presentation may evolve out of the presence of unusual experiences, with a critical factor being how these experiences are interpreted. Psychosis is associated with experiences such as being interpreted as negative, threatening, and external, and with hypervigilance and safety behaviors. For example, an individual who "hears a voice" and decides that this perceptual experience is due to a lack of sleep is likely to have a different outcome than an individual who decides that the Devil is speaking to him or her with bad intent.

While many of the treatment implications of these two models may overlap, one of the key theoretical distinctions is the extent to which the core unusual experiences are "normal" or anomalous biologically based phenomena. Whereas Garety et al. (2001) refer to the potential role of a genetic vulnerability in the propensity for some of these experiences, Morrison focuses on the extent to which these phenomena are normal and stresses that it is the interpretation of these experiences that is critical. In particular, Morrison focuses on the role of common "intrusive experiences," such as intrusive thoughts and images that may form the basis of an unusual experience for some individuals. However, both models highlight the critical role of the appraisal of the unusual experience in determining whether an individual arrives at a "psychotic" explanation. Therefore, while incorporating the generic cognitive model of anxiety and depression, these models also enable the formulation of the development of psychotic symptoms. A major strength is that these models incorporate a wide range of psychological processes associated with psychosis and have the potential to be flexible enough to enable the formulation of a heterogeneous range of psychotic presentations.

Clinical Implications

Although little is known about who is likely to benefit most from CBT for psychosis (CBTp), the intervention is highly flexible and appropriate for patients working toward a wide range of goals. The initial aim for the clinician is to engage and educate the patient about the broad framework of the cognitive-behavioral approach (i.e., collaborative, goal focused and time-limited). Given that CBT usually involves a certain amount of homework and the need to build on the contents of previous sessions, care should be taken to ascertain whether any cognitive functioning deficits interfere with this process. Should this be the case, wherever possible adaptations should be made. This is likely to include repetition of the contents of a session and making sessions shorter. As CBT interventions are short term, it is useful to include other professionals involved in the long-term care of the patient in the process, especially toward the end of treatment. This is essential if the sessions have focused on implementing some form of relapse prevention or crises plan, if required, in the future.

Once engagement has been established and the goals of any potential intervention have been discussed collaboratively, the therapist should ensure that the client has at least a basic understanding of the principles of the therapeutic approach to be adopted. The principles of CBTp are the same as those for any other form of CBT. Therefore, assessment covers how events and experiences ("unusual" or otherwise) are interpreted in a manner that results in emotional distress. The therapists goes into some detail about the various bits of "evidence" to which an individual attends when interpreting an event. As described earlier, the "events" that are assessed within a cognitive-behavioral analysis may include hearing a voice or experiencing an involuntary intrusive phenomenon. Neither event is automatically distressing, but either may become so if interpreted in a negative and threatening way. However, relevant "events" may also include seemingly benign daily occurrences, such as being looked at by a stranger, which may also be interpreted in a negative and threatening way. Such interpretations may contribute to the maintenance of a paranoid belief (e.g., "Government agents are trying to kill me").

As the assessment develops, it is important that the therapist maintain an empathic, nonjudgmental stance and not attempt to challenge beliefs at an early stage. As with other forms of CBT, the therapist needs to extend the assessment from how an individual interprets specific events to cover (1) any patterns within the interpretation of a wide range of events, (2) when this pattern of interpretation started, and (3) any significant life events associated with the onset of this pattern of interpretation. For example, a sexual assault during adolescence may be associated with the development of the core belief "I am vulnerable." Such a core-belief will be deeply engrained and determine the interpretation of a wide range of ambiguous daily events. Thus, ambiguous situations such as being looked at by a stranger, may trigger thoughts of being in danger and an associated feeling of threat and anxiety. Such thoughts and emotions may serve to develop the underlying generic core belief into a more specific paranoid belief. The role of core beliefs within psychosis has been highlighted in the research (Fowler et al., 2006).

Once a basic "formulation" has been established, the therapist hopes to maneuver the patient into understanding that while his or her own version of events is one possibility, it is not the only possibility. The cognitive formulation then acts as a basis for a collaborative exploration of how to test out which version of events has the most evidence. During this process the therapist should be aware that if the patient begins to entertain alternative beliefs, this may be associated with dilemmas (e.g., "How could I have been so stupid as to believe I was being persecuted by the government?").

It should be noted that CBTp includes various interventions that have evolved in an attempt to deal with the wide range of presentations associated with a psychotic disorder. Whereas some of the published treatment manuals describe a flexible intervention aimed at all forms of presentation (Chadwick, Birchwood, & Trower, 1996; Fowler, Garety, & Kuipers 1995; Morrison, 2002; Morrison, Renton, Dunn, Williams, & Bentall, 2003), others focus on a specific form of the disorder, such as command hallucinations (Byrne, Birchwood, Trower, & Meaden, 2006). Also, while some clinicians may focus on a formulation that includes a developmental history, as described earlier, others place more emphasis on the maintaining factors, such as looking for information that is consistent with our current beliefs and behaving in a way that prevents us from challenging them. These factors are, of course, not unique to those diagnosed with a psychotic disorder, and they serve to maintain current beliefs within all of us. However, it is norm to wait until a patient has some cognitive flexibility with regard to his or her psychotic beliefs before focusing on maintenance factors.

The Evidence Base for CBT

Although single case reports of psychological interventions for psychosis date back more than 50 years (e.g., Beck, 1952), significant developments in this area did not occur until the 1980s. Early behavioral interventions were aimed at symptom management and predominantly embedded in the traditional psychiatric view of schizophrenia. During the mid-1990s a small number of mainly U.K.-based researchers conducted the first trials in CBTp. The encouraging results led to clinical trials in other countries and to large-scale randomized controlled trials funded within the United Kingdom. The rapid growth in the number of clinical trials aimed at evaluating CBTp has led to an increasing number of meta-analyses. The most recent and comprehensive review has been able to incorporate a large-enough number of clinical trials to investigate the role of a number of variables that may be associated with outcome (Wykes, Steel, Everitt, & Tarrier, 2008). Thirty-four trials met inclusion criteria, 22 of which were individual CBTp aimed at the positive symptoms of psychosis. The overall effect sizes for CBTp were moderate and broadly similar (around 0.4) whether the analysis was based on outcome in relation to positive symptoms, negative symptoms, mood, or social functioning.

The evidence to date predominantly provides support for CBTp as an intervention for individuals suffering from "treatment-resistant" psychosis in a chronic but stable phase. However, most trials have adopted a generic approach to CBTp. Despite being aimed at the positive symptoms of psychosis, there has been little differential impact between psychotic and nonpsychotic symptoms. Consequently, relatively little is known about the effectiveness of CBTp for other phases of the disorder. Also, little is known about which elements of CBTp are the most important in producing change, and there are few markers as to who would benefit most from this intervention.

The modest overall outcomes of most CBTp trials may, in part, be a product of the choice of measure for the assessment of outcome. As discussed earlier, the most widely used assessment tool has been the PANSS (Kay et al., 1989), which is predominantly a symptom-based measure developed for use in drug trials. It has been shown to be a poor measure of the psychological distress associated with psychotic symptoms (Steel et al., 2007). Use of the PANSS contrasts the view that CBTp should be seen not as a quasi-neuroleptic (i.e., targeting symptoms) but as an intervention aimed at reducing emotional distress (Birchwood & Trower, 2006). Also, the use of a generic form of CBTp aimed at a heterogeneous population may contribute to limited effect sizes. This limitation seems all the more significant given that a large number of clinical researchers question the scientific validity of the diagnosis of schizophrenia (Bentall, 2004) upon which most trials are based. Of interest, the study which exhibited the largest effect size within the Wykes et al. (2008) review, adopted a specific protocol for a specific from of psychotic presentation (command hallucinations) and used an appropriate outcome measure (Trower et al., 2004).

Family-Based Theories

There is a long history of theories suggesting that the family may be the cause of schizophrenia. These include the double-bind theory (Bateson, Jackson, Haley, & Weakland, 1956), in which contradictory information from parents (usually mothers) produced unavoidable conflict from which the child mentally withdrew. The parent who could induce the symptoms of psychosis was embodied in the concept of the schizophrenogenic mother, characterized as cold and alienating to her children (Fromm-Reichmann, 1948). These theories lacked evidence and resulted in family members of individuals diagnosed with schizophrenia feeling blamed by psychiatry.

A more recent and useful concept is that of "expressed emotion" (EE), which refers to the emotional atmosphere of a family, and how this appears to be associated with the relapse of psychotic symptoms. Early research in this area revealed that individuals with schizophrenia were more likely to return to hospital for further treatment if they were discharged to live with members of their family than if they lived in separate lodgings (Brown et al., 1958). Later studies refined this result and showed that relapse of positive symptoms was specifically associated with family environments that were hostile, critical, or overinvolved (i.e., high EE; Kavanagh, 1992). Such families tend to have inflexible styles of coping with the problems associated with schizophrenia and a tendency to attribute the blame for the symptoms of psychosis to the patient.

Clinical Implications

The concept of EE lends itself directly to an intervention for those individuals diagnosed with schizophrenia who have families or caretakers. These family interventions are based on psychoeducation and improving communication. Psychoeducation is aimed at providing the family with basic information about the disorder (which they often have not been offered before), and using this as the basis of a family discussion. During discussions the clinicians defuse conflict and improve communication through strategies such as asking family members to talk directly to each other rather than in the third person. Individuals are then given time to comment on how they feel about statements made by other family members.

It is unclear whether high levels of EE in a family occur before a patient's relapse or as a response to an increased level of symptoms. However, interventions aimed at reducing EE have been shown to reduce rates of relapse significantly (Hogarty et al., 1986).

Social Theories

While most clinicians will work with clients in an individual or family context, it is important to be mindful of the wider social issues associated with a diagnosis of schizophrenia. The social stigma associated with such a diagnosis is deeply embedded, and a lack of mental health knowledge within the general public means that this is unlikely to change in the near future. While the public is likely to view the "schizophenic" as dangerous and unpredictable, individuals who have been diagnosed are also likely to make assumptions about themselves, or to adopt a "label" of being mentally ill (Scheff, 1974). Such self-labeling may include "I am unable to work" and "People will look down on me if they know my diagnosis."

Clinical Implications

Self-labeling can have a powerful negative impact on a patient and serve to maintain a state of depression (Birchwood, Iqbal, & Upthegrove, 2005). There are two broad forms of intervention. First, individuals diagnosed with a psychotic disorder and their families are often very ill-informed about the clinical implications of a psychotic disorder and the frequently prescribed antipsychotic medication. One basic intervention is the provision of psychoeducation, in which relevant clinical information is provided and discussed. This may help with problems, such as individuals (and their families) thinking of themselves as lazy and useless because they are lying in bed most of the day. Increased awareness of the side effects of medication, as well as a medication review, may allow for reduced self-blame in this context.

For some individuals the negative self-view adopted after a diagnosis of psychosis may be the product of an underlying vulnerability to depression; that is, they may have had low self-esteem before the onset of psychosis. This form of presentation is likely to require a longer-term intervention, such as CBT, but patients may also receive some benefit from psychoeducation.

GENERAL TREATMENT ISSUES

The content of this chapter should alert the clinician to a range of issues to consider when conducting a full assessment. It is likely that an individual diagnosed with schizophrenia will suffer a range of emotional and functional problems, and the clinician should be cautious not to assume which of these are the most significant. Although this chapter focuses on positive symptoms, any initial assessment should also cover physical health, social and occupational functioning, and suicidality. Any therapeutic intervention should begin with a collaborative development of treatment goals, so that the patient feels some ownership of the process. This process will be of particular importance for those who have experienced many years of coercion within the psychiatric system (i.e., involuntary sections and forced medication). These individuals are likely to be suspicious of any offer of help from a professional they consider to belong to that system, and extra effort must be made to create a collaborative therapeutic relationship.

Clinicians should be alert to the possibility of patients trying to get them to offer help they cannot provide. For example, this may include wanting therapists to help them get the police to arrest neighbors using a thought-stealing machine on them. Clinicians should adopt an empathic position, but they are unable to act before hearing more about the problems. Many inexperienced therapists are fearful of saying anything that may seem to collude with the contents of patients' symptoms, out of fear of reinforcing their "madness." However, the therapist who states that he or she (currently) simply does not know enough about the situation to be sure what is going on is likely to maintain the therapeutic relationship, without committing to any specific belief.

It is advised that the initial assessment be conducted in a flexible manner, and in an environment where the patient feels most comfortable. This may mean going for a walk while the patient has a cigarette, or meeting in the patient's own home. There are many areas to cover in an assessment, and it may help to let the patient start with the area he or she feels is most important. This may be current symptoms, current social problems, or earlier life events. The clinician can guide the conversation toward those issues that have been missed in later sessions. During the early sessions, the therapist should be building a model of how the patient constructs his or her position. There are many possible models the patient may endorse. These include believing that one has a genetic vulnerability to the current mental health problem, that medication does help, that stress can exacerbate symptoms, and that he or she does not believe the delusional beliefs when well. Another individual may believe his or her condition is purely stress-related and not biologically based, and that medication is useless. Still another may believe there is nothing wrong except that he or she hears voices that *sometimes* are troubling, and he or she would like some coping strategies for this. It is important to consider what clinicians and patients need to agree on, in order to help patients achieve their goals. Patients do not need to believe they are suffering from a biologically based illness called schizophrenia in order to benefit from a therapeutic intervention. Attempting to induce such "insight" is likely to cause many patients to drop out of the process. Therefore, the clinician can be flexible regarding the model of mental illness he or she shares collaboratively with the patient, in order to help the patient achieve his or her goals. During the course of therapy, new information and reconsideration of old information may cause this model to evolve.

In summary, a nonexpert, empathic, flexible approach should enable the clinician to engage with most people who have received a diagnosis of a psychotic disorder. Most clinicians should then, as part of a wider assessment, be able to picture how the patients understand their current position. This information is crucial in the development of an intervention package that may well draw on the skills of a wide range of professionals, including clinical psychologists, psychiatric nurses, social workers, occupational therapists, and psychiatrists.

REFERENCES

American Psychiatric Association. (2013). *Diagnostic and statistical manual of mental disorders* (5th ed.). Arlington, VA: Author.

Aylward, E., Walker, E., & Bettes, B. (1984). Intelligence in schizophrenia: Meta-analysis of the research. *Schizophrenia Bulletin, 10,* 430–459.

Bateson, G., Jackson, D., Haley, J., & Weakland, J. (1956). Toward a theory of schizophrenia. *Behavioral Science, 1,* 251–264.

Bebbington, P. E., Bhugra, D., Brugha, T., Farrell, M., Lewis, G., Meltzer, H. et al. (2004). Psychosis, victimisation and childhood disadvantage: Evidence from the Second British National Survey of Psychiatric Epidemiology. *British Journal of Psychiatry, 185,* 220–226.

Bebbington, P., Wilkins, S., Jones, P., Foerster, A., Murray, R., Toone, B., et al. (1993). Life events and psychosis: Initial results from the Camberwell Collaborative Psychosis Study. *British Journal of Psychiatry, 162,* 72–79.

Beck, A. T. (1952). Successful outpatient psychotherapy of a chronic schizophrenic with a delusion based on borrowed guilt. *Journal for the Study of Interpersonal Processes, 15,* 305–312.

Bell, M. D., Zito, W., Greig, T., & Wexler, B. E. (2008). Neurocognitive enhancement therapy with vocational services: Work outcomes at two-year follow-up. *Schizophrenia Research, 105,* 18–29.

Bentaleb, L., Beauregard, M., Liddle, P., & Stip, E. (2002). Cerebral activity associated with auditory verbal hallucinations: A functional magnetic resonance imaging case study. *Journal of Psychiatry and Neuroscience, 27,* 100–115.

Bentall, R. P. (2004). *Madness explained: Psychosis and human nature.* New York: Penguin.

Bentall, R. P., Corcoran, R., Howard, R., Blackwood, N., & Kinderman, P. (2001). Persecutory delusions: A review and theoretical integration. *Clinical Psychology Review, 21,* 1143–1192.

Birchwood, M., Iqbal, Z., & Upthegrove, R. (2005). Psychological pathways to depression in schizophrenia: Studies in acute psychosis, post psychotic depression and auditory hallucinations. *European Archives of Psychiatry and Clinical Neuroscience, 255,* 202–212.

Birchwood, M., & Trower, P. (2006). The future of cognitive-behavioural therapy for psychosis: Not a quasi-neuroleptic. *British Journal of Psychiatry, 188,* 107–108.

Bleuler, E. (1908). Die Prognose der Dementia praecox (Schizophreniegruppe). *Allgemeine Zeitschrift fur Psychiatrie, 65,* 436.

Brebion, G., Amador, X., David, A., Malospina, D., Sharit, Z., & Gorman, J. (2000). Positive symptomatology and source monitoring failure in schizophrenia: An analysis of symptom specific effects. *Psychiatry Research, 95,* 119–131.

Brown, G., Carstairs, G., & Topping, G. (1958). Post-hospital adjustment of chronic mental patients. *Lancet, 2,* 685–668.

Byrne, S., Birchwood, M., Trower, P. E., & Meaden, A. (2006). *A casebook of cognitive behavioural therapy for command hallucinations.* Hove, UK: Routledge.

Cannon, M., Caspi, A., Moffitt, T. E., Harrington, M. L., Taylor, A., Murray, R., et al. (2002). Evidence for early-childhood, pan-developmental impairment specific to schizophreniform disorder: Results from a longitudinal birth cohort. *Archives of General Psychiatry, 59,* 449–456.

Chadwick, P., Birchwood, M. J., & Trower, P. (1996). *Cognitive therapy for delusions, voices and paranoia.* Chichester, UK: Wiley.

Cohen, J. D., & Servan-Schreiber, D. (1992). Context, cortex, and dopamine—a connectionist approach to behavior and biology in schizophrenia. *Psychological Review, 99,* 45–77.

Cuesta, M. J., & Peralta, V. (1995). Cognitive disorders in the positive, negative, and disorganization syndromes of schizophrenia. *Psychiatric Research, 58,* 227–235.

Curran, C., Byrappa, N., & McBride, A. (2004). Stimulant psychosis: Systematic review. *British Journal of Psychiatry, 185,* 196–204.

Ehlers, A., & Clark, D. M. (2000). A cognitive model of posttraumatic stress disorder. *Behaviour Research and Therapy, 38,* 319–345.

Fowler, D., Freeman, D., Smith, B., Kuipers, E., Bebbington, P., Bashforth, H., et al. (2006). The Brief Core Schema Scales (BCSS): Psychometric properties and associations with paranoia and grandiosity in non-clinical and psychosis samples. *Psychological Medicine, 36,* 749–759.

Fowler, D., Garety, P., & Kuipers, E. (1995). *Cognitive behaviour therapy for psychosis: Theory and practice.* Chichester, UK: Wiley.

Freeman, D., Garety, P. A., Bebbington, P. E., Smith, B., Rollinson, R., Fowler, D., et al. (2005). Psychological investigation of the structure of paranoia in a non-clinical population. *British Journal of Psychiatry, 186* 427–435.

Frith, C. (1992). *The cognitive neuropsychology of schizophrenia.* Hove, UK: Erlbaum.

Fromm-Reichmann, F. (1948). Notes on the development of treatment of schizophrenics by psychoanalytic therapy. *Journal for the Study of Interpersonal Processes, 11,* 263–273.

Garety, P. A., Kuipers, E., Fowler, D., Freeman, D., & Bebbington, P. E., (2001). A cognitive model of the positive symptoms of psychosis. *Psychological Medicine, 31,* 189–195.

Goldman-Rakic, P. S. (1991). Prefrontal cortical dysfunction in schizophrenia: The relevance of working memory. In B. J. Carroll & J. E. Barrett (Eds.), *Psychopathology and the brain.* New York: Raven Press.

Gottesman, I. I., McGuffin, P., & Farmer, A. (1987). Clinical genetics as clues to the "real" genetics of schizophrenia (a decade of modest gains while playing for time). *Schizophrenia Bulletin, 13,* 23–47.

Gray, R., Leese, M., Bindman, J., Becker, T., Burti, L., David, A., et al. (2006) Adherence therapy for people with schizophrenia—European multicentre randomised controlled trial. *British Journal of Psychiatry, 189,* 508–514.

Grubaugh, A. L., Zinzow, H. M., Paul, L., Egede, L. E., & Frueh, B. C. (2011). Trauma exposure and posttraumatic stress disorder in adults with severe mental illness: A critical review. *Clinical Psychology Review, 31,* 883–899.

Haddock, G., McCarron, J., Tarrier, N., & Faragher, E. (1999). Scales to measure dimensions of hallucinations and delusions: The Psychotic Symptom Rating Scales (PSYRATS). *Psychological Medicine, 29,* 879–889.

Hardy, A., Fowler, D., Freeman, D., Smith, B., Steel, C., Kuipers, E., et al. (2005). Trauma and hallucinatory experience in psychosis. *Journal of Nervous and Mental Disease, 193,* 501– 507.

Harrow, M., Rattenbury, F., & Stoll, F. (1988). Schizophrenic delusions: An analysis of their persistence, of related premorbid ideas, and of three major dimensions. In T. E. Oltmanns & B. A. Maher (Eds.), *Delusional beliefs.* New York: Wiley.

Hemsley, D. (1987). An experimental psychological model for schizophrenia. In H. Hafner, W. Gattaz, & K. Jansair (Eds.), *Search for the causes of schizophrenia.* Berlin: Springer-Verlag.

Hemsley, D. R. (1994). Cognitive disturbance as the link between schizophrenic symptoms and their biological bases. *Neurology, Psychiatry and Brain Research, 2,* 163–170.

Heston, J. J. (1966). Psychiatric disorders in foster home reared children of schizophrenic mothers. *British Journal of Psychiatry, 112,* 819–825.

Hogarty, G., Anderson, C., Reiss, D., Kornblith, S., Greenwald, D., Jauna, C., et al. (1986). Family psychoeducation, social skills training, and maintenance chemotherapy in the aftercare treatment of schizophrenia: I. One-year effects of a controlled study on relapse and expressed emotion. *Archives of General Psychiatry, 43,* 633–642.

Janssen, I., Krabbendam, L., Bak, M., Hanssen, M., Vollebergh, W., de Graaf, R., et al. (2004).

Childhood abuse as a risk factor for psychotic experiences. *Acta Psychiatrica Scandinavica, 109,* 38–45.

Jaspers, K. (1913). *Allgemeine Psychopathologie. Ein Leitfaden für Studierende, Ärzte und Psychologen.* . Berlin: Springer.

Johns, L., Cannon, M., Singleton, N., Murray, R., Farrell, M., Brugha, T., et al. (2004). Prevalence and correlates of self-reported psychotic symptoms in the British population. *British Journal of Psychiatry, 185,* 298–305.

Johnson-Selfridge, M., & Zalewski, C. (2001). Moderator variables of executive functioning in schizophrenia: Meta-analytic findings. *Schizophrenia Bulletin, 27,* 306–316.

Jones, P. B., Barnes, T. R., Davies, L., Dunn, G., Lloyd, H., Hayhurst, K. P., et al. (2006). Randomized controlled trial of the effect on quality of life of second- vs first-generation antipsychotic drugs in schizophrenia: Cost Utility of the latest antipsychotic drugs in Schizophrenia Study (CUtLASS 1). *Archives of General Psychiatry, 63,* 1079–1087.

Kahn, R. S., Fleischhacker, W. W., Boter, H., Davidson, M., Vergouwe, Y., Keet, I. P., et al. (2008). Effectiveness of antipsychotic drugs in first-episode schizophrenia and schizophreniform disorder: An open randomised clinical trial, *Lancet, 371,* 1085–1097.

Kapur, S. (2003). Psychosis as a state of aberrant salience: A framework linking biology, phenomenology, and pharmacology in schizophrenia. *American Journal of Psychiatry, 160,* 13–23.

Kavanagh, D. J. (1992). Recent developments in expressed emotion and schizophrenia. *British Journal of Psychiatry, 160,* 601–620.

Kay, S. R., Opler, L. A., & Lindenmayer, J. P. (1989). The Positive and Negative Syndrome Scale (PANSS): Rationale and standardisation. *British Journal of Psychiatry, 155,* 59–65.

Kemp, R., Hayward, P., Applewhaite, G., Everitt, B., & David, A. (1996). Compliance therapy in psychotic patients: Randomised controlled trial. *British Medical Journal, 312,* 345–349.

Kumari, V., Das, M., Zachariah, E., Ettinger, U., & Sharma, T. (2005). Reduced prepulse inhibition in unaffected siblings of schizophrenia patients. *Psychophysiology, 42,* 588–594.

Leucht, S., Corves, C., Arbter, D., Engel, R. R., Li, C., & Davis, J. M. (2009). Second-generation versus first-generation antipsychotic drugs for schizophrenia: A meta-analysis. *Lancet, 373,* 31–41.

Lewis, S., Barnes, T. R., Davies, L., Murray, R. M., Dunn, G., Hayhurst, K. P., et al. (2006). Randomized controlled trial of effect of prescription of clozapine versus other second-generation antipsychotic drugs in resistant schizophrenia. *Schizophrenia Bulletin, 32,* 715–723.

Lewis, S., & Lieberman, J. (2008). CATIE and CUtLASS: Can we handle the truth? *British Journal of Psychiatry, 192,* 161–163.

Lieberman, J. A., Stroup, T. S., McEvoy, J. P., Swartz, M. S., Rosenheck, R. A., Perkins, D. O., et al. (2005). Effectiveness of antipsychotic drugs in patients with chronic schizophrenia. *New England Journal of Medicine, 353,* 1209–1223.

Maher, B. (2001). Delusions. In P. B. Sutker & H. E. Adams (Eds.), *Comprehensive handbook of psychopathology* (3rd ed.). New York: Kluwer Academic/Plenum.

McGurk, S. R., Mueser, K. T., Feldman, K., Wolfe, R., & Pascoris, A. (2007). Cognitive training for supported employment: 2–3 year outcomes of a randomized controlled trial. *American Journal of Psychiatry, 164,* 437–441.

McGurk, S. R., Twamley, E. W., Sitzer, D. I., McHugo, G. J., & Mueser, K. T. (2007). A meta-analysis of cognitive remediation in schizophrenia. *American Journal of Psychiatry, 164,* 1791–1802.

Medalia, A., Revheim, N., & Casey, M. (2000). Remediation of memory disorders in schizophrenia. *Psychological Medicine, 30,* 1451–1459.

Morrison, A. P. (2001). The interpretation of intrusions in psychosis: An integrative cognitive approach to psychotic symptoms. *Behavioural and Cognitive Psychotherapy, 29,* 257–276.

Morrison, A. P. (Ed.). (2002). *A casebook of cognitive therapy for psychosis.* Hove, UK: Routledge.

Morrison, A. P., Frame, L., & Larkin, W. (2003). Relationships between trauma and psychosis: A review and integration. *British Journal of Clinical Psychology, 42*, 331–353.

Morrison, A. P., Renton, J. C., Dunn, H., Williams, S., & Bentall, R. P. (2003). *Cognitive therapy for psychosis: A formulation based approach.* Hove, UK: Routledge.

O'Leary, D. S., Flaum, M., Kesler, M. L., Flashman, L. A., Arndt, S., & Andreasen, N. C. (2000). Cognitive correlates of the negative, disorganized, and psychotic symptom dimensions of schizophrenia. *Journal of Neuropsychiatry and Clinical Neurosciences, 12*, 4–15.

Peters, E., Day, S., McKenna, J., & Orbach, G. (1999). Delusional ideation in religious and psychotic populations. *British Journal of Clinical Psychology, 38*, 83–96.

Read, J., Perry, B. D., Moskowitz, A., & Connoly, J. (2001). The contribution of early traumatic events to schizophrenia in some patients: A traumagenic neurodevelopmental model. *Psychiatry, 64*, 319–345.

Romme, M., & Escher, S. (1989). Hearing voices. *Schizophrenia Bulletin, 15*, 209–216.

Scheff, T. J. (1974). The labeling theory of mental illness. *American Sociological Review, 39*, 444–452.

Shaw, K., McFarlane, A., Bookless, C., & Air, T. (2002). The aetiology of postpsychotic posttraumatic stress disorder following a psychotic episode. *Journal of Traumatic Stress, 15*, 39–47.

Shevlin, M. Dorahy, M. J., & Adamson, G. (2007). Trauma and psychosis: An analysis of the National Comorbidity Survey. *American Journal of Psychiatry, 164*, 166–169.

Steel, C., Fowler, D., & Holmes, E. A. (2005). Trauma-related intrusions and psychosis: An information processing account. *Behavioural and Cognitive Psychotherapy, 33*, 139–152.

Steel, C., Garety, P., Freeman, D., Craig, E., Fowler, D., Bebbington, P., et al. (2007). The multidimensional measurement of the positive symptoms of psychosis. *International Journal of Methods in Psychiatric Research, 16*, 88–96.

Trower, P., Birchwood, M., Meaden, A., Byrne, S., Nelson, A., & Ross K. (2004). Cognitive therapy for command hallucinations: Randomised controlled trial. *British Journal of Psychiatry, 184*, 312–320.

Van Os, J., Linscott, R. J., Myin-Germeys, I., Delespaul, P., & Krabbendam, L. (2009). A systematic review and meta-analysis of the psychosis continuum: Evidence for a psychosis proneness–persistence–impairment model of psychotic disorder. *Psychological Medicine, 39*, 179–195.

Walker, E., & Diforio, D. (1997). Schizophrenia: A neural diathesis–stress model. *Psychological Review, 104*, 667–685.

Wykes, T., Huddy, H., Cellard, C., McGurk, S., & Czobor, P. (2011). A meta-analysis of cognitive remediation for schizophrenia: Methodology and effect sizes. *American Journal of Psychiatry, 168*, 472–485.

Wykes, T., Reeder, C., Corner, J., Williams, C., & Everitt, B. (1999). The effects of neurocognitive remediation on executive processing in patients with schizophrenia. *Schizophrenia Bulletin, 25*, 291–307.

Wykes, T., Reeder, C., Landau, S., Everitt, B., Knapp, M., Patel, A., & Romeo, R. (2007). Cognitive remediation therapy in schizophrenia: Randomised controlled trial. *British Journal of Psychiatry, 190*, 421–427.

Wykes, T., Reeder, C., Williams, C., Corner, J., Rice, C., & Everitt, B. (2003). Are the effects of cognitive remediation therapy (CRT) durable?: Results from an exploratory trial in schizophrenia. *Schizophrenia Research, 61*, 163–174.

Wykes, T., Steel, C., Everitt, B., & Tarrier, N. (2008). Cognitive behaviour therapy for schizophrenia: Effect sizes, clinical models and methodological rigor. *Schizophrenia Bulletin, 34*(3), 523–537.

Zubin, J., & Spring, B. (1977). Vulnerability: A new view on schizophrenia. *Journal of Abnormal Psychology, 86*, 103–126.

CHAPTER 12

The Negative Symptoms of Schizophrenia

Ann M. Kring
David A. Smith

By any standard schizophrenia is among the most severe of the formally recognized psychological disorders. The symptoms of schizophrenia influence everything that makes us human: the way we think, the way we feel, and the way we behave. In Chapter 11, Steel and Wykes considered the positive symptoms of schizophrenia that manifest in thinking and behaving. In this chapter, we consider the negative symptoms of schizophrenia that manifest in feeling and behaving. "Negative symptoms" are labeled as such because they involve absences of or deficits in something that is typically present in healthy people. For example, the symptom blunted affect is an absence of emotion expression. Most of the negative symptoms involve difficulties in emotion (e.g., lack of outward expression, diminished motivation), though they also involve difficulties in social relationships, goal-directed behavior, and communication.

In this chapter, we describe the current and future schizophrenia diagnostic criteria. We then review recent data on the epidemiology of schizophrenia, including the number and the types of people affected (i.e., their gender, ethnicity, socioeconomic status), and recent data on schizophrenia's typical course, comorbidities, and prognosis. Positive symptoms of schizophrenia, including delusions and hallucinations, are reviewed in Chapter 11, which also covers etiology and issues associated with intervention. Building on this foundational material, the bulk of this chapter is devoted to descriptions of schizophrenia's negative symptoms and the ways in which translational research has illuminated the nature of these symptoms. It will become clear that research translating the theory, methods, and measures from affective science, cognitive neuroscience, and behavioral neuroscience has enabled us more precisely than ever before to pinpoint the nature of the negative symptoms. This increased explanatory precision has in turn informed the next generation of negative symptom assessment measures and psychosocial treatments for schizophrenia. In addition to covering these assessment tools and interventions, the chapter derives clinical implications from psychopathology research and general principles of change from effective and promising treatments.

TYPICAL SYMPTOMS AND CLASSIFICATION

To meet the diagnosis for schizophrenia in DSM-5 (American Psychiatric Association, 2013), a person must demonstrate at least two symptoms from five symptom domains (hallucinations, delusions, disorganized speech, disorganized behavior or catatonia, and negative symptoms) for at least 1 month. In addition, these symptoms must persist either in their "active phase" or in attenuated form for 6 months. Though DSM-IV contained several subtypes of schizophrenia (disorganized, catatonic, paranoid, undifferentiated, residual), these were removed from DSM-5, because of their limited reliability and validity.

An empirical alternative to the DSM consensus-driven approach to characterizing the symptoms of schizophrenia is to factor-analyze symptom ratings. Fortunately, there is some convergence between the two approaches, especially with respect to DSM-5. Although the findings are not entirely consistent, the bulk of factor-analytic studies demonstrate three underlying factors schizophrenia symptoms (for review see Blanchard & Cohen, 2006; Peralta & Cuesta, 2001): positive (hallucinations, delusions), disorganization (disorganized speech and behavior), and negative. Of course, factor-analytic studies are constrained by the representativeness and psychometric properties of the items entered into the analysis (Smith, 1998) and, unfortunately, many existing schizophrenia symptom rating scales have conceptual and psychometric limitations that undermine confidence in factor-analysis findings (Smith, Mar, & Turoff, 1998).

EPIDEMIOLOGY

The lifetime prevalence of schizophrenia is nearly 1%, and it affects men slightly more often than women (Kirkbride et al., 2006; Walker, Kestler, Bollini, & Hochman, 2004). Schizophrenia is more prevalent in developed than in developing nations (Saha, Chant, Welham, & McGrath, 2005), but the incidence (i.e., number of new cases in a particular time period) does not vary according to the economic status of the country (Saha, Welham, Chant, & McGrath, 2006), suggesting that factors other than socioeconomics may account for the prevalence differences across countries. In the United States, schizophrenia is diagnosed more frequently among some racial groups, such as African Americans, than among others, though it remains unclear whether this reflects an actual difference among groups or diagnostic bias among clinicians (Kirkbride et al., 2006; US Department of Health and Human Services, 2001).

COURSE, ASSOCIATED CLINICAL FEATURES, AND COMORBIDITY

The typical age of schizophrenia onset is between 18 and 25, usually somewhat earlier in men than in women. Some evidence suggests that an earlier age of onset is associated with more negative symptoms and a poorer prognosis (Tandon, Nasrallah, & Keshavan, 2009). Perhaps related to their later age of onset, women with schizophrenia tend to have an overall better prognosis than men, including better functioning prior to the onset of the first episode, fewer hospitalizations, fewer negative symptoms, better response to treatment, and better social and occupational functioning (Salem & Kring, 1998). People with schizophrenia typically have a number of more severe acute episodes with less severe but still debilitating symptoms, including negative symptoms, between these episodes. Some estimates suggest that about 1 in 5 people with schizophrenia have an optimal course of illness, meaning that they are able to live independently, hold a job, and have meaningful relationships. Most people with this disorder, however, have multiple episodes and more serious deficits in social and occupational functioning (Cancro, 1989).

Comorbid substance abuse occurs in as many as 50% of people with schizophrenia, complicating treatment efforts (Blanchard, Brown, Horan, & Sherwood, 2000). Anxiety disorders, including panic disorder, obsessive–compulsive disorder, and social anxiety are also commonly comorbid with schizophrenia (Braga, Petrides, & Fifueira, 2004). Depression is also common in people with schizophrenia, though it can be difficult to distinguish between clinical depression and side effects of medications commonly used to treat schizophrenia (Tandon et al., 2009). Perhaps related to the high comorbidity with depression, people with schizophrenia are more likely than people in the general population to die from suicide (Palmer, Pankratz, & Bostwick, 2005), Sadly, for reasons that are not fully understood, people with schizophrenia are also more likely to die from any cause (Saha, Chant, & McGrath, 2007). Results from a meta-analysis of over 300 people with schizophrenia found that sleep difficulties, including sleep inefficiency, decreased total sleep time, and increased sleep latency, are also common, even among people not being treated with antipsychotic medications (Chouinard, Poulin, Stip, & Godbout, 2004).

Clinical Implications

Given the key gender differences in schizophrenia, consideration of gender is important for both assessment and treatment. In addition, it is important to do a thorough diagnostic assessment to identify any comorbid conditions that also require clinical intervention. Of particular importance is consideration of suicide risk among people with schizophrenia.

Diagnostically, there are some important clinical considerations as well. DSM requires the presence of at least two symptoms from its set of five domains. Because only one of the DSM domains includes negative symptoms, a person evidencing negative symptoms without positive symptoms would not qualify for a diagnosis of schizophrenia. Conversely, a patient with positive symptoms (say, delusions and hallucinations) without negative symptoms, *could* be diagnosable with schizophrenia. Because, establishing the 6-month duration of illness criterion can also be a challenge clinically, especially with people who characteristically lack insight into their difficulties, outside consultations with family members and others might be especially valuable when schizophrenia is suspected. The negative symptoms themselves, because they are evidenced by the *absence* of ordinary functions, such as emotional expressivity, can pose unique diagnostic challenges, making refined assessment instruments and thorough training in this area very important. Finally, as suggested by Steel and Wykes in Chapter 11, people with schizophrenia may not appear to be experiencing strong subjective distress, so the DSM psychosocial impairment diagnostic criterion takes on added importance.

NEGATIVE SYMPTOMS: CLINICAL DESCRIPTIONS AND SIGNIFICANCE

A 2006 National Institute of Mental Health (NIMH) consensus statement on negative symptoms posited five negative symptoms: asociality, avolition, anhedonia, blunted affect, and alogia (Kirkpatrick, Fenton, Carpenter, & Marder, 2006). What follows are descriptions of each of these symptoms based on the work of the Collaboration to Advance Negative Symptom Assessment in Schizophrenia (CANSAS; Blanchard, Kring, Horan, & Gur, 2010). The CANSAS group has developed the next generation of negative symptom assessment measures, the Clinical Assessment Interview for Negative Symptoms (CAINS, 2011; Horan, Kring, Gur, Reise, & Blanchard, 2011; Kring, Gur, Blanchard, Horan, & Reise, 2013), following the recommendations of the NIMH consensus statement.

Asociality

"Asociality" involves decreased interest in forming close relationships with others and/or reduced social activity. People with this symptom may not desire close relationships with family, friends, or romantic partners. Instead, they may wish to spend much of their time alone. When around others, people with this symptom may interact only superficially and briefly, and appear aloof or indifferent to these social interactions. People with asociality may believe that close, intimate relationships are not important or valuable, and they may not have any desire to establish close relationships with family, friends, or romantic partners. People with asociality may report frequently being alone, yet they do not report feeling lonely. Asociality is distinct from social skills deficits or conditions that limit the opportunity to interact with other people (e.g., living far away from friends or family members).

Avolition

"Avolition" refers to diminished motivation and difficulty in initiating and persisting in what are usually routine activities, such as work or school, hobbies, or social activities. For example, a person with avolition may not be motivated to seek out work or to keep up with household chores or hobbies, and may instead spend much of the time at home doing nothing. Like asociality, avolition involves both an experience component (i.e., motivation) and a behavioral component (i.e., goal-directed behavior). Therefore, failure to be working is not an indicator of avolition in a non-working person who is otherwise motivated to work.

Anhedonia

"Anhedonia" involves a reduction in the experience of pleasure. People with anhedonia may report diminished pleasure in different domains, such as social activities, physical activities (e.g., food, sex, exercise), work or school, hobbies, and so forth. Anhedonia is the most commonly occurring negative symptom, with as many as three-fourths of people with schizophrenia having this symptom (Fenton & McGlashan, 1991).

As we discuss in more detail below, recent research suggests that it is important to distinguish consummatory or "in-the-moment" pleasure from anticipatory pleasure (Kring & Caponigro, 2010). People with schizophrenia appear to have a deficit in anticipatory but not consummatory pleasure; that is, when people with schizophrenia are asked about expected future situations or activities that are pleasurable to most people (e.g., good food, recreational activities, social interactions), they report that they anticipate less pleasure from these sorts of activities than people without schizophrenia (Gard, Kring, Germans, Gard, Horan, & Green, 2007). However, when presented with actual pleasant activities, such as amusing films or tasty beverages, people with schizophrenia report experiencing as much pleasure as do people without schizophrenia (Kring & Moran, 2008).

Blunted Affect

"Blunted affect" (also called "flat" or "restricted affect") refers to a lack of outward expression of emotion. A person with this symptom may stare vacantly, the muscles of the face motionless, the eyes lifeless. When spoken to, the person may answer in a flat and toneless voice and not look at his or her conversational partner. Of people with schizophrenia, two-thirds or more exhibit flat affect (Fenton & McGlashan,

1991; Sartorious, Shapiro, & Jablonsky, 1974). Importantly, this symptom refers only to the outward expression of emotion and not to reported experience of emotion, which is not impoverished at all (Kring & Moran, 2008).

Alogia

"Alogia" refers to a significant reduction in the amount of speech. Simply put, people with this symptom do not talk much. People with alogia answer questions with one or two words and elaborate on their answers with only the minimum of additional detail. About half of people with schizophrenia exhibit alogia (Fenton & McGlashan, 1991).

Structure of Negative Symptoms

As described earlier, negative symptoms emerge as a distinct factor in factor-analytic studies of schizophrenia symptoms. Moreover, this negative symptom factor is not strongly correlated with the other factors that emerge (positive, disorganization). Studies that have focused on the structure of the negative symptoms themselves typically report two distinct negative symptom factors (Blanchard & Cohen, 2006; Horan et al., 2011; Messinger et al., 2011). The first factor is *expression*, and includes blunted affect and alogia; the second factor, *experience*, includes avolition, asociality, and anhedonia.

Clinical Significance of the Negative Symptoms

The negative symptoms tend to endure beyond acute episodes and have profound effects on the lives of people with schizophrenia, as well as their family members. Cross-sectional and longitudinal studies have shown that the presence of many negative symptoms is a strong predictor of a poor clinical outcome (Fenton & McGlashan, 1991; Ho, Nopoulos, Flaum, Arndt, & Andreasen, 1998; Milev, Ho, Arndt, & Andreasen, 2005). Negative symptoms are also prognostic of functional outcomes, including poor occupational attainment, financial dependence, and impaired social adjustment (Siegel et al., 2006). Negative symptoms can also have a major impact on family members. They are a significant source of caregiver burden (Dyck, Short, & Vitaliano, 1999; Perlick et al., 2006; Provencher & Mueser, 1997) and may also contribute to family conflict, which in its own right is related to poor prognostic outcomes for patients (e.g., Hooley, 2007; Weisman, Nuechterlein, Goldstein, & Snyder, 2000).

ASSESSING NEGATIVE SYMPTOMS IN SCHIZOPHRENIA

There are many methods for assessing negative symptoms in schizophrenia. We briefly review two methods here: clinical interviews and self-report measures. We discuss laboratory methods for assessing negative symptoms later in a section on translational research.

Clinical Interviews

Perhaps the most typical way to assess negative symptoms is the clinical interview and rating scale. Clinical interviews are designed to aid diagnosis by assessing the severity of specific symptoms. They typically focus on symptoms over a particular time interval (e.g., the last week, last month, last year), and symptom severity is indicated on a rating scale that corresponds to the interview. Some measures, such as the Brief Psychiatric Rating Scale (BPRS; Lukoff, Nuechterlein, & Ventura, 1986; Overall & Gorham, 1962), assess general psychiatric symptoms, including those observed in schizophrenia, anxiety, and mood disorders. The negative symptoms comprise only a small part of these measures.

Two clinical rating scales designed specifically to assess negative symptoms in schizophrenia are the Scale for the Assessment of Negative Symptoms (SANS; Andreasen, 1982) and the Positive and Negative Syndrome Scale (PANSS; Kay, Fiszbein, & Opler, 1987). Though widely used, these measures have a number of problems, such as inclusion of processes that are not actually negative symptoms (e.g., inattention) and assessment of behavioral referents for symptoms that are essentially experiential deficits (e.g., lack of pleasure, lack of interest, lack of motivation).

This tradition of privileging interviewer observations over patient reports may reflect the dogma that people with schizophrenia have limited insight or awareness of their illness and cannot reliably report on their own experiences (e.g., Amador et al., 1994; Selten, Gernaat, Nolen, Wiersma, & van den Bosch, 1998). For example, to explain the mismatch between psychiatrists' and patients' reports of flat affect and anhedonia, the authors of one study considered the patient reports to be "less realistic" (Selten et al., 1998, p. 353). Reconciling two discrepant reports is never an easy task, but such discrepancies may reflect something other than lack of insight or limited self-awareness on the part of the person with schizophrenia. For example, asking people with schizophrenia whether they generally experience pleasure (or even to describe what kinds of things they find pleasurable) might elicit a different response than asking whether they derive pleasure from consuming a favorite meal; that is, the context in which questions about emotional experiences are asked can lead to different responses. As a result, people with schizophrenia may look different as not so much the result of their different experiences as the result of their different responses to the context in which these experiences are assessed. Moreover, and in some ways more importantly, the tendency to interpret mismatches between patient and other reports as patient error conveys the message that patient subjective reports are not meaningful. Yet subjective reports are the cornerstone of current conceptualizations of negative symptoms (Blanchard et al., 2011).

In response to these complexities, next-generation negative symptom clinical interview rating scales include assessments of both observable behavior and reported experience of emotion, motivation, and desire for close relationships. The CAINS (Horan et al., 2011; Kring et al., 2013) includes items for each of the five negative symptoms, and the interviewer is instructed to consider multiple perspectives (experience, behavior) and to resolve inconsistencies by using follow-up questions.

Although clinical interviews and rating scales effectively assess negative symptoms, they do not necessarily capture emotion, motivation, and close relationships. First, the behavioral sample upon which these interviews are based may not be representative, because the ratings are typically made at a single time point, such as during hospitalization, that may not be representative. Second, the format of these interviews, which demand a certain degree of clinical skill, may systematically fail to elicit appropriate emotional material, and may not provide an opportunity for people to express or experience a wide range of emotions. Finally, most uses of the rating scales require tabulation of a total score rather than specific subscale scores. Knowing the total score is informative with respect to overall symptomatology, but it does not provide any specific information about emotional, motivational, or relationship symptoms. Thus, self-report and laboratory measures can be a useful means for augmenting clinical interviews when assessing negative symptoms.

Self-Report Measures

Although there is currently only one self-report measure of negative symptoms (Park, Llerna, McCarthy, Couture, Bennett, & Blanchard, 2012), the myriad self-report measures assessing emotion expression, pleasure, motivation, and relationships may capture a person's perspective on domains affected by negative symptoms. In fact, self-report measures may have an advantage over clinical interview rating scales in such cases, because they are not affected by social skills deficits or other interpersonal factors that may influence the process of gathering information from patients within the context of a clinical interview (Dworkin, 1992).

Somewhat surprisingly, self-report measures have not often been used in the study of schizophrenia. This may be due to a general misperception that people with schizophrenia cannot reliably and accurately complete such measures. However, research employing a variety of paradigms documents the ability of people with schizophrenia to provide reliable and valid reports of anhedonia, emotion expression, motivation, and other constructs related to negative symptoms (e.g., Barch, Yodkovik, Sypher-Locke, & Hanewinkel, 2008; Horan, Green, Kring, & Nuechterlein, 2006; Horan, Kring, & Blanchard, 2006).

That people with schizophrenia produce valid self-reports of emotion is less remarkable when we understand that they do not approach such measures with different underlying conceptualizations or knowledge structures of the constructs. For example, a study using multidimensional scaling techniques demonstrated that people with schizophrenia use the same two-dimensional structure (valence and arousal) as people without schizophrenia when completing emotion ratings (Kring, Barrett, & Gard, 2003). Self-report measures are also related to other measures, such as physiology and behavior (Kring & Moran, 2008). In short, there is considerable evidence that people with schizophrenia self-report their emotion and other internal states and motivations related to negative symptoms in reliable and valid fashion.

Insofar as specific negative symptom processes are concerned, an illustrative study by Barch and colleagues (2008) examined self-reports of motivation using the Motivational Trait Questionnaire, a 42-item measure that assesses intrinsic motivation related to personal mastery, competition, and anxiety (Kanfer & Ackerman, 2000). People with schizophrenia differed from healthy controls only on the subscale capturing motivation related to anxiety, suggesting that people with schizophrenia might exhibit less motivation for situations in which they worry about falling short or failing. Notably, there has been little research on motivation and schizophrenia using any type of measure (Barch et al., 2008). In the past few years, however, laboratory measures of motivation have been usefully deployed for the study of schizophrenia, a point to which we turn in the next section.

Perhaps the most widely used negative symptom self-report measures are of anhedonia. In particular, two measures developed in the 1970s by Loren and Jean Chapman at the University of Wisconsin, the Physical Anhedonia Scale (Chapman & Chapman, 1978) and the Social Anhedonia Scale (Eckblad, Chapman, Chapman, & Mishlove, 1982), have been used in many, many studies (the article describing initial versions of these scales [Chapman, Chapman, & Raulin, 1976] has been cited nearly 600 times). These studies indicate that people with schizophrenia (1) score higher than healthy controls and (2) score higher than people with bipolar disorder, but (3) they do not differ from people with depression. However, whereas scores on these scales wax and wane with depression episodes, they remain elevated among people with schizophrenia, suggesting a more trait-like anhedonic disturbance. Indeed, scores on these scales show stability across not only time but also treatment status (Horan, Kring, & Blanchard, 2006). While the Chapman scales are useful self-report measures of anhedonia that have been widely used in schizophrenia research, their content is somewhat outdated, and more recent research suggests that it is important to consider distinct components of anhedonia that are not necessarily reflected on these scales (Kring & Caponigro, 2010).

A more contemporary anhedonia measure, which takes into consideration the time course of emotion in its conceptualization of anhedonia in schizophrenia, is the Temporal Experience of Pleasure Scale (TEPS; Gard, Germans, Gard, Kring, & John, 2006). This trait measure assesses consummatory physical pleasure (i.e., extent to which a person gets pleasure from physical activities; e.g., food and the outdoors) and anticipatory physical pleasure (i.e., extent to which a person experiences pleasure in anticipation of future physical activities). Studies in the United States (Gard et al., 2007), China (Chan et al., 2010), and France (Favrod, Ernst, Giuliani, & Bonsack, 2009) have shown that patients with schizophrenia can reliably and validly complete this measure, and that they score lower than people without schizophrenia on the Anticipatory but not the Consummatory subscale.

Clinical Implications

The myriad ways in which negative symptoms may be assessed suggest a few key treatment implications. First, the clinical interview itself may be viewed as a form of "therapeutic assessment" (Finn, 2007); that is, simply by engaging a person with schizophrenia in a careful and detailed discussion of emotions, social relationships, and motivations, the clinician may be helping to identify treatment targets or, in cognitive-behavioral therapy parlance, to develop the problem/treatment goals list (Beck, Rector, Stolar, & Grant, 2009). Second, because there are strengths and weaknesses to any assessment approach, routine use of both interview and self-report measures (as well as laboratory measures, discussed in the next section) may be the only way to ensure comprehensive coverage of domains that treatment needs to target. Third, no matter what assessments are used, it will be important to consider whether a specific person exhibits particular negative symptoms, as opposed to reliance on a global rating or total score that sums across negative symptoms. Although the incremental contribution of finer-grained assessments to the delivery of more effective treatment remains an empirical matter, it would seem that consideration of particular symptoms guides treatment decisions more effectively and efficiently than lumping all the negative symptoms together.

TRANSLATIONAL RESEARCH ON NEGATIVE SYMPTOMS

The aim of translational research is to convert basic laboratory findings into clinically useful knowledge, moving them from "bench to bedside." Our clinical understanding of the negative symptoms of schizophrenia is a good example of translational research, because it has been enhanced by researchers who adopt the methods and theories developed in affective science, social psychology, personality psychology, and neuroscience to study emotion, motivation, and to a lesser extent, personal relationships in schizophrenia. With respect to emotion, these methods include laboratory studies in which emotionally evocative stimuli are presented to people with and without schizophrenia while measures of facial expression, reported experience, physiology, and brain activation are obtained. With respect to motivation, these methods include laboratory presentation of cues signaling reward, along with assessments of motivated or goal-directed behavior to obtain those rewards (or avoid losses). In the social domain, laboratory-based interpersonal interactions and social perception tasks create opportunities for assessing social behavior and cognition. Below, we briefly review examples of such translational research as it pertains to blunted affect, anhedonia, and avolition. Apart from the direct applications of findings in this literature, it is worth pointing out that many laboratory measures that are part and parcel of translational research can also be used effectively in clinical assessments of negative symptoms, as well as in gauging the effectiveness of interventions targeting negative symptoms.

Blunted Affect and Alogia

For years, clinicians relied solely on clinical interviews to assess blunted affect. This had the unfortunate consequence of encouraging the belief that people with schizophrenia who had blunted affect also did not experience emotion. However, a remarkably consistent pattern of findings has emerged from translational research studies over the past 20 years (see Kring & Moran, 2008, for review): In the presence of emotionally evocative stimuli—whether they be films, pictures, foods, odors, or sounds—people with schizophrenia are less outwardly expressive of positive and negative emotion than are people without schizophrenia. However, people with schizophrenia report *feeling* emotions as strongly as, if not stronger than, people without schizophrenia.

Research has also shown that people with schizophrenia are not literally expressionless. In fact, they do contract their facial muscles in response to emotional stimuli, albeit at a micro or unobservable level. Electromyographic studies of facial muscle activity find that people with schizophrenia contract the cheek (zygomatic) muscle when seeing something positive (smiling face, funny film clip) and contract the brow muscle (corrugator) when seeing something negative (frowning face, fearful or disgusting film clip) in much the same way as people without schizophrenia (e.g., Kring, Kerr, & Earnst, 1999). Thus, facial expressive behavior is not completely deficient among people with schizophrenia: They are actually expressing (i.e., contracting the facial musculature) but at an intensity level that is undetectable by unaided observers.

There have been far fewer translational research studies of alogia. However, narrative studies that focus on how people with schizophrenia tell stories or narrative events in their lives can be informative for understanding alogia. In these studies, participants are asked to tell stories about different sorts of events, including emotional events, and the resulting narratives are then coded for the language used to describe the event, the temporal sequencing of its elements, and the social context of the event (e.g., Burbridge & Barch, 2002). One might expect people with schizophrenia who have alogia not to provide much detail or elaboration in their narrative accounts. Unfortunately, no study has yet looked at this directly. Interestingly, one narrative study that asked people with and without schizophrenia to recount narratives about positive, negative, and neutral life experiences found only minimal differences between groups in word usage. People with schizophrenia tended to use fewer words than people without schizophrenia when recounting stories of positive life events, but they did not differ from people without schizophrenia in the words used for their negative and neutral narratives (Gruber & Kring, 2008).

Anhedonia

Over the past 10 years, researchers have taken a closer look at emotional experience in schizophrenia. Results from studies using physiological measures of emotion (e.g., skin conductance, facial muscle activity, startle modulation) underscore laboratory findings that emotional experiences in people with and without schizophrenia are largely the same, rendering especially unlikely the possibility that people with schizophrenia are reporting feelings according to the demands of the experimental situation.

As noted earlier, as much as 75% of people with schizophrenia receive a clinical rating of anhedonia, indicating that they have diminished experience of positive emotion. Yet in the presence of emotionally pleasant things, such as films, pictures, tastes, or just day-to-day life, people with schizophrenia report experiencing as much pleasure as do people without schizophrenia (Kring & Moran, 2008). Translational research has helped to resolve this paradox. Specifically, neurobehavioral models that distinguish between components of hedonic experience (e.g., Berridge & Robinson, 1998, 2003; Depue & Collins, 1999; Knutson, Adam, Fong, & Hommer, 2001; Schultz, 2002; Wise, 2002) point to an important distinction between pleasure experienced when directly engaged in an enjoyable activity (i.e., "consummatory pleasure") and pleasure experienced in anticipation of future activities (i.e., "anticipatory pleasure"). Anticipatory pleasure can be further parsed into two components: (1) predicting the future experience of pleasure, and (2) the concurrent experience of pleasure in knowing that a future activity is going to occur—that is, the pleasure experienced *in anticipation* of things to come. Behavioral and functional magnetic resonance imaging (fMRI) evidence now support the contention that, compared to people without schizophrenia, because people with schizophrenia appear less likely to anticipate that future events will be pleasurable and to experience pleasure in anticipation of things to come, they may be less likely to seek out experiences they might find equally pleasurable (e.g., Gard et al., 2007, 2011; Juckel et al., 2006).

Avolition

More recent translational research has turned to unpacking the nature of avolition. There is a growing but still small body of evidence at both the behavioral and neural levels that people with schizophrenia have difficulty translating reward information (picking up on cues of reward, maintaining information about forthcoming reward, parsing out costs and benefits to action) into goal-directed or motivated, reward-seeking behavior (for a review, see Barch & Dowd, 2010). Heerey and Gold (2007) showed emotionally evocative pictures to people with and without schizophrenia in two conditions, asking them to press a button quickly either to see it again (for positive images) or not to see it again (for negative images). In the first, called the representational responding condition, button pressing took place after the image was removed from view for 3 seconds. In the second, called the evoked responding condition, button pressing commenced during picture viewing. Interesting group differences emerged in the representational condition, in which participants presumably needed to maintain a representation of the pictures to guide their button pressing. Healthy individuals exhibited a pattern of button pressing that was distinguishable by valence (i.e., they pressed the button more frequently for emotional compared to neutral pictures); participants with schizophrenia did not show such differentiation, suggesting a deficit in motivated behavior that required maintaining representation of the forthcoming reward (in this case, to see a picture again).

Clinical Implications

What are the treatment implications of translational research findings? First, when treating a person with schizophrenia who is not very outwardly expressive, whether facially, vocally, or gesturally, it is important to recognize that the person likely *feels* strong emotions. Inasmuch as levels of subjective distress contribute to impairment of judgments that are necessary for psychiatric diagnosis, mistaking lack of expression for a lack of distress needs to be avoided, perhaps through special efforts to understand emotional experience, when making diagnostic decisions. Second, people with schizophrenia can express emotion facially if instructed to do so (e.g., Kohler et al., 2008; Putnam & Kring, 2007). Thus, interventions built around training expressive behavior may be effective. Third, blunted affect might account for myriad family and interpersonal difficulties, inasmuch as the social consequences of unexpressive behavior are likely great, disrupting interactions with both familiar and unfamiliar people (e.g., Hooley, Richters, Weintraub, & Neale, 1987; Krause, Steimer-Krause, & Hufnagel, 1992).

Fourth, assuming, based on a clinical interview or self-report measures of anhedonia, that people with schizophrenia experience no pleasure would be a mistake. Clinical interviews and self-report measures in themselves would have to cause consummatory pleasure to expose genuine variability in hedonic capacity. Fifth, it is important to assess both anticipatory and consummatory pleasure, perhaps borrowing directly from laboratory-dependent measures to do so. Finally, existing cognitive-behavioral interventions for depression, such as pleasure predicting, may be useful for people with schizophrenia who have a deficit in anticipatory pleasure.

TREATMENT

Treating negative schizophrenia symptoms is notoriously difficult. In fact, according to the American Psychiatric Association's *Practice Guidelines for the Treatment of Schizophrenia* (2004), "There are no treatments with proven efficacy for primary negative symptoms" (p. 15). The reason the NIMH sponsored its Consensus Development Conference in 2006 was to facilitate the development and implementation of effective treatments for the negative symptoms of schizophrenia. The evidence in support of medication treatments is underwhelming, with studies showing only minor benefit from pharmacological treatment of negative symptoms (e.g., Leucht et al., 2009; Murphy, Chung, Park, & McGorry, 2006). In the United States, the Food and Drug Administration, the body that approves new medication treatments for all illnesses, has yet to approve any medication with an indication for negative symptoms (Laughren & Levin, 2006). Psychosocial interventions show more promise than do current pharmaceuticals, but there is still an urgent need for more, and more effective, negative symptom treatments. In what follows, we consider how currently available treatments do (or, in most cases do not) effectively treat negative symptoms.

Medication Treatment

In the 1950s, the serendipitous discovery of the class of antipsychotic drugs known as phenothiazines, especially the drug chlorpromazine (e.g., Thorazine), revolutionized the way schizophrenia was treated. Indeed, in less than 20 years, these drugs became the primary form of treatment for schizophrenia. Other early antipsychotics include the thioxanthenes (e.g., thiothixene/Navane) and the butyrophenones (e.g., haloperidol/Haldol). Collectively, these drugs are referred to as first-generation antipsychotics, because they came out of the first "wave" of significant, empirically supported medication treatments for schizophrenia. These first-generation antipsychotic drugs are most effective with the positive and disorganization symptoms, but as many as 30% of people with schizophrenia do not respond favorably to the first-generation antipsychotics. As well, about half the people who take any antipsychotic drug quit after 1 year, and up to three-fourths quit before 2 years, because of unpleasant side effects such as sedation, dizziness, blurred vision, restlessness, and sexual dysfunction (e.g., Lieberman et al. 2005). Other more serious side effects include "extrapyramidal side effects" (e.g., tremors of the fingers, a shuffling gait, and drooling), "dystonia" (rigid muscles), "akathesia" (inability to remain still), and "tardive dyskinesia" (involuntary and unstoppable movements of the mouth area). Because of these side effects, current clinical practice guidelines from the American Psychiatric Association (2004) call for treating people with the smallest possible doses of drugs. Notably, and unfortunately, the first-generation antipsychotic drugs are not very effective in treating negative symptoms (e.g., Leucht et al., 2009).

In order to remedy the deficiencies of first-generation antipsychotics, a second wave of research produced a group of drugs referred to as the second-generation antipsychotics. Heralded at the time as drugs that would have fewer side effects and be more effective than first-generation drugs in treating negative symptoms (e.g., Kane, Honigfeld, Singer, Meltzer, & the Clozapine Study Group, 1988), these medications have their own troubling profile of side effects, such as pancreatitis (Koller, Cross, Doraiswamy, & Malozowski, 2003) and weight gain, which has been linked to the development of type 2 diabetes (Leslie & Rosenheck, 2004). Furthermore, there is no strong evidence that these drugs are more effective for negative symptoms. An early meta-analysis of 124 studies comparing first- and second-generation antipsychotic drugs found that some, but not all, second-generation drugs were modestly more effective than the first-generation drugs in reducing negative symptoms and improving cognitive deficits (Davis, Chen, & Glick, 2003). However, a later meta-analysis of 150 studies, including over 21,000 patients, failed to find an advantage for second-generation over first-generation drugs in the treatment of negative symptoms (Leucht et al., 2009). In addition, nearly three-fourths of people taking second-generation drugs discontinue them due to side effects (Jones et al., 2006; Lieberman et al., 2005).

Psychosocial Treatments for Negative Symptoms

The current treatment recommendation for schizophrenia from the Patient Outcomes Research Team (PORT) is for medication plus psychosocial intervention (Lehman et al., 2004). The PORT recommendation is based on extensive reviews of treatment research. For example, a review of 37 prospective studies of people after their first episode of schizophrenia found that the combination of medication and psychosocial treatment predicted the best outcome (Menezes, Arenovich, & Zipursky, 2006).

Cognitive-Behavioral Therapy

As discussed by Steel and Wykes (Chapter 11, this volume) a growing body of evidence demonstrates that the maladaptive beliefs of some people with schizophrenia can benefit from cognitive-behavioral therapy (CBT; Garety, Fowler, & Kuipers, 2000; Wykes, Steel, Everitt, & Tarrier, 2008). People with schizophrenia can be encouraged to test out their delusional beliefs in much the same way as do people without schizophrenia. Through collaborative discussions (and in the context of other modes of treatment, including antipsychotic drugs), some people with schizophrenia have been helped to attach a nonpsychotic meaning to paranoid symptoms and thereby reduce their intensity and aversive nature, similar to what is done for depression and panic disorder (Beck & Rector, 2005; Beck et al., 2009).

But does CBT help with the negative symptoms? Studies offer a tentative "yes" (e.g., Sensky et al., 2000; Turkington et al., 2006), even with medication-refractory cases. CBT formulations targeting negative symptoms may include challenging belief structures tied to low expectations for success (avolition) and low expectations for pleasure (anticipatory pleasure deficit in anhedonia) (Rector, Beck, & Stolar, 2005; Wykes et al., 2008). A meta-analysis of 34 studies of close to 2,000 people with schizophrenia, across eight different countries, found small to moderate effect sizes for CBT in treating positive symptoms, negative symptoms, mood, and general life functioning (Wykes et al., 2008).

Initial indications of successful treatment of negative symptoms with CBT suggest some exciting prospects for future developments in this area (Tai & Turkington, 2009). CBT exists within an extremely active and creative research community that not only values empirical research but also aggressively pursues innovative means of effecting change. Recently, CBT has embraced mindfulness-based approaches, acceptance and commitment therapy, emotion theory, and meta-cognitive concepts, among others. Collectively, these are sometimes referred to as third-wave approaches, because they follow behavioral, then cognitive-behavioral approaches. CBT is also studied in the context of nearly every other form of psychopathology, creating ample opportunity for cross-fertilization of theories and methods.

Cognitive Training

Another form of treatment involving cognition is referred to broadly as "cognitive training" (sometimes also called "cognitive remediation" or "cognitive enhancement therapy"). These interventions are designed to improve or enhance basic cognitive functions such as problem solving, verbal learning, perceptual learning, memory, and the like. Cognitive training typically involves repeated administration of cognitive tasks, often via computer, over the course of weeks, to train and promote practice on targeted skills. Perhaps because these treatments were not designed to ameliorate negative symptoms, the extent to which they do so varies a good bit across studies. Indeed, many studies of cognitive training do not assess symptoms at all, because treatment focuses on a highly specific cognitive process.

A 2007 meta-analysis of cognitive training studies in schizophrenia found only a small effect size for symptom reduction (McGurk et al., 2007). Unfortunately, this review did not distinguish among positive, negative, and disorganized symptoms when presenting the effects on symptoms. A more recent qualitative review noted that only one of 11 studies on cognitive training conducted since the 2007 meta-analysis reported an improvement in negative symptoms following cognitive training (Wykes & Huddy, 2009). Taken together, the specific benefits of cognitive training do not appear to encompass the negative symptoms as well, though it is possible that similarly intensive training targeting negative symptoms directly may hold more promise (e.g., Russell, Chu, & Phillips, 2006).

Social Skills Training

Social skills training is designed to teach people with schizophrenia how to manage successfully a wide variety of interpersonal situations, such as discussing their medications with the psychiatrist, interviewing for jobs, and reading bus schedules (Heinssen, Liberman, & Kopelowicz, 2000; Liberman, Eckman, Kopelowicz, & Stolar, 2000). Social skills training typically involves role playing and other group exercises to practice skills, both in a therapy group and in actual social situations. As might be expected, social skills training has its largest impact on social skills, but it also has significant impact on negative symptoms. In a meta-analysis, Kurtz and Mueser (2008) report moderate effects (effect size [ES] = 0.40) across six studies (N = 363) of social skills training on negative symptoms. Interestingly, these effect sizes exceed those for other psychiatric symptoms (ES = 0.15), though they are substantially smaller than those found for actual social skills (ES = 1.20).

Adapted Meditation

It is easy enough to advocate basing new and innovative treatments on the best contemporary translational science. It is somewhat harder actually to do so. Nevertheless,
this work has already begun. For example, preliminary data from an emotion-focused
meditation treatment targeting anticipatory pleasure and motivation difficulties in
schizophrenia show some promise (Johnson et al., 2009, 2011). This group treatment
was developed as an extension and adaptation to schizophrenia of loving-kindness
meditation (LKM). Similar to other meditation practices, LKM involves quiet contemplation and attention to the here and now. Participants follow a guided meditation
that asks them direct their attention to their heart region and contemplate a person
for whom they already feel warm, tender, and compassionate feelings, or a situation
in which they felt warm feelings. They are then asked to extend these warm feelings
to themselves, using such internally spoken phrases as "May I be safe" or "May I be
at peace," to help generate these feelings. As the practice continues, participants are
asked to radiate these warm, tender, and compassionate feelings to others: first to
a few people they know well, then to all their friends and family, and finally to all
people with whom they have a connection.

In the emotion-focused meditation, two groups of nine participants with schizophrenia attended 1-hour weekly sessions for 6 weeks, as well as a review session 6
weeks after the final session. The weekly group sessions incorporated three major
components: discussion, skills teaching, and practice. At the beginning of each
session the participants were encouraged to discuss something they learned from
doing the meditation or a perceived benefit of the meditation. Problems, challenges,
or questions about the practice were then addressed by the group, with advice given
by the therapist to meet participants' needs and reinforce positive aspects of the
practice. Next, a mindfulness activity such as mindful eating, walking, listening,
or body movement, was taught and practiced. Next, the group facilitator led participants in 5- to 10-minute meditation practice during the session, gently reminding participants to redirect their attention nonjudgmentally to the feeling of loving-
kindness and positive emotions when their attention wandered. Participants were
encouraged to practice at home and were given a CD with guided meditations.

Although this was a completely uncontrolled study and the findings are
extremely preliminary, the attendance of people with schizophrenia was over 90%,
and feedback suggested that participants enjoyed and benefited from the treatment.
The treatment was associated with a decrease in anhedonia and asociality, and an
increase in positive emotions at posttreatment and at 3-month follow-up assessments (Johnson et al., 2011).

Preliminary data from five people with schizophrenia who completed a skills-
based treatment targeting anticipatory pleasure were also promising. For this treatment, the therapist worked with patients to develop a personalized list of pleasurable activities. Next, mindfulness meditation was taught, and participants were
instructed to imagine a series of standard future events (e.g., eating an apple, going

for a walk), while focusing closely on the sensory experiences. Participants were directed to anticipate pleasurable feelings. The sessions then moved to imagining past pleasurable events participants had experienced and to future, hoped-for pleasurable experiences. Though, again, extremely preliminary, participants reported benefiting from the treatment and demonstrated an increase in the TEPS Anticipatory subscale posttreatment (Favrod, Giuliani, Ernst, & Bonsack, 2010).

It remains to be seen whether these two interventions can be effective treatments for negative symptoms when put to a more rigorous test, but these early results, at a minimum, suggest that such rigorous tests ought to be conducted. In the coming years, additional efforts to develop treatments that selectively target the specific emotional, motivational, and social relationship difficulties in schizophrenia will likely yield additional insights, thus realizing the potential of translational research.

Principles of Change

Although clinical implications of negative symptoms have been discussed at various points throughout this chapter, it is perhaps also worth attempting to delineate some more general principles of change. Foremost among these is the proposition that psychosocial and biological interventions complement rather than contradict each other. Just as medications have psychosocial effects so, too, do psychosocial interventions have biological effects. A completely deterministic biological accounting for the etiology of schizophrenia will not change this any more than a biological account of learning would eliminate the need for formal education. Similarly, fundamentally psychosocial phenomena may be affected by biological interventions. Unlike other disorders, such as depression, the symptoms of schizophrenia— especially the negative symptoms—are far enough from ordinary experience that it is tempting to assume there must be something wrong neurobiologically with patients and that a biological intervention is therefore necessary. Both assumptions are based on faulty logic that researchers must avoid.

It may also be the case that the effective treatments are aimed not at schizophrenia or the negative symptoms per se but at circumscribed problems associated with schizophrenia. For instance, social skills training has its greatest effects on social skills, anhedonia and asociality appear to be affected by emotion-focused meditation, and anticipatory pleasure seems to be improved by interventions specifically targeting this phenomenon. Changes may be most likely when basic symptom and translational research processes are targeted for intervention.

CONCLUSION

The limitations of contemporary treatments are as heartbreaking as they are well known. Clearly, the search for effective negative symptom treatments continues. To the extent that the search for next-generation schizophrenia treatments leverages contemporary translational research, there is cause for optimism that this tragic disorder will one day be tractable.

REFERENCES

Amador, X. F., Flaum, M., Andreasen, N. C., Strauss, D. H., Yale, S. A., Clark, S. C., et al. (1994). Awareness of illness in schizophrenia and schizoaffective and mood disorders. *Archives of General Psychiatry, 51*, 826–836.

American Psychiatric Association. (2004). *Practice guidelines for the treatment of patients with schizophrenia* (2nd ed.). Available at *www.psych.org.*

American Psychiatric Association. (2013). *Diagnostic and statistical manual of mental disorders* (5th ed.). Arlington, VA: Author.

Andreasen, N. C. (1982). Negative symptoms in schizophrenia: Definition and reliability. *Archives of General Psychiatry, 39*, 784–788.

Barch, D. M. (2005). The relationships among cognition, motivation, and emotion in schizophrenia: How much and how little we know. *Schizophrenia Bulletin, 31*, 875–881.

Barch, D. M., & Dowd, E. C. (2010). Goal representations and motivational drive in schizophrenia: The role of prefrontal–striatal interactions. *Schizophrenia Bulletin, 36*(5), 919–934.

Barch, D. M., Yodkovik, N., Sypher-Locke, H., & Hanewinkel, M. (2008). Intrinsic motivation in schizophrenia: Relationships to cognition, depression, anxiety, and personality. *Journal of Abnormal Psychology, 117*, 776–787.

Beck, A. T., & Rector, N. A. (2005). Cognitive approaches to schizophrenia: Theory and therapy. *Annual Review of Clinical Psychology, 1*, 577–606.

Beck, A. T., Rector, N. A., Stolar, N., & Grant, P. (2009). *Schizophrenia: Cognitive theory, research, and therapy.* New York: Guilford Press.

Berridge, K. C., & Robinson, T. E. (1998). What is the role of dopamine in reward: Hedonic impact, reward learning, or incentive salience? *Brain Research Reviews, 28*(3), 309–369.

Berridge, K. C., & Robinson, T. E. (2003). Parsing reward. *Trends in Neuroscience, 26*(9), 507–513.

Blanchard, J. J., Brown, S. A., Horan, W. P., & Sherwood, A. R. (2000). Substance use disorders in schizophrenia: Review, integration, and a proposed model. *Clinical Psychology Review, 2*, 207–234.

Blanchard, J. J., & Cohen, A. (2006). The structure of negative symptoms within schizophrenia: Implications for assessment. *Schizophrenia Bulletin, 32*, 238–245.

Blanchard, J. J., Kring, A. M., Horan, W. P., & Gur, R. (2011). Toward the next generation of negative symptom assessments: The collaboration to advance negative symptom assessment in schizophrenia. *Schizophrenia Bulletin, 37*(2), 291–299,

Braga, R. J., Petrides, G., & Fifueira, I. (2004). Anxiety disorders in schizophrenia. *Comprehensive Psychiatry, 45*, 460–468.

Burbridge, J. A., & Barch, D. M. (2002). Emotional valence and reference disturbance in schizophrenia. *Journal of Abnormal Psychology, 111*(1), 186–192.

Cancro, R. (1989). Schizophrenia. In *Treatments of Psychiatric Disorders: A Task Force Report of the American Psychiatric Association,* (1–3:1485–606). Washington, DC: American Psychiatric Association.

Chan, R. C. K., Wang, Y., Huang, J., Yanfang, S., Wang, Y., Hong, X., et al. (2010). Anticipatory and consummatory components of the experience of pleasure in schizophrenia: Cross-cultural validation and extension. *Psychiatry Research, 175.* 181–183.

Chapman, L. J., & Chapman, J. P. (1978). *The Revised Physical Anhedonia Scale* [Unpublished test]. Madison: University of Wisconsin.

Chapman, L. J., Chapman, J. P., & Raulin, M. L. (1976). Scales for physical and social anhedonia. *Journal of Abnormal Psychology, 85,* 374–382.

Chouinard, S., Poulin, J., Stip, E., & Godbout, R. (2004). Sleep in untreated patients with schizophrenia. *Schizophrenia Bulletin, 30,* 957–967.

Clinical Assessment Interview for Negative Symptoms [CAINS; Clinical rating scale and manual]. Unpublished measure.

Davis, J. M., Chen, N., & Glick, I. D. (2003). A meta-analysis of the efficacy of second-generation antipsychotics. *Archives of General Psychiatry, 60,* 553–564.

Depue, R. A., & Collins, P. F. (1999). Neurobiology of the structure of personality: Dopamine, facilitation of incentive motivation, and extraversion. *Behavioral and Brain Sciences, 22*(3), 491–517.

Dworkin, R. (1992). Affective deficits and social deficits in schizophrenia: What's what? *Schizophrenia Bulletin, 18,* 59–64.

Dyck, D. G., Short, R., & Vitaliano, P. P. (1999). Predictors of burden and infectious illness in schizophrenia caregivers. *Psychosomatic Medicine, 61,* 411–419.

Eckblad, M. L., Chapman, L. J., Chapman, J. P., & Mishlove, M. (1982). *The Revised Social Anhedonia Scale* [Unpublished test]. Madison: University of Wisconsin.

Favrod, J. Ernst, F., Giuliani, F., & Bonsack, C. (2009). Validation of the Temporal Experience of Pleasure Scale (TEPS) in a French-speaking environment. *L'Encéphale, 35,* 241–248.

Favrod, J., Giuliani, F., Ernst, F., & Bonsack, C. (2010). Anticipatory pleasure skills training: A new intervention to reduce anhedonia in schizophrenia. *Perspectives in Psychiatric Care, 46,* 171–181.

Fenton, W. S., & McGlashan, T. H. (1991). Natural history of schizophrenia subtypes: II. Positive and negative symptoms and long-term course. *Archives of General Psychiatry, 48,* 978–986.

Finn, S. E. (2007). *In our clients' shoes: Theory and techniques of therapeutic assessment.* Mahwah, NJ: Erlbaum.

Gard, D. E., Cooper, S., Fisher, M., Genevsky, A., Mikels, J. A., & Vinograduv, S. (2011). Evidence for an emotion maintenance deficit in schizophrenia. *Psychiatry Research, 187,* 24–29.

Gard, D. E., Germans Gard, M., Kring, A. M., & John, O. P. (2006). Anticipatory and consummatory components of the experience of pleasure: A scale development study. *Journal of Research in Personality, 40,* 1086–1102.

Gard, D. E., Kring, A. M., Germans Gard, M., Horan, W. P., & Green, M. F. (2007). Anhedonia in schizophrenia: Distinctions between anticipatory and consummatory pleasure. *Schizophrenia Research, 93,* 253–260.

Garety, P. A., Fowler, D., & Kuipers, E. (2000). Cognitive behavioral therapy for medication-resistant symptoms. *Schizophrenia Bulletin, 26,* 73–86.

Gruber, J., & Kring, A. M. (2008). Narrating emotion events in schizophrenia. *Journal of Abnormal Psychology, 117,* 520–533.

Heerey, E. A., & Gold, J. M. (2007). Patients with schizophrenia demonstrate dissociation between affective experience and motivated behavior. *Journal of Abnormal Psychology, 116,* 268–278.

Heinssen, R. K., Liberman, R. P., & Kopelowicz, A. (2000). Psychosocial skills training for schizophrenia: Lessons from the laboratory. *Schizophrenia Bulletin, 26,* 21–46.

Ho, B. C., Nopoulos, P., Flaum, M., Arndt, S., & Andreasen, N. C. (1998). Two-year outcome in first-episode schizophrenia: Predictive value of symptoms for quality of life. *American Journal of Psychiatry, 155,* 1196–1201.

Hooley, J. M. (2007). Expressed emotion and relapse of psychopathology. *Annual Review of Clinical Psychology, 3,* 329–352.

Hooley, J. M., Richters, J. E., Weintraub, S., & Neale, J. M. (1987). Psychopathology and marital distress: The positive side of positive symptoms. *Journal of Abnormal Psychology, 96,* 27–33.

Horan, W. P., Green, M. F., Kring, A. M., & Nuechterlein, K. H. (2006). Does anhedonia in schizophrenia reflect faulty memory for subjectively experienced emotions? *Journal of Abnormal Psychology, 115,* 496–508.

Horan, W. P., Kring, A. M., & Blanchard, J. J. (2006). Anhedonia in schizophrenia: A review of assessment strategies. *Schizophrenia Bulletin, 32,* 259–273.

Horan, W. P., Kring, A. M., Gur, R. E., Reise, S. P., & Blanchard, J. J. (2011). Development and psychometric validation of the Clinical Assessment Interview for Negative Symptoms (CAINS). *Schizophrenia Research, 132*(2–3), 140–145.

Johnson, D. J., Penn, D. L., Fredrickson, B. L., Kring, A. M., Meyer, P. S., Catalino, L. I., et al. (2011). A pilot study of loving-kindness meditation for the negative symptoms of schizophrenia. *Schizophrenia Research, 129,* 137–140.

Johnson, D. J., Penn, D. L., Fredrickson, B. L., Meyer, P. S., Kring, A. M., & Brantley, M. (2009). Loving-kindness meditation to enhance recovery from negative symptoms of schizophrenia. *Journal of Clinical Psychology 65,* 499–509.

Jones, P. B., Barnes, T. R. E., Davies, L., Dunn, G., Lloyd, H., Hayhurst, K. P., et al. (2006). Randomized controlled trial of the effect on quality of life of second- vs first-generation antipsychotic drugs in schizophrenia: Cost Utility of the Latest Antipsychotic Drugs in Schizophrenia Study (CUtLASS 1). *Archives of General Psychiatry, 63,* 1079–1087.

Juckel, G., Schlagenhauf, F., Koslowski, M., Wustenberg, T., Villringer, A., Knutson, B., et al. (2006). Dysfunction of ventral striatal reward prediction in schizophrenia. *NeuroImage, 29*(2), 409–416.

Kane, J., Honigfeld, G., Singer, J., Meltzer, H., and the Clozapine Collaborative Study Group. (1988). Clozapine for treatment resistant schizophrenics. *Archives of General Psychiatry, 45,* 789–796.

Kanfer, R., & Ackerman, P. L. (2000). Individual differences in work motivation: Further explorations of a trait framework. *Applied Psychology: An International Review, 49,* 470–482.

Kay, S., Fiszbein, A., & Opler, L. (1987). The Positive and Negative Syndrome Scale (PANSS) for schizophrenia. *Schizophrenia Bulletin, 13,* 261–276.

Kirkbride, J. B., Fearon, P., Morgan, C., Dazzon, P., Morgan, K., et al. (2006). Heterogeneity in the incidence of schizophrenia and other psychotic illnesses: Results from the 3–center Aesop study. *Archives of General Psychiatry, 63,* 250–258.

Kirkpatrick, B., Fenton, W., Carpenter, W. T., & Marder, S. R. (2006). The NIMH-MATRICS Consensus Statement on Negative Symptoms. *Schizophrenia Bulletin, 32,* 296–303.

Knutson, B., Adams, C. M., Fong, G. W., & Hommer, D. (2001). Anticipation of increasing monetary reward selectively recruits nucleus accumbens. *Journal of Neuroscience, 21*(RC159), 1–5.

Kohler, C. G., Martin, E. A., Milonova, M., et al. (2008). Dynamic evoked facial expressions of emotions in schizophrenia. *Schizohprenia Research, 105,* 30–39.

Koller, E. A., Cross, J. T., Doraiswamy, P. M., & Malozowski, S. N. (2003). Pancreatitis associated with atypical antipsychotics: from the Food and Drug Administration's MedWatch surveillance system and published reports. *Pharmacotherapy, 23,* 1123–1130.

Krause, R., Steimer-Krause, E., & Hufnagel, H. (1992). Expression and experience of affects in paranoid schizophrenia. *European Review of Applied Psychology, 42,* 131–138.

Kring, A. M., Barrett, L. F., & Gard, D. E. (2003). On the broad applicability of the affective circumplex: Representations of affective knowledge in schizophrenia. *Psychological Science, 14,* 207–214.

Kring, A. M., & Caponigro, J. M. (2010). Emotion in schizophrenia: Where feeling meets thinking. *Current Directions in Psychological Science, 19,* 255–259.

Kring, A. M., Gur, R. E., Blanchard, J. J., Horan, W. P., & Reise, S. P. (2013). The Clinical Assessment Interview for Negative Symptoms (CAINS): Final development and validation. *American Journal of Psychiatry, 170,* 165–172.

Kring, A. M., Kerr, S. L., & Earnst, K. S. (1999). Schizophrenic patients show facial reactions to emotional facial expressions. *Psychophysiology, 36,* 186–192.

Kring, A. M., & Moran, E. K. (2008). Emotional response deficits in schizophrenia: Insights from affective science. *Schizophrenia Bulletin, 34,* 819–834.

Kurtz, M. M., & Mueser, K. T. (2008). A meta-analysis of controlled research on social skills training for schizophrenia. *Journal of Consulting and Clinical Psychology, 76,* 491–504.

Laughren, T., & Levin, R. (2006). Food and Drug Administration perspective on negative symptoms in schizophrenia as a target for a drug treatment claim. *Schizophrenia Bulletin, 32,* 220–222.

Lehman, A. F., Kreyenbuhl, J., Buchanan, R. W., Dickerson, F. B., Dixon, L. B., & Goldberg, R. (2004). The schizophrenia patient outcomes research team (PORT): Updated treatment recommendations 2003. *Schizophrenia Bulletin, 30,* 193–217.

Leslie, D. L., & Rosenheck, R. A. (2004). Incidence of newly diagnosed diabetes attributable to atypical antipsychotic medications. *American Journal of Psychiatry, 161,* 1709–1711.

Leucht, S., Corves, C., Arbter, D., Engel, R. R., Li, C., & Davis, J. M. (2009). Second-generation versus first-generation antipsychotic drugs for schizophrenia: A meta-analyis. *Lancet, 373,* 31–41.

Liberman, R. P., Eckman, T. A., Kopelowicz, A., & Stolar, D. (2000). *Friendship and intimacy module.* Available from Psychiatric Rehabilitation Consultants, PO Box 2867, Camarillo, CA 93011.

Lieberman, J. A., Stroup, T. S., et al. (2005). Effectiveness of antipsychotic drugs in patients with chronic schizophrenia. *New England Journal of Medicine, 353,* 1209–1223.

Lukoff, D., Nuechterlein, K. H., & Ventura, J. (1986). Manual for the Expanded Brief Psychiatric Rating Scale. *Schizophrenia Bulletin, 12,* 594–602.

McGurk, S. R., Twamley, E. W., Sitzer, D. I., McHugo, G. J., & Mueser, K. T. (2007). A meta-analysis of cognitive remediation in schizophrenia. *American Journal of Psychiatry, 164,* 1791–1802.

Menezes, N. M., Arenovich, T., & Zipursky, R. B. (2006). A systematic review of longitudinal outcome studies of first-episode psychosis. *Psychological Medicine, 36,* 1349–1362.

Messinger, J. W., Tremeau, F., Antonius, D., Mendelsohn, E., Prudent, V., Stanfore, A. D., et al. (2011). Avolition and expressive deficits capture negative symptom phenomoenology: Implications for DSM-5 and schizophrenia research. *Clinical Psychology Review, 31,* 161–168.

Milev, P., Ho, B. -C., Arndt, S., & Andreasen, N. C. (2005). Predictive values of neurocognition and negative symptoms on functional outcome in schizophrenia: A longitudinal first-episode study with 7-year follow-up. *American Journal of Psychiatry, 162,* 495–506.

Murphy, B. P., Chung, Y.-C., Park, T.-W., & McGorry, P. D. (2006). Pharmacological treatment of primary negative symptoms in schizophrenia: A systematic review. *Schizophrenia Research, 88,* 5–25.

Overall, J. E., & Gorham, D. R. (1962). The Brief Psychiatric Rating Scale. *Psychological Reports, 10,* 799–812.

Palmer, B. A., Pankratz, V. S., & Bostwick, J. M. (2005). The lifetime risk of suicide in schizophrenia: A reexamination. *Archives of General Psychiatry, 62,* 247–253.

Peralta,V., & Cuesta, M. J. (2001). How many and which are the psychopathological dimensions in schizophrenia?: Issues influencing their ascertainment. *Schizophrenia Research, 49,* 269–285.

Perlick, D. A., Rosenheck, R. A., Kaczynski, R., Swartz, M. S., Canive, J. M., & Lieberman, J. A. (2006). Components and correlates of family burden in schizophrenia. *Psychiatric Services, 57,* 1117–1125.

Provencher, H. L., & Mueser, K. T. (1997). Positive and negative symptom behaviors and caregiver burden in the relatives of persons with schizophrenia. *Schizophrenia Research, 26,* 71–80.

Putnam, K. M., & Kring, A. M. (2007). Accuracy and intensity of posed emotional expressions in unmedicated schizophrenia patients: Vocal and facial channels. *Psychiatry Research, 151,* 67–76.

Rector, N. A., Beck, A. T., & Stolar, N. (2005). The negative symptoms of schizophrenia: A cognitive perspetive. *Canadian Journal of Psychiatry, 50,* 247–257.

Russell, T. A., Chu, E., & Phillips, M. L. (2006). A pilot study to investigate the effectiveness of emotion recognition remediation in schizophrenia using the micro-expression training tool. *British Journal of Clinical Psychology, 45,* 579–583.

Saha, S., Chant, D., & McGrath, J. (2007). A systematic review of mortality in schizophrenia: Is the differential mortality gap worsening over time? *Archives of General Psychiatry, 64,* 1123–1131.

Saha, S., Chant, D., Welham, J., & McGrath, J. (2005). The systematic review of the prevalence of schizophrenia. *PLoS Medicine, 2,* 413–433.

Saha, S., Welham, J., Chant, D., & McGrath, J. (2006). Incidence of schizophrenia does not vary with economic status of the country: Evidence from a systematic review. *Social Psychiatry and Psychiatric Epidemiology, 41,* 338–340.

Salem, J. E., & Kring, A. M. (1998). The role of gender differences in the reduction of etiologic heterogeneity in schizophrenia. *Clinical Psychology Review, 18,* 795–819.

Sartorius, N., Shapiro, R., & Jablonsky, A. (1974). The international pilot study of schizophrenia. *Schizophrenia Bulletin, 2,* 21–35.

Schultz, W. (2002). Getting formal with dopamine and reward. *Neuron, 36*(2), 241–263.

Selten, J. P., Gernaat, H. B., Nolen, W. A., Wiersma, D., & van den Bosch, R. J. (1998). Experience of negative symptoms: comparison of schizophrenic patients to patients with a depressive disorder and to normal subjects. *American Journal of Psychiatry, 155,* 350–354.

Sensky, T., Turkington, D., Kingdon, D., Scott, J. L., Scott, J., & Siddle, R. (2000). A randomized controlled trial of cognitive–behavioural therapy for persistent symptoms in schizophrenia resistant to medication. *Archives of General Psychiatry, 57,* 165–172.

Siegel, S. J., Irani, F., Brensinger, C. M., Kohler, C. G., Bilker, W. B., Ragland, J. D., et al. (2006). Prognostic variables at intake and long-term level of function in schizophrenia. *American Journal of Psychiatry, 163,* 433–441.

Smith, D. A. (1999). Shooting the messengers: What meta-analysis can and cannot do. *Schizophrenia Research, 39,* 243–246.

Smith, D. A., Mar, C. M., & Turoff, B. K. (1998). The structure of schizophrenic symptoms: A meta-analytic confirmatory factor analysis. *Schizophrenia Research, 31,* 57–70.

Tai, S., & Turkington, D. (2009). The evolution of cognitive behavior therapy for schizophrenia: Current practice and recent developments. *Schizophrenia Bulletin, 35,* 865–873.

Tandon, R., Nasrallah, H. A., & Keshavan, M. A. (2009). Schizophrenia, just the facts: 4. Clinical features and conceptualization. *Schizophrenia Research, 110,* 1–23.

Turkington, D., Kingdon, D., Rathod, S., Hammond, K., Pelton, J., & Mehta, R. (2006). Outcomes of an effectiveness trial of cognitive-behavioural intervention by mental health nurses in schizophrenia. *British Journal of Psychiatry, 189,* 36–40.

U.S. Department of Health and Human Services. (2001). *Mental health: Culture, race, and ethnicity—a supplement to mental health: A report of the Surgeon General.* Rockville, MD: U. S. Department of Health and Human Services, Substance Abuse and Mental Health Services Administration, Center for Mental Health Services.

Walker, E., Kestler, L., Bollini, A., & Hochman, K. (2004). Schizophrenia: Etiology and course. *Annual Review of Psychology, 55,* 401–430.

Weisman, A. G., Nuechterlein, K. H., Goldstein, M. J., & Snyder, K. S. (2000). Controllability perceptions and reactions to symptoms of schizophrenia: A within-family comparison of relatives with high and low expressed emotion. *Journal of Abnormal Psychology, 109,* 167–171.

Wise, R. A. (2002). Brain reward circuitry: Insights from unsensed incentives. *Neuron, 36*(2), 229–240.

Wykes, T., & Huddy, V. (2009). Cognitive remediation for schizophrenia: It is even more complicated. *Current Opinion in Psychiatry, 22,* 161–167.

Wykes, T., Steel, C., Everitt, T., & Tarrier, N. (2008). Cognitive behavior therapy for schizophrenia: Effect sizes, clinical models, and methodological rigor. *Schizophrenia Bulletin, 34,* 523–537.

CHAPTER 13

Marital and Relational Discord

David A. Sbarra
Mark A. Whisman

P roblems in interpersonal relationships are core or associated features of most forms of psychopathology. Mental illness occurs in a social context, and this observation dates back well over a century (see Sullivan, 1953). Far from being anecdotal, a large body of empirical research supports this claim, with evidence indicating that relational processes play a role in the etiology, maintenance, and relapse, for a range of different disorders in adulthood (Beach, Wamboldt, Kaslow, Reiss, & Heyman, 2006); it hardly seems necessary to note that family relationships provide the context for most forms of psychopathology that occur in childhood and adolescence (Wamboldt & Wamboldt, 2000). Furthermore, there is strong evidence that relationship-focused treatment approaches (by either including significant others in the treatment itself, or targeting patterns of interpersonal functioning within individual treatment) can yield outcomes as effective as individually focused treatments for psychiatric disorders (Barbato & D'Avanzo, 2008; Powers, Vedel, & Emmelkamp, 2008). Beyond these observations, there is little doubt about the importance of relationships for physical well-being (House, Landis, & Umberson, 1988; Kiecolt-Glaser & Newton, 2001).

In this chapter, we review what is known about the presentation, classification, prevalence and course, comorbidities, and available treatment options for *marital and relational discord* (MRD). For our purposes in this chapter, we limit the scope of our review on MRD to adult marital or long-term partnerships, which we call "marriage-like relationships," given that the most immediate and relevant interpersonal context for adults is marriage or a marriage-like partnership. We note that the topic of relational discord in general can be cast much more widely to consider other family and close relationships (see Beach et al., 2006), but space limitations prohibit a thorough discussion of each of these topics independently. From our perspective, the inclusion of a chapter on marital and relational discord in a volume on psycho-pathology–psychotherapy integration is a positive sign of the times; it is inarguable that MRD is associated with considerable suffering, both in its own right and in its association with other forms of psychopathology.

Although MRD can be understood in many of the same ways we typically think about individual psychopathology, MRD also contains at least two major elements that make it distinct from the other disorders considered in this volume. First, MRD is inherently dyadic (First et al., 2002): People cannot have marital or relational dis-cord unless they are in a relationship, although they can be diagnosed with every other disorder in the table of contents (of this book) without a partner in their lives. Because of this dyadic focus, it is important to think about MRD as a systemic prob-lem when considering assessment, etiology, and treatment. We address these issues, which may be distinct to MRD and other relational-based problems, throughout the chapter. Second, the relationships that define the context for MRD are—in most of the Western industrialized world—based on choice. Most love relationships hinge on free will and the choice two people make to live together. A corollary of this point, then, is that people can choose to greatly mitigate the psychological toll of MRD by ending the relationship. Romantic breakups and divorce can introduce an entirely different set of stressors, especially when children are involved, but when someone wants to put an end to relational conflict, bitterness, and consternation, separating from a partner is an option that must be considered. It is clear that same cannot be said for major depression or panic disorder, for example; we cannot dis-avow the part of ourselves that causes us to feel sad and guilty in the same way we can attempt to solve MRD by distancing ourselves from a dysfunctional relation-ship (Emery & Sbarra, 2002). We return to this point at the end of the chapter when reviewing literature on the available treatments for MRD.

TYPICAL SYMPTOMS

MRD is a heterogeneous and broad construct. In DSM-5 (American Psychiatric Association, 2013), MRD is included under "Other Conditions That May Be a Focus of Clinical Attention," listed as V code 61.10 "Relationship Distress With Spouse or Intimate Partner," and defined in terms of negative or distorted communication or noncommunication (e.g., withdrawal behavior) that is associated with clinically significant impairment to one or both partners. Classification of MRD is discussed in greater detail below, but it is important to note here that with the exception of relationship violence, MRD is defined not a priori by the behaviors of one partner toward another but by the consequent sentiments that emerge about the relation-ship and one's partner as a result of repeated interactions. At the broadest level, one may feel a global sense of satisfaction or dissatisfaction with the relationship, and this sense manifests itself in at least two specific ways: persistent negative feeling states (e.g., frustration, anger, desire to escape a partner) and negative attributions about a partner's actions/intentions (that he or she is uncaring, thoughtless, too messy, too rigid, etc.). These feeling states and negative attributions underpin many negative behaviors that in turn corrode relationship satisfaction and reverberate back to intensify negative emotions and thoughts. This positive feedback toward worsened distress is one of the most typical features of MRD, and many couple therapists speak anecdotally about interrupting vicious cycles of negative thoughts and behaviors (e.g., Gottman, Driver, & Tabares, 2002).

No available data suggest that intimate partner violence is a *typical* feature of MRD, although, as one might expect, higher rates of physical aggression are more common among couples reporting low levels of marital satisfaction (Cascardi, Langhinrichsen, & Vivian, 1992). Although marital adjustment may play a role in the emergence of physical aggression for some individuals, this role must be understood in the context of a multivariate constellation of other risk factors (e.g., jealously, emotion regulation, power imbalances, perceived stress) that ultimately lead to violence (O'Leary, Smith Slep, & O'Leary, 2007). Relative to women in nonabusive but still discordant relationships, women who report being physically abused by report more fear of their partners and that their spouses are more coercive and psychologically aggressive (Cascardi, O'Leary, Lawrence, & Schlee, 1995). Thus, even among highly discordant couples, physical and sexual violence have a unique set of correlates (O'Leary & Woodin, 2009). Because marital violence presents its own treatment considerations (e.g., most manualized couple interventions consider ongoing physical or sexual violence to be contraindications for treatment; see Gurman, 2008), we omit a thorough discussion of this topic but point the interested reader to more in-depth coverage elsewhere (e.g., Martin, Taft, & Resick, 2007; O'Leary & Gurman, 2008).

Clinical Implications

A detailed description of assessing MRD and couple functioning is beyond the scope of this chapter; the interested reader is referred to Snyder, Heyman, and Haynes (2005) for a description of evidence-based approaches to assessing couple functioning. Minimally, an assessment of couple functioning usually includes a self-report assessment of overall relationship quality, such as is provided with the Dyadic Adjustment Scale (DAS; Spanier, 1976), the Quality of Marriage Index (QMI; Norton, 1983), and the Marital Satisfaction Inventory—Revised (MSI-R; Snyder, 1997). These measures provide a global evaluation of the degree to which a person is satisfied with the quality of his or her relationship. As noted by Snyder, Castellani, and Whisman (2006), several other domains are routinely included in a thorough assessment of relationship functioning, in addition to measuring global relationship quality. First, couple-based assessment evaluates relationship behaviors, including partners' ability to communicate and successfully solve problems and resolve conflict. Second, couple-based assessment examines relationship cognitions, such as causal and responsibility attributions for partner behavior, and relationship assumptions, standards, and expectancies. Third, couple-based assessment evaluates relationship affect, including partners' intensity, duration, and reciprocity of negative feelings about each other and their relationship.

A thorough couple-based assessment incorporates assessment of individual distress and psychopathology (as discussed in other chapters of this volume), as well as enduring characteristics of each individual, such as personality characteristics and attachment styles (both of which are addressed later in this chapter). A variety of interview, observational, and self-report measures are available for assessing these domains (see Snyder et al., 2006). We should note no set of measures is appropriate for all couples or for a given couple at all times in their relationship. Instead, a valid couple-based assessment needs to consider the demographic characteristics of both members of a couple (e.g., differences in religions and/or religiosity, racial differences, and other family-of-origin differences that may impact marital functioning), as well as the theoretical orientation of the assessor, in order to tailor the assessment to best meet the needs of the couple and clinician. It is also worth noting that the assessment of symptoms and clinical features should be done regularly during the course of treatment, not just at the onset of treatment. Repeated assessment allows clinicians to evaluate whether partners continue to exhibit individual distress, even after the relationship has improved, which may suggest the need for extending treatment or supplementing couple-based treatments with individual-based treatments.

ASSOCIATED CLINICAL FEATURES

One of the most common clinical features of MRD is high rates of psychopathology, and we consider this topic later in the section on comorbidity. In this section, we address issues of quality of life, physical health, and sexual problems, all of which are important associated clinical features of MRD.

First, MRD is associated with lower quality of life as operationalized in terms of lower subjective well-being. For example, in a large-scale, nationally representative sample of middle-aged adults in the United States, marital satisfaction demonstrated the strongest association with overall life satisfaction, surpassing the associations obtained for finances, children, health, work, sexuality, and contributions to others (Fleeson, 2004). MRD is also associated with quality of life as operationalized in terms of distress and impairment. For example, Whisman and Uebelacker (2006) evaluated the association between MRD and multiple measures of distress and impairment in a population-based sample of married and cohabiting adults (N = 2,677). Results indicated that MRD was significantly associated with (1) higher levels of general distress, (2) poorer perceived health, (3) suicide ideation, (4) greater social role impairment with relatives and friends, and (5) greater work role impairment. Importantly, with the exception of suicide ideation, each of the associations between MRD and distress and impairment remained significant when controlling for current (i.e., 12-month) diagnosis of mood, anxiety, and substance use disorders.

These results suggest not only that is MRD associated with distress and impairment but also that this association is incremental to the effects of active psychiatric disorders. Furthermore, longitudinal studies have shown that MRD is predictive of changes in distress and functional impairment over time (e.g., Choi & Marks, 2008). For example, MRD was a better predictor of job satisfaction over time than job satisfaction was in predicting MRD in a 12-year panel survey (Rogers & May, 2003).

Second, marital quality is associated with health-relevant indicators in healthy adults (Kiecolt-Glaser & Newton, 2001; Robles & Kiecolt-Glaser, 2003), and evidence also indicates that marital quality plays a role in the morbidity of disease processes (e.g., Rohrbaugh, Shoham, & Coyne, 2006). Among the most profitable and widely used paradigms for investigating the mechanisms connecting these associations are laboratory-based marital interaction tasks that track physiological responding while or after couples engage in discussions of relationship problems (typically referred to as "conflict" or "problem-solving interactions"). In a study of 90 newlywed couples, for example, Kiecolt-Glaser and colleagues (1993) found that couples exhibiting more negative behavior during a problem-solving discussion task showed greater immunological changes over a 24-hour hospitalization period than couples low in negative behavior; similar response patterns were observed for endocrine markers of stress during the 30-minute marital conflict discussion (Malarkey, Kiecolt-Glaser, Pearl, & Glaser, 1994). In their review of over 20 studies assessing marital interaction and physiological responses, Kiecolt-Glaser and Newton (2001) concluded that a key theme in the literature is that women demonstrate greater physiological reactivity than men, and women show a greater persistence in physiological responses after tasks end.

Although it is clear that laboratory-based paradigms show a strong association between indicators of MRD (e.g., high hostility, criticism, demand–withdrawal interaction patterns), the mechanisms through which these processes contribute to poor health are just beginning to come into relief. Robles et al. (2003) proposed four processes through which marital functioning may have a detrimental effects on health. The first pathway is repeated "hits" to biological systems by novel stressors; the key idea here is that frequent, high-levels of physiological reactivity spurred by frequent conflicts can exert a detrimental wear and tear on regulatory systems. The second pathway is a failure of physiological systems to adapt, or habituation to the same stressor; the key idea here is that adults who show the same high levels of physiological responses to repeated arguments about finances, children, work, and so forth, are most susceptible to illness, because their bodies are subject to repeated cardiovascular, neuroendocrine, and immunological changes that have deleterious consequences over time. The third pathway is a failure to shut off physiological responses following an exposure to a stressor; the key idea here is that in situations of high MRD, people may have difficulty letting go of conflicted interactions or not ruminating on their partners' behaviors, which in turn maintains high levels of physiological stress responses. The final pathway is an inadequate response to stress; the key idea here is that, over time, the cumulative effects of abrasive marital interactions may impair the body's ability to mount an effective response to stressors in general, which in turn makes people more susceptible to disease. Rather than steeling the body against future stressors, repeated wear and tear associated with MRD can compromise the deployment of physiological responses in other stressful situations. Within a given couple, one, some, or all of these processes may be in play to impair long-term health.

Third, MRD is also associated with increased risk of sexual problems. For example, in a population-based sample of people in the United States, marital difficulties were associated with elevated risk of arousal problems, orgasmic dysfunction, and inhibited enjoyment in women; no association between marital difficulties and sexual problems was obtained for men (Dunn, Croft, & Hackett, 1999).

Clinical Implications

A primary implication that emerges from considering the clinical features associated with MRD is the need to assess a wider range of functioning than MRD alone. Quality of life, work functioning, physical health, and sexual difficulties, for example, affect and are affected by MRD, and clinicians should consider all of these issues when assessing the broader context of MRD. A useful tool for assessing these domains is the Treatment Outcome Package (TOP; Kraus, Seligman, & Jordan, 2004), which provides clinical cutoff scores in a variety of different domains of functioning. When assessing these domains, a critical issue for clinicians to consider is whether the associated features exacerbate or are exacerbated by MRD. In most cases, it is likely that the causal arrow of effect is reciprocal and operates in both directions. Consider, for example, sleep disturbance, which was found to be associated with marital quality in a large, community-based study of over 2,000 women (Troxel, Buysse, Hall, & Matthews, 2009). Whereas sleep disturbance in one partner can follow from MRD, insomnia can also be a leading indicator of a major depressive disorder (Sbarra & Allen, 2009), which suggests that in some situations where MRD and sleep disturbances co-occur, MRD is likely driven at least in part by mood disturbances (consequent to sleep problems) in one partner. To date, there are no established algorithms for determining the order in which clinicians should attend to these issues, but thorough assessment and critical thinking about the cause/correlate issue will help clinicians determine precisely where and how they should intervene. If a clinician determines that the presenting complaint of MRD appears to be driven largely by sleep problems in one partner, it makes sense to target this symptom cluster first via established methods (e.g., Smith & Perlis, 2006), then assess potential changes in MRD.

CLASSIFICATION

DSM-5 classifies MRD as a V code among other conditions that may be the focus of clinical attention. The relegation of MRD to a V code is viewed by some as a peripheral inclusion of family diagnosis in DSM-IV (Kaslow & Patterson, 2006), and the approach is criticized on many fronts (Denton, 2007), with the largest points of contention being that the DSM system falls short in its mission to facilitate reliable communication between clinicians when it comes to relational disorders. However, we note that relative to DSM-IV, DSM-5 includes a breakdown of the behavioral, cognitive, and affective dimensions through which relationships may become discordant.

Recently, Beach et al. (2006) proposed a classifying system for relational processes, based on two broad distinctions that result in four mutually exclusive categories. At the broadest level, this approach distinguishes (1) relational characteristics as disordered versus nondisordered, and (2) the effects of relationship functioning as general versus specific. General disordered relationships might include problems such as marital discord and intimate partner abuse, whereas specific disordered relationships might include problems such as coercive family interactions in conduct disorder or sexual disorders; in contrast, general nondisordered relationship problems might include topics such as expressed emotion and conflict avoidance in marriage (which, by themselves, are not characteristic of disturbed relationships but can worsen distress in other areas), whereas nondisordered specific relationship problems might include peer group influences on conduct disorder or interpersonal problems in depression and anxiety disorders. This approach has the benefit of classifying all possible types of relational distress, as well as specifying the ways that relationships impact other forms of psychopathology.

From a practice perspective, one of the promises of the four-category classification system is that clinicians can distinguish between explicit and embedded relational disorders (First et al., 2002), with the former comprising those problems encompassed within the disordered/general category. Presently, there is no adequate means in the DSM system for specifying that MRD is the primary presenting problem for a given couple, and the four-category proposal elevates these problems to the status of a diagnostic category warranting clinical attention. At the same time, this approach also raises an important taxonomic question, one that has bearing on both research and practice: Can MRD be considered a diagnostic category, and, if so, what is the appropriate threshold for placing couples in or out of the category?

Categorizing individuals or couples as discordant implies that there is a meaningful qualitative distinction between discordant and nondiscordant individuals or couples, and that currently available measures can correctly assign individuals or couples to the appropriate category. For example, individual or couples are commonly defined as discordant using the cutoff point of 97 on the DAS (Spanier, 1976); this cutoff point was selected because it is halfway between functional (married) and dysfunctional (divorced) populations on this measure (Jacobson et al., 1984).

Two studies have evaluated whether dimensional measures of relationship discord are reflective of an underlying discrete entity or taxon. If they are, then it would make sense to categorize people as being in discordant and nondiscordant relationships that differ in kind, as well as in degree of discord. Addressing this question involves the use of taxometric procedures that examine the covariation among indicators (i.e., measures of relationship discord), seeking patterns that are diagnostic of either latent categories (i.e., taxa) or dimensions. Beach, Fincham,

Amir, and Leonard (2005) examined the taxometric structure of MRD in a sample of newlywed couples (N = 447) and found evidence of a marital discord taxon. More recently, Whisman, Beach, and Snyder (2008) replicated and expanded on the earlier study by evaluating the taxometric structure of MRD based on a multidimensional measure of marital quality completed by a representative sample of couples (N = 1,202) from across the United States. Results from this study also suggested the presence of a marital discord taxon.

Clinical Implications

If MRD is taxonic, then methods are needed for identifying individuals or couples that are members of the taxon and therefore may need treatment. Whisman, Snyder, and Beach (2009) developed a 10-item, reliable, and easy to use screen that represents a nonarbitrary way of classifying relationships as discordant, thereby identifying couples who may be in need of treatment. A briefer self-report version of the MSI screening measure (the MSI-B) is available from Western Psychological Services (*www.wpspublish.com*), and an interview version can be found in Whisman et al. (2009). Both versions can be administered by people with minimal expertise in family psychology, and the measures are scored by counting the number of coded responses, with couples scoring more than 4 classified as discordant and therefore potentially in need of treatment.

The availability of a clinical cutoff on the MSI-B has obvious implications for couple therapists focused on MRD, but it also has implications for primarily individual therapists who wish to know, for example, whether a mood disorder is primarily driven by *intrapersonal* (limited, for the most part, to the client) or *interpersonal* problems. Within individual treatment, the presence of MRD above the clinical cutoff can alert the therapist to proceed with the relationship in mind during the course of intervention. Presently, no clear-cut decision tree indicates when individual therapists should consider referring the individual to couple therapy (or when to bring the partner into to the treatment), largely because it is often unclear whether MRD is a cause or consequence of the individual problems. As we discuss later in this chapter, we do know that couple interventions are effective in treating mood disorders, but given the expertise of a specific therapist, a move to couple treatment might not always be advisable. Thus, the easiest enacted clinical recommendation is for individual therapists to track MRD and to determine whether clinically relevant discord precedes or follows the primary presenting problem, and if the former, then incorporate couple-based interventions or refer out for couple-based treatment.

EPIDEMIOLOGY, COURSE, AND OUTCOMES

Understanding the epidemiology of MRD hinges on understanding the general epidemiology of marriage and romantic relationships. According to data from the National Health Interview Survey, which conducted over 127,000 interviews with adults 18 and over from 1999 to 2002, 58.2% of respondents described themselves as married, 6.6% as widowed, 10.4% as divorced or separated, 19% as never married, and 5.7% as living with a partner (Schoenborn, 2004). In terms of incidence, there are roughly 2,200,000 new marriages each year (7.1 new marriages per 1,000 adults in the U.S.; Tejada-Vera & Sutton, 2009). The incidence of divorce has decreased over, the last 35 years, from 5.0/1,000 marriages in 1970 to 3.5/1,000 in 2008 (Bramlett & Mosher, 2002; Tejada-Vera & Sutton, 2009). Using data from the National Survey of Family Growth, which involved face-to-face interviews with 10,847 women ages 15 to 44 years, Bramlett and Mohser (2002) estimated the divorce rate for first marriages in the United States to be 43%. Among adults who do divorce, 15% remarry within 1 year, 39% within 3 years, and 75% with 10 years; close to 40% of second marriages break up within 5 years (Bramlett & Mosher, 2002).

In the preceding section, we reviewed two taxometric studies that found evidence for a marital taxon (i.e., that marital discord is best represented as a category; Beach et al., 2005; Whisman et al., 2008). Taxometric analyses can also be used to estimate the base rate of the taxon. In their study of newlywed couples, Beach et al. (2005) estimated the base rate of the taxon to be approximately .20. In the study of couples with different lengths of marriage, Whisman et al. (2008) estimated the base rate of the taxon to be approximately .31 across the full sample of participants; the base rate of the taxon among recently married couples was .26, which approximates the base rate of the Beach et al. (2005) study of newlyweds.

In summary, the results from these two studies suggest that approximately three out of every 10 couples are likely to experience MRD (i.e., are likely to be members of the taxon), and as such, are likely to differ in kind, as well as degree, from couples in nondiscordant relationships. Insofar as it is estimated that over 90% of Americans will marry in their lifetime (Kreider & Fields, 2001), and that most people who do not marry will form other types of committed, intimate partnerships (e.g., cohabiting relationships), these results suggest that a large percentage of the population is likely to be exposed to clinically significant MRD at least sometime in a lifetime.

Although future research needs to determine the rate and predictors of movement into (or out of) the MRD taxon, it is informative to consider normative changes in continuous measures of martial satisfaction over time (see Karney & Bradbury, 1995). Normatively, marital satisfaction declines over time, with the steepest declines in marital satisfaction occurring during the earliest and latest years of marriage (Van-Laningham, Johnson, & Amato, 2001). This window coincides with the greatest rates of marital dissolution (Bramlett & Mosher, 2002), and some evidence indicates that women's marital satisfaction declines faster than men's (Kurdek, 2005). Also, it appears that marital distress is a chronic condition for distressed couples, at least for couples seeking therapy. For example, Baucom, Hahlweg, and Kuschel (2003) examined the effect sizes for distressed couples who were placed in waiting-list control groups and found that across 17 investigations, couples typically showed no improvement and, on average, exhibited a small amount of deterioration during the waiting period.

Finally, there is some evidence that marital satisfaction varies by gender and race. For example, in an analysis of data from the 1973–2006 General Social Survey,

Corra, Carter, Carter, and Knox (2009) found independent effects for both race and gender, with whites and husbands reporting greater marital satisfaction than blacks and wives. Furthermore, they found that when comparing four subgroups (white husbands, white wives, black husbands, and black wives) over time, although white husbands consistently report the highest level of marital satisfaction, the difference between groups has been steadily declining.

Clinical Implications

The emerging taxometric data suggest that marital discord is widespread, affecting approximately 30% of all couples, and 20–25% of newly married couples. This suggests that clinicians should anticipate that a sizable proportion of partnered individuals are likely to be unhappy with their relationship and, therefore, they should routinely assess level of relationship quality. Furthermore, given that relationship quality seems to decline over time, the assessment of relationship quality may be particularly important for people whose relationship is of longer duration. Finally, the chronic nature of relationship discord in couples seeking treatment underscores the importance of obtaining a history of relationship quality, including information about the onset of relationship problems. Such information may be useful in helping clinicians determine whether MRD preceded or followed the onset of psychopathology. In situations in which MRD is believed to be an important contributing factor in the etiology or maintenance of psychopathology, couple therapy may be indicated, either by itself or in combination with individual-focused treatments such medication or individual therapy. In a later section of this chapter, we review evidence that couple-based interventions have been shown to be effective in treating depression and substance use disorders, and compared to individual-based treatments, have the added benefit of improving relationship quality.

COMORBIDITY

A large and growing body of research indicates that MRD is comorbid with a variety of manifestations of psychopathology. For example, early research by Brown and Harris (1978) indicated that the lack of an intimate, confiding relationship with a romantic partner is a risk factor for depression. Since then, several studies have shown that people in treatment for mental health problems report higher levels of MRD than people who are not in treatment. Results from epidemiological studies, however, suggest that the majority of people with an active (i.e., 12-month) psychiatric disorder are not in treatment (Wang et al., 2005). Therefore, to make sure that the association between relationship functioning and psychopathology is not limited only to people in treatment—a minority of all people with psychopathology—researchers have more recently studied the association between MRD and psychopathology in representative (i.e., population-based) community samples.

MRD has been shown to covary with psychiatric disorders in several population-based samples. For example, in a population-based sample from Ontario, Canada, 24.5% of people with a current psychiatric disorder were likely to report troubled relationships with their spouse, compared to only 8.9% of people without a current psychiatric disorder (Whisman, Sheldon, & Goering, 2000). Similarly, in two population-based samples of people across the 48 coterminous United States, MRD was associated with DSM-III (Whisman, 1999) and DSM-IV-based (Whisman, 2007) definitions of mood, anxiety, and substance use disorders, defined in terms of broad-band classification of groups of disorders, and narrow-band classification of specific disorders. Results from other population-based surveys have similarly found greater MRD among people with specific psychiatric disorders, including people with mood disorders (e.g., McLeod, 1994; Weissman, 1987) and anxiety disorders (e.g., Markowitz, Weissman, Ouellette, Lish, & Klerman, 1989; McLeod, 1994).

MRD has also been shown to be associated with personality disorders. For example, in a population-based survey, Whisman and Schonbrun (2009) examined the association between borderline personality disorder (BPD) symptoms and relationship outcomes, and found that BPD symptom severity was positively associated with marital distress, perpetration of minor and severe marital aggression, and marital disruption; these associations remained significant when they controlled for other past-year mental disorders. South, Turkheimer, and Oltmanns (2008) evaluated a broader array of personality disorder symptoms as assessed by self- and spouse reports in a community sample of married couples. They found that personality disorder symptoms, particularly symptoms of BPD and dependent personality disorder, were associated with lower levels of marital satisfaction and higher levels of verbal aggression and perpetration of physical violence. They also found that spouses' reports of personality disorder symptoms added incrementally to self-report in predicting marital functioning.

Longitudinal studies evaluating MRD and psychopathology have found that MRD predicts increased risk for psychiatric symptoms and onset of psychiatric disorders. For example, a meta-analysis of prospective studies evaluating the longitudinal association between MRD and subsequent depressive and anxiety symptoms obtained a weighted mean effect size (r) of .25 (Proulx, Helms, & Buehler, 2007). Furthermore, researchers who have evaluated MRD and psychiatric symptoms over time have found that the longitudinal association between MRD and depressive symptoms is comparable in magnitude to the longitudinal association between depressive symptoms and MRD (e.g., Davila, Karney, Hall, & Bradbury, 2003; Whisman & Uebelacker, 2009). With respect to onset of psychiatric disorders, a 12-month prospective study involving a community sample of adults who did not meet criteria for the corresponding disorder at baseline revealed that MRD at baseline predicted incidence of a major depressive episode (Whisman & Bruce, 1999) and alcohol abuse or dependence (Whisman, Uebelacker, & Bruce, 2006) at 12-month follow-up; these associations remained significant when researchers controlled for sociodemographic variables and prior history of the respective disorder. Similarly, spouse problems predicted 1-year onset of major depression in female twins (Wade & Pevalin, 2004); neither spouse support nor family or friend problems or support predicted incidence of depression. In a community sample from the Dutch general population, MRD predicted 2-year incidence of broad-band diagnosis of mood, anxiety, and substance use disorders, and narrow-band diagnosis of major depressive disorder, dysthymia, social phobia, and alcohol abuse (Overbeek et al., 2006).

Clinical Implications

Evidence that MRD often co-occurs with mental disorders and predicts increases in psychiatric symptoms and the onset of mood and substance abuse disorders has important clinical implications. First, it is reasonable to assume that people who are unhappy with their relationship may be less likely to respond to individually oriented treatment for mental health problems. Indeed, MRD predicts poorer outcomes for individually based treatments for a variety of disorders. For example, in a sample of depressed individuals who received medication, cognitive therapy, or interpersonal psychotherapy as part of the Treatment of Depression Collaborative Research Project, (1) greater pretreatment MRD was associated with more depressive symptoms (i.e., poorer outcome) at the end of treatment and at 6-month follow-up, and (2) greater posttreatment MRD was associated with more depressive symptoms at 6-, 12-, and 18-month follow-up (Whisman, 2001). Similarly, MRD predicted poorer outcome to treatment (i.e., greater likelihood of relapse, fewer days abstinent, and shorter time to relapse) for men with substance use disorder (Fals-Stewart, O'Farrell, & Hooley, 2001), and greater marital tension predicted poorer treatment outcome for people with generalized anxiety disorder (Durham, Allan, & Hackett, 1997). Second, as reviewed in greater detail later in this chapter, couple therapy may be effective when people present for treatment with both psychiatric disorders and MRD. Third, in the case of people presenting for treatment with both personality disorders and MRD, development of greater insight into their behavior may be an important goal in therapy, because they may fail to recognize that some of their relationship unhappiness is due to how they process and interact with the world (South et al., 2008).

ETIOLOGY

Most marriages begin happily and are characterized by a great deal of optimism. Baker and Emery (1993) conducted a study to reveal just how optimistic people are about their marriage. One hundred thirty-seven adults who had recently filed for a first marriage license were surveyed about their knowledge of the general divorce rate and their estimate of the likelihood that *their own marriage* would end in divorce. In terms of the general divorce rate, participants accurately reported that 50% of marriages (in the early 1990s) would end in divorce, but the median response was 0% when assessing the likelihood that *they personally* would divorce (Baker &

Emery, 1993). This finding illustrates a foundational point for considering the etiology of MRD: The transition from an optimistic beginning to teetering on the brink of divorce is a developmental process that unfolds over time (Bradbury & Karney, 1993). Gottman (1994) referred to this process as the "cascade model of marital dissolution." Here we detail three of the major approaches to understanding the cascade into MRD. It is important to recognize that deterioration of marital quality and emergence of MRD occur at multiple levels, including interactions between partners, psychological processes within individuals, and contextual demands and stressors that impact both between- and within-person dynamics. Following our review of the different etiological models of MRD, we describe the treatments that stem from cognitive-behavioral and attachment frameworks.

Cognitive-Behavioral Models of Relationship Functioning

The cognitive-behavioral model of relationship functioning emphasizes partner behaviors, as well as people's interpretations and evaluations of their own and their partners' behavior. Regarding partners, this approach focuses on two major aspects of behavior. First, this approach emphasizes the frequency and range of reciprocal positive reinforcers exchanged between partners: Relationship satisfaction is high when rates of relationship rewards (or reinforcers) outweigh relationship costs, and when rates of actual rewards exceed one's expectations for the rate of rewards (Kelley & Thibaut, 1978). Second, this approach emphasizes a couple's ability to communicate, successfully negotiate behavior change, and resolve problems and conflict in their relationship. For example, compared to people who are satisfied with their relationship, dissatisfied partners are more likely to engage in (1) negative verbal and nonverbal communication, including negative reciprocity (i.e., the tendency for negative behavior by one person to be followed by negative behavior by the partner; Gottman, 1979, 1994); (2) corrosive behaviors, such as criticism and contempt (Levenson, Carstensen, & Gottman, 1994); and (3) demand–withdraw communication, in which one person pressures the partner with demands, complaints, or criticisms and the partner withdraws with defensiveness and inaction (Christensen & Heavey, 1990).

The cognitive-behavioral approach emphasizes not only partner and relationship behavior but also partners' interpretation of this behavior. For example, compared to people who are satisfied with their relationship, dissatisfied partners are more likely to attribute each other's negative behavior to broad and stable traits, and to view negative partner behavior as selfishly motivated and worthy of blame (Bradbury & Fincham, 1990). Dissatisfied partners are also more likely to hold dysfunctional, extreme, or unreasonable assumptions (i.e., beliefs about how things are), standards (i.e., beliefs about how things should be), and expectations (i.e., beliefs about how things will be) with respect to themselves, their partners, and their relationship (Baucom, Epstein, Sayers, & Sher, 1989). Satisfied partners are more likely than dissatisfied partners to hold positive cognitive biases. For example, individuals who are satisfied with their relationship view their partners in a more positive light than their partners view themselves, and people who idealize their partners, and have their partners idealize them are happier in their relationships (Murray, Holmes, & Griffin, 1996).

Attachment Theory and MRD

A great deal is written about the role of attachment theory and relationship distress (e.g., Kobak, Ruckdeschel, Hazan, Johnson, & Greenberg, 1994; Mikulincer & Shaver, 2007; Simpson & Rholes, 1998). Basic research has demonstrated that individual differences in attachment styles are associated with MRD. A large body of evidence indicates that adults' behaviors and emotional responses to attachment-related threats can be understood along two dimensions—anxiety and avoidance—with people high in anxiety engaging in *hyperactivating* responses and people high in avoidance engaging in *deactivating* responses (Mikulincer & Shaver, 2007). Although it is widely believed that attachment anxiety and avoidance serve the adaptive function of helping people regulate the experience of felt security, adults with high anxiety and/or avoidance dimensions are at-risk for MRD, because they are at times either too engaged and enmeshed in attachment themes (hyperactivating) or too distant and disconnected (deactivating). Another way of understanding this process is that what may be an adaptive and functional means of regulating emotions outside of a relationship does not easily translate to relational dynamics; the larger the attachment discrepancy between partners, the greater the risk for MRD (cf. Banse, 2004; Treboux, Crowell, & Waters, 2004).

In one of the first mechanistic studies of attachment styles and marital satisfaction, Davila, Bradbury, and Fincham (1998) found that "negative affectivity," which they defined as the stable tendency to experience and express negative emotion, mediated the association between husbands' and wives' attachment anxiety (about abandonment) and marital satisfaction. The results of this study also revealed an interesting partner effect, in which husbands' satisfaction was negatively associated with wives' anxiety (with no effect from husbands' to wives); in this study, men's marital satisfaction was associated with their partners' attachment style but not the other way around, suggesting that it is important to consider sex-specific effects when studying the link between attachment and marital satisfaction or discord (Davila et al., 1998). Other research suggests that high levels of attachment security associated with high levels of marital satisfaction promote positive perceptions of one's partner, which, in turn, are associated with greater social support behavior (Cobb, Davila, & Bradbury, 2001).

Contextual Variables and MRD

Although a great deal can be learned about the etiology of MRB by considering within- and between-person processes, most of the work discussed earlier says little about the contextual circumstances that increase risk for MRD. The last 10 years

have witnessed a surge of research dedicated to understanding how life circumstances are associated with relational quality (Karney & Bradbury, 1995, 2005; Story
& Bradbury, 2004). It is well-established that financial hardship and daily stress
increase risk for divorce (Lavee, McCubbin, & Olson, 1987), and a major focus of
the research in this area is to understand how external forces are associated with
decreases in marital quality and increases in MRD. Important distinctions in this
area include whether the stressors are chronic (e.g., job loss) or acute (e.g., a heavy
workload), and whether individuals and couples can adjust to these demands (Story
& Bradbury, 2004). An excellent example of the stress–adjustment process was
observed in a study by Thompson and Bolger (1999), who investigated daily moods
and feelings about the relationship in 68 couples for 1 month while one member of
the couple prepared for the New York State Bar Exam. The findings revealed that
between-partner rates of emotional transmission were strongest at the start of the
study, but diminished significantly as the bar exam approached, which the authors
argued might reflect a recognition of the potential emotional transmission as the
stressful event became more salient. When external stressors decay relationship
quality, how do these *spillover* processes operate? Neff and Karney (2004) assessed
82 newlywed couples every 6 months for the first 4 years of marriage and found
that wives who experienced the highest levels of stress spillover demonstrated the
greatest declines in marital satisfaction over the study. Importantly, as reported of
stress levels increased, wives reported a corresponding increase in the perceptions
of specific relationship problems, and these negative cognitions mediated the association between stress and relationship quality. Neff and Karney noted, "Stress may
lead to lower satisfaction by hindering spouses' ability to separate negative specific
relationship perceptions from their global relationship satisfaction" (p. 145). Story
and Repetti (2006) provided a conceptual replication of the spillover effect, demonstrating that negative mood mediated the association between wives' daily workload and marital anger. Building on this research, Neff and Karney (2007) provided
another replication of the spillover effect and also found evidence for a dyadic *crossover* effect, whereby husbands reported lower satisfaction when their wives experienced higher stress. This latter finding demonstrates that mediating processes linking contextual variables and relationship quality must be considered in terms of
moderating processes that include different effects for husbands and wives.

One of the best-studied contextual factors impacting marital satisfaction is the
transition to parenthood, especially for couples having their first child (Cowan &
Cowan, 2000). Cowan and Cowan (1995) reported that following the birth of a first
child, about 15% of men and women move from above to below the clinical cutoff
for marital distress on standard self-report assessment instruments. A meta-analysis of studies on parenthood and marital satisfaction found that parents report
lower marital satisfaction compared to nonparents, and that marital satisfaction
was negatively correlated with the number of children (Twenge, Campbell, & Foster, 2003). However, the effect sizes obtained from the meta-analysis were small in
magnitude and moderated by individual differences: The effect of parenthood on

marital satisfaction was stronger for younger couples and people from higher socio-economic groups. Recent evidence suggests that these declines are *more* pronounced in couples who are highly satisfied with the first 6 month of marriage relative to less satisfied couples (Lawrence, Rothman, Cobb, Rothman, & Bradbury, 2008).

Clinical Implications

The brief overview of etiological models of MRD offers several directions for treatment that may help in preventing or treating MRD. For example, the cognitive-behavioral model suggests that increasing rates of positive relationship behaviors, improving communication and problem-solving skills, and recognizing and modifying unrealistic or distorted cognitions should improve relationship quality. Indeed, research has shown that cognitive-behavioral couple therapy is effective in decreasing negative communication behaviors and cognition, and increasing relationship satisfaction (e.g., Halford, Sanders, & Behrens, 1993).

The attachment theory suggests that helping couples change their emotional engagement, responsiveness, and soothing behaviors should improve the quality of their relationship. Changing these patterns of relating is the focus of emotion-focused couple therapy (EFCT; Johnson, 1996). Process-level research demonstrates that changes in these patterns of relating are associated with positive outcomes in EFCT. Using a task analysis methodology, Greenberg, Ford, Alden, and Johnson (1993), for example, reported on three EFCT studies demonstrating that couples were significantly more supportive, affirming, and understanding with each other at the end of treatment than at the beginning; that greater affiliation and depth of experiencing was highly associated with couple-rated "peak" session events, as were self-focused disclosing and expressions of emotion; and that therapist-facilitated intimate self-disclosures increased affiliative behaviors within a couple. Together, these findings suggest that EFCT exerts its effects in a manner consistent with attachment theory; although more comprehensive mechanistic studies are needed, it appears that teaching partners to use each other as a secure base and to engage in behaviors that soften and deepen the emotional connection within the relationship are among the key elements for the successful treatment of MRD.

Finally, helping couples during times of stress, including the transition to parenthood, should result in improving the quality of their relationship. Indeed, there is evidence that declines in marital quality during the transition to parenthood are preventable. In the largest prevention trial to date, Schulz, Cowan, and Cowan (2006) reported that relative to a control group, a 24-week couple group that included support, communication training, parenting discussions, and specific attention to the issues and events that affect satisfaction in new parents buffered against declines in satisfaction up to 66 months after the birth of a first child. These findings are promising and demonstrate that preventive interventions can forestall the onset of MRD for couples over the transition to parenthood. An issue for further investigation is the therapeutic dosing needed to achieve these effects. Over 2 hours of weekly meetings for 6 months is burdensome for participants; whether this amount of time is required to achieve long-term benefits remains to be determined.

TREATMENT OUTCOME

In a meta-analysis of 20 couple therapy outcome studies (specifically targeting couple distress), Byrne, Carr, and Clark (2004) reported large effect sizes for behavioral couple therapy (BCT) and EFCT. Specifically, the mean effect size for posttreatment couple distress was 0.95 for BCT and 1.27 for EFCT, indicating that couples in BCT and EFCT fared better at the end of treatment than 83 and 89% of untreated couples, respectively. In BCT, the mean percentage of couples falling into the nondistressed range of functioning 6 months to 4 years after treatment was 54%; across four studies, recovery rates for EFCT were similar, with 53% of couples falling into the nondistressed range of functioning 2 months to 2 years after treatment (Byrne et al., 2004). These effect sizes are comparable to (if not stronger than) the effects frequently observed for the treatment of other disorders (Smith & Glass, 1977). Consistent with the evidence on the effectiveness of couple therapy for relational discord is research demonstrating that couple-level interventions are effective for a range of disorders. In couple therapy, it is important to recognize that clinically significant change *in both partners* is often hard to demonstrate. Christensen and Heavey (1999) reviewed data from multiple studies indicating that only 35–41% of couple treatments were successful in moving from distressed to nondistressed levels. More recent evidence suggests higher recovery rates in other treatments (Christensen et al., 2004; Johnson, Hunsley, Greenberg, & Schindler, 1999; Snyder et al., 2006), but systematic analyses of clinically significant change are needed before these more recent investigations can be said to improve upon well-established rates of change.

Related to the question of recovery and clinically significant change is the durability of treatment effects for MRD. Early studies of couple therapy often failed to include follow-up data beyond 6 months. In the first follow-up studies of BCT spanning 1- and 2-year marks, many couples deteriorated below their pretest levels of functioning, but the active behavioral therapy treatment package performed consistently better than its two major component comparison treatments (Jacobson, 1985; Jacobson, Schmaling, & Holtzworth-Munroe, 1987). At the 2-year follow-up, for example, 30% of participants in the active treatment had relapsed (relative to 78 and 57%, respectively, in the comparison treatments). In one of the longer follow-up studies to date, Snyder, Wills, and Grady-Fletcher (1991) found that insight-oriented couple therapy (IOCT) led to fewer divorces at 4-year follow-up than BCT; specifically, 38% of the couples in BCT divorced, compared with only 3% of the couples in IOCT. Snyder et al. also noted that at 4-year follow-up, 58% of couples in BCT were unchanged or had deteriorated from their pretreatment levels. More recent analyses suggest that the treatment gains of BCT can be maintained for at least 2 years. In a comparison of BCT to integrative behavioral couple therapy (IBCT), more than half the participants in both groups (69% of IBCT couples and 60% of BCT couples) showed *clinically significant* improvements 2 years posttreatment (Christensen, Atkins, Yi, Baucom, & George, 2006). This durability finding is especially significant, because couples in the BCT–IBCT trial were selected for being chronically distressed and dissatisfied with their relationship (see Christensen et al., 2004).

Clinical Implications

When looking across the multiple efficacious treatments for couples, what factors can be derived that would be considered general principles, or unifying themes, of change? Although entire volumes are dedicated to different perspectives on this issue (e.g., Gurman, 2008), efforts have been made to integrate diverse themes in the treatment of MRD. Sprenkle and Blow (2004), for example, highlight three nonspecific (general) treatment variables that are common to marriage and family therapies: behavioral regulation (i.e., changing interactional patterns among and between people), cognitive mastery (i.e., clients gaining new perspectives about themselves and their partners, as well as new insights into interaction processes), and emotional experiencing (i.e., clients changing the way their experience and respond to emotional events. These therapeutic processes are common to many individual interventions as well, and Sprenkle and Blow further suggest three common factors unique to couple and family treatments: relational conceptualizations (i.e., a view of family problems as relational in nature and embedded in the relationship context), expanded direct treatment system (i.e., a push in most couple treatments to treat the couple over the individual), and the expanded therapeutic alliance (i.e., the therapist must form a strong alliance with both members of the couple). As another example, Snyder, Schneider, and Castellani (2003) proposed an organizational model for sequencing and pacing couple interventions using a pluralistic approach that draws on diverse theoretical perspectives and interventions. In short, these authors proposed six levels of intervention that progress across three broad domains. This model begins with the use of interventions that establish a collaborative alliance, contain crises (e.g., physical aggression, infidelity), and strengthen the couple's relationship. This is followed by behavioral techniques (e.g., communication skills training) that promote relevant relationship skills. Finally, the model encourages the use of cognitive and insight-oriented approaches to address intrapersonal factors (e.g., unrealistic standards, previous relationship injuries) linked to relationship functioning.

Beyond these common factors, one way to think about unifying principles for treating MRD is to consider what changes need to occur for most couples who experience clinically significant MRD. Of course, there exists no mean or modal couple, and functional analytic assessment of idiographic, controlling variables plays as important a role in couple treatment as in individual treatment. The dangers of generalities notwithstanding, the most common reasons that couples give for seeking couple therapy are problematic communication and lack of emotional affection (Doss, Simpson, & Christensen, 2004). Similarly, couple therapists report that the most common problems in couples presenting for therapy are communication, power struggles, and unrealistic expectations in the relationship one's partner (Whisman, Dixon, & Johnson, 1997). Consequently, regardless of the treatment approach a therapist chooses, we believe skilled clinicians typically target the following areas for decreasing MRD: (1) negative attributions about a partner and his or her intentions during relationship events; (2) difficulties understanding, tolerating, and accepting a partner's affective experiences; (3) difficulties expressing and sharing affective experiences in a satisfying way; and (4) difficulties engaging in behaviors that promote and do not deteriorate relationship quality, including experiencing and engaging in relationship conflicts, or fights, in a manner that does not leave lasting emotional hurt.

We make no claim that addressing these problem areas is necessary *or* sufficient for decreasing MRD, only that these are a few of the most fundamental areas addressed by couple therapists. It is beyond the scope of this chapter to spell out the specific techniques therapists use to address these areas, but we do note that—just as in many individual treatments—successful outcomes often hinge on instructing couples to do more or less of specific behaviors. For example, when couples complain of too little intimacy (not enough shared activities and/or too little emotional expression), each person is invited to change what he or she is doing in a way that seems acceptable to the partner. Once one or both members of the couple attempt to change specific behaviors, the question of behavioral deficits or performance difficulties is paramount. Said differently, does each individual have the skills necessary to enact agreed-upon changes, or does time need to be spent in therapy learning about specific modes of communication, emotional sharing and deepening, ways of disarming a heated fight? Like individual treatments, successful outcomes in couple therapy hinge on identifying the major problem areas, then solidifying behavioral changes through the repeated actions of one or both partners that support the desired changes.

General Contributions to Treatment

Research on client's variables has also provided evidence that might help clinicians decide who might benefit from MRD, and newly emerging data are beginning to shed light on the moderators of treatment durability effects. Baucom, Atkins, Simpson, and Christensen (2009) investigated the predictors of 2-year outcomes in the BCT–IBCT trial discussed earlier. Moderation analyses revealed that none of the intrapersonal distress (e.g., overall mental health, high neuroticism) or interpersonal variables (e.g., commitment, sexual satisfaction, power bases) predicted long-term treatment outcome, nor did any of the self-reported communication variables (e.g., demand–withdraw patterns, constructive communication); instead, several of the behavioral communication variables interacted with type of treatment to predict long-term treatment response (Baucom et al., 2009). For example, the use of "soft influence" tactics (i.e., couple-level patterns of language that reflect a collaborative style free of manipulation and pressure for change) predicted improved response in IBCT, with high influence tactics predicting an increased likelihood of a couple being classified as having deteriorated functioning at the follow-up. Influence patterns were not associated with treatment response within BCT. These findings are among the first long-term aptitude 1 × 1 treatment interactions in couple therapy research (see Shoham & Rohrbaugh, 1995), and this approach should be used as a model for future studies.

Furthermore, because MRD predicts the onset and/or course of some forms of psychopathology, it is also reasonable to assume that improving relationship functioning may improve the mental health and well-being of partners more generally. Indeed, there is good evidence that couple therapy can be effective in terms of improving not only relationship quality but also mental health outcomes. In a mega-analysis of 20 meta-analyses of different couple therapies, Shadish and Baldwin (2003) reported that the average person receiving treatment for couple therapy was better off at the end of treatment than 80% of the no-treatment control group. A more focused meta-analysis of 30 studies comparing BCT to a no-treatment control found a smaller effect size ($d = 0.59$) but clearly demonstrated that BCT is effective over a range of clinical representative conditions (Shadish & Baldwin, 2005).

There are two specific forms of psychopathology for which couple therapy has been shown to be effective. First, couple therapy has been shown to be an effective treatment for depression. Results from a meta-analysis of eight controlled trials reported no differences between couple therapy and individual psychotherapy in the treatment of depression (measured in terms of either depressive symptoms or persistence of depression) and that couple therapy was more effective than individual psychotherapy in improving MRD, particularly among couples in distressed relationships at the beginning of treatment (Barbato & D'Avanzo, 2008). Second, BCT has been shown to be an effective treatment for substance use disorders. A meta-analysis of 12 controlled trials reported that couple therapy was more effective than individual-based treatments in improving relationship satisfaction at posttreatment, and more effective than individual-based treatments in impacting frequency of use, consequences of use, and relationship satisfaction at follow-up (Powers et al., 2008). Other reviews have concluded that compared to individual-based treatments for substance abuse, BCT results in significantly higher reductions in partner violence, greater improvements in psychosocial functioning of children, and better cost–benefit results and cost-effectiveness (Fals-Stewart, O'Farrell, Birchler, Cordova, & Kelley, 2005).

CONCLUSION

Humans are naturally motivated to form and maintain interpersonal bonds, and most people spend much of their adult life married or in a marriage-like relationship. Consequently, many people experience relationship discord, and the associated emotional and behavioral sequelae, at least some time in their life. In this chapter, we have provided an overview of the presentation, classification, prevalence and course, comorbidities, and available treatment options of MRD. It is our hope that continued research on the onset, prevention, and treatment of MRD will help with respect to not only improved interpersonal relationships but also greater quality of life, and improved physical and mental health.

REFERENCES

American Psychiatric Association. (1994). *Diagnostic and statistical manual of mental disorders* (4th ed.). Washington, DC: Author.

American Psychiatric Association. (2013). *Diagnostic and statistical manual of mental disorders* (5th ed.). Arlington, VA: Author.

Baker, L. A., & Emery, R. E. (1993). When every relationship is above average. *Law and Human Behavior, 17*(4), 439–450.

Banse, R. (2004). Adult attachment and marital satisfaction: Evidence for dyadic configuration effects. *Journal of Social and Personal Relationships, 21*, 273–282.

Barbato, A., & D'Avanzo, B. (2008). Efficacy of couple therapy as a treatment for depression: A meta-analysis. *Psychiatric Quarterly, 79*, 121–132.

Baucom, B. R., Atkins, D. C., Simpson, L. E., & Christensen, A. (2009). Prediction of response to treatment in a randomized clinical trial of couple therapy: A 2-year follow-up. *Journal of Consulting and Clinical Psychology, 77*, 160–173.

Baucom, D. H., Epstein, N., Sayers, S., & Sher, T. G. (1989). The role of cognitions in marital relationships: Definitional, methodological, and conceptual issues. *Journal of Consulting and Clinical Psychology, 57*, 31–38.

Baucom, D. H., Hahlweg, K., & Kuschel, A. (2003). Are waiting-list control groups needed in future marital therapy outcome research? *Behavior Therapy, 34*, 179–188.

Beach, S. R. H., Fincham, F. D., Amir, N., & Leonard, K. E. (2005). The taxometrics of marriage: Is marital discord categorical? *Journal of Family Psychology, 19*, 276–285.

Beach, S. R. H., Wamboldt, M. Z., Kaslow, N. J., Reiss, D., & Heyman, R. E. (2006). Describing relationship problems in DSM-V: Toward better guidance for research and clinical practice. *Journal of Family Psychology, 20*, 359–368.

Bradbury, T. N., & Fincham, F. D. (1990). Attributions in marriage: Review and critique. *Psychological Bulletin, 107*, 3–33.

Bradbury, T. N., & Karney, B. R. (1993). Longitudinal study of marital interaction and dysfunction: Review and analysis. *Clinical Psychology Review, 13*, 15–27.

Bramlett, M. D., & Mosher, W. D. (2002). *Cohabitation, marriage, divorce, and remarriage in the United States.* Hyattsville, MD: National Center for Health Statistics.

Brown, G. W., & Harris, T. (1978). *Social origins of depression: A study of psychiatric disorder in women.* London: Tavistock.

Byrne, M., Carr, A., & Clark, M. (2004). The efficacy of behavioral couples therapy and emotionally focused therapy for couples distress. *Contemporary Family Therapy, 26*, 361–387.

Cascardi, M., Langhinrichsen, J., & Vivian, D. (1992). Marital aggression: Impact, injury, and health correlates for husbands and wives. *Archives of Internal Medicine, 152*, 1178–1184.

Cascardi, M., O'Leary, K. D., Lawrence, E. E., & Schlee, K. A. (1995). Characteristics of women physically abused by their spouses and who seek treatment regarding marital conflict. *Journal of Consulting and Clinical Psychology, 63*, 616–623.

Choi, H., & Marks, N. F. (2008). Marital conflict, depressive symptoms, and functional impairment. *Journal of Marriage and Family, 70*, 377–390.

Christensen, A., Atkins, D. C., Berns, S., Wheeler, J., Baucom, D. H., & Simpson, L. E. (2004).

Traditional versus integrative behavioral couple therapy for significantly and chronically distressed married couples. *Journal of Consulting and Clinical Psychology, 72,* 176–191.

Christensen, A., Atkins, D. C., Yi, J., Baucom, D. H., & George, W. H. (2006). Couple and individual adjustment for 2 years following a randomized clinical trial comparing traditional versus integrative behavioral couple therapy. *Journal of Consulting and Clinical Psychology, 74,* 1180–1191.

Christensen, A., & Heavey, C. L. (1990). Gender and social structure in the demand/withdraw pattern of marital conflict. *Journal of Personality and Social Psychology, 59,* 73–81.

Christensen, A., & Heavey, C. L. (1999). Interventions for couples. *Annual Review of Psychology, 50,* 165–190.

Cobb, R. J., Davila, J., & Bradbury, T. N. (2001). Attachment security and marital satisfaction: The role of positive perceptions and social support. *Personality and Social Psychology Bulletin, 27,* 1131–1143.

Corra, M., Carter, S. K., Carter, J. S., & Knox, D. (2009). Trends in marital happiness by gender and race, 1973 to 2006. *Journal of Family Issues, 30,* 1379–1404.

Cowan, C. P., & Cowan, P. A. (1995). Interventions to ease the transition to parenthood: Why they are needed and what they can do. *Family Relations, 44,* 412–423.

Cowan, C. P., & Cowan, P. A. (2000). *When partners become parents: The big life change for couples.* Mahwah, NJ: Erlbaum.

Davila, J., Bradbury, T. N., & Fincham, F. (1998). Negative affectivity as a mediator of the association between adult attachment and marital satisfaction. *Personal Relationships, 5,* 467–484.

Davila, J., Karney, B. R., Hall, T. W., & Bradbury, T. N. (2003). Depressive symptoms and marital satisfaction: Within-subject associations and the moderating effects of gender and neuroticism. *Journal of Family Psychology, 17,* 557–570.

Denton, W. H. (2007). Issues for DSM-V: Relational diagnosis: An essential component of biopsychosocial assessment. *American Journal of Psychiatry, 164,* 1146–1147.

Doss, B. D., Simpson, L. E., & Christensen, A. (2004). Why do couples seek marital therapy? *Professional Psychology: Research and Practice, 35,* 608–614.

Dunn, K. M., Croft, P. R., & Hackett, G. I. (1999). Association of sexual problems with social, psychological, and physical problems in men and women: A cross sectional population survey. *Journal of Epidemiology and Community Health, 53,* 144–148.

Durham, R. C., Allan, T., & Hackett, C. A. (1997). On predicting improvement and relapse in generalized anxiety disorder following psychotherapy. *British Journal of Clinical Psychology, 36,* 101–119.

Emery, R. E., & Sbarra, D. A. (2002). What couples therapists need to know about divorce. In A. Gurman & N. Jacobson (Eds.), *Clinical handbook of couple therapy,* (3rd ed., pp. 502–532). New York: Guilford Press.

Fals-Stewart, W., O'Farrell, T. J., Birchler, G. R., Cordova, J., & Kelley, M. L. (2005). Behavioral couples therapy for alcoholism and drug abuse: Where we've been, where we are, and where we're going. *Journal of Cognitive Psychotherapy, 19,* 229–246.

Fals-Stewart, W., O'Farrell, T. J., & Hooley, J. M. (2001). Relapse among married or cohabiting substance-abusing patients: The role of perceived criticism. *Behavior Therapy, 32,* 787–801.

First, M. B., Bell, C. C., Cuthbert, B., Malison, R., Reiss, D., Widiger, T., et al. (2002). Personality disorders and relational disorders: A research agenda for addressing crucial gaps in DSM. In T. Widiger & K. L. Wisner (Eds.), *A research agenda for DSM-V* (pp. 123–199). Washington, DC: American Psychiatric Association.

Fleeson, W. (2004). The quality of the American life at the end of the century. In O. G. Brim, C. D. Ryff, & R. C. Kessler (Eds.), *How healthy are we?: A national study of well-being at midlife* (pp. 252–272). Chicago: University of Chicago Press.

Gottman, J. M. (1979). *Marital interaction: Experimental investigations.* San Diego: Academic Press.

Gottman, J. M. (1994). *What predicts divorce?: The relationship between marital processes and marital outcomes.* Hillsdale, NJ: Erlbaum.

Gottman, J. M., Driver, J., & Tabares, A. (2002). Building a sound marital house: An empirically derived couple therapy. In A. S. Gurman & N. S. Jacobson (Eds.), *Clinical handbook of couple therapy* (3rd ed., pp. 373–400). New York: Guilford Press.

Greenberg, L. S., Ford, C. L., Alden, L. S., & Johnson, S. M. (1993). In-session change in emotionally focused therapy. *Journal of Consulting and Clinical Psychology, 61,* 78–84.

Gurman, A. S. (2008). *Clinical handbook of couple therapy* (4th ed.). New York: Guilford Press.

Halford, W. K., Sanders, M. R., & Behrens, B. C. (1993). A comparison of the generalization of behavioral marital therapy and enhanced behavioral marital therapy. *Journal of Consulting and Clinical Psychology, 61,* 51–60.

House, J. S., Landis, K. R., & Umberson, D. (1988). Social relationships and health. *Science, 241,* 540–545.

Jacobson, N. S. (1985). A component analysis of behavioral marital therapy: 1–year follow-up. *Behaviour Research and Therapy, 23,* 549–555.

Jacobson, N. S., Follette, W. C., Revenstorf, D., Baucom, D. H., Hahlweg, K., & Margolin, G. (1984). Variability in outcome and clinical significance of behavioral marital therapy: A reanalysis of outcome data. *Journal of Consulting and Clinical Psychology, 52,* 497–504.

Jacobson, N. S., Schmaling, K. B., & Holtzworth-Munroe, A. (1987). Component analysis of behavioral marital therapy: 2-year follow-up and prediction of relapse. *Journal of Marital and Family Therapy, 13,* 187–195.

Johnson, S. M. (1996). *The practice of emotionally focused marital therapy: Creating connection.* Philadelphia, PA US: Brunner/Mazel.

Johnson, S., Hunsley, J., Greenberg, L., & Schindler, D. (1999). Emotionally focused couples therapy: Status & challenges. *Clinical Psychology: Science & Practice, 6,* 67–79.

Karney, B. R., & Bradbury, T. N. (1995). The longitudinal course of marital quality and stability: A review of theory, method, and research. *Psychological Bulletin, 118,* 3–34.

Karney, B. R., & Bradbury, T. N. (2005). Contextual influences on marriage: Implications for policy and intervention. *Current Directions in Psychological Science, 14,* 171–174.

Kaslow, F., & Patterson, T. (2006). Relational diagnosis—a brief historical overview: Comment on the special section. *Journal of Family Psychology, 20,* 428–431.

Kelley, H. H., & Thibaut, J. W. (1978). *Interpersonal relations: A theory of interdependence.* New York: Wiley.

Kiecolt-Glaser, J. K., Malarkey, W. B., Chee, M., Newton, T., Cacioppo, J. T., Mao, H. Y., et al. (1993). Negative behavior during marital conflict is associated with immunological down-regulation. *Psychosomatic Medicine, 55,* 395–409.

Kiecolt-Glaser, J., & Newton, T. L. (2001). Marriage and health: His and hers. *Psychological Bulletin, 127,* 472–503.

Kobak, R., Ruckdeschel, K., Hazan, C., Johnson, S. M., & Greenberg, L. S. (1994). From symptom to signal: An attachment view of emotion in marital therapy. In S. M. Johnson & L. S. Greenberg (Eds.), *The heart of the matter: Perspectives on emotion in marital therapy* (pp. 46–71). Philadelphia: Brunner/Mazel.

Kraus, D. R., Seligman, D. A., & Jordan, J. R. (2004). Validation of a behavioral health treatment outcome and assessment tool designed for naturalistic settings: The Treatment Outcome Package. *Journal of Clinical Psychology, 61,* 285–314.

Kreider, R. M., & Fields, J. M. (2001). *Number, timing, and duration of marriages and divorces: Fall 1996* [Current Population Reports, P70-80]. Washington, DC: U.S. Census Bureau.

Kurdek, L. A. (2005). Gender and marital satisfaction early in marriage: A growth curve approach. *Journal of Marriage and Family, 67,* 68–84.

Lavee, Y., McCubbin, H. I., & Olson, D. H. (1987). The effect of stressful life events and transitions on family functioning and well-being. *Journal of Marriage and the Family, 49,* 857–873.

Lawrence, E., Rothman, A. D., Cobb, R. J., Rothman, M. T., & Bradbury, T. N. (2008). Marital satisfaction across the transition to parenthood. *Journal of Family Psychology, 22,* 41–50.

Levenson, R. W., Carstensen, L. L., & Gottman, J. M. (1994). The influence of age and gender on affect, physiology, and their interrelations: A study of long-term marriages. *Journal of Personality and Social Psychology, 67,* 56–68.

Malarkey, W. B., Kiecolt-Glaser, J. K., Pearl, D., & Glaser, R. (1994). Hostile behavior during marital conflict alters pituitary and adrenal hormones. *Psychosomatic Medicine, 56,* 41–51.

Markowitz, J. S., Weissman, M. M., Ouellette, R., Lish, J. D., & Klerman, G. L. (1989). Quality of life in panic disorder. *Archives of General Psychiatry, 46,* 984–992.

Martin, E. K., Taft, C. T., & Resick, P. A. (2007). A review of marital rape. *Aggression and Violent Behavior, 12,* 329–347.

McLeod, J. D. (1994). Anxiety disorders and marital quality. *Journal of Abnormal Psychology, 103,* 767–776.

Mikulincer, M., & Shaver, P. R. (2007). *Attachment in adulthood: Structure, dynamics, and change.* New York: Guilford Press.

Murray, S. L., Holmes, J. G., & Griffin, D. W. (1996). The benefits of positive illusions: Idealization and the construction of satisfaction in close relationships. *Journal of Personality and Social Psychology, 70,* 79–98.

Neff, L. A., & Karney, B. R. (2004). How does context affect intimate relationships?: Linking external stress and cognitive processes within marriage. *Personality and Social Psychology Bulletin, 30,* 134–148.

Neff, L. A., & Karney, B. R. (2007). Stress crossover in newlywed marriage: A longitudinal and dyadic perspective. *Journal of Marriage and Family, 69,* 594–607.

Norton, R. (1983). Measuring marital quality: A critical look at the dependent variable. *Journal of Marriage and the Family, 45,* 141–151.

O'Leary, K. D., & Gurman, A. S. (2008). Couple therapy and physical aggression. In A. S. Gurman (Ed.), *Clinical handbook of couple therapy* (4th ed., pp. 478–498). New York: Guilford Press.

O'Leary, K. D., Smith Slep, A. M., & O'Leary, S. G. (2007). Multivariate models of men's and women's partner aggression. *Journal of Consulting and Clinical Psychology, 75,* 752–764.

O'Leary, K. D., & Woodin, E. M. (2009). *Psychological and physical aggression in couples: Causes and interventions.* Washington, DC: American Psychological Association.

Overbeek, G., Vollebergh, W., de Graaf, R., Scholte, R., de Kemp, R., & Engels, R. (2006). Longitudinal associations of marital quality and marital dissolution with the incidence of DSM-III-R disorders. *Journal of Family Psychology, 20,* 284–291.

Powers, M. B., Vedel, E., & Emmelkamp, P. M. G. (2008). Behavioral couples therapy (BCT) for alcohol and drug use disorders: A meta-analysis. *Clinical Psychology Review, 28,* 952–962.

Proulx, C. M., Helms, H. M., & Buehler, C. (2007). Marital quality and personal well-being: A meta-analysis. *Journal of Marriage and Family, 69,* 576–593.

Robles, T. F., & Kiecolt-Glaser, J. K. (2003). The physiology of marriage: Pathways to health. *Physiology and Behavior, 79,* 409–416.

Rogers, S. J., & May, D. C. (2003). Spillover between marital quality and job satisfaction: Long-term patterns and gender differences. *Journal of Marriage and Family, 65,* 482–495.

Rohrbaugh, M. J., Shoham, V., & Coyne, J. C. (2006). Effect of marital quality on eight-year survival of patients with heart failure. *American Journal of Cardiology, 98,* 1069–1072.

Sbarra, D. A., & Allen, J. J. B. (2009). Decomposing depression: On the prospective and reciprocal dynamics of mood and sleep disturbances. *Journal of Abnormal Psychology, 118,* 171–182.

Schoenborn, C. (2004). *Marital status and health: United States, 1999–2002* [Advance data from vital and health statistics, No. 351]. Hyattsville, MD: National Center for Health Statistics.

Schulz, M. S., Cowan, C. P., & Cowan, P. A. (2006). Promoting healthy beginnings: A randomized controlled trial of a preventive intervention to preserve marital quality during the transition to parenthood. *Journal of Consulting and Clinical Psychology, 74*, 20–31.

Shadish, W. R., & Baldwin, S. A. (2003). Meta-analysis of MFT interventions. *Journal of Marital and Family Therapy, 29*, 547–570.

Shadish, W. R., & Baldwin, S. A. (2005). Effects of behavioral marital therapy: A meta-analysis of randomized controlled trials. *Journal of Consulting and Clinical Psychology, 73*, 6–14.

Shoham, V., & Rohrbaugh, M. J. (1995). Aptitude × treatment interaction (ATI) research: Sharpening the focus, widening the lens. In M. Aveline & D. Shapiro (Eds.), *Research foundations for psychotherapy practice* (pp. 73–95). Sussex, UK: Wiley.

Simpson, J. A., & Rholes, W. S. (1998). *Attachment theory and close relationships.* New York: Guilford Press.

Smith, M. L., & Glass, G. V. (1977). Meta-analysis of psychotherapy outcome studies. *American Psychologist, 32*, 752–760.

Smith, M. T., & Perlis, M. L. (2006). Who is a candidate for cognitive-behavioral therapy for insomnia? *Health Psychology, 25*, 15–19.

Snyder, D. K. (1997). *Manual for the Marital Satisfaction Inventory—Revised.* Los Angeles: Western Psychological Services.

Snyder, D. K., Castellani, A. M., & Whisman, M. A. (2006). Current status and future directions in couple therapy. *Annual Review of Psychology, 57*, 317–344.

Snyder, D. K., Heyman, R. E., & Haynes, S. N. (2005). Evidence-based approaches to assessing couple distress. *Psychological Assessment, 17*, 288–307.

Snyder, D. K., Schneider, W. J., & Castellani, A. M. (2003). Tailoring couple therapy to individual differences: A conceptual approach. In D. K. Snyder & M. A. Whisman (Eds.), *Treating difficult couples: Helping clients with coexisting mental and relationship disorders* (pp. 27–51). New York: Guilford Press.

Snyder, D. K., Wills, R. M., & Grady-Fletcher, A. (1991). Long-term effectiveness of behavioral versus insight-oriented marital therapy: A 4–year follow-up study. *Journal of Consulting and Clinical Psychology, 59*, 138–141.

South, S. C., Turkheimer, E., & Oltmanns, T. F. (2008). Personality disorder symptoms and marital functioning. *Journal of Consulting and Clinical Psychology, 76*, 769–780.

Spanier, G. B. (1976). Measuring dyadic adjustment: New scales for assessing the quality of marriage and similar dyads. *Journal of Marriage and the Family, 35*, 15–28.

Sprenkle, D., & Blow, A. (2004). Common factors and our sacred models. *Journal of Marital and Family Therapy, 30*, 113–129.

Story, L. B., & Bradbury, T. N. (2004). Understanding marriage and stress: Essential questions and challenges. *Clinical Psychology Review, 23*, 1139–1162.

Story, L. B., & Repetti, R. (2006). Daily occupational stressors and marital behavior. *Journal of Family Psychology, 20*, 690–700.

Sullivan, H. S. (1953). *The interpersonal theory of psychiatry.* New York: Norton.

Tejada-Vera, B., & Sutton, P. (2009). *Births, marriages, divorces, and deaths: Provisional data for July 2008* [National Vital Statistics Reports, Vol. 57, No. 13]. Hyattsville, MD: National Center for Health Statistics.

Thompson, A., & Bolger, N. (1999). Emotional transmission in couples under stress. *Journal of Marriage and the Family, 61*, 38–48.

Treboux, D., Crowell, J. A., & Waters, E. (2004). When "new" meets "old": Configurations of adult attachment representations and their implications for marital functioning. *Developmental Psychology, 40*, 295–314.

Troxel, W. M., Buysse, D. J., Hall, M., & Matthews, K. A. (2009). Marital happiness and sleep disturbances in a multi-ethnic sample of middle-aged women. *Behavioral Sleep Medicine, 7*, 2–19.

Twenge, J. M., Campbell, W. K., & Foster, C. A. (2003). Parenthood and marital satisfaction: A meta-analytic review. *Journal of Marriage and Family, 65*, 574–583.

VanLaningham, J., Johnson, D. R., & Amato, P. (2001). Marital happiness, marital duration, and the U-shaped curve: Evidence from a five-wave panel study. *Social Forces, 78*, 1313–1341.

Wade, T. J., & Pevalin, D. J. (2004). Marital transitions and mental health. *Journal of Health and Social Behavior, 45*, 155–170.

Wang, P. S., Lane, M., Olfson, M., Pincus, H. A., Wells, K. B., & Kessler, R. C. (2005). Twelve-month use of mental health services in the United States: Results from the National Comorbidity Survey Replication. *Archives of General Psychiatry, 62*, 629–640.

Wamboldt, M. Z., & Wamboldt, F. S. (2000). Role of the family in the onset and outcome of childhood disorders: Selected research findings. *Journal of the American Academy of Child and Adolescent Psychiatry, 39*, 1212–1219.

Weissman, M. M. (1987). Advances in psychiatric epidemiology: Rates and risks for major depression. *American Journal of Public Health, 77*, 445–451.

Whisman, M. A. (1999). Marital dissatisfaction and psychiatric disorders: Results from the National Comorbidity Survey. *Journal of Abnormal Psychology, 108*, 701–706.

Whisman, M. A. (2001). Marital adjustment and outcome following treatments for depression. *Journal of Consulting and Clinical Psychology, 69*, 125–129.

Whisman, M. A. (2007). Marital distress and DSM-IV psychiatric disorders in a population-based national survey. *Journal of Abnormal Psychology, 116*, 638–643.

Whisman, M. A., Beach, S. R. H., & Snyder, D. K. (2008). Is marital discord taxonic and can taxonic status be assessed reliably?: Results from a national, representative sample of married couples. *Journal of Consulting and Clinical Psychology, 76*, 745–755.

Whisman, M. A., & Bruce, M. L. (1999). Marital distress and incidence of major depressive episode in a community sample. *Journal of Abnormal Psychology, 108*, 674–678.

Whisman, M. A., Dixon, A. E., & Johnson, B. (1997). Therapists' perspectives of couple problems and treatment issues in couple therapy. *Journal of Family Psychology, 11*, 361–366.

Whisman, M. A., & Schonbrun, Y. C. (2009). Social consequences of borderline personality disorder features in a population-based survey: Marital distress, marital violence, and marital disruption. *Journal of Personality Disorders, 23*, 410–415.

Whisman, M. A., Sheldon, C. T., & Goering, P. (2000). Psychiatric disorders and dissatisfaction with social relationships: Does type of relationship matter? *Journal of Abnormal Psychology, 109*, 803–808.

Whisman, M. A., Snyder, D. K., & Beach, S. R. H. (2009). Screening for marital and relationship discord. *Journal of Family Psychology, 23*, 247–254.

Whisman, M. A., & Uebelacker, L. A. (2006). Impairment and distress associated with relationship discord in a national sample of married or cohabiting adults. *Journal of Family Psychology, 20*, 369–377.

Whisman, M. A., & Uebelacker, L. A. (2009). Prospective associations between marital discord and depressive symptoms in middle-aged and older adults. *Psychology and Aging, 24*, 184–189.

Whisman, M. A., Uebelacker, L. A., & Bruce, M. L. (2006). Longitudinal association between marital discord and alcohol use disorders. *Journal of Family Psychology, 20*, 164–167.

CHAPTER 14

Psychopathology Research and Clinical Interventions

Broad Conclusions and General Recommendations

Louis G. Castonguay
Thomas F. Oltmanns

O ur goals for this book were twofold. First, we aspired to provide the field with expert reviews of the research literature on psychopathology, particularly as it pertains to the most commonly treated psychological disorders. With graduate students and residents (as well as experienced clinicians and researchers) in mind, we intended to offer an overview of what we know, scientifically, regarding how these problems manifest themselves, the clinical issues frequently related to them, and the specific vulnerabilities that may be involved in their origin and/or maintenance. Second, we asked the authors to tackle the difficult but exciting challenge of deriving clinical implications from the basic research. Our thought was that these implications (delineated by recognized psychopathology and/or psychotherapy scholars) could provide clinicians with useful guidelines for assessment and treatment interventions, irrespective of their theoretical orientation, professional background, and level of experience. We reasoned that by providing a rigorous and distinctive source of knowledge, basic research could enrich and expand current efforts toward evidence-based practice.

A number of conclusions, some obvious and others less so, can be drawn by taking a broad perspective on the information presented in the previous chapters. First, when described purely in terms of symptoms, it is clear that psychopathology takes many different forms. The disorders covered in this book, let alone the entire list of clinical problems included in the *Diagnostic and Statistical Manual of Mental Disorders* (DSM) or *International Classification of Diseases* (ICD) categorization systems, do involve a wide array of maladaptive ways of being or reacting. While it is true that some symptoms overlap across disorders, those described in this book reflect fairly distinguishable diagnostic profiles. The symptomatic features of posttraumatic stress disorder (PTSD), for example, are largely distinct from those of substance use or eating disorders.

The obvious implication of such diversity is that clinicians, researchers, and students must be aware of the various ways in which different disorders can become manifest, in order to practice clinically, conduct research in abnormal behavior, or simply to learn about psychopathology. In other words, they must be able to assess, measure, and/or retain the distinctive prototypical criteria by which psychological disorders have been identified in our diagnostic classifications.

It is also clear, however, that as clinical and theoretical constructs, each of these disorders represents much more than a list of symptoms (Morey, 1991). Understanding depression, for instance, also requires knowledge about its associated (nonsymptomatic) clinical features, epidemiology and, of course, etiology. Interestingly, a second broad conclusion that can be drawn from this book is that basic research has revealed considerable convergence across disorders with regard to these and other core aspects of psychopathology. Furthermore, and in line with one of the main goals of this book, several specific clinical implications have been derived from these issues for each of the problems covered in this book.

Although the particular foci (in terms of target of assessment or interventions) of these clinical implications and particular ways of implementing them vary across clinical problems, a number of general recommendations can be formulated from them. Among these are the following:

1. Basic research clearly demonstrates that psychopathology appears within relational contexts. All clinical problems covered in this book have been associated with interpersonal (including marital) and social difficulties. These relational difficulties have been identified as consequences of the individual psychopathology and, in some cases, as factors that may cause, maintain, or exacerbate a person's suffering. Accordingly, clinicians should assess clients' interpersonal situations and functioning (in terms of needs, gratification, skills, environmental opportunities, and support), irrespective of clients' reported symptoms. Such assessment should be made early in therapy, as well as during and before termination of treatment. Unmet needs, lack of resources, adversities (e.g., neglect, rejection, and hostility), and/or personal deficiencies (with regard to how an individual seeks, receives, and provides support, validation, and affection) should be the target of clinicians' interventions and/or referral to other appropriate services.

2. Even if the focus is limited to symptomatology, research shows that psychopathology is quite complex. None of the clinical problems covered in this book stands alone: Comorbidity appears to be an intrinsic characteristic of most, if not all,

diagnostic conditions. The most frequent "comrades in arms" are depression, anxiety disorders, substance abuse, and personality disorders. Far from being mere statistical trivia, the high likelihood of comorbidity carries important clinical implications.

It warns against the limitation and potential inadequacy of a brief assessment. One short intake session is not likely to provide a comprehensive evaluation of all the symptoms that define and are most typically associated with disorders commonly seen in practice, and that may require therapeutic attention. Comorbidity also complicates assessment and case formulation. Once the various problems experienced by clients are identified, it behooves clinicians to establish whether and how these difficulties are functionally related. The relationship between disorders can, of course, be bidirectional: While the impairment and distress associated with substance abuse, for example, can lead to depression, the reverse may also take place. Moreover, multiple problems can be caused by the same underlying factor. Although stated within the context of substance use disorders, Pihl and Stewart's (Chapter 8, p. 249, this volume) criticism may also be relevant to the assessment of other disorders: "Perhaps the most significant error in current practice is the pervasive blindness to common underlying vulnerabilities."

Comorbidity also raises important questions with regard to treatment plans: If therapy is to focus primarily on one issue, what should it be? If two clinical problems need to be addressed, what should receive attention first, and how might treatment be conducted so that other clinical difficulties are not ignored and do not interfere with therapeutic progress? Comorbidity also alerts clinicians that therapy may be less effective (or may need to last longer) than might be anticipated, because it has been associated with treatment complications or worse prognoses for several disorders (e.g., Beutler, Blatt, Alimohamed, Levy, & Angtuaco, 2006; Newman, Stiles, Janeck, & Woody, 2006).

Furthermore, comorbidity points to the importance of ongoing assessment. While the successful treatment of a predominant problem might lead to the reduction of other difficulties, this may not always be the case. Even if one clinical problem has been precipitated by another (e.g., the use of a substance to abate anxiety), with time it may have become functionally independent from its initial determining factor. Therefore, an evaluation of clients' difficulties during and before the end of therapy is indicated to increase the probability that all serious problems are sufficiently and adequately addressed. Finally, the frequency of some comorbid conditions may not be suspected by many clinicians. As described in this book, for example, both the high rate of sexual abuse and traumatic experience of acute psychotic symptoms may contribute to the relatively high level of PTSD for individuals diagnosed with schizophrenia, which, of course, impose serious considerations in terms of how to provide them the best possible care. As simple and straightforward as it may first seem, comorbidity dictates upon clinical practice not only the acquisition of extensive knowledge but also the integration of sophisticated clinical skills.

3. Importantly, sleep problems and sexual dysfunction are found in addition to (or, in some cases, as part of) the symptomatic picture of many disorders covered

in this book. These difficulties may frequently go undetected by many clinicians, either because of a lack of attention to these issues as part of their training or lack of time for comprehensive evaluation during intake and therapy sessions. Nevertheless, these issues increase distress and impairment, and they can also prevent an individual (and his or her significant other) from achieving full life satisfaction. Because clients may not always think about (or be comfortable with) reporting such difficulties, it falls to clinicians to assess them (verbally and/or via self-report measures) at different time points of their treatment and to provide (or refer to) appropriate interventions to address them.

4. Also directly related to a client's quality of life are work functioning and medical health. These are not always sufficiently emphasized in theoretical models underlying many psychological treatments of psychopathology. Because these problems may prevent, delay, or otherwise interfere with use of many traditional forms of psychological therapies, a full understanding of these factors should be part of clinicians' case formulation and treatment plan, in order to guide choices of what interventions to implement, how and when to conduct them, and what other services (occupational and medical services) a client should receive and when.

5. A most unfortunate but inescapable reality associated with psychopathology is the possibility of suicide. Although the danger of suicide attempt or completion is well known for some disorders such as depression, bipolar disorder, and schizophrenia, increased risk of suicidal ideation and/or attempts has also been associated with most of the anxiety disorders, marital discord, eating disorders, and personality disorders. As a consequence, the possibility of suicide should never be underestimated by clinicians—even when working with "less severe" forms of psychopathology and/or highly functioning clients. Signs or reports of suicidal ideation, intention, and attempts must be the focus of attention and intervention. Monitoring of suicidal risk (perhaps as part of routine use of brief, noninvasive, and valid self-report measures) should also be encouraged in clinical practice.

6. Basic research clearly demonstrates that for most forms of psychopathology, a limited amount of suffering, distress, and impairment is more the exception than the norm. The course of some disorders may vary (e.g., PTSD, eating and substance use disorders), but most of the clinical problems covered in this book have been described as chronic conditions. Many of them are characterized by frequent recurrence and substantial rates of relapse after treatment. For clinicians, this suggests that, in addition to inquiring about the presence of symptoms at the beginning of treatment, it is also important to examine the history of the symptoms reported by the client. For some disorders the duration of the problem is associated with poor prognosis (e.g., Newman et al., 2006) and may thus suggest longer and/or more intense treatment. Moreover, the high rates of relapse in many disorders should lead clinicians to (a) do a systematic assessment of symptoms before ending a treatment (to make sure that residual problems are adequately addressed), (b) ensure that clients have acquired skills (e.g., relapse prevention strategies) to cope with future triggers of maladaptive reactions, as well as (c) inform clients that booster

sessions and/or additional incidences of therapy can be anticipated and are likely to be beneficial.

7. Demographics matter. Empirical findings related to a factor as global as gender can provide useful clinical prediction and even explanation. Research informs clinicians that when working with clients who suffer from bipolar disorder, for example, they should expect that their female clients will have more episodes than their male clients. On the other hand, when working with individuals diagnosed with schizophrenia, they should anticipate that the prognosis of their male clients will be worse than that of their female clients. Moreover, gender appears to the primary risk factor for eating disorder, as well as a robust marker of one etiological pathway for depression (i.e., rumination—which has been found to explain, at least in part, why women are two times more vulnerable to depression than men). Furthermore, as indicated in a number of chapters in this book, the manifestations of psychopathology (e.g., the content of worry) may differ across gender, age, education, religion, ethnicity, and/or sexual orientation. These sociocultural components, which in part define who we are, should be taken into account when conducting assessment, as well as when building case formulation and treatment plans.

8. Psychopathology research provides indisputable evidence that biological vulnerabilities are involved, more or less extensively, with all clinical problems reviewed in this book (including marital discord). Although this might dispel the hope, if there ever was one, that psychological and/or social treatments might eventually lead to a cure of psychiatric difficulties (or problems of living), it does not imply that nonbiological interventions have negligible impact on abnormal behavior. A more nuanced conclusion that might be drawn is that psychosocial interventions are likely to have boundaries in terms of the change that they can foster, at least for some individuals. Such a "therapeutic ceiling" may in part explain why some clients either do not respond (fully or at all) to or relapse from psychological treatments (even those that are empirically supported).

Although very tentative, one recommendation that could be derived from what we know about biological vulnerabilities and correlates is that it may be wise for the clinician to inquire about the extent of psychopathology in a client's relatives (past and current), and be prepared to provide longer treatment (and/or arrange for the prescription of medication) if the incidence of psychological disorders is extensive in the client's pedigree. We should also mention, however, that even for disorders with firmly established biological vulnerabilities, current biological treatments are far from being panaceas. As noted in this book, medication is typically not sufficient as an effective and comprehensive treatment of bipolar disorders and schizophrenia, and research suggests that psychosocial interventions can help to reduce symptoms and risk for relapse for people with these severe and chronic problems. Similarly, while medication is an effective form of therapy for depression (another disorder for which there is strong evidence of biological determinants), the relapse rate observed after its discontinuation is higher than what has been found following cognitive therapy (Hollon & Dimidjian, 2009).

9. Also dispelled by research is the contention (some may say "the myth") that psychiatric disorders are purely, and simply, medical diseases. For each of the disorders covered in this book, several psychological and social vulnerabilities have been identified, including *cognitive* (e.g., dysfunctional views of self, world, and future; biases or deficits in attention, information processing, and/or memory; maladaptive attributions; deficits in inhibition and cognitive control; worry; intolerance of uncertainty; low self-efficacy expectations; difficulties in anticipating pleasure), *emotional* (e.g., maladaptive emotional regulation strategies; fear of emotional contrasts; emotional avoidance; deficits in emotional expression), *interpersonal* (e.g., parental neglect and/or abuse; attachment problems; family interaction patterns, such as high level of hostility expression; dysfunctional interpersonal styles, e.g., excessive reassuring seeking), *personality traits* (e.g., neuroticism, perfectionism, impulsivity, sensation seeking, and antagonism), *maladaptive learning* (operant and classical conditioning, modeling), *skills deficits* (e.g., social and communication skills; problem solving and stress coping skills), and *sociocultural* (e.g., stress, traumatic life events and conditions, low social support; financial difficulties; social pressures, e.g., cultural views of beauty and cultural norms about substance use) variables. Biological factors are, of course, more than likely to be involved in, or related to, these psychosocial issues. What the massive amount of research on psychosocial risk factors clearly conveys, however, is that genetic predispositions, as well as biochemical and anatomical abnormalities, cannot explain all the variables playing a role in the onset, maintenance, recurrence, and/or relapses of psychiatric disorders.

Fortunately, and as illustrated in this book, a number of empirically supported treatments address some of the psychosocial vulnerabilities investigated by basic researchers. While most of these treatments have been tied to particular theoretical models (especially but not exclusively cognitive-behavioral), all of the authors in this book have also derived principles of change underlying their respective techniques and procedures. Formulated without jargon, these general principles of change provide guidelines that therapists of all orientations should seriously consider assimilating (even if specialized training may in some cases be required for them to do so) into their intervention repertoires. Interestingly, the principles identified in this book converge with and expand upon another set of empirically based change principles that emerged from a previous initiative co-led by one the authors of this chapter (Castonguay & Beulter, 2006). However, neither of these efforts has remotely encompassed all of the clinical implications highlighted in the previous chapters of this book. We hope the implementation of these new recommendations and guidelines will help to increase the validity of our assessment and the effectiveness of our treatments.

10. Perhaps the main implication that one can derive from the rich empirical findings on the etiology factors (biological, psychological, and social) presented in this book is that with regard to psychopathology, many roads lead to Rome, and most pathways to get there intersect. None of the previous chapters has identified a unique, isolated vulnerability factor in the onset and maintenance of abnormal

behavior, and most of the authors who wrote these chapters have explicitly mentioned that different risk factors interact with each other. Practically, this suggests that clinicians are likely to benefit from assessing all possible determinants (and their functional and/or synergetic relationships) of their clients' difficulties and focusing their interventions on what are likely to be the most important and current determining factors, yet also assessing and targeting other variables that are likely to be involved in the onset and maintenance of the problems experienced by their clients.

Needless to say, such practical suggestions assume a difficult balance of focus (or cohesiveness) and flexibility (and comprehensiveness on the part of a psychotherapist). If based on a firm grasp of empirical and theoretical knowledge, as well as sophisticated clinical skills, maintaining this delicate balance may improve our efforts to decrease distress and suffering, and reduce the probability of relapse, while also trying to increase coping skills, level of functioning, and overall quality of life (in terms of not only satisfaction and accomplishment but also meaning, purpose, affiliation, and attachment). Considering the advances made in our understanding of the variables related to effective treatments (client, therapist, relationship, and technical factors; see Castonguay & Beutler, 2006), as well as the implications that can be derived from psychopathology (and other basic) research, Rome (however beautiful it is metaphorically) does not have to be a long-lasting destination.

While these 10 general recommendations are far from being comprehensive and do not do justice to the rich and detailed clinical implications described in the previous chapters, they do, as a whole, allow for a third broad conclusion: Basic psychopathology research can be clinically relevant. By adding another avenue for evidence-based practice, it is our hope that the clinical implications derived from such research will further enrich the integration of science and practice that is crucial for future progress in the field of mental health.

REFERENCES

Beutler, L. E., Blatt, S. J., Alimohamed, S., Levy, K. N., & Angtuaco, L. A. (2006). Participant factors in treating dysphoric disorders. In L. G. Castonguay & L. E. Beutler (Eds.), *Principles of therapeutic change that work* (pp. 13–63). New York: Oxford University Press.

Castonguay, L. G., & Beutler, L. E. (Eds.). (2006). *Principles of therapeutic change that work*. New York: Oxford University Press.

Hollon, S. D., & Dimidjian, S. (2009). Cognitive and behavioral treatment of depression. In I. H. Gotlib & C. L. Hammen (Eds.), *Handbook of depression* (2nd ed., pp. 586–603). New York: Guilford Press.

Morey, L. C. (1991). Classification of mental disorders as a collection of hypothetical constructs. *Journal of Abnormal Psychology, 100,* 289–293.

Newman, M. G., Stiles, W. B., Janeck, A., & Woody, S. R. (2006). Integration of therapeutic factors in anxiety disorders. In L. G. Castonguay & L. E. Beutler (Eds.), *Principles of therapeutic change that work* (pp. 187–202). New York: Oxford University Press.

Index

An *f* following a page number indicates a figure; a *t* following a page number indicates a table.